The Biodynamic Heart

"The wisdom and invitations of this book are compelling! Compassion serves as one's compass and map. Our bodies have an innate capacity to heal. Discover what is possible for you!"

DALE G. ALEXANDER, PH.D., CERTIFIED INTEGRATED AWARENESS TEACHER

"In *The Biodynamic Heart*, Shea unveils his traumatic journey and how to uncover the courage of the heart to heal. You cannot read this book and not touch into your own heart as his words resonate within. It is more than a book on craniosacral therapy; it is a deep dive into one's own inner world of the heart and the ideas and beliefs within it."

LISA UPLEDGER, DC, CST-D, FELLOW OF THE
INTERNATIONAL ACADEMY OF MEDICAL ACUPUNCTURE

"Michael Shea's latest book, *The Biodynamic Heart*, may be his masterpiece. Drawing on many years of experience, this journey of the heart is enriched by fascinating stories of birth, death, and the semi-embodied in-between shamanic states."

CHERIONNA MENZAM-SILLS, PH.D., AUTHOR OF *THE PRENATAL SHADOW*

"Michael Shea provides transformative practices to release deep emotional wounds, realign the physical and spiritual heart, and awaken compassion as an embodied presence. This book is invaluable for those committed to heart-centered healing and the restoration of love in our world."

WENDY ANNE MCCARTY, PH.D., AUTHOR OF *WELCOMING CONSCIOUSNESS*

"Michael brings the wide perspective of how trauma contributes to heart disease, which is directly linked to one's own spiritual healing of the most painful wounds. This book brings the urgency of healing the world's traumas that affect our hearts and the heart of planet Earth."

EFU NYAKI, AUTHOR OF *HEALING TRAUMA THROUGH FAMILY
CONSTELLATIONS AND SOMATIC EXPERIENCING*

"This transformative guide empowers holistic practitioners to embrace the physical and spiritual dimensions of healing, birth, loss, and life itself, giving practitioners invaluable tools to guide and support the healing journeys of others."

CISSI WILLIAMS, AUTHOR OF *YOUR HEART KNOWS HOW TO HEAL YOU*

"My first experience with Michael was during a biodynamic heart course. Through the deepening of the anatomy and physiology of the heart, I experienced a new approach to my physical and spiritual heart. A wonderful journey began that has not yet ended."

SUSANNA HERRGESELL, MD,
CRANIOSACRAL OSTEOPATHY PRACTITIONER, AUSTRIA

"As an integrative physician, I appreciate how Shea's work serves as a bridge between the scientific and spiritual aspects of health, providing valuable insights for both practitioners and patients."

C. DANIELLE DiPIERO, DO, BOARD-CERTIFIED FAMILY PHYSICIAN

"This book will ignite the practitioner to a sense of awe, wonder, and love for the connection between our hearts and hands that flows through biodynamic cardiovascular therapy."

SARAH NESLING, BIODYNAMIC CRANIOSACRAL THERAPIST

"This book offers tremendous value! What an incredible read!"

ELLEN GROESSER, MSc, RCST, TEACHER AT
BIOSTILLNESS INTERNATIONAL SCHOOL

"An invaluable gem for all readers on the path to connecting deeply with their own heart or the hearts of those they touch."

JÖRG SCHÜRPF, COAUTHOR OF *OSTEOTHAI, THE POETRY OF TOUCH*

"*The Biodynamic Heart* is a manual for advanced healers seeking to penetrate beneath the surface of symptoms into the heart itself."

WILL JOHNSON, AUTHOR OF *BREATHING THROUGH THE WHOLE BODY*

"This is a book destined to become a reference for craniosacral therapy as well as for traditional osteopathy and other disciplines."

ÓSCAR SÁNCHEZ MARTÍNEZ, OSTEOPATH AND
BIODYNAMIC CRANIOSACRAL THERAPIST, MADRID

"This book is a wonderful combination of biodynamic cardiovascular therapy and spirituality, all underpinned by Michael Shea's love for people. This book is a must-read for any bodyworker who wants to grow in compassion."

CARLOS RODEIRO HP,
BIODYNAMIC CARDIOVASCULAR THERAPY TEACHER, EUROPE

"Shea has provided a strong impulse in this book to finally set the foundations for the long-awaited bridge between Western and Eastern health practices."

LUISA BRANCOLINI, CHAIR OF THE
ASSOCIATION CRANIOSACRAL THERAPY ITALY (ACSI)

The Biodynamic Heart

Somatic Compassion Practices for a Clear and Vital Heart

A Sacred Planet Book

Michael J. Shea, Ph.D.

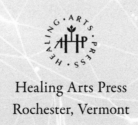

Healing Arts Press
Rochester, Vermont

Healing Arts Press
One Park Street
Rochester, Vermont 05767
www.HealingArtsPress.com

Healing Arts Press is a division of Inner Traditions International

Sacred Planet Books are curated by Richard Grossinger, Inner Traditions editorial board member and cofounder and former publisher of North Atlantic Books. The Sacred Planet collection, published under the umbrella of the Inner Traditions family of imprints, includes works on the themes of consciousness, cosmology, alternative medicine, dreams, climate, permaculture, alchemy, shamanic studies, oracles, astrology, crystals, hyperobjects, locutions, and subtle bodies.

Note to the reader: This book is intended as an informational guide. The remedies, approaches, and techniques described herein are meant to supplement, and not to be a substitute for, professional medical care or treatment. They should not be used to treat a serious ailment without prior consultation with a qualified health care professional.

Cataloging-in-Publication Data for this title is available from the Library of Congress

ISBN 979-8-88850-062-0 (print)
ISBN 979-8-88850-063-7 (ebook)

Printed and bound in India by Nutech Print Services

10 9 8 7 6 5 4 3 2 1

Text design and layout by Debbie Glogover
This book was typeset in Garamond Premier Pro with Acherus Grotesque, Gill Sans MT Pro, and Source Sans Pro used as display typefaces

Photograph in chapter 3 by Cathy Shea
Photographs in chapter 24 by Amanda Roxborough of Kylar Productions, K. Michelle Doyle, Beatrice Fischer, Claudine Laabs (1944–2016), Evelyn Stetzer Jagesar, Robert James Cutter, L.Ac., and Catherine Vitte
Photographs in chapter 26 by Beatrice Fischer, Evelyn Stetzer Jagesar, and Amanda Roxborough of Kylar Productions
Photographs in chapter 26 by Victoria Kereszi
Photographs in chapter 27 by Amanda Roxborough of Kylar Productions and Evelyn Stetzer Jagesar
Photographs in chapter 28 by Evelyn Stetzer Jagesar and Claudine Laabs (1944–2016)
Photographs in chapter 29 by Evelyn Stetzer Jagesar, K. Michelle Doyle, Claudine Laabs (1944–2016), Amanda Roxborough of Kylar Productions, and Robert James Cutter, L.Ac.
Photographs in chapter 31 by Amanda Roxborough of Kylar Productions and Evelyn Stetzer Jagesar
Artwork in color insert by Friedrich Wolf

To send correspondence to the author of this book, mail a first-class letter to the author c/o Inner Traditions • Bear & Company, One Park Street, Rochester, VT 05767, and we will forward the communication, or contact the author directly at **SheaHeart.com**.

Scan the QR code and save 25% at InnerTraditions.com.
Browse over 2,000 titles on spirituality, the occult, ancient mysteries, new science, holistic health, and natural medicine.

To my mom and dad,
couldn't have done this without your love.

To my sister, Sheila, and my brothers, Dan and Brian,
couldn't have done this without your love.

To my wife, Cathy,
couldn't have done this without your love, and love, and love.

To all my students and teachers, alive and dead,
from John Upledger to Jim Jealous,
from Wilhelm Blattner to April Hamatake,
couldn't have done this without your love.

To the Dalai Lama,
without your voice whispering in the ears of my heart,
there would be no book. This is your book.

To the feminine principle of originality,
Green Tara, Mary, Demeter, and the Dakini,
you entered my marrow, I absorbed your potency,
I wrote it all down fearlessly.

Contents

PART 1

Ignition of Life and Death, Conception and Birth

PART 2

Mindfulness and Awareness,
Empathy and Compassion

PART 3

Instincts, Metabolism, and Embodiment

PART 4
A Ministry of Laying On of Hands

Foreword

MARY BOLINGBROKE

I first met Dr. Michael Shea several decades ago. He was teaching a course in London called "Spirals of Life." For some time prior to this, I'd been drawn to the image and symbolism of the spiral and its appearance throughout the natural world, so Michael's course immediately appealed. By that time, I'd been practicing as a craniosacral osteopath for many years and had begun my biodynamic training with Dr. James Jealous. However, I'd recently stepped back; my mind, body, and spirit felt dejected, my self-confidence felt battered, and my spirit yearned for guidance. Michael's spiral course was instantly restorative. I signed up for his next one, which was more biodynamic in nature, more about working in a slow tempo with Primary Respiration.

Of course, these concepts were not new to me, but Michael's way of teaching them was a revelation. He taught quite complex, often esoteric subjects with great clarity, and he shared insights of personal difficulty and suffering with generosity, and throughout the days he would tell us what phase the Tide was in. Consequently, by the end of the course we had all experienced our beings being breathed. We had all been met by and acquainted with this beautiful gift as stillness seemed to bring the light of the natural world into the practice room. I was struck, too, by the accepting, gently compassionate, good-humored open-heartedness of my fellow students. In those days in Great Britain there was rather a rift between the craniosacral osteopaths and craniosacral therapists, and yet it seemed to me that although our practices had grown from the same roots, they had grown apart. There was animosity where there could have been sharing, yet we each had gifts and insights we could be teaching each other. My feeling was that the whole would be greater than the sum of these two parts. I decided there and then that in some small way I would make it part of my journey to try to bring our "separate" disciplines closer.

In a similar but more magnificent way, Michael Shea has brought not just the disciplines of osteopathy, craniosacral therapy (CST), and manual therapy closer together but has seamlessly interwoven Eastern and Western medicine and spirituality.

He shows us how to incorporate Indo-Tibetan five element practice and the use of sound, color, and light visualization with Western-based anatomy, embryology, and physiology. Throughout, he uses the intuitive gift of the Breath of Life as the guiding principle that holds the mix so beautifully together in heart-based compassion.

The book itself is a combination of three different distillation processes. The first is the distillation of the works of the founders of osteopathy and thus the founders of CST. The second is the distillation of the thousands of years of medicine, philosophy, and spirituality from the East and West. The third is the distillation of Michael's own life experience. The result is this book, *The Biodynamic Heart*, a combination of the biodynamic wisdom combined with the divine love of the heart.

The names *biodynamic craniosacral osteopathy* and *craniosacral therapy* were defined by three founding fathers: Dr. Andrew Taylor Still, Dr. William Garner Sutherland, and Dr. James Jealous. Each passed the baton on to the next, and each, often after years of hardship, experimentation, soul searching, and revelation, brought a new dimension of insight. It was Still who coined the term *osteopathy* but was clear that "no human hand had framed its laws" (Lewis 2012). He turned the medical understanding of the time completely on its head by saying the role of the doctor was to find the Health, adding, "Anyone can find disease." He had arrived at this understanding following many years of grief. He had lost three of his children in an epidemic, he had lost his career as a medic, he had lost his professional standing and the respect of his colleagues. Yet as Michael Shea says, out of sorrow comes the ferment of grief, and from there the wisdom and spiritual resource that is alchemized by such suffering and heartfelt seeking. For Andrew Taylor Still, the wisdom he found was in what he termed "Health," implying a divine connection between living beings and something greater that, regardless of the presence of disease, dysfunction, or injury, would work constantly to bring us back to wholeness, perfection, and harmony. Still taught that given the proper conditions, the body, mind, and spirit had the capacity to self-regulate, to heal itself and to be healed. In this regard, one of his most basic principles is "the Rule of the Artery is Supreme" (Lewis 2012). Michael Shea has delivered an invaluable exposition and deep exegesis of this rule.

In 1899, W. G. Sutherland was studying at Stills's school of osteopathy when he was struck by the revelation that the temporal bones of the skull were shaped like the gills of a fish, implying for him a respiratory movement. From then until his death in 1956 he explored this insight, often practicing on himself to gain knowledge through firsthand experience, adding that if he had simply observed the effect of his experiments on another, he would have gained only information (very similar to the principle of interoceptive awareness explored by Michael Shea). He gained many insights this way, including the recognition that the cranial bones do indeed exhibit a breathing motion, as does the sacrum; that there is more power or potency in the stillness of a fulcrum around which things move than is found in the movement itself; and that the stillness is dynamic and is being motivated by the same respiratory movement.

Sutherland termed this breathing Primary Respiration or the Breath of Life (BOL). He understood that the BOL or Tide was more essential to life than the respiration of the lungs (which he called secondary respiration), as it appeared life couldn't exist at all without the BOL. He began to see sparks and liquid light within the tissues. The more afferent his palpation, the greater his perception. He said, "Be away from the sensation of physical touch wherein you have the Knowing touch. In a state of Stillness be receptive, afferent, humble and reverent" (Sutherland 1993). The stillness had taught him so much that he asked to have carved on his gravestone the words "Be Still and know."

Dr. Rollin Becker was a student of Sutherland and one of Dr. James Jealous' teachers. He, too, taught about listening in stillness, saying, "How can the body report to you if you keep doing something to it during your examination? Let the tissues tell you their story. Be quiet and listen" (Becker 2000). Dr. Jealous took Sutherland and Becker's work forward and added the term *biodynamic* when he realized that the unfolding, spiraling, creative forces he could feel within the tissues were identical to the embryological forces and movements that were being discovered by the German embryologist Erich Blechschmidt, who had used the term *biokinetics* to describe the embryological forces of the developing body and *biodynamic* to describe the movement of the whole embryo over time. Dr. Jealous recognized that the forces and movements of growth and development in the embryo continued throughout our lives, becoming the forces of healing, repair, and renewal in all dimensions of mind, body, and spirit. Recognizing that these forces cannot be controlled, only revered, he said, "To acknowledge a Higher wisdom is the Soul of Osteopathy. The Breath of Life permeates through all form and ignites all function without diminishing its own force. It is non vectorial and nonlinear, It cannot be controlled and is unaffected by disease" (Jealous 2001). As Michael says, he was fortunate indeed to be mentored by Dr. Jealous.

In his introduction, Michael says he needed to write this book "to save my own life" and goes on to describe his experience with post-traumatic stress disorder (PTSD). He recognizes that the journey to "heal the gun" in his heart begins with loss and the ignition of sorrow, saying, "Sorrow is the capacity to bear all things, but especially loss. . . . Sorrow is not grief but helps ferment grief into an expanded capacity to love and potentize compassion." In traditional Chinese medicine, the emotions of sorrow, grief, loss, and loss of control over one's life are governed by the lung and large intestine meridians and the element of metal. Metal is the element of transmutation; it can take the deepest of griefs and, through an almost alchemical process, transform the trauma of loss into the resource of clarity and wisdom. For metal alchemy, there is no cloud so dark that it cannot have a silver lining. Through many years of practice, Michael did indeed alchemize his experience of PTSD and has then further distilled his insights so that he not only heals his own life but helps us all save our own and that of the world, currently ravaged by all dimensions of heart dis-ease. In the Jewish Talmud, Sanhedrin 37A says, "Whosoever saves a single life is considered by scripture to have saved the whole world."

Michael seems to have had several lifetimes of experience and study in one life. He has had many careers, clients, spiritual practices, exercises, diets, and gardening disciplines. He has taught, written, loved, worked, explored, and defined so much that it seems impossible to have fit it all into one such relatively short life, and yet he has with this book. It is the distillation of his insights, wisdom, practices, trials, and errors.

One of the most heartfelt prayers of my life arose in my early twenties. I was living in New Orleans, where Michael got his first university degree. As the Mardi Gras festival reached its climax and the Crescent City seemed to be awash with a revelry bordering on insanity, I was at a loss, desperate for guidance, insight, and direction. Nothing made any sense. What was the point of all of this, of life, of my life? Where were the grown-ups to guide me? Where and who were the wise elders? In the early hours beside the Mississippi, beneath the Easter full moon of rebirth, I opened my heart and asked God for help, for teachers to show me the way. In the forty years since then, my prayer has been answered many, many times over. I have been blessed with many brilliant teachers who have illuminated my life and career path like guiding stars.

Michael Shea is such a teacher, an answer to mine and many people's prayers. My prayer was for spiritual guidance and wisdom. I was fortunate enough to be guided by Providence toward a career in osteopathy, which historically had its roots firmly growing from the soil of the sacred. However, today's practice is more profane than sacred, and the same is true for most of us. At home, at work, and at play, all our lives are more profane and less sacred than they may have ever been. We are starved of the divine in our lives, and hungering for we know not what, we fill the ache in our hearts with the quick fixes and junk foods of contemporary life. We all become unwell, and we all require the life of our heart to be saved. Michael's book is beautifully, generously, unashamedly about multifaith spirituality. It is the equivalent of being taken by the hand and our deepest heart of hearts being ministered to. Read it and know that your heart's prayer has been answered.

MARY BOLINGBROKE is a craniosacral osteopath with thirty years of practical and teaching experience. She also works as an animal communicator and remote healer.

Preface

All of my writing is born from my heart. Now is the time to use our heart and hands to bless all sentient beings. The spirit, the sacredness that lives within our heart and pulses through our blood to every cell in our body, is hidden in our civilization. The ancient Confucian philosopher Mencius once noted that when people lose their chickens or dogs, they have the good sense to go look for them, but when they lose their heart, they don't. Indeed, too often such common sense is missing when it comes to the loss of the heart, the loss of our purpose and our joy. Consider the fact that the demand for heart transplants is at an all-time high in the United States, with thousands of people on waiting lists to receive a new heart. Somewhere between the physical heart and the spiritual heart is a living experience of deep meaning that everyone can perceive without polarization or argument. A spiritual heart replacement requires contemplation. What does that mean? This book explores contemplative science as an embodied art that begins by simply sensing our own heartbeat and belly breathing. It continues with a full-spectrum exploration of the heart, moving step by step from the metabolic to the spiritual.

The metabolism of the body is the bridge to the subtle body of spirit. The contemplative arts awaken the heart and allow the subtle emotions of kindness, empathy, gratitude, acceptance, and humility to sprout and grow. These are the effects of contemplative practice. Solitude and silence are the essence. We must weed the inner garden with solitude and silence to allow these aspects of our preexisting sacred nature to flourish.

Recognizing the internal state of emotional and cognitive upset is imperative to being able to shift attention to the state of open awareness, one of the ten thousand faces and names of the divine. Open awareness is free of conflict and located in the heart both physically and subtly. It is formlessly woven together in our metabolism, with its trillions upon trillions of molecular interactions every moment. It requires diligent contemplative practice.

Weeding the garden includes and integrates acknowledgment of grief and loss. Change is our must valuable asset internally and externally because we all will die and do so throughout our life, with trillions of cells in our body dying in every moment. In order to convey the deep nature of our heart and its loving mind, I share my own personal experience of compassion igniting while I was in military service and had a near-death experience in a terrorist bombing attack. I was ordained in that explosion as a warrior-priest. I was baptized in the blood of the dead and wounded. I then transferred to pediatric practice and was trained in compassion by the many infants and children I worked with who had severe developmental disabilities. This allowed a deeper sense of self-compassion, and its predecessor empathy, to be aroused in my being. I learned that broken heart syndrome is a side effect of trauma, and that it can be repaired and restored in the fullness of its own prophetic nature of acknowledged embodied suffering connected to the sacred. The heart has an innate capacity to expand with love in the midst of loss. This requires a divine commitment to relieve all suffering in one's self and other, and to call it out as the prophets did.

I am an expert in the manual therapeutic arts, and this book presents an art form I have developed called biodynamic cardiovascular therapy (BCVT). Simply put, BCVT is the application of biodynamic craniosacral therapy to the cardiovascular system. While the spiritual aspects of having a body were surgically removed in the Renaissance and split off from medicine into the European religion of that time, our hands and heart-mind are both designed to perform benediction and offer a blessing with every client we see, even if we are not touch therapists. Like the blood coursing through our vascular tree, the seed of divinity lives in the heart of all sentient beings, whether we call it Buddha nature, Christ consciousness, or Shen. The focus of bio-dynamic cardiovascular therapy is restoration of the heart, meaning an integration of its metabolic function and its sacred nature, and as a practice it can be undertaken by anyone, regardless of profession, and applied to everyone.

The Breath of Life spoken of in all traditional cultures and modern religions is a sacred light that radiates from the human heart. In Eastern traditions, this light appears as rainbow forms, like the human body. Light, color, and appearance are all medicine, as is demonstrated herein, and offer an optimal prognosis for the planet and its inhabitants. The universe on both sides of our skin is explored through the five elements of the Indo-Tibetan medical tradition: space, wind, fire, water, and earth. Those five elements are present at conception and dissolve in reverse order during the dying process. Many visionary experiences made possible during the dying process are incredibly profound and healing. The practice of Buddhist tantra is all visualization, and its medical aspect is a foundation of this book. The subtle body described in Eastern traditions is much more than chakras, central channel, side channels, and so forth. And visualizing those levels of a subtle body embedded within our physical body is preparation for the moment after death when the subtle body is still present. It is a vast playground and that's why holy people are left to lie in a state for many days without tinkering with their corpse. Their heart is still warm with the clear light of innate divinity. We are designed to dissolve into our heart at death.

The natural world here on planet Earth is a vast exploration of the five elements and their interaction. I live in Florida and have been through many hurricanes. I now worship the wind and its power. I also worship the ocean and the majesty of her waves and tides; she moves the Earth. Having grown up with sunburn, I've had many skin cancers. The sun is very hot. I worship him. I worship Earth; dust to dust, we shall return to her, and the pleasure the Great Mother gives us with her endless bounty is magical. The most ancient traditional medicine found all over this planet has its foundation in such worship. This is the most practical solution to restoring our original Health. The medicine is in our backyard.

I offer a multifaith exploration of using contemplative practices and hands-on spiritual healing to find our individual and collective hearts. There is no dogma. This book transcends theology. There is only each person's unique aptitude for spiritual formation. How each of us brings meaning to life as a sacred experience is the path of spiritual maturation. Spiritual maturation leads to spiritual authority and the capacity to be a blessing to all beings. All sentient beings have the capacity to invoke the Holy Spirit. This spiritual aptitude depends on the perception of slowness, stillness, and light. It is so simple and yet incredibly profound when direct spiritual authority unfolds internally through the contemplative practices found in this book. It naturally awakens to offer profound love to everyone and all sentient beings.

Compassionate love is an innate natural responsiveness ignited by contemplative wisdom practices in every tradition. In this way the sacred heart, our sacred heart in the middle of our chest, can flourish.

With 93 percent of Americans having metabolically unhealthy hearts and the rest of the world not far behind (O'Hearn, Wong, and Kim et al.), we must begin to cultivate compassion with wisdom through contemplative practice. And that is not enough. Compassion, the knowing of our own pain that we share with all beings, must be followed with love in action; they are ultimately the same. It is a spiritual maturation formed through trial and error over many years.

Our mind can cause us to ignore our body with too many thoughts, concepts, and unrealistic world views taking our attention. Consequently we lose embodied safety and inner peace on a daily basis. The ordinary mind is constantly changing with endless variations and distortions. Thoughts of the past and thoughts of the future can be challenging sometimes. Obsessing about the past leads to depression, according to the literature, and obsessing about the future leads to anxiety. Concepts about the nature of the present moment of experience must be embodied through contemplative practice for integration, stability, and mental and emotional resilience. Analytical meditation, which leads to the special insight of no separation, is the essence of wisdom. Contemplative practice is just the development of an ethical onboard neutral observer of our behavior. We have the ability to contemplate the past and the future in terms of growth and development while being neutral. And this leads to a different state in the mind of complete self-knowing awareness with no observer. This is always present. As is proclaimed in Christianity, the sacred heart of Jesus lives in everyone and can be visualized for deep healing. The Buddha and Jesus were both medical doctors, and that capacity is preexisting in our hearts, waiting to be awakened. Our inner physician is discovered through contemplative practices. We can learn to see the inside of our body and that of others for self-healing.

The foundation of spiritual maturity is the contemplation of wisdom and awe as an essential mystery. Wisdom and wonder constantly manifest in our visible and invisible heart, without separation, and without rejection of the shady neighborhoods that challenge us. These neighborhoods are always present, but we can turn the car around. We can be the driver rather than the passenger. It is an inside job. All the spiritual metaphors, all of the awe, wonder, and nonthinking, must personally unfold in each person's perception derived from contemplative practices. The metabolism of the body inside is as vast as the entire universe outside and is affected by the subtle aspects of stillness, light, and color, from the scientific to the mystical. We can only perceive the outside universe with our internal mind-body senses. These senses require interoceptive awareness of how our heart and other organs express their needs in relation to the universe. There is no universe without our senses, and it is therefore the heart that constantly radiates the universe we see and hear and taste and feel. Biodynamic cardiovascular therapy explores the heart that radiates the light of love in action. This is the universe we perceive. We are the center of the universe located in our heart. Therefore, this book and everyone who reads it is love in action.

Acknowledgments

My wife, Cathy, sacrificed so much of our intimate time for the sake of this book. Her heart is in this book. Her passion moves me and moves through this book. My writing station for the book was in the living room of our home, and as I worked there, often Cathy was preparing food in the kitchen to sustain and nourish me, as is one of her passions. The smells and sounds of her kitchen and her love infuse this book.

Joshua Horwitz inspired my previous book on the immune system, and yet again his spiritual mastery ignited my desire and capacity to both begin and finish this book. I am indebted to his inspiration as a practitioner and human being.

Without Bill Harvey for constant spiritual Ignition, this book would not have been possible. His inspiration that manual therapy must evolve into a spiritual discipline creates the core exploration of this book.

My thanks to April Hamatake, who died while I was finishing this book. You showed me your heart as a student, and I am a better human being and biodynamic practitioner because of you and your reflection of grace and radiant love.

Thanks to the contributors to this book, my wife Cathy, Mary Monro, Ann Weinstein, Michelle Doyle, Friedrich Wolf, and Bill Harvey. I am speechless in your display of generosity.

Thanks to Jeanie Burns, who for many years has been able to capture with her vision the numerous images seen in my written work. Your aesthetic refined the edges of this book into a portrait of the heart that I could never have imagined.

Thanks to Kathy Weaber, who shaped the text into a coherent whole and gave me peace of mind knowing that this project would get done. Thanks also to Richard Grossinger for his clarity and vision of the world of bodies, politics, and the multidimensional nature of the human embryo; I am deeply grateful for your courage.

Thanks to the entire osteopathic profession of men and women, from the very beginning, with Andrew Taylor Still "the rule of the artery," Sutherland "must be capable of respiratory motion," Becker "trust the Tide," Jim Jealous "wait, watch, and wonder," and my brother Brian, an inspired biodynamic osteopath. The mystical origins of osteopathy permeate this book.

Carlos Rodeiro, your blood carries a passion and commitment to love. I am full of joy knowing you, and your heart knowledge, your skill in teaching, and your radiance, shining brightly from your heart, inspire me.

Almut Althaus, my business partner for the past twenty years and a naturopathic healing practitioner, you created the opportunity for every single perception, theory, and palpation unfolded in this book to be able to take place with hundreds of students over the past fifteen years. Everything in this book has been tested in our classroom and the students' offices. Without your skill in the management and feedback on what works and what doesn't work clinically, this book would not be possible. I thank the teaching teams you assembled, including Bettina Ravanelli, Ursula Walke, and Joachim Lichtenberg, all of whom are incredible therapists. You all gave me rich and rewarding feedback regarding everything in this book to polish it and embed safety throughout.

Thanks to Margery Chessare and the teaching teams in Saratoga Springs, through whom I was able to explore the basic cardiovascular work and get invaluable feedback. It was a blessing to have Margery set up the classes and assemble teaching teams consisting of Andraly Horn, Kelli Foley, Sarah Rosensweet, and Bill Harvey, all of whom created equanimity and feedback to build the core of this book into a blossom of heartfulness. Almut and Margery's help ensured that everything taught in this book is clinically safe.

Thanks to Jörg Schürpf, my friend, my teacher, my assistant, my therapist, and my French wine consultant and genuine lover of the world. You inspire me with every word and every action. Your hands and your thoughts and ideas about theory, perception, and palpation fill this book and make it more whole, more complete, and certainly much deeper than I could have imagined.

Thanks to my translators in Europe, especially Beate Kircher, Claudia Oliveri, and Birte Heissenberg. Without your skill in giving my words to the students and giving the students' words to me, I would not know the potential of this book and its poetry and richness. The effort you put in to translating my crazy American jokes is worthy of spending your next lifetime in heaven.

Thanks to Thalbert Allen, my Chi Kung teacher and a master Chi Kung instructor; your sage advice on the advanced protocols in this book polished the diamond into a radiance that sometimes is blinding and certainly is healing. Thanks to Dale Alexander and Therese Panchura, who kept my body relaxed and blood pumping to my brain; your hands and extraordinary skills made this book happen.

To my spiritual advisers Annalis Prendina, Annette Saager, Catherine Vitte, and Sarajo Berman, thank you for seeing my heart and helping to shape it with balance and integrity. Thanks to my office manager, Lisa Fay, who is also a spiritual adviser and kept the organization of this book in impeccable shape, especially at the end. Thanks also to Todd McLaughlin, a spiritual adviser, friend, and yogi and the owner of Native Yoga here in Juno Beach, Florida, who gave me his studio to perfect the contemplative practices taught herein. I am grateful to you all, and to the entire family of friends, students, and teachers who made this possible.

Finally, this book is a miracle because of the work of Nancy Ringer, the copy editor, and Beth Wojiski, the project editor. Their help, care, and enormous effort shaping and massaging this book brought it to perfection. I have never worked with a more dedicated and compassionate editorial team on this, the biggest and most complicated book I have ever written. I am beyond gratitude in my admiration for their skill and the whole team at Inner Traditions, especially Richard Grossinger, who saw my potential—my embryo so to speak—and gave me the opportunity to publish with him. Thank you all of you! May compassion and wisdom perfectly arise in your hearts and all hearts on the planet.

The Four Intentions

The first intention of this book is to save lives. Following the publication of my previous book, *The Biodynamics of the Immune System*, I was interviewed many times and always asked the same question: Why did I write the book? My answer was simple and, for some of the interviewers, surprising: to save lives.

That same intention inspired this book, *The Biodynamic Heart*. While setting out to save lives is altruistic, and certainly the intention is to see our world with more compassion, through the process of writing I came to realize that this work is also about saving my own life. The reader will see, starting with chapter 1, how I narrowly escaped death and the work I have subsequently put in to save my own life by every means possible. I have received a lot of love and support along the way, especially from the infants and children I worked with. It is by saving my own life that I can share my learning that can save other lives.

The second intention is to teach practitioners and all health care providers that biodynamic cardiovascular therapy (BCVT) is a ministry of laying on of hands. It is a ministry of using our hands to bless every client. The terminology used in biodynamic practice lends itself to mysticism and direct experience of the sacred regardless of religious affiliation. We can no longer avoid this reality, as many clients cannot make the changes necessary to relieve their metabolic syndrome and thus biodynamic work becomes palliative care in which we make our offering and our blessing for its potential to assist the client in waking their instinct for self-transcendence. Through palliative care, we help clients bear their sorrow and joy. This is the work of compassion and the essence of this book. The felt sense of sorrow is warmth and coziness. It is the music of the heart. It exists on a continuum with joy, the felt sense of brightness and clarity. It is with contemplative practice that sorrow and joy become a single continuum. They are as inseparable as the different movements in a piano concerto. They are inseparable because neither state is superior or inferior to the other. In its essence of infinite equality, the present moment of awareness, awakened by contemplative practice, provides this insight of beauty that is always there, waiting to be recognized and remembered as the preexisting condition of life and death. This is the deeper meaning of biodynamic practice.

This is a book about multifaith spirituality rather than furthering concepts about

God, male or female, who lives in the natural world or heaven, and whose depictions are based on the need of different cultures and the fashion of the times. The premise of this book is that everyone can experience their very subtle nature and essence of spirituality as clear light, color, and form without fear. These are the doorways that contemplative practice provides so that we can experience essence and spirit. Such metaphors are still conceptual, though, and deep contemplative practice allows the disappearance of concept, leaving the felt sense of sorrow and joy. Contemplative practice is about turning inward and learning to love one's self by feeding oneself internally as the basis for being a compassionate, social human being. Said another way, the second intention of this book is to view biodynamic practice as spiritual practice based on the emerging field of contemplative neuroscience.

The third intention is to help readers form a contemplative relationship with their thoughts, emotions, concepts, and life views. To recognize, reframe-release, and relax mental and emotional afflictions are the skills necessary for spiritual resilience. Contemplative practice invokes each individual's spiritual formation and leads to spiritual maturation. Gradually spiritual maturation fulfills itself as direct knowing of the sacred without an interpreter. This book provides a framework for a multifaith direct knowing of the sacred. Contemplative practice is the key to self-transcendence of self and other.

The purpose of contemplative practices is, first, to be able to recognize challenging or disruptive internal states of mind associated with thoughts, emotions, concepts, and views. Such recognition comes through mindfulness and awareness practices. Next, upon recognition, there is an immediate reframing or empathetic response to one's own internal state. Finally, one simply relaxes into such freedom that contemplative practice gives by the enhancement of nonreferential awareness and nonattachment to internal states. Over time this type of contemplative practice develops spiritual resilience and allows thoughts, emotions, and concepts to reside in the heart, as they are transmuted into loving kindness and compassion. This is called heart-mind. In this way, contemplative practice is food for our heart.

The fourth intention is to help readers feel the physical and spiritual nature of the human heart as one thing. The heartbeat and the stillpoint at the back of the heart are the home of our spiritual essence, the heart inside the heart. The overall intention of this book is to help readers find their heart, and to do this, we will discuss the heart in numerous ways, from the physical to the spiritual.

OVERVIEW

This book describes the categories of conceptual and spiritual knowing that support the professional practice of BCVT. BCVT is a contemplative manual therapeutic art form in which the priority is kindness and sublime gentleness radiating from the heart of the practitioner as light. BCVT is initiated by the application of biodynamic craniosacral therapy to the cardiovascular system. It integrates skills derived from Eastern and Western cosmologies and human embryology. It originates partly with Andrew Taylor Still, the late nineteenth-century founder of osteopathy, who said, "The rule of the artery is supreme." This tradition was moved forward by William Garner Sutherland, a student of Still who claimed the osteopathic tradition to be religious or spiritual in its essence. Its core foundations further derive from all ancient animistic and shamanistic medical traditions. And as a ministry of laying on of hands, BCVT is derived from all spiritual traditions involving hands-on healing or "spiritist passe" (Carneiro, Moraes, and Terra 2016; Carneiro et al. 2017). Yet it is an emergent knowing rather than an eclectic or mixed-bag therapeutic approach for the contemporary client.

This book elaborates a comprehensive set of perceptual and palpation competencies for the contemporary practitioner and client for integrating mind-body-spirit. The palpation skills are derived from a variety of sources including osteopathy and its derivatives, traditional cultural methods as just mentioned, and especially spontaneous knowing from contemplative practice. This book clarifies the core principles and scope of clinical practice for the international community of biodynamic practitioners, and especially biodynamic cardiovascular therapy practitioners, who are interested in the spiritual domain of making meaning around pain and suffering in the contemporary world, which faces significant civilizational issues.

BCVT is a contemplative art form that explores a range of subtle motions, forms, and colors that are expressed within and around the body. A practitioner's ability to visualize them is considered a spiritual aptitude, as is the ability to perceive stillness and Primary Respiration (PR). The exploration of these biodynamic spiritual aptitudes is associated with optimizing metabolic function. This book explores the Indo-Tibetan system of wisdom colors from which the elements of space, wind, fire, water, and earth emerge in the evolution of universes big and small. BCVT further differentiates the use of yogic mudras, classical Chinese medicine meridians, and the Sino-Tibetan system of elements. BCVT creates bridges to ancient systems of healing that recognize the innate unity of mind-body-spirit in all sentient beings. Consequently, BCVT practitioners are expected to cultivate a personal contemplative practice that supports their spiritual maturation and leads to a direct experience of the sacred. There is a need for an inner practice to develop emotional resilience and an outer practice that connects practitioners to the natural world as both sentient and medicinal. I introduce biodynamic healing practices that apply to both the client and the practitioner's spiritual formation without dogma. This traditional medical capacity predates all formal Eastern and Western medical practices. BCVT is animistic-shamanistic, mystical, and practical without romanticizing traditional ways of knowing and healing or politicizing its origins. No one has the right to claim dominion over such healing practices.

The emphasis in BCVT is for practitioners to hold themselves and their client as an interconnected whole extending to the horizon in order to harmonize the forces of Health in the natural world with the inner forces of Health that organize the subtle body with the metabolism of structure and function. The inner and outer organization of Health is uniformly scaled across the universe as colors, their associated elements, and states of mental clarity. Practitioners synchronize their attention with the immutable Health that is preexisting inside and outside the human body as a single continuum ultimately free of a perceptual reference point. It can be called nonreferential awareness or God and numerous other metaphors because of a multifaith orientation in BCVT. Health in the context of a biodynamic session is the potency of PR, a deep wisdom expression of the wind and fire elements that drive all life expressions and the instincts discussed thoroughly in this book. All BCVT processes and life experiences are perceived from within a person's heart and soma as a sacred center extending to the edge of the universe. All origins are located in the heart inside the heart of every sentient being. It is within this universal context of manifestation arising from subtle perception of the heart-mind of love that change process constantly takes place. This includes death and dying, since our body is constantly igniting its death at the cellular level. The inability to accept natural and constant change leads to disease.

BCVT palpation skills are discussed in the context of the term *synchronization*. As osteopath Anne Wales wrote in 1953, "The first step in the management of this [biodynamic] fluid action is to establish a contact without disturbing its activity. This may be compared to the problem of a rider who desires to mount a horse in motion" (Wales 1953, 35–36). This means that practitioners are constantly synchronizing with the activity of PR in themselves and in their client. BCVT is an essential inquiry into an embodied interconnected harmony with all things that are constantly changing. We can call this the *cycle of attunement*. The cycle of attunement is the first step in synchronizing with the universe with care and mindfulness of where one's attention is located and how to automatically shift attention to the subtle and sublime nature of PR and the stillness. This requires skill at recognizing the three spiritual aptitudes of PR, stillness, and visualization of the sacred.

BCVT relies on the perceptual exploration of Health based on a core set of spiritual principles set forth in the chapters of this book. The lineage holders of osteopathy in the cranial field were Christian mystics. However, as mentioned, BCVT is a multifaith approach for the contemporary client who is suffering. Furthermore, BCVT is an experientially based contemplative practice in which practitioners are empowered to apply these principles in accordance with their own spiritual formation and level of spiritual maturation.

BCVT includes interoceptive awareness as a critical embodied practice for the development of body knowing—that is, recognition of the body as an intelligence that speaks to us and reveals its needs from the inside. As such, the principles contained herein are available for exploration and evolution in each practitioner in order for all to realize a reliable sovereignty over their body and mind while acknowledging the human heart as the center of the universe. This is what is offered to the client as a blessing from the hands and heart of the practitioner.

PART I: IGNITION OF LIFE AND DEATH, CONCEPTION AND BIRTH

There are four parts to this book. In part 1, the journey of the heart begins with loss and the ignition of sorrow. Without sorrow, it is difficult to experience deep love and deep grief. These core elements of compassion require the ability to integrate constant change and loss from the mundane moment by moment to the extraordinary social and tribal conditions on our planet. This first part includes my own story and that of others finding their heart in the midst of loss. My experience is that compassion is based on a heart of sorrow. Sorrow is the capacity to bear all things, but especially loss. And it is the very nature of being human to experience constant loss, whether personally or impersonally through the media. Sorrow is not grief but helps ferment grief into an expanded capacity to love and potentize compassion.

Part 1 contains nine chapters. Chapter 1 begins with my near-death experience in a terrorist bombing attack on May 11, 1972, while I was in the military. It is here where I was given a baptism of life and death, and the ignition of a compassionate life that brought me to this book and all the books I have written. Chapter 2 describes my career in pediatric craniosacral therapy for more than forty years. I worked with children and infants with moderate to severe developmental disabilities. These children and their parents taught me a deeper nature of compassion and its relationship to sorrow and loss. Chapter 3 is a contemplation on death as an ignition and in particular my mother's death. Chapters 4 and 5 were written by professional colleagues of mine, Ann Weinstein and Barry Williams; Ann describes her experience in losing a grandchild, and Barry describes his own experience as a parent losing his child who was born in a persistent vegetative state and lived to the age of 26. These gifts that awaken a heart of sorrow—gifts given to all of us—also grant us the capacity to expand our heart and form a pillar of BCVT. While not usually seen as a gift in the immediacy of grief, sorrow allows grief to ferment a very deep and ever-expanding love for the lost one. The first part continues with a chapter on pregnancy as a great act of compassion. This is followed by two chapters from Mary Monro on the metabolic nature of pregnancy and birth. Finally, Michelle Doyle, a gifted midwife, shares her experience with helping to deliver a stillborn baby. With a genuine heart of sorrow balanced with a genuine heart of joy, I continue to the second part.

PART 2: MINDFULNESS AND AWARENESS, EMPATHY AND COMPASSION

Part 2 begins an in-depth look at the way of healing self and others with a compassionate heart. I begin with chapter 10 and the formal diagnosis of a PTSD disability that I was given by the Veterans Administration (VA) after a year of rigorous evaluation. I then turn to the healing ceremonies I underwent while apprenticing with John Nelson, a Diné medicine man on a reservation in Arizona. During one such ceremony, spirit revealed to John that a gun in my heart was blocking my healing. My heart needed to melt away its blockages, and so we transition to chapters 11 and 12, which discuss self-awareness and the Buddhist concept of the Four Immeasurables, which together relate to loving kindness and compassion as applied to recognizing one's state of mind for self-healing and helping others. It includes an outline of how to create one's own origin story. Origin stories as personal mythologies are opportunities to integrate life experience. If we can frame each of our lives in a context of an originality, we can be of greater service to others. This begins a crucial discussion of the necessity of contemplative practices for self-healing and igniting compassion.

Chapter 13 discusses the four foundations of mindfulness and begins to take a deeper look at the nature and necessity of contemplative practice for dealing with mental and emotional challenges of all kinds. It is critical to be able to recognize debilitating states of mind in order to reframe the experience and relax. Contemplative practice is both medicine and food for emotional and cognitive challenges. It is said that biodynamic practice is a study of perception, and chapter 14 is oriented toward therapeutic relationships and how to work heart-to-heart with the perception of Primary Respiration (PR) and the dynamic stillness. PR and stillness are the two foundational perceptual practices at the core of biodynamic cardiovascular therapy. Chapter 14 ends with a thorough review of interpersonal neurobiology and the necessity of maintaining awareness of one's own state of mind, not only in therapeutic practice with clients, but throughout life. Here awareness is differentiated from mindfulness and compassion. It is directly related to nonduality and consequently the essence of appropriate compassionate responses.

Chapter 15 discusses the deep nature of care for self and other. It is an in-depth discussion of the nature of health, from both a physical and a spiritual point of view. Spiritual health is spelled Health. It introduces the reader to the manner in which past and present forms of biodynamic practice perceive the Breath of Life described in the Book of Genesis in the Bible.

At this point in the book, I begin to pivot toward understanding these processes through the lens of the Indo-Tibetan elements of space, wind, fire, water, and earth. Chapter 16 discusses the five Indo-Tibetan elements and their importance in working biodynamically with clients who have metabolic problems. The five elements are directly related to biodynamic perceptual processes, especially PR, the stillness, and the Breath of Life as a light. I introduce visualization practices to support and enhance biodynamic practice with self and other. I finish chapter 16 with a personal experience of how my auditory and visual hallucinations resulting from my PTSD transformed into apparitions of Buddhist deities in order to relieve a core of fear and terror in my heart and body. Once the gun was removed from my heart and home, the deep states of fear and terror could be reckoned with. And thus in part 3 I delve deeply into the reduction of fear and terror in transmuting trauma.

PART 3: INSTINCTS, METABOLISM, AND EMBODIMENT

Chapters 17, 18, and 19 develop a profound view of the origin of our human metabolism being rooted in three primary instincts: self-preservation, self-healing, and self-transcendence. To understand metabolism and trauma, it is important to have a thorough embodied understanding and felt sense of these three instincts. Interoception is key to our human instincts and here is differentiated from exteroception, which involves the five senses. I create a bridge to my own instinctual processes in healing my symptoms related to complex PTSD. Trauma in all of its forms must now be understood in its relationship to human metabolism and the influence of instinctual drives. All clients have a trauma story, and this section of the book presents a new model of working with trauma.

Chapter 20, which I wrote together with my wife Cathy, explores the deep metabolism of the enteric nervous system (ENS). The ENS derives from the vagus nerve in embryology and is of critical importance due to its relationships with the gut, the spinal cord, the heart, and the brain. The ENS is a major player in linking the acquired and innate immune systems, pain mediation, and the gut microbiome. This chapter also contains an important discussion of the pelvic floor and its neurovascular relationships with the abdominal viscera. Chapter 21 introduces the reader to important terminology used in biodynamic practice associated with ignition, midline, and spiritual aptitude. Part 1 began with spiritual ignition, and in this chapter I go much deeper and show how it relates to clinical practice and life in general. I begin exploring embodied spirituality, and especially how to develop the biodynamic spiritual aptitude of visualization practice. Finally, chapter 22 is a thorough exploration of synchronization. This involves a much deeper understanding of the perceptual processes involved in developing biodynamic spiritual aptitudes and introduces the reader and clinician to the cycle of attunement, the root perceptual biodynamic practice. An entire outline of the biodynamic cardiovascular therapy model is presented.

It is within these chapters that the purpose for including the color images in the insert comes to light, for here I have the great good fortune to introduce you to the embryology of the human heart. My good friend Friedrich Wolf, a biodynamic instructor from Germany, made twenty-four watercolor drawings of the development of the heart, which you'll find in the color insert. We worked together to write the captions, and these together with the illustrations are designed to give the reader a sense of the unfolding of the heart and vascular system. The images themselves are important contemplations for seeing and feeling the heart. They are healing images. Following these drawings are ten images that offer a complete mapping of the entire arterial system of the human body. These images come from European anatomy texts and use Latin nomenclature for the individual arteries. In addition, there is a beautiful illustration of the vascular tree, set up as if it were the Tree of Life from the Book of Genesis. It is. At the bottom of this image readers will find a picture of the artery wall, which is essential to its palpation. This is important in terms of the visualization practices taught in parts 3 and 4. Furthermore there are ten images of cardiovascular anatomy of the adult depicted as a labyrinth as well as an image of the Sacred Heart of Jesus to investigate visually in order to find one's heart as an embodied experience.

PART 4: A MINISTRY OF LAYING ON OF HANDS

Part 4 offers a complete exploration of clinical practice with BCVT. Chapter 23 begins with the basic guidelines for integrating perception and palpation of the cardiovascular system. Starting with chapter 24, I present four basic protocols in sequential order for optimal effectiveness in helping the client self-regulate their cardiovascular system at a metabolic level. Chapter 25 presents the four intermediate levels and their protocols with the same intention to improve metabolism. Chapter 26 presents the first of several advanced protocols. Michelle Doyle, who contributed chapter 9, here demonstrates how to safely work metabolically with a pregnant client.

Chapter 27 explores three protocols for the fire element based on Tibetan medicine. It also includes a lengthy discussion of potency, another key osteopathic concept. The potency of PR is directly related to the fire element and is a marker for an optimal outcome at the end of a BCVT session. Chapter 28 explores three protocols for the water and earth elements based on Tibetan medicine. All of these advanced protocols involve visualization practices, and chapters 27 and 28 introduce the biodynamic practitioner and all health care providers to important guidelines for visualizing Health as discussed in chapter 15. In these advanced protocols, Health is associated with color, form, and light. Visualization practices, as I teach them, are medicine and food for the inner work of recovering harmony in the three major instincts discussed in part 3.

Chapter 29 contains three advanced protocols for working with concussions and mild traumatic brain injuries. This level of trauma is becoming more common in our culture and is linked to a breakdown in the metabolic barrier function of the intestines. It is a basic premise of this book that all trauma negatively affects the gut.

Chapter 30, written by Bill Harvey, explores a deep spiritual ignition of the heart. To end the book, chapter 31 takes a deep dive into the heart inside the heart, where spirit lives, and the phenomenon of spiritual heart ignition. I present three protocols to contact the spiritual essence of the heart and its radiance of virtue through the blood to every single cell in the human body.

In this book, I recognize the evolution of biodynamic practices and their various roots in the human embryology of morphology and the cosmology of a variety of ancient world traditions. This evolution meets the needs of the contemporary client suffering with metabolic problems. BCVT is the emergence of a new and constantly evolving biodynamic approach. It is a spiritual practice to wake up the instincts for self-healing and self-transcendence. BCVT is a contemplative practice leading to appropriate compassionate responsiveness. It is now time to find our multidimensional heart centered in spirit.

PART 1

IGNITION OF LIFE AND DEATH, CONCEPTION AND BIRTH

1

5/11

I commend you for your actions on the evening of 11 May 1972 when a terrorist bomb exploded at the Officers' and Civilians' Open Mess in Frankfurt, West Germany. Your presence of mind and self-assured manner contributed to the orderly evacuation of the mess and were instrumental in preventing panic among the employees and patrons.

LT. GENERAL WILLARD PEARSON

I woke that morning like so many others, just before sunrise, as the night surrendered to day. I looked out the window and was glad to see the weather would be good for my mile run around Gruneberg Park before going to work in my office at V Corps, the second largest American military headquarters in Europe. I was prepping for rigorous testing required to earn the German Sports Fitness Medal, despite my troop's doubts. As I headed out, the early morning fog was filled with a smell of ancient trees, all hiding in their magnificent shadows, now only minutes before sunrise. A seeming mirage of other humans appeared out of the fog and as quickly disappeared, each of us attending our wilderness church, hoping the darkness would lift from our minds. I remember them like it was yesterday. The overweight guy who ran with a red hat. The woman with a slight limp. The pretty woman I always waved to. All these souls wanting a moment of peace. They were just bodies moving through the fog, complete strangers to each other.

As the sun began to rise, I arrived back at my pad in the bachelor officer's quarters (BOQ). After a quick shower, two eggs, German rye toast, and Italian coffee, I was off to work at 9 a.m. at the IG Farben Building in Frankfurt, a squat five-story ellipse and a Corps-level Army headquarters housed in a World War II Nazi building. Its history made it a harrowing presence in our lives; we all knew it had been previously owned by a chemical manufacturer that, we all were certain, supplied the four thousand Nazi concentration death camps, spread throughout Germany and its conquered territories in World War II. As an officer I was required to visit the concentration camps to look directly into the face of evil, as if it might motivate me instead of haunt my dreams for the rest of my life. But I went more often than required, again and again, to stand in the gas chambers and peer into the cremation ovens. The images of evil percolated through my being night and day for my entire tour of duty in the IG Farben Building and beyond.

The building was built like a brick shithouse, as we liked to say. It had a unique elevator system consisting of a large, continuously running dumbwaiter without a door, requiring good timing to step on and off it. It was the office for 175 staff officers, including the commanding three-star general, Lieutenant General Willard Pearson, who was fresh from the Vietnam War, where he had commanded the 82nd Airborne Division. In my role as morale and welfare expert, I frequently wrote some of his speeches extolling the virtues of our troops and our foreign policy. Often, I frequented the US Consulate in Frankfurt with him. Sometimes I got to hold his briefcase and hand him his papers.

After work, which was so inconsequential that, despite how intensely that day still sits in my memory, I can't remember a shred of it, I arranged to meet my friend Lieutenant Smythe for dinner at seven o'clock that night at the Terrace Club, an officer's club at the back of the IG Farben Building. I had a date later that same night with my girlfriend, Cindy. We were having the best sex I'd ever had in my life, and I had asked her to marry me. We were going to get together to do some planning.

First I went home, changed, and put in another run in Gruneberg Park, this time with the late-afternoon intoxicating smell of grass and trees. Whereas in the mornings I connected to the fog, in the afternoons I connected to the trees, though in some thoughtless, simplistic way, like a schoolkid knowing that we breathe out carbon dioxide and inhale oxygen, and the trees do the opposite, binding us forever together in a shared act of respiration.

I cleaned up and drove to the Terrace Club. A parking spot—the best parking spot—was reserved for the second lieutenant (meaning me) directly in front of the entrance to the club. The Terrace Club was part of that Nazi configuration of office buildings where I worked and fortunately, as it turns out, was also built like a brick shithouse. It had a magnificent hotel-style ballroom, a second floor where the general had his private dining room, a basement bar called the Keller for beer and wine, and numerous other appointments like a hair salon for the wives of the officers. The night before I had helped host what was called a hail-and-farewell party in the ballroom of the club. Hail-and-farewell parties happened often as officers came and went with their families. Each departing officer was given a silver plaque engraved with their name and time of duty at V Corps Headquarters in Frankfurt. So it was not unusual to have suitcases by the front door of the Terrace Club on any day of the week. Somebody was always coming and going to the airport, having their last two or three or seven drinks before heading out.

C-4 is an extremely powerful plastic explosive. And I loved it. I was trained as a combat engineer officer at Fort Belvoir, Virginia, just down the street from the Pentagon. I learned how to blow stuff up in my training. Lots of neat stuff to blow up. I knew how to shape C-4 around a cement piling on a bridge, a building, or whatever, place the blasting cap in it, and either hardwire it to a detonator, which required a lot of cable, or use a radio-operated detonator, which is the best way to go if you're a combat engineer or a terrorist. The blast is extraordinary no matter what size or amount of C-4 is being used, and the smell of burnt plastic is intoxicating. I loved the size of the fireball, the sound, the smell. It is a whole package of destruction. It's better than any Fourth of July fireworks. I wonder how I can still enjoy classical music when we never used earplugs for our practice bombings.

I pulled into my convenient second lieutenant parking space next to several suitcases. I walked into the club, and immediately around the corner was the cashier, who helped me change dollars for Deutsche Marks, which were still the coin of the realm in the early 1970s. I went into the dining room and could smell the steaks, the burgers, the bratwurst, the cordon bleu, and all my favorites being prepared in the kitchen. I sat down, and two bombs placed on the front steps of the IG Farben Building across the street detonated, and in that millisecond, I thought to myself, that is C-4. And in the moment of that thought, the bomb next to my car exploded. A suitcase by the front door had been filled with C-4—a lot of it, as you can see from the damage in figure 1.1. It detonated with a timer inside the suitcase itself. Brilliant. Kaboom.

The bombing of the Terrace Club formally inducted me into the new age of terrorism that began on 5/11/1972 in Heidelberg, not on 9/11/2001 in New York

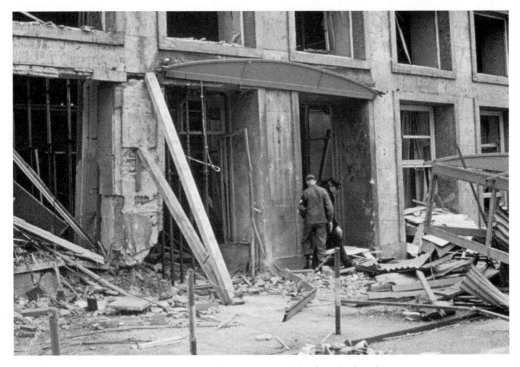

Fig. 1.1. The front of the Terrace Club after the bombing

City with the World Trade Towers going down. The attack was the work of the Baader-Meinhof gang, a large anarchist organization named for its founders, Andreas Baader and Ulrike Meinhof, whose members were responsible for bombings targeting German banks and US military bases throughout the 1970s and early '80s, ostensibly as protests against the politics of American imperialism and the German banking system. Just the week before, a US Army captain and enlisted man had been killed by the same group and same type of bomb in the parking lot of Army headquarters in Heidelberg, Germany. That same year, the Palestinian militant group known as Black September murdered Israeli athletes at the Munich Olympics. The IRA (Irish Republican Army) were bombing Northern Ireland. And on and on the list continues. It was the inaugural year of international terrorist bombings, and the beginning of a predicament filled with hatred and rage that is now continually faced around the world.

The blast in front of the Terrace Club was so powerful it concussed my brain and knocked me off my chair. My head hit the floor, which knocked me out. In that state of unconsciousness, something I never would have believed happened. I've read about it a thousand times since then. I saw a white light, and it was joyful, liberating, and freeing. It was the direction home, and when I moved my attention toward that light, and it got brighter, and I felt bliss. And like in some near-death narratives, a voice rang out: "Go back, it is not your time. Go back, it is not your time. Go back, it is not your time." As the voice faded out, my eyes popped open. Around me on the floor were numerous civilian employees, shocked, terrified, stunned, and immobilized. I got up and started helping people get to their feet: "Come on, let's get up, let's get out of here to a place that's safer." I stumbled into the kitchen and found the chefs on their knees or hunched under their stainless-steel food prep tables, cooking interrupted. I missed my cordon bleu that evening. One by one I helped them up, holding their arms, putting my hands around their waists, lifting them, getting them moving, making sure they could walk out of the building (see fig. 1.2).

The dust from the fake ceiling that had collapsed throughout the building was a choking mix of asbestos, debris, and burnt C-4 (see figs. 1.3–4). It hung in the air, a violent mixture of evil, the smell of blood mixed in a cloud of horror. As I shifted into the lobby, numerous people, mostly civilians, were moving out of the collapsed facade of the front door, climbing over the hellish obstacle course of concrete rubble. I saw brave soldiers stay behind to direct traffic, blood streaming down their faces, arms, and torsos. Most of the front of the Terrace Club was glass, and it had flown like a million sharp-edged bullets in all directions. Those who were closest to the blast got a faceful of it; some lost their eyes. I've never seen that much blood—it spilled everywhere on the floor, like it had just rained red water inside the building. Coagulated blood caked up on my shoes. I was baptized in blood that day.

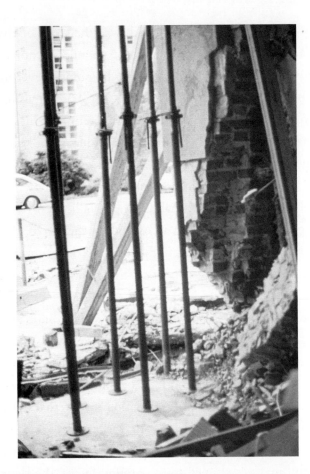

Fig. 1.2. The back of my car, seen through what was once the front door of the Terrace Club

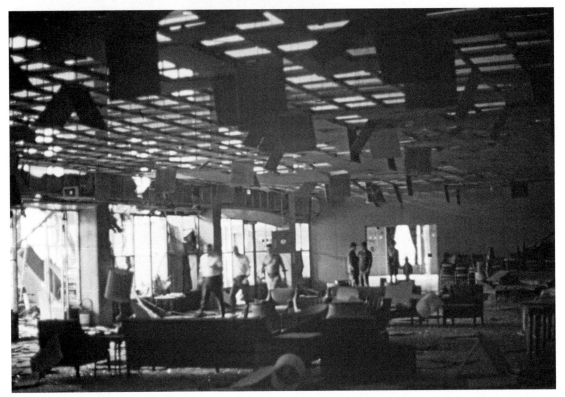

Fig. 1.3. Blown-out ceiling panels in the lobby of the club

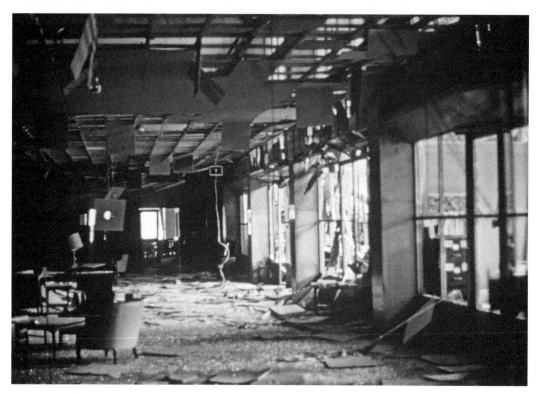

Fig. 1.4. The collapsed lobby

I staggered into the destroyed lobby of the building where Major Smith was directing the evacuation. I asked him where I could help. He told me go down to the Keller and get the civilians down there up and out. So down I went into the basement bar. It was dark. The blast had knocked out the power. I grabbed a flashlight from behind the bar. And sure enough, civilians were huddled under the bar, under the tables, all shaking and trembling like leaves in a tree during a squall. One by one, I helped them up the stairs so they could be escorted out the front of the building. "I'm here to help you," I told them. "Everything is going to be okay."

When all the civilians were out of the Keller, I found Major Smith again as he had moved closer to the entrance to the building. Streams of blood still poured from his face, dripping down his neck and covering over the already dried blood on his shirt. He too was baptized in blood. Major Smith directed me to exit the building and secure space for the ambulances to take away the casualties. Outside, the evening air was fresh. I felt a cool breeze that did not know or care about what had just happened. I felt like I was floating in a timeless realm without feeling or body weight. I looked around and up at the sky to orient and release whatever I had accumulated from inside. Impossible. Many onlookers had gathered, and one ambulance was already there. I could see a body on the ground, and several men preparing to lift the body up into the ambulance. The victim who I had never met until just this moment was Colonel Bloomquist. Dead. I immediately went over and found a place by his shoulder to help lift his dead body. Colonel Bloomquist had walked directly into the bomb when it went off. The shrapnel partially decapitated his head. All that held his head to his torso were his neck bones and shredded muscles. He had bled out on the pavement, and I stared into the eyes of a dead man, my shoes in his blood, and as I knelt down in his blood to lift him, it felt like kneeling to pray in a Roman mithraeum, sacrificing a bull to honor the war god Apollo. My hands became covered in fresh blood.

I partially lost consciousness again, momentarily. I entered a beautiful mysterious place that appeared as another bright tunnel, except this time my eyes were wide open. Now I know it was the Holy Spirit descending on that killing field. I could see Colonel Bloomquist's spirit, his consciousness, hovering on those gorgeous old-growth trees in Gruneberg Park. I could see and feel his presence like an apparition, a purely mystical experience. He was surrounded by the halo of the Holy Spirit. He was sitting on a tree limb, seeming not at all surprised by his apparent condition. And he looked at me and said: "Go forward with compassion, as I did."

Colonel Bloomquist was a highly decorated Vietnam medevac pilot. He transported nine thousand wounded American soldiers from combat zones back to surgical hospital units in Vietnam. He also transported eight thousand dead American soldiers from combat zones to morgues, where the bodies would be identified, put into plastic bags, stacked in a transport plane, and flown home to the United States. He knew something about compassion, and in that moment of being baptized in blood, the heart of compassion was birthed in me. It would need time—a lot of time, indeed the rest of my life—to gestate. It would need time for the divine in all its forms to take up residence in my heart.

More ambulances were arriving, picking up the wounded. Army medics helped clean up the blood from the baptism. Blood was everywhere. As I looked down, my hands and clothes were covered in Colonel Bloomquist's blood. The blood of a hero. We became blood brothers for life that night.

I did eventually make it to my girlfriend's house, even without a car. My car was destroyed since I parked it next to the bomb. Colonel Bloomquist's hat landed in the backseat of my car. The car was totaled. But my girlfriend and I didn't have sex that night or, as it turns out, very often in the weeks and months that followed. Our relationship began to crumble from that point on.

The next morning my boss, Colonel Gregory, called me into his office. He closed the door. I stood at attention. He slowly came around from his position behind his desk. I turned and faced him at attention. He got twelve inches away from my face, his eyes piercing into mine. He asked, "Lieutenant Shea, how was your first taste of action last night?"

I thought for a moment and said, "Sir, I've been trained as a combat engineer, and

I've blown up a lot of bombs, big and small, but that suitcase had a lot of C-4 in it last night. Thank God the Terrace Club was built by Nazis!"

He smiled. Then I said, "Sir, we lost a hero last night, and that's affected me the most. Colonel Bloomquist was a hero. How do you replace heroes who die a senseless death?"

Colonel Gregory said, "Lieutenant Shea, the general staff has already met this morning, and the best we can do at this moment is to name one of our airfields in southern Germany after him. We are then going to create a fund for a museum, celebrating his life of military heroism in his hometown in Idaho. Lieutenant Shea, there is a potential hero in everyone, and you can use this experience to become a hero whether you pursue this military career or not. You are dismissed and can get back to work now, Lieutenant. Thank you, sir. Have a good day."

Have a good day. I ponder having a good day every day of my life since then. I continually ponder getting back to work.

At the time, NATO war exercises took place every several months, and V Corps was a major player to prevent the Russians from bringing their tanks through the Fulda Gap, a lowland corridor running between what was then East and West Germany. To stop the tanks, we had Pershing missiles carrying small-yield tactical nuclear weapons. These nukes were very small and not harmful to the environment—or at least that's what the military had me tell the European press when I was the briefing officer for NATO war games. So, a month later after 5/11, orders were given for a five-day NATO war exercise. The IG Farben Building cleared out, except one officer had to stay behind on each floor as a kind of guard for the duration of the exercises. You just never know when some crazy German national might want to break in and steal one of the many IBM Selectric typewriters. I was chosen to stay behind with my Colt .45 holstered at my waist to guard and live in the office for five days. I was in the morale and welfare division of the headquarters, an ironic name given my state of mind. I was assigned an enlisted man for whatever duties might be needed, which basically entailed getting me food. I was hungry after the bombing. Really hungry. I began eating five meals a day. I sent out my enlisted man, Gary, all through the day and into the evening to retrieve brats and beer for both of us. I could've won a bratwurst eating contest with the amount of sausage I was stuffing into my belly. It was as if I was reinforcing the solidity of my sorrow and sadness.

It was midnight on day three. I was ready for my next exercise in overeating and wondering where Gary was. I walked down the hallway in the suite of offices, and there he was with his feet up on the colonel's desk, smoking a pipe. Gary's pipe was filled with a potent mixture of opiated hash and tobacco. It smelled terrible and filled the office with a huge ball of smoke that thankfully was not setting off any fire alarms. I looked at him, and he looked at me, and then he said, "Lieutenant Shea, sir, do you want a hit?" I did not hesitate to partake. That was the point at which I turned down the path of recreational drug use to relieve the deep inner fear that had grabbed hold of my heart. Compassion had been born entangled with terror. What a screwed-up partnership to unwind. Relief, however temporary, was one quick hit away.

Since the bombing, my BOQ, the IG Farben Building, and many other American facilities in Frankfurt, and Germany in general, had been ringed with fully armed combat infantry soldiers. Outside the window of my BOQ was an American soldier with a loaded rifle to protect me for the next three months. My sense of hearing became more acute, and every time the metal front door of the BOQ banged closed, it sounded like a small explosion, rattling the windows and metal frames echoing throughout the building. It was a constant reminder, a perpetual wake-up call, day and night, of the horror. The bomb began to explode regularly, at full volume, in my dreams, shocking me awake with a racing heart and a sweat-drenched bed. Still does after all these years.

At the same time that combat soldiers appeared outside my BOQ window, every entrance and exit to the Autobahn superhighway system in West Germany was closed and each car inspected. Within a week, Andreas Baader and Ulrike Meinhof were captured and put in jail, and they mysteriously committed suicide by hanging themselves in their jail cells a month later. And in figure 1.5 you can see the medal I received.

That baptism of blood left me with a sense of unresolved grief, but I did not know that I had a mental health problem for almost twenty years after I got out of the Army. Every soldier who has survived a killing field carries sorrow buried deep

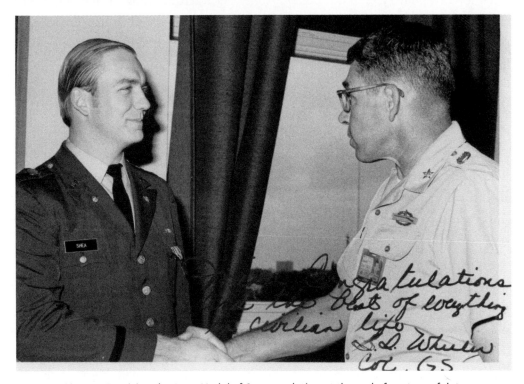

Fig. 1.5. Receiving the Army Medal of Commendation at the end of my tour of duty

in the heart. I do. Yet I ingested my grief without mixing it with my sorrow and became bloated and obese physically. PTSD is one thing; unresolved grief is another. My heart hardened like a prison cell block, as you will see in chapter 10, and forty years later began exhibiting atrial fibrillation. It's been my work to activate the spiritual enzyme of sorrow in order to ferment and digest my grief with an open heart. Through my work with children experiencing moderate to severe developmental delays, I was gradually able to begin this process, as you will see in the next chapter.

I welcome all of you to *The Biodynamic Heart*.

2

Igniting Compassion

Working with Babies

This chapter describes my forty-year history of pediatric practice and in particular my experience with trauma and cerebral palsy in young children. In 1980 I began working with children who suffered from traumatic brain injury (TBI). At that time, I was practicing Rolfing, a reorganization of the fascial connective tissue system of the body around a central axis. I remember flying to Cincinnati at the invitation of a pediatric physical therapist. I was invited to evaluate twenty infants and children with a diagnosis of cerebral palsy. I had given a series of Rolfing sessions to her, and she thought that Rolfing or what might now commonly be called myofascial release would be a wonderful adjunct to her manipulation and movement therapy. She was right. And my pediatric career was launched.

In the years since, I've worked with young children with moderate to severe developmental disabilities and many in a persistent vegetative state. Usually that includes no walking or speech. My first learning was that no matter how severe or life-threatening the diagnosis, their personalities and communication styles were intact. Compromised infants and children have a communication system that doesn't take too long to figure out, and it's collaborative and reciprocal. My Jungian analyst Barry Williams had a child who survived twenty-six years in a persistent vegetative state. I was around this child while he was in his mother Renata's womb because I treated her during her pregnancy, and Barry and Renata brought this child home for care after a horrendous birth in which Rafael did not breath for more than five minutes. Because they are also trained as shamans in the Huichol tradition, they flew him to all the best shamans in the world; Barry tells the story in chapter 5. I attended and facilitated one of these shamanic sessions on the Diné reservation in Arizona. Barry and Renata were always told the same thing: This child is a shaman; he is a healer. Such children live partly in the divine realm and only partially in the human realm. They have a foot in both worlds. They are special; they are facilitators of great compassion in those who care for them.

It's important to let go of all expectations about the form and function of a human being over a lifetime. Development unfolds differently for every human being, especially for a child born prematurely. In a human embryo, every part of the body has a different timing for growth—and it's different from human to human, even in identical twins. Traditional developmental maps of humans miss this important piece. Working with children with severe developmental disabilities teaches us to be with them as they are, not according to what a developmental science map says about everyone being in the same box at the same time of life. Working with this population for so many years taught me that the client was the teacher, and what I was being taught was compassion. Does that not make these kids enlightened beings because they clearly have a foot in two worlds?

Cerebral palsy is a form of TBI caused by a variety of traumas (prenatal, birth-related, or postnatal) that result in significant developmental delays. These can include anything from an inability to walk or eat to cognitive and sensory deficits. A prenatal trauma can be on a spectrum from intrauterine growth restriction from a wide variety of factors, many of which are associated with a poor diet, to physical abuse coming from a partner who kicks or punches the pregnant mother's abdomen or rages constantly at the mother. I worked with many such children who sustained prenatal violence from their mom's partner. Birth trauma can result from overuse of forceps, vacuum extraction, and/or subsequent loss of oxygen to the brain (anoxia). Health outcomes can be disastrous from obstetrical racism, which is well documented (Bryant et al. 2010). It may include the shock and trauma of cesarean sections and premature cutting of the umbilical cord. (And yes, emergency C-sections are necessary to save lives but are overused.) Postnatal trauma to the brain can come about through a wide spectrum of experiences, from physical abuse to the consequences of insecure and disorganized attachments with caregivers that disrupts the autonomic nervous system of the infant, resulting in numerous downstream psychological and physical problems.

In my early years of working with TBI, I used Rolfing techniques on a category of these children called *high toned*. These children had extensive spasticity in the musculoskeletal/fascial system, preventing them from standing and walking properly. They also had problems with feeding and sensory deficits. The physical manipulation of Rolfing allowed these children to stand up and stabilize with their feet on the ground and establish a better and more stable movement pattern. It also helped with feeding issues, especially with physical manipulation around the gut and administration of a ketogenic diet to improve brain health. (Ketogenic diets have been used with children since the 1920s with excellent results, and it is comical that there is such controversy today about using keto diets to improve adult brain health.) These improvements allowed the brain to become more plastic and adaptive. These changes could be sustained over time with other adjunct therapy, such as movement therapy done by a pediatric team of physical therapists, occupational therapists, and speech therapists.

CRANIOSACRAL THERAPY

Having seen success in treating children with severe developmental delays using the physical manipulation of Rolfing, I gradually developed protocols and courses for the Easterseals organization and several pediatric clinics associated with the medical schools at Wake Forest University, the University of Florida, and Ohio State University. I also developed protocols for children with TBI who had fetal alcohol and fetal cocaine syndromes, which cause brain seizures and significant developmental delays. I traveled extensively around the United States and Canada to consult and teach at numerous pediatric clinics. I love working with these kids. It is a great way to ignite compassion. Children are the best spiritual teachers.

I began studying craniosacral therapy and combining it with myofascial release. The results were quite remarkable. There was a significant reduction or elimination of seizure activity in many children, a noticeable increase in cognition and learning, improved feeding (which is critical), and a reduction in hyperarousal.

I began consulting for different state institutions housing children with very severe developmental delays. They included infants with shaken baby syndrome, in which a caretaker violently shakes the baby to stop it from crying, thus severely damaging the infant's fragile brain, as well as children who had been heinously abused. One such child whom I will never forget had boiling oil poured over her face and into her mouth to stop her from crying when she was a baby. The resulting neurological insult was devastating. Even she, at the age of nine when I first saw her, gained a greater degree of cognition and communication from the therapeutic protocol I'd put together.

I learned through these experiences that all children have an intact communication system. All I had to do was synchronize with it, and then I could start negotiating with the child on what was needed. No matter what age or trauma, every child has the capacity to indicate a yes and a no. In many cases the children guided my hands and mind to form a safe therapeutic container and safe relationship. I must also say that these brave little ones and their caregivers taught me so much about the power of compassion and the family love.

I was invited to develop a program called Integrative Touch Therapy at the Miami Children's Hospital, Dan Marino Center, in Westin, Florida. I worked there in conjunction with pediatric neurologists and pediatric physical therapists for a year. I developed protocols for children with a wide variety of issues, but especially for infants with anomalies of the cranium, such as craniosynostosis, which is a birth defect involving premature fusion of the cranial sutures, and pediatric encephalopathy or plagiocephaly, which is a misshapen head resulting from compression during a vaginal delivery. The pediatric physical therapists I worked with were already utilizing craniosacral therapy to a large degree, including at summer camps for children with cerebral palsy in which the children would receive multiple-hands craniosacral therapy.

I began to see the value of craniosacral therapy more and more when the principal challenge was with the head itself. It greatly relieved entrapment neuropathies of the cranial nerves, thus normalizing the suck-swallow-breathe reflex in children and improving digestion and elimination. I started to form a postdoctoral research committee to study the value of craniosacral therapy with these children, but at the end of the year, the hospital decided to go in a different direction with the program and so I left. I then decided to focus exclusively on the use of biodynamic craniosacral therapy for the children I was seeing. This work evolved into a five-level training in pediatric craniosacral therapy and a six-level training in trauma resolution for adult clients. I taught those programs throughout Europe and North America.

Until the onset of COVID in 2020, I was seeing several children with TBIs in Italy and Germany. Leo, in Germany, had been in a very bad car accident at the age of six months; he'd suffered a severe concussion, his tongue was severed and had to be surgically reattached, and the insult to his brain caused him to become quadriplegic. Leo's mother, who had been the driver, needed three years of rehabilitation to repair all her broken bones. The father, who had not been in the car with them, was a completely amazing caregiver (a phenomenon I've seen over and over again with the parents of these children). Leo was on a respirator but was able to speak and very communicative. He gradually became very responsive to biodynamic craniosacral therapy and the perception of a slow therapeutic movement in the brain and body called Primary Respiration. I taught his mother how to perceive Primary Respiration and sense it in Leo therapeutically. After the first session in which I worked on him, his parents told me that I was the first male therapist Leo had allowed to contact him since his hospitalization. I attribute this to the work with Primary Respiration, which creates a safe space for children with brain injuries.

More often in these past few years, I see biodynamic therapy helping children such as Leo become much more able to self-regulate, both emotionally and physiologically, regarding feeding and communication, including speech improvement. In addition, while working with a severely neurologically damaged child in Italy several years ago, I came to appreciate the value of metabolic testing. I now advise that any child with a TBI have metabolic testing for specific intolerances of foods such as gluten, sugar, and dairy. Children with TBIs who have proper metabolic testing and are fed a ketogenic diet that matches their metabolism get better across all parameters of development compared to other children with the same problems but no dietary changes (Wells et al. 2020). This is especially true in conjunction with the use of biodynamic craniosacral therapy because of the support for the suck-swallow-breathe reflex. I now feel that even my adult clients with TBI should be metabolically tested for inflammation caused by eating processed food. It simply speeds up the healing process in the brain and body.

Perhaps the most common problem I am presented with nowadays is infants with feeding issues. Through the pediatric osteopaths I studied with, I learned to evaluate the suck-swallow-breathe reflex before working on the head. This is because feeding issues may arise from the respiratory diaphragm, as the esophagus passes through it, and intestinal tone in general.

I have also worked with children who are dying. This is a great gift and one more story that will lift your heart. I treated a little one near death at the request of the family's therapist, who knew me and was taking a class with me at the time. I ended up treating this child several times in class, with the child's extended family present. You cannot know the rare gift that children who are dying give us when they look in your face with complete acceptance. The child died the night after a session. The next morning, the therapist reported that the parents had been completely awestruck to see that, as the child lay there dying, he broke out into a smile. He died with that smile on his face, beaming for the world to see his happiness and relief. That is when I learned about the power of the Breath of Life in my subsequent work with adults in end-of-life care. When I place my hands on dying patients, whether in hospice, at home, or at a hospital, the gift of biodynamics is pure grace. We must remember how lucky we are to have this practice. These children helped melt my fearful heart and ignite compassion for myself and the world.

EMPATHY AND COMPASSION

The primary intention in Buddhism is to directly relate with and acknowledge one's own suffering. This is followed by realizing how it is shared with all of humanity. This means getting to know one's mind through thoughts, feelings, perceptions, and conceptualizations from a witness perspective. Upon looking more closely at the nature of one's mind, it is clear that we are all on a roller-coaster ride of ups and downs, moods and emotions, and lots of thoughts. In general, this is considered suffering because of its compulsive and afflictive emotional and cognitive states, and all sentient beings share in this style of suffering. It is suffering because it prevents us from seeing the world clearly.

Relating to one's own suffering and then recognizing how other people suffer similarly develops the instinct for compassion. Sometimes a specific event ignites the development of compassion, like the bombing attack I was in during my military service in Germany; I was twenty-four years old when that happened, and I had fifty years of gestating and ripening this opportunity to be compassionate into a spiritual maturity thanks to so many children who taught me. It takes time to develop compassion because we are the experiment; we are the laboratory of trial and error. In this way, compassion requires a spiritual formation process that leads to a spiritual maturation that leads to the embodiment of a direct connection to the sacred that lives in the human heart.

Empathy

Empathy can be called ordinary compassion because it simply and yet profoundly involves feeling what another person is feeling. We live in a day and age in which the lack of empathy is pandemic. And again, before we can feel what another person is feeling, we must have a relationship with our own suffering and neurotic compulsive mind. Otherwise, as one teacher of mine called it, we have idiot compassion, or, as it's known in the psychological literature, codependency. Consequently, empathy for oneself is necessary, and it is trending right now in the literature under the term "self-compassion."

Empathy has three categories: somatic, emotional, and cognitive. For many years I had a full practice of Rolfing, and frequently when I was walking to the office in the morning my body would take on the aches and pains of the clients I was about to treat—somatic empathy. That became obvious to me early in my career.

During treatments, one hears the stories clients tell about their experience. I always ask: "How did this happen?" This generates emotional empathy and softens the heart with a felt sense of sorrow about the other person's condition. It can also amuse you, which is also empathy. There are two sides to the empathy coin—sadness and joy (great!).

The hardest empathy to realize is cognitive empathy. This is the transition to a deeper knowing in which we begin to set aside our own thoughts, feelings, and emotions through our meditation practice or other therapeutic skills. We do this in order to literally place ourselves in the mindset or shoes of another person and truly see the world from their eyes and body. And again, what we experience is a sense of sorrow, elation, or neutrality. This depends of course on what the other person's experience is about and the condition of our preset filters, mentally and emotionally, for hearing and seeing complex psychoemotional situations and stories of spiritual dilemmas. Self-compassion requires the ability to look at yourself from open awareness.

A lot of our work is to deconstruct our own filters and beliefs about life and inhabit a neutral space in the therapeutic relationship, mentally and emotionally. Knowing our own motivation clearly is vital. We all create identities around life experience. Hi, I'm Michael and I have PTSD was my identity for many years.

If we are immersed in a dramatic and draining situation—for example, if we are working at a hospital and seeing devastating disease and trauma—we can enter empathetic distress, which is also related to moral distress when we don't agree with decisions about whether or how a patient lives or dies. Therefore, the loop starts with our own inner perception and our own mind states. Empathetic distress is natural, but once we recognize it, we need a vacation as soon as possible to recharge and build up the potency of self-compassion.

Compassion

Deep compassion or great compassion, as it is called in Buddhism, is based on all the foregoing conversation about the development of empathy and recognizing mental-emotional sources of suffering. Fundamentally, compassion involves an appropriate response first to one's own suffering and then toward that of our clients or family, friends, and loved ones. The determination of an appropriate response rather than a knee-jerk reaction, like the sympathetic desire to be of help or to ignore, is challenging. So many of our reactions do not come from a place of compassion because we really don't know the depth of what others carry.

That is why getting to know our own mind, especially when we encounter fear, the fear of not knowing how to be with another person, is so important. Once we come to grips with our own fear, we are able to transition to a more relaxed state of bearing witness.

Compassion is the glue of love, the spiritual nature of the connection we have with a client. We can regularly practice the three types of empathy—somatic, emotional, and cognitive—to fully engage our own compassionate instinct. Our client is experiencing pain and suffering. Our innate compassion metabolizes the client's feelings with our perception in the present moment. Physical pain or emotional distress is no longer limited to the client's body and mind but becomes a shared sensation in the present moment of a safe two-person biology. This makes suffering less deep and anchored. The next step is watching Primary Respiration (PR) and stillness do their work, connecting to the energetic source of life, the universal intelligence that lives in our heart and from which we all derive. A divine source created by love is the heart inside the heart of every human being. Connecting with the help of PR and in stillness to that part of our heart enables deep connection with all of life in the moment. We may feel grateful and humble for the creation of life as a function of our own heart, the pure essence of being. In that space and in that moment, the client gets access to healthy versions of their higher self. As therapists, we observe PR and stillness guiding the client with compassion as a radiance from our own heart. The connection to PR and its guidance takes place in the stillness.

Biodynamic practice involves a lot of waiting for the appropriate response under the guidance of PR and dynamic stillness. For me, PR and dynamic stillness are the circulatory processes of loving kindness and compassion. Empathy and compassion fit within a larger framework of spiritual maturation because they take time to develop, like all instincts do.

WISDOM

From a Buddhist point of view, to properly develop compassion one must have a wisdom practice. One must cultivate mindfulness and awareness through meditation practice, of which many styles are now taught. A side effect of meditation practice is gaining insight called vipashyana. This relates to discovering the lack of a solid self that in reality is simply one's personality. This examination and realization that there is no solid self under our personality leads to compassion. Such solidity is simply built from thoughts building concepts and concepts building unrealistic world views and interpretations of body and mind. It is not solid at all. Meditation disassembles such seemingly solidness into a natural flow and acceptance of a constantly changing process called life. One's motivation for meditation practice must also be explored because the territory that is investigated with meditation can be profound on a spectrum from difficult to blissful. It offers a full-on look at one's self as it has been built over one's lifetime.

A large category of Buddhist teachings is based on meditation practice. You start with either shamatha from the Indo-Tibetan system or zazen from the Chinese-Japanese system. I've done both and currently prefer shamatha, which matches the study I am undertaking with Tibetan medicine and medical tantric yoga practice. Eastern traditions study the bridge between the ordinary body physiology and the subtle body of the channels, winds, and subtle energies. These traditions say that there is also a very subtle body, the body of the primordial Buddha, the awakened mind in which all sentient beings are the primordial Buddha. It is the essence of nonduality and its lived experience. It is built into the package of having a human body and defines the nature of great compassion as seeing all sentient beings as Buddha or God or Holy Spirit. The fundamental notion is the development of a nonconceptual meditation practice to calm the mind and see reality clearly, without polarization. Compassion requires such wisdom in order to arise naturally and spontaneously in any given situation.

For my own basic meditation practice to ignite wisdom, I sit in the following posture:

- The spine is upright, with a natural curve.
- The hands are resting palms down on the thighs.
- The arms and shoulders are relaxed.
- The chin is slightly tucked.

- The eyelids are half closed, and the eyes have a soft gaze.
- The face and jaw are natural and relaxed.
- If I'm sitting on a cushion, the legs are loosely crossed, with the knees below the plane of the hips.

When meditating, our mind tends to move around constantly. And there are consistent patterns to such movement called the six factors. Whenever my mind wanders toward these six factors, I bring myself back to the last point to overcome solidity:

> *Don't recall. Let go of what has passed.*
> *Don't imagine. Let go of what may come.*
> *Don't think. Let go of what is happening now.*
> *Don't examine. Don't try to figure anything out.*
> *Don't control. Don't try to make anything happen.*
> *Rest. Relax, right now, and rest.*

COMPASSION SCIENCE

The science of compassion is its own academic field. The *Oxford Handbook of Compassion Science* (Seppälä et al. 2017) is its bible. In addition, the Center for Compassion and Altruism Research and Education (CCARE) at Stanford University does excellent work bridging the world of compassion science and Buddhism.

It's important to remember that empathy and compassion are instincts that require development over time. Contemplative neuroscience is an emerging field that studies the manner in which contemplative practices, such as those that explore empathy and compassion in the pursuit of wisdom, affect the brain. Research in this field is showing that regular practice of prayer, meditation, and other mindfulness practices can promote neuroplasticity, meaning the ability of the brain's neural networks to change, adapt, and grow.

Once upon a time mirror neurons were seen as the neurological map of compassion. However, that notion was disproved some years ago as the original research was done on monkeys and somehow did not translate to humans. It was an elegant theory and I lectured on it, but no longer.

The fields of interpersonal neurobiology and interpersonal cardiovascular systems based on affective neuroscience are also related to the embodied development of compassion. The hearts and brains of mom and baby are synchronized through pregnancy and beyond. This template of interpersonal connectedness extends to everyone following birth and perhaps even before birth. The foundation for compassion can be linked to the social interaction between caregiver and baby. In fact, compassion's broad developmental context includes the prenatal and neonatal time. I wrote a piece for Ann Weinstein's 2016 book *Prenatal Development and Parents' Lived Experiences: How Early Events Shape Our Psychophysiology and Relationships* in which I postulated that pregnancy itself is the greatest act of compassion—you'll find that piece in chapter 6.

In a chapter in *The Oxford Handbook of Compassion Science,* Stephen Porges makes a case for polyvagal theory being a compassion-based model in which social safety ignites the desire to care for another person. From this perspective, to be compassionate means to reduce our own defensive physiology safely, feel the other person empathetically, and wait to engage in an appropriate response. We have learned unconscious patterns of physiological defensiveness depending on our trauma history and early attachment experience with a caregiver. This means each of us has a set point of defensive physiology that needs to be softened for trusting the world and feeling safe with another person. Consequently, the first responsibility of a therapist is to promote safety and know the moment when a client's nervous system and heart has reduced its defensive physiology. Porges lays out four points for his polyvagal compassion model. The first two involve the passive and active vagal pathways, but in number three he calls for "extensive contemplative training; and [number four] the emergent properties of contemplative practices, including the capacity to experience and express compassion" (Porges 2017, 201). He contends that this capacity to express compassion depends on the brain stem, where the vagus nerve originates, and requires the interoceptive awareness to know that one's heartbeat is elevated and the skills to put on the vagal brake, which slows the heart.

Thus, compassion is about the heart both literally and figuratively, and emotional empathy and deep cardiac compassion is necessary to be a full human being. And to know the heart at this depth requires having a contemplative practice.

3

Understanding Sorrow and Death

*When the true practitioner dies, he is like a beggar in the street, alone
with no hope and no one taking care, like an infant who does not even
have conceptions about birth and death.*

LONGCHENPA, FOURTEENTH-CENTURY TIBETAN
BUDDHIST SCHOLAR (NORBHU 1999, 78)

We are all standing at the edge of an incredible opportunity. We create the world
based on our inner perception. We have the capacity to transform our inner space,
emotionally and spiritually, and thus also to transform the outside world. If we can
accept the necessity of turning inward and facing our inner reality, we can then
turn outward—toward our home, our family, our friends, and our clients—and be a
force for transformation via the kindness of the *life force of the tide* coming from our
heart. The osteopathic community over the years has used different metaphors for
this life force. *The Tide* and *Primary Respiration* are most frequently used and are
interchangeable.

The life force is a movement and a felt sense coming from the heart as a bright
light and a sacred image. It opens the whole spiritual spectrum of healing, bridging the span between the realm of the divine and the realm of the natural world. It
offers completion, containment, and integration of the heart inside the heart. This is
the place in our heart where all good, wholesome qualities and virtues reside. Some
traditions say this place is formless and call it the fifth chamber of the heart. Other
traditions claim it is in the left ventricle of the heart.

SORROW IGNITION

Tonglen is an important Tibetan Buddhist compassion meditation. In the Kagyu tradition of Tibetan Buddhism, Tonglen requires an initiation from a qualified master; I
myself received the transmission of Tonglen from Pema Chodron in an afternoon ceremony at the Karma Dzong Meditation Center in Boulder, Colorado, in 1981, before
I took the Bodhisattva Vow. The short version of the Bodhisattva Vow that I recite

every day is: As long as space remains, as long as sentient beings remain, until then may I remain to dispel the miseries of the world.

Tonglen, as I learned it, ignites sorrow. It is always preceded by shamatha-vipashyana (calm abiding) meditation, which initiates a very deep purification of the heart and cardiovascular system and allows the self to dissolve. The practitioner then traditionally generates a felt sense of sorrow, perhaps by bringing to their mind's eye one particular memory that evokes sorrow for them. That is the start of the practice to acknowledge our preexisting sorrow and allow it to ferment with grief.

Sorrow is the ground of compassion and the preexisting condition of our human heart. When our heart experiences sorrow, it relaxes and expands into its original condition in the embryo. The embryonic heart, especially the ventricles, grows in what is called a dilation field, in which, without ribs in front of it, it has an incredible capacity to expand and enlarge. When the left ventricle first forms, it is like watching a balloon blowing up (consequently, it is called ballooning). The act of engaging our sorrow actually relaxes and opens the heart so that we are better able to contain more and metabolically process challenges—not just our own but those of others as well. When it comes to taking on grief, this expandable ballooning quality of the heart increases, and specifically the left ventricle, allowing the felt sense of love to continue to grow while less blood is ejected from the left ventricle. Imagine that the left ventricle of the heart is the center of love and its many permutations in our whole body. By igniting sorrow, we ignite our capacity for love and humility and the recognition and felt sense of our own suffering and the suffering of other people. This level of humility breaks down barriers between humans and helps us understand our shared humanity.

Sorrow is an expression of love. It is not sadness. Sadness is a relatively generic psychological state that may or may not be connected to love. Sadness is transitory; it passes or becomes depression and pathological. In contrast, sorrow informs us physically, by the interoception of our heartbeat and its potency, about how big our heart really is—and how big love really is. If our heart is so vast that it can hold deep sorrow, then the space of the heart is large enough to house the sacred, as is held in all major world religions. Jesus lives in your heart. Buddha lives in your heart. These are metaphors for the way the sacred incubates in our sorrow, which feels like it is happening in a huge empty void. This is your left ventricle. Visualize a divine figure living in your heart in the recesses of your left ventricle. Convert Tonglen meditation into a compassion practice in which you visualize the Breath of Life, the Buddha, Jesus, the Breath of Life, or simply a clear light literally housed in your left ventricle. Then visualize the person—and maybe it is you—who is suffering. Allow an image of Jesus (or any sacred figure) to rest over the head and body of the suffering person. Allow bright light to radiate from the heart of Jesus into the suffering person. How simple and how profound. It takes only a minute and requires only a quiet space to practice.

All human beings have a heart of sorrow that connects us to a spiritual essence. Our heartbeat is powered by the sacred. Our blood is moved by the sacred. It is possible to see the sacred if we can sense our heartbeat and its potency. If we have emptied our heart space of toxic emotions, the spirit can reside in its true home inside our body and inside our heart.

At this time on the planet, driven by social and news media, we have become more sensitive to our fears. Consequently, now is the time to use all of our inner spiritual-contemplative skills to reduce our own fears and the fears of others. If not now, when? Some years ago, the Dalai Lama requested that anyone who knows the practice of Tonglen please begin immediately teaching it to as many people as possible, without any need to have received the initiation of the Bodhisattva Vow. (You can find the instructions for Tonglen in my previous book, *The Biodynamics of the Immune System*.) More recently, Pema Chodron said that when we practice the giving aspect of compassion meditation, we can make it simple: Inhale the bad, exhale the good.

As biodynamic practitioners, we give the life force of the tide from our heart, which is free from fear. It is a very deep level of healing. But everyone can learn to give from their heart in one way or another. We can visualize, intend, or think about giving simple things to other people to reduce their fear. If my brother, who absolutely loves coffee, is having some anxiety or other challenge, I visualize offering him a fantastic cup of coffee. Sometimes the best thing we can give someone else is our smile. That is all. That is enough.

When we feel the life force of the tide moving from the back of our heart, extending everywhere in the world or to specific people, in whatever way, we are offering everyone a second heart, the heart within the heart that I discuss throughout this book. It is a metaphor for compassion, and a practice for our time.

DEATH IGNITION

The biggest imprint on the embryo is death anxiety. Creation automatically generates its partner, so to speak. This is the most fundamental polarity of life. There is always an ending to match the beginning. The embryo has been surrounded by death from the moment of its original differentiation into an egg. Millions of eggs die in the course of development. Most embryos die and never make it to birth. Something must end for something to begin. Once the infant is born, his umbilical cord is cut, and he must die to himself as his external body of the placenta dies. Thus, birth is also about death.

One intention of biodynamic cardiovascular therapy is to reconnect the client to the natural world. The natural world does not fear death but sees it as an instinctual phase of existence. I cannot know what a client carries, but in the phases of Primary Respiration I can hold the client and support the client if they choose to let go of a pattern or need to hold it to clarify and understand the meaning of their own life. For me, Primary Respiration is a zone of descent and deliberation. It seems so close to death that I am convinced that Primary Respiration on its phases of expansion and contraction gives us a glimpse of our own death and last breath as well as a space to examine death at many different levels, from the mundane letting go of anger and resentment to a clear space to examine any fear around our actual death.

Death ignition is related to the programmed cell death in our body called apoptosis. At the same time it is an intimate experience of self-transcendence, a deep inner knowing of the ultimate reality that our body will cease to exist. This instinctual knowing is linked to an innate part of our metabolic identity and must be considered in the therapeutic process. Death surrounds the embryo and fills the embryo as a metabolic and spiritual reality. We all live with an "inner corpse."

In each of us is an inner corpse struggling to be exhumed. Unlike the corpse you will one day become, this shadow corpse is alive. It is the living presence of death that you carry within you. It is more than your certain knowledge of death's ultimate triumph; it is your portal to nothingness, the other ocean of Being. If you can find the courage to unearth and embrace your inner corpse, you can lead a more vivid, expansive, and authentic life. But if you keep your inner corpse buried away, you live a great lie. You distort your search for truth into a project of false immortality. You deny the most solemn core of your being, condemning yourself to premature cheerfulness. To the outside world you might seem healthy, happy, and successful—but your inner corpse might just as well be dead.

My inner corpse is not dead.*

In some ways, it is a gift to be able to contemplate death as closely and easily as opening the news app on our phone, as often as we please, to see one disaster after another up close and personal. Our work now is to contemplate death, to ignite sorrow and understand the imminence of death, and we now receive daily reminders of the dying to come in every corner of the world. How close is our own death? This is real food for our heart within our heart!

The Buddha said there is suffering and there is joy. Let us all remember to stay

---

*From: "Embracing Your Inner Corpse" from: *Daily Afflictions: The Agony of Being Connected to Everything in the Universe* by Andrew Boyd. Copyright © 2002 by Andrew Boyd. Used by permission of W. W. Norton & Company, Inc.

balanced in these times. They will end. And our lives will end too. We all will experience a last breath. Make being conscious of this reality a priority for spiritual transformation. How do we want to die? Right now, we have the present moment, which is a profound spiritual teacher.

May all the breaths left in our individual lifetimes be holy. May we constantly contemplate our inhalation as life and our exhalation as death. May we allow ourselves to admit spirit into the deepest recesses of our hearts.

The Four Reminders

The four reminders are based on a beautiful traditional story in Buddhism about a lone billion-year-old blind turtle who lives at the bottom of the ocean. Every one hundred years it comes to the surface of the ocean to take a breath. Floating on the surface of the entire ocean is only one cattle yoke. The chances of the turtle popping its head through the cattle yoke when surfacing is said to be greater than the chances of becoming a human being. Being born human is luckier than the probability of this blind turtle popping its head through a cattle yoke on the vast ocean. This lends itself to a recent conversation by the scientist Richard Dawkins. According to him, the very unlikely chance of being born is 1 in 400 trillion. This is because the amount of available DNA so vastly outnumbers the number of actual people. The four reminders are a contemplation on how lucky we are and how quickly our life is over. Consequently we are reminded that it is time to lead the spiritual life.

First, contemplate the preciousness of having a human body, with its sensory capacity, and being free from war and oppression, being well-favored with time and health, and having access to sacred teachings and an authentic teacher. Human birth is rare: difficult to gain, easy to lose. Now I must do something meaningful for the benefit of all sentient beings.

Second, the whole world and its inhabitants are impermanent. Change is constant. Every day is a roller coaster of thoughts and emotions. Even this ordinary mind exhausts itself. Whatever appears will disappear. I have the same nature. The life of all sentient beings is like a temporary bubble. Death can come without warning; this body will be a corpse. At that time, the dharma of self-knowing wisdom awareness of open space and relaxation will be my only help; I must practice not-knowing, simplicity, and humility with exertion 24/7 to overcome fear. I must learn non-thinking by allowing my thoughts to self-liberate, on their own, without stimulating them.

Third, when death comes, I will be helpless to prevent it. Fear, anxiety, and pain may accompany my dying. Now is the time to tame my mind of fear, anxiety, and pain. I make friends with my inner demons and do not kick the can of avoidance down the road. Because I create karma, I must discern compulsive ill-intentioned actions and always devote my time to recognizing innate virtue. Contemplating this, every day I will exert mindfulness toward my mental, emotional, and physical behavior.

Fourth, social media, junk food, debt, negative thoughts, emotional afflictions, and cognitive confusion result in unrealistic life views and ironically become the comforts of samsara (hell). They are a constant spiritual torment. Yet by cultivating nonreferential awareness, I may perceive the inescapable vision of samsara and nirvana (heaven) being one and the same thing. It is all good. The present moment is the supreme spiritual teacher.

MY MOTHER TAUGHT ME SORROW

My mother forgave me for every way in which I had ever failed her. It was one of my Christmas presents in the mid-1990s. She had been intubated the year before and lived on a respirator and a feeding tube, with occasional catheterization, in a nursing home called Whitehall (see fig. 3.1). She remained lucid throughout these interventions, which gave her almost a decade more of life.

It happened so easily and suddenly that it caught me by surprise. I was getting ready to leave, and my mother was getting ready for the twenty-minute ritual that it took for the nursing home staff to put her into bed. As the nurses brought in the Hoyer lift, a crane that lifts a person out of a wheelchair and into bed, my mother asked me to wait. I usually go home at this point, but she said, "If you wait, I'll forgive you for everything you ever did to me." This staunch Roman Catholic Irish woman held grudges for a lifetime, but this offer—well, I believed her. Her voice and her eyes told me she meant it, and as she lay there with eight breaths per minute being pumped into her by machine, her yellow gown and the white collar around the stoma of the trachea, looking much like a bow tie, gave an air of formality to her statement. I quipped that I'd be lucky to go three days before I did something new to piss her off, but I stayed. I wondered why my mother's love seemed conditional. *I'll forgive you if you stay with me.* I could not know her inner sorrow.

Eventually I left to go home. From Whitehall to Powerline Road to Glades Road to the Florida Turnpike north to Juno Beach, the whole trip takes fifty minutes. This was the time in which I would contemplate my visits with my mom. This was the time in which I shed my tears for her dilemma and mine. I played Mozart, especially the overture to *The Magic Flute.* On this trip, I thought about her forgiveness, after all these years, for me not going to the right college, not being in the right profession, not wearing the right clothes, not cutting my hair right, not crossing my legs in public, not telling her the truth. She really meant it, and I somehow really needed it.

My mother had just returned to the nursing home from the intensive care unit at Boca Raton Community Hospital the week before. She'd been hospitalized because her blood gases weren't normalizing. She had begun to hallucinate ("Michael, what is that green grass doing on the shelf over there?") and was constantly drowsy, staying in bed all day, feeling anxious, and having no appetite. These are all symptoms of retaining carbon dioxide. I watched it for two days and then the nursing home staff inflated the collar on the inside of her tracheostomy. The internal collar makes it impossible for oxygen being pumped into her lungs by the ventilator to escape up and out her mouth and nose. Inflating the cuff also narrows the esophagus against the trachea so that swallowing becomes difficult and in general the feeling is that someone has their hands around your throat and is trying to choke you. Also, you can't talk. After several years on a respirator, she still hadn't gotten used to it. Could you ever get accustomed to being choked and gagged? She had conned all the respiratory therapists and nurses into deflating the cuff, so when they had to inflate it for such emergencies, she got anxious and they medicated her with Xanax or Ativan, and the side effects made her shake like a tree in a storm. The medication reduced her natural ability to breathe. And Xanax gives rebound anxiety. It was a vicious circle. Imagine a permanent case of not being able to catch your breath. The small portable ventilator did not get anxious with her. It just did eight breaths a minute—good for watching TV or a ballgame, but not for being anxious.

On this occasion the staff decided they couldn't stabilize her blood gases at the nursing home. My mom lived on the subacute wing, next to the dementia unit. They were drawing a "blood gas" every thirty minutes. This was done with a 10-gauge 4-inch needle into the artery in her arms, which had started to look like a cratered moon that had been pockmarked with a blowtorch. The needle was inserted and then used to search with a twisting motion until it hit an artery. It hurt like hell, and if she flinched in the slightest, they'd have to start over again, thus prolonging her agony. In watching all that I wondered again and again where Mom got her courage. It was certainly not God, I deduced. The clergy had rarely been to see her, and she didn't like the priest assigned to her anyway. It had to be her Irish genes.

After consulting with the on-call pulmonologist, the staff decided to hospitalize her and called the paramedics. I told Mom I would go with her to the emergency room. The transfer of a ventilator patient to anywhere outside the subacute wing of her nursing home is done with a minimum of six people. Two paramedics worked the gurney and a heart monitor, a respiratory therapist worked the ventilator, an aide worked at keeping all the tubes and hoses untangled, and a nurse and another aide made the transfer of my mother from the bed to the gurney.

My eyes began to tear up. She was in obvious distress. I held back from crying. It was so pathetic to see my mother heavily medicated, strapped down on the gurney, surrounded by machines. Life is not meant to be this way. And why her, anyway? Well, I kept it together because she was making strong eye contact with me. Even though she'd been through this before, it was a terrifying journey of no breath, breath, no breath. From bed to ambulance, it was a forty-five-minute job. Door to door, it was a five-minute ride.

I wasn't permitted into the emergency room for an hour and a half. As I sat in the waiting room, I called my brother, Brian, an osteopath, to calm my nerves and watched a parade of traumatized children and their equally traumatized parents passing through. I figured if the kids walked in, they couldn't be that bad off. I watched Frank Sinatra's eightieth birthday celebration on TV. Now it was Bruce Springsteen singing. Now it was Natalie Cole, and on and on. Finally the staff let me into the ER and there she was, stabilized and pissed.

She let me have it. "You lied to me about coming here! You've lied to me all your life!" Et cetera. She was steamed. So, I kept steady eye contact with her, and I was grateful for my master's degree in contemplative psychotherapy that I could draw upon for steadiness in this moment.

They had her plugged into one of those big Puritan Bennett 7200 ventilators. It looked and sounded like a commercial cement mixer. Her blood gases were fine. The attending physician came in and recommended that she stay overnight for observation. Before they took her upstairs to cardiac intensive care unit (CICU) she asks me to call the nurses station at Whitehall and let them know she was OK. I did so, and she accused me of lying again. She was really steamed about something.

It wasn't until much later that she told me what happened that night in the ER. When her blood gases began to stabilize, she woke up and became more aware of her surroundings. No one was talking to her, though they were poking and prodding her, and nobody responded to her requests for water or information. She said she was suddenly overcome by a feeling that she was in an evil place surrounded by evil people, and it was horrifying—like waking up *into* a nightmare rather than *from* a nightmare.

Well, the nightmare continued up in the CICU. The first respiratory therapist to come in was a young woman who was cold and impersonal and not willing to get my mother into a more comfortable position in bed. When I protested, I was told to mind my own business or leave the unit. I left. It was late. I was tired. I returned the next day and my mother barely recognized me. I knew I had to get her out of there. Her blood gases were normal, though she was weak, and everyone figured at this point that she was just getting over a cold. I looked at her and told her she had to eat something to get her strength back up. I fed her a bowl of soup, one spoonful at a time. I wiped her lips and then put Chapstick on them. I cleaned her face and combed her hair. Then I called the doctor and requested that she be taken back immediately to Whitehall. What I found out was that insurance companies don't like to pay for a single overnight in the hospital. Staying for just one night might make it look like the visit was unnecessary, and to really make it look good, the doctor would like to keep her there for at least four days. I said, "No effing way." We came to a compromise: If she ate today and got some of her strength back, she could go back to Whitehall the following morning.

She was cognizant enough to understand this. Even though she didn't want to eat—and believe me, this woman would not eat if she didn't want to (she had the Irish potato famine imprint)—she ate. I fed her. The next morning she was sent back to Whitehall. This is the stuff forgiveness is made of.

I don't think my mother ever really knew I cared about her. The last time I saw her alive, she seemed to know she would never see me again. When I looked at her and said "I love you, Mom," just as I always did before leaving, she looked at me and said, "Get closer to my face, look me in the eye, and say that like you mean it." I did. And then I knew I would never see her alive again. I would dream for the rest of my life about being on my way to visit her or being unable to save her.

Being in that emergency room for that brief period of time was a mystical transformative experience for me. In addition to the blood gases and weakness, she had been developing a bedsore at the tip of her coccyx. For relief, I would massage that area, and the best way to do that was with her underwear off. I came face to face with where I came from. I came from her out of her womb, and there it was, the place where I was made and birthed. My love for her includes all of her now. It is a place of forgiveness and great sorrow. If she had died several years before, when they first put her on a ventilator and gave her six months to live, it would indeed have been a tragedy. I would never have known all of my mother and her character. It's taken these years of being her health care surrogate and maintaining lucidity in the face of the insanity of heroic death prevention biomedicine to facilitate my spiritual transformation of knowing the place I came from physically and developing a deep and profound appreciation for that place called my mother.

In the Catholic church, Mary, the mother of Jesus, is also called Our Lady of the Seven Sorrows. The teaching is that Mary has seven sorrows arising from her love for her son. The lesson is that all humans have a heart of sorrow because the power of love needs to be fertilized by sorrow and the felt sense of the heart. Sorrow is not grief. Sorrow is the birthplace of compassion. My mother's last lesson for me as a healer was to ignite a heart of sorrow.

What follows are four poems I wrote about my mom's condition during her years on the respirator, including two death poems.

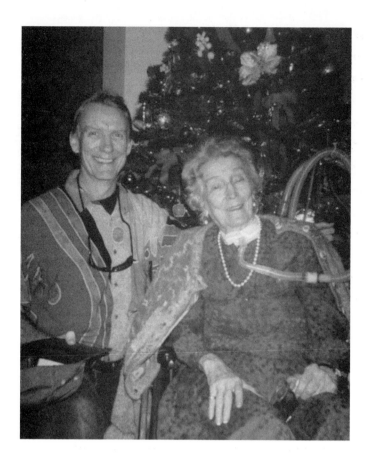

Fig. 3.1. My mom with her respirator and me at Christmas in December 2000

To Mom's Respirator

I wrote this after watching my mother's respiratory therapists suction out her lungs several times a day. I watched her suffocate each time.

> *This grip that life*
> *has on us*
> *IS vicious, unrelenting,*
> *restless. Turns us*
> *INTO astronauts in*
> *need of a tether to a*
> *machine and another machine*
> *as though back to the*
> *BREAST we could go,*
> *but no, it is somewhere*
> *else to rest we resist*
> *flying in circles as*
> *buzzards in need of*
> *rotting flesh plucked*

AWAY and pressed
forward to one
inevitable conclusion
to rest to sleep
to die
AND our death
will be so sweet
without the fury of
pounding demons
we invent to
torture our fleshly
SPIRIT let go! Is
the call, the trumpet
of SANITY

JANUARY 1993

Yellow Band

I wrote this poem after watching my mother be tube-fed for a decade. Every attempt to eat orally resulted in aspiration of food down into her lungs.

My mother
Wears a yellow
Band on her wrist,
A fragile canary
That says:
No Oral Feeding.
No eating
No drinking
No chewing.

Something wants to
Wail from your
Son's soul like
A screech owl
In the damp night
Of an overcast moon.

My placenta my blood
Is drying up.
What will I eat,
My toothless canary?
Will I learn to love
Through a frozen childhood?

Is this heart of mine capable
Of being alone on
The windswept mountain
Of bitterness?
I die in your death.
I starve in your starvation.

Who will hold me
In the cold dark stillness
When my demons
Swallow me alive?

SEPTEMBER 2003

Cremation Prep

I wrote this upon viewing my mother's body in the mortuary. She struggled with a bad bedsore for many years, and her body was frozen in the position of trying to lift her pelvis away from that pain.

Dark yellow stripes
Banding her face
Mustard barber pole
To the toes
A setting sun
Glowing in the day
Glowing in the bed
Glowing all night
Glowing on the gurney
Eyes circled white
Lungs bubbling fluid
Rattling broken
Suction pump
fountain of death

trembling
at the core
half here
half there
all there
swept through with death
washed by its hand
rigor mortis in mustard yellow
cremation prepped
surgical tape covering
precisely drained blood
below the subclavian
twisted
right hip swiveled
hinged
around the ageless bedsore
arms pockmarked from
a thousand and one
blood
draws
time-lapsed photo
frozen
in a moment of
anguish
hers and ours
face buttressed against
torment
of purgatory
no remorse
no regret
no teeth
no life
no serenity
empty shell
eyebrows trimmed
hair combed
one last
view
I touch the cold toes

I hold the cold hand
I kiss the cold face
One last
caress
Separated at last
Ready
for the crematorium

MAY 2004

On the Death of My Mother

I wrote this after I viewed her body, frozen in time, getting ready for cremation, in the mortuary.

After Ginsberg
She's gone gone gone
Won't be back again
Yes she's gone
Gone far away
Gone gone gone
To some other shore
No more free ride from AARP
She's gone gone gone
No more cakes and cookies
Lima beans and lamb chops
She's gone gone gone
won't ever be back again
no more Uncle Morrie Aunt Alice
and train rides to New York
gone gone gone
no more baseball Tom Brokaw
or Entertainment Tonight
no more bridge hands
fishing or swimming
for she's gone gone gone
gone far away
no more Mounds club
Cole Porter or Rex Harrison
Gone gone gone

Gone far away
No more suctioning
tube feeding
bedsores
And catheters
Finally gone at last
Gone gone gone away
No more negative mother
No more positive mother
No more mom
She's gone gone gone
Won't ever be back again
For she's gone gone gone

LOVE, MICHAEL
APRIL 3, 2004

MEDITATIONS ON THE GREAT MOTHER AND THE HEART

When my mother was dying, I developed a great ache and pain in the middle of my belly. I closed my eyes when I was with her, and I saw the umbilical cord running from her uterus to my umbilicus slowly dissolving. With the help of PR, I spent many weeks practicing the following three meditations daily. I have offered practice to many clients, and all report that it brought them relief and grace. You are ready for these meditations once you have begun to be able to sense the slow tempo of PR moving between your body and the horizon and back.

These contemplations involve active engagement and perception of the three embryonic fulcrums that are important points of organizing growth and development. The first is the umbilicus and umbilical cord connection. The second is the heart-to-heart connection between two people, such as between someone and their spiritual teacher or a friend. The third is the perception of movement from the third ventricle to horizon and back, which I detailed in the last chapter. Now we will begin to work more closely with the umbilicus and heart. These contemplations can be done seated or in a side-lying position. They can also be practiced in bed.

∞

Umbilical Meditation

This umbilical meditation can be particularly valuable for someone who has lost or is losing their mother. It can formally dissolve the umbilical cord between the mother and child and reconnect the umbilical cord to the Great Mother of the Earth or ocean.

To begin, I ask a client to visualize their mother sitting close to them. Then I proceed as follows.

Now I would like you to bring your attention to your umbilicus. [*Pause.*]

I'd like you to sense the whole space and shape of your abdomen as though it had only a very warm living fluid in it. In the middle of this fluid is a slow movement going toward your umbilicus. [*Pause.*]

Imagine there is an umbilical cord connected between your umbilicus and your mother's umbilicus. [*Pause.*]

Perhaps your umbilical cord actually goes from your umbilicus into your mother's womb. Either way is fine. [*Pause.*]

Which image works for you in terms of sensing the connection to your mother? [*Pause.*]

Begin to sense the stream that moves for about a minute out through your umbilical cord into your mother. [*Pause.*]

Let's wait until it reverses direction, and now the movement of this slow nurturing tide comes from your mother, deep in her core, through the umbilical cord and into your belly and body. [*Pause.*]

Originally all sorts of nourishment came through to you from your mother. Her own cells and molecules and even her genes floated into you through this cord. Likewise, your cells and genes floated into your mother in this unspoken communication. Now let's repeat this cycle at least three times, sensing this slow tide of sharing food and parts of each other through the cord. [*Pause.*]

Now I'd like you to imagine that this umbilical cord is starting to dissolve at a point that is halfway to your mother. Your now mother slowly disappears, piece by piece and part by part, fading away, leaving your umbilical cord suspended in space. Let her go because her cells and genes are still inside of you and you no longer need her to feed you. [*Pause.*]

Where does this umbilical cord attach itself now? Does it go down into the Earth? [*Pause.*]

Does it go down into the ocean? [*Pause.*]

Let it go into the Great Mother, either the Earth or the ocean. Allow the Earth or the ocean to send its flow of love and generosity through the umbilical cord very slowly into the depths of your belly and body. [*Pause.*]

Now sense your whole being as a fluid entity streaming out the umbilical cord, perhaps with bright colors, going right down into the Earth or ocean. [*Pause.*]

Repeat this cycle adding a color visualization three times. [*Pause.*]

Now wait for the stillness, and let yourself rest in the greater womb of Mother Earth and Mother Ocean.

꙰
Heart-to-Heart Meditation

This meditation is a heart-to-heart connection using PR. I like to practice it while sitting with a picture of my spiritual teacher, His Holiness the Dalai Lama, on a table directly in front of me. It can also be done sitting outside in nature. The contemplation proceeds as follows.

Settle yourself into a stillpoint. This stillpoint sits in the pericardium that surrounds your heart, or perhaps deep inside the heart between the atrium and the ventricles. It is the deepest stillness in the body, centered in and around the heart. Here is the starting point. [*Pause.*]

Next, allow yourself to feel a genuine sense of warmth generated by the heart and circulated by the blood. Imagine love and affection as though your own spiritual teacher or your own spiritual essence is actually present. [*Pause.*]

Now imagine that your chest cavity is slowly opening, exposing your entire heart, and imagine the color red moving like a slow ocean current in a canal or channel directly to the heart of your spiritual teacher or the horizon or a cloud if you are sitting in nature. [*Pause.*]

Wait for this spiritual blood transfusion to switch directions, and allow the blood of your spiritual teacher as the color red to move slowly into your heart and surround and support your body. Imagine the deepest love possible, even more profound than that of a mother for her child, a love that seeks only for your total spiritual fulfillment. [*Pause.*]

Let more and more of your chest cavity open, all the way down through the abdomen to the pubic bone. Surrender all the contents of your body, starting with the heart, as the color red moving toward the heart of your spiritual teacher. [*Pause.*]

At the tempo of PR, this tide of blood changes directions and begins to move into your body. Allow the entire inside of your body to be completely rebuilt and renovated with the highest known spiritual principle of loving kindness and compassion. [*Pause.*]

Repeat this cycle of sensing the change of phase of PR three times. [*Pause.*]

Wait for a deep stillpoint to emerge and fill your body and the space all the way out to the horizon. Imagine the very edges of the universe are clear light.

4

What's Inside?

ANN DIAMOND WEINSTEIN

ANN DIAMOND WEINSTEIN, PH.D., is a Preconception, Prenatal, and Early Parenting specialist with a doctorate in Prenatal and Perinatal Psychology.

I have a knot in my stomach. My mother used to say that. I wasn't quite sure what she meant. I think I do now. I am curious about the waves of anxiety that draw me inside following the incrementally slow-moving, multilayered grief I've experienced for more than three years now. The felt sense of anxiety and nausea, arising in the background several times a day, sends a muted message of a desire to vomit. To forcefully expel these painful emotions. The grief feels like it has morphed into an actual substance that, in doing so, can be thrown up and out.

The experience of losing my grandchild Enzo, born fifteen weeks premature and living in the neonatal intensive care unit (NICU) for only six days, has become a symbol, an image representing a file folder in my heart where many experiences of loss in my life reside. But now I am beginning to feel more acutely than at other times in my life, and am increasingly afraid to feel, the losses my children have experienced and are experiencing and anticipate experiencing. The resonance in their cells that still circulate within me, the resonance of shared energy, the vibration as memory that can still be activated by voice, sight, proximity, and nonlocal heart connection, reflects my whole organism's absolute recognition that these humans are different, unique from all others, having grown and come into being within my physical body and all that it has held, carrying forward the energy and vibrations of my parents and ancestors. I am compelled to see and hear and feel and be with them. Only them. Not my other relatives. Only my children. It is through this heart connection, no matter where we are in physical space, that I sense and understand the intensity and depth of my children's grief.

Experiences of past trauma, loss, and grief are triggered by the current loss, compounding the intensity and traumatic impact associated with it. Each family member's past experiences of trauma, loss, and grief impact their capacity to support other family members through their current loss and grief. One family member's current loss may trigger another family member's past trauma as well as their fear of similar or anticipated loss and grief, which may lead to disconnection between family members. Disruptions in attachment between family members resulting from current and past triggered trauma may be very difficult to repair.

We are a fragmented family, having lost the connections that, in some fantasized conception of "family," grief would be held and supported together as a family, or in some cultures as a tribe, through existing rituals or ones newly created. We are no longer connected as a whole immediate family and therefore have not participated in grief rituals in which we have all been present at the same time in the same place. Some of us have been together for some rituals and some of us have created solitary ones. A ritual where my son spread some of Enzo's ashes in the sea in Baja. Rituals where some of us found release at the ocean's edge with other grieving strangers. Rituals where some of Enzo's ashes have been buried at the base of a huge rock high on a hill in a cemetery. Rituals where some of Enzo's ashes have been buried at the base of rose bushes and on a hill in a rose garden. My heart experiences this as incomplete grieving—missing people, missing hearts, missing arms to hold each other and the ritual space. Perhaps this is also the fantasy—the gut feeling that if our whole family was connected, some aspect of the grief would be less painful.

Rituals do not cure grief. They provide some relief for a short time. They provide an opportunity to acknowledge our loss to ourselves, to honor the love that preceded the grief and the love that endures, and a space where we may be able to release our tears and the sound of our heart pain. Our individual experiences of grieving are different. In some ways, we are isolated from each other in silos of grief. The loss of Enzo exacerbated already difficult interpersonal dynamics between members of my immediate family. It brought into focus how few skills and resources my family as a whole had to cope with grief. We have not yet been able to all come together again, to hug, to hold, to cry, to laugh, to talk, to sing, to eat, even though we are blood relatives who share unique cells and energy and years of experience together. Another huge loss in the file folder in my heart.

My family of origin was also fragmented intermittently over many years. There were reasons, secrets about traumatic experiences and deep wounds left unnamed and unspoken. As a child, the secrets were confusing, incongruous, and overwhelming, creating double-binds. The only coping strategy was disconnection. Unspoken and unnamed wounds do not get addressed within a family. The risk of doing so and experiencing more harm can be too great. I now understand my mother's grief over the fragmentation of her immediate family. Perhaps in some way this tendency to disconnect from family to protect oneself from the trauma experienced within it was passed from one generation to the next. I ask myself: Is this karma?

My parents died years ago. The opportunity to heal my family of origin's wounds together, in this realm, has passed. With the support of plant medicine, the concept of unconditional forgiveness emerged in my heart. I was able to reconnect with the one living member of my family of origin around our present experiences and some shared memories of our parents and grandparents, without expectation or need for acknowledgment of harm done or an apology.

This was the most easeful, healing, and heart-liberating interaction I have had around the trauma I experienced in my family of origin, following decades of therapeutic work. I wonder if this repair will, in some way, have transgenerational, asynchronous healing benefits for my immediate family.

The opportunity to heal the wounds and rifts my immediate family is experiencing is still possible but will not be forever. I hold down the scream that wants to escape, to get my immediate family's attention, to warn them that, someday, it will be too late and we do not know when that time will be.

It's 3:00 a.m. I'm awake with a pain in my belly. Perhaps it is the solidification of grief, the hardening of broken attachment, unrepaired misattunements, and unprocessed and unresolved grief. I keep busy during the day, distracting myself, avoiding looking directly at this entity or even using other senses to begin to know it and feel it. Loss and grief feel like life threat as the ties of love in the physical realm are no longer available, nor the felt sense of safety within that connection. Panksepp and Biven (2012) call it the Panic/Grief system, which describes the experience of Panic that arises in response to our separation from our caregivers, ideally loving ones who kept us safe; this is the basis for which grief feels life-threatening. Because it could have been. Way back then. And we remember that at the deepest levels.

I am aware that I am much more anxious about losing my kids since Enzo died. In my mind, the sequence was not supposed to happen this way. I would become a grandmother. I would die before my children and their children. I now understand that the sequence of who dies when has no set order. Anything can happen. If my son can lose his son, I can lose my children. I CAN LOSE MY CHILDREN. And the cells and energy within my heart that recognize them as MY children could experience an intensity of grief beyond all others—intolerable, unbearable.

My whole being reverberated with the fear and panic of my son and his partner as they witnessed Enzo's suffering in the NICU in the hours following his birth and the days that preceded his impending death. Prenatal and perinatal experiences are imprinted on prenates and newborns. Their experience in the womb is drastically different from their experience in the NICU. Having been born at twenty-five weeks, incredibly fragile and extremely vulnerable, Enzo was not fully developed or prepared to sustain life outside his mother's womb. The sudden transition can only be described as shocking, abrupt, brutal, overwhelming, and traumatic. It is impossible to imagine that the NICU environment is experienced by premature babies as safe on any level. Parents who have experienced an arduous journey that brought them to the NICU with their very premature baby do not feel safe, nor do they perceive their baby to be safe. They may have experienced prior prenatal and perinatal losses and carry unprocessed trauma and unresolved grief, layers of loss which shaped the current pregnancy and add to the fear that they may also lose this baby. They often experience their baby as being in danger or near death and try to understand the medical providers' assessments, their baby's statistical chances of survival, and the prognosis if their baby lives. Parents careen through days when NICU and postpartum unit visiting may be restricted, without the holding, the support, or the resources they might want and need to be able to be fully present and grounded with calm energy for their baby in the isolette connected to tubes and wires.

Parents are vigilant; their nervous systems are on high alert as alarms on the machines monitoring their baby's heart rate and breathing go off periodically. Babies must sense their parents' fear and the tightrope they are on. The chaotic energy of the NICU environment—the parents' stress and trauma, the perceived stress and trauma of the premature baby, the sights and sounds of mechanical devices, the quality of presence of medical providers, the medical procedures, the anxiety, the anticipated grief—would shock and overwhelm any human being. Healthy full-term babies are more prepared, more resourced, to make the transition between womb and world than very premature and extremely premature babies, whose nervous systems are not fully developed and do not have the same capacity to cope with stress outside the womb, much less the overwhelming experiences in the NICU. They are trapped in the harsh NICU environment on which their life depends. One must wonder, do the babies want to be saved? Enzo's parents (the only ones allowed in the NICU during COVID) observed his responses to the invasive assault of medical technology in the doctors' well-intentioned, desperate attempts to save his life.

The interpersonal neurobiological exchange between parents and their very premature baby in the NICU is restricted by limitations on physical contact and masks. My grandson couldn't be held in his parents' arms or skin-to-skin until the day he died. His parents (and all the medical staff who cared for Enzo around the clock) were required to wear masks, so their facial expressions would only have been communicated through their eyes, if in fact he had opened his eyes to see them before he died. We do not know the color of Enzo's eyes. His father's eyes are brown, his mother's blue. I believe our love reached him in the realm beyond his embodied presence.

My son's description of witnessing his son's experience in the NICU was heartbreaking. My son's and Enzo's mother's feelings of helplessness were extremely intense in part due to the fact that they could not hold and comfort him in their arms. There was so little action they could take to help their son. Love and comfort were communicated by touch through the portals of Enzo's isolette, amidst the tubes, tape, and wires, the sound of their voices and the healing prayers of all who supported him and his parents from a distance.

My son and his partner held their son for the first and last time on the morning Enzo died. I watched my grandson slip away in my son's arms, on the only day my husband and I were allowed in the NICU. I watched my son carry Enzo in his arms, wrapped in a sheepskin bought earlier in the pregnancy in anticipation of bringing him home, as he walked on a stone ledge in a rooftop garden outside Enzo's room, his first and last contact with the blue sky, bright sun, and cool breeze, the world outside the NICU. Dreams of shared experiences, of showing the world to a child, are also lost. Witnessing sweet interactions between my son and other young children bring tears to my eyes as they provide a glimpse of the father my son would have been to Enzo. As a parent, I know the joy of seeing the world through my children's eyes, of feeling the wonder in watching small things, the micro world we as adults do not often slow down enough to take in, but shift our tempo and our gaze when sharing them with a young child who may be seeing these for the first time. The sadness that my son and Enzo will not share that experience wells up inside my chest and throat. I will not share the experience of seeing the world through my grandson's eyes. This trauma, this grief, the heart pain of deep loss across generations, is what's inside.

I have felt the vibration of my son's grief. I have sensed the resonance of Enzo's mother's grief.

I was a grandmother for six days. Am I still a grandmother? Although I cannot physically hold my grandson now, I learned so very much from him during his brief time here and afterward. He has been a gift to our family. His physical body streaked across our physical bodies like a shooting star. He bathed us in love, softened our hearts, came tethered to his umbilical cord, and left us forever connected to him by the felt-sense memory of him in our arms, fleeting as it was.

Those of us who have suffered perinatal loss don't know how to answer seemingly simple questions posed by acquaintances, even health care providers. When your child or grandchild lived for only six days and then died, what do you say when asked, "Do you have children? Do you have grandchildren?" Why do I hesitate to answer that question? I find myself weighing the burden of dealing with the reaction of an acquaintance or health care provider, the oblivious individual who couldn't imagine that I could have lost a child or grandchild. Anticipating the person's response if told—the blank stare, the pained facial expression, the averted gaze—I have to decide in an instant whether to take the chance and be honest about the trauma that has happened in my life, not knowing whether I will receive a compassionate response or have to bear the awkward discomfort of the person with whom I have shared this. To withhold the truth of Enzo's life and death feels disrespectful to Enzo, his parents, and myself. It treats his existence as a secret, which evokes a sense of incongruence, confusion, and internal dissonance. Why is it difficult to acknowledge perinatal loss in our culture?

As Markin and Zilcha-Mano acknowledge, "There is a cultural taboo against the public recognition and expression of perinatal grief that hinders parents' ability to mourn and their psychological adjustment following a loss" (2018, 20). As a result, parents and families are not adequately supported in the aftermath of perinatal loss.

Anticipatory grief, my own and my children's, also has its place in the folder in my heart. Anticipatory grieving for children and grandchildren who may never be conceived or born.

I am aging. I have lived many years. I may have more wisdom, but I have less resilience. I am wrinkled, have less muscle mass and less bone density, am missing connective tissue between joints, and survived breast cancer twice in my left breast over my heart. My eyes see less sharply, my ears hear less acutely. I have been asked to carry, to support, to hold space for and with, more and more over time with a body that is less solid, except for the solidified impaction of grief in my belly. It is more and more difficult to hold on and show up for all that is asked of me. And for my children, I am compelled to continue to do so even as I feel I am less able, and it takes a greater and greater toll over time because of the shared energy, because my body held them safe within while they grew enough to live on the outside. I did it. They made it. Enzo did not grow enough on the inside. He didn't make it. Some do and some don't. My son and Enzo's mother had to let him go. Some grandchildren never arrive.

Since Enzo died, I pay more attention to my heartbeat. I wonder how long it will continue. I ask why my heartbeat has lasted this long and Enzo's stopped so soon. For the weeks before Enzo was born and six days after, both of our hearts were beating, and then Enzo's slowed and stopped. The heartbeat is the signal, the rhythm that distinguishes life ongoing from life ended. Enzo struggled on life support, each breath and beat mechanically stimulated. I have taken my breath and heartbeat for granted for more than seventy years.

Singing and drumming move the anxiety and nausea; it is the rhythm that softens my heart and draws my attention out of my body as I listen, sing and drum along with the voices and hands of others who do not know the grief I hold. I feel part of an instant community in a field on a hill under the sky and clouds with a view of a distant mountain when I join in creating the repetitive, hypnotic rhythms that begin to ease the grief in my belly. I imagine the others with whom I sing and drum can sense the grief in the sound of my voice and the tone of my drum.

It is the rhythm of my steps that soothes my heart as I walk near the gentle bay waves. The expanse of the water all the way to the mountain on the other side makes more room for the feelings crammed in my belly and provides relief for a time.

Sometimes I feel Enzo's spirit in the wind, the sound of the water, the movement of the clouds at the water's edge.

In the dark at 3:00 a.m. I do not sing. I do not walk. There are no wave sounds nearby. I lie still wondering if I can slip back into sleep where my grief is transformed into dreams. Puzzles with messages I to try to understand when I awake. Sometimes my mother visits me in my dreams. My mother whose prenatal losses preceded my conception. Losses that included an illegal abortion, decades before *Roe v. Wade* became law, only to be overturned decades later. Two miscarriages, the second of which threatened my mother's capacity to conceive again. And then she conceived me. The resonance of her unresolved trauma, grief, and fear from her three prenatal losses, pulsed in her womb accompanying her heartbeat as I grew. The trauma of prenatal losses was not acknowledged back then. My mother's unprocessed grief was carried forward in dissociative moments in the postnatal period and shaped the quality of my attachment relationship with her. When I conceived my first child, my mother's reaction was strikingly solemn. To me it appeared to be heavily laden with a fear of me losing my prenate.

My mother's mother, whose husband was an Orthodox Jew, lost her first child at a year old from pneumonia, following eight years of trying to conceive. The trauma she experienced of prolonged infertility in a culture where having children was an expectation and then losing her first child has been passed down through the generations, to my mother, me, and my children. And then my son loses his child.

The belly pain continues. Perhaps it's the energy of generations of loss and grief, not just my own. It's sore, like scarred tissue. They say scarred tissue is stronger. I'm not sure about that. I know one thing: It hurts.

I am the matriarch. I have searched for an answer, a way, a process that could support the healing of the wounds and rifts that have fragmented our family's connection. I have come to understand I do not have the solution, nor can I impose one on my family if I did. Although that eases the pressure I have put on myself to solve this problem, it does not ease the pain of the loss of my immediate family's connection to each other that is layered on top of the pain of losing Enzo. The fear of sensing into the deep well of this multilayered grief and despair keeps me skirting above it in the sea of anxiety and nausea.

Each day I open my eyes and reach for my glasses, it takes only milliseconds to recognize that the grief is not an arm's length away but inside my belly still. Each day I am challenged to accept the "isness" of losing Enzo and the current fracture in our immediate family. Each day I reach to hold the possibility that, someday, we will repair the rift that disconnects us from each other. I remind myself to make a heart connection with Enzo through nature on my daily walks. Feeling the love that endures helps me accept these losses and hold in my heart the possibility of healing and change.

5

The Boy and the Medicine Are One

BARRY WILLIAMS

BARRY WILLIAMS, M.DIV., PSY.D., is a Diplomate Jungian Analyst living and practicing in the mountains near Taos, New Mexico. Along with his wife and late son, he is a fully initiated mara'akame, or healer in the tradition of the Huichol people of the Sierra Madre in Central Mexico. He has a particular interest in dreams, healing, wilderness, and the reality of the psyche as the world.

I want to tell a story that is still as raw and as close to me as my breath or heartbeat. No theory or concept can soften or contain it enough so that I can say I understand it. It is the story of a little boy and his now twenty-three-year passage into and through the world. His ongoing life is more like an unfolding story of meaning and realization than a narration of events, although those events both contain and are also the meanings themselves. By accepting what has happened as it has come in its own mysterious manifestation, what can seem so foreign and other as a life event can reveal itself as an aspect of the Self trying to emerge into consciousness. This is my personal, somewhat confessional story of parenting, together with my wife, a profoundly disabled child, so injured in a catastrophic birth that his path through life has been most unusual, to say the least. My wife's story is so different in kind as a woman and mother that I will leave it to her to tell. I also want to acknowledge that many, if not most, of you readers have some version of this story in your lives: of illness, trauma, tragedy, despair, loss, shattered expectations or disability, in which you have experienced the becoming of an other to yourself, to your family, community, culture, or seemingly even God. Love, care, anguish, darkness, and heartbreak travel through the events of lives and can present themselves in unimaginable otherness. The events might differ, but the intrinsic patterns are all similar. This story is without outcome, except for the crucial and all important goal of seeing and realizing just what happens if, instead of angrily fighting against the fatefulness of the situation, succumbing to despair, doubt, and questioning, or seeming to comprehend or fall into easy explanatory theories and concepts of what this means, we simply accept and follow the lead of the Self as it presents itself in a kind of numinous otherness—in this case, of a child as an embodied reality of the psyche. If we allow ourselves to be taught, shaped, molded, and transformed by this manifestation of life in its wildest formation, it can lead to our destiny.

I recently had one of those significant milestone birthdays, the kind that had me asking myself whether I have done anything substantial with my life—the decisive and telling question of a life. Has there been anything of substance that could tell me, as Jung would ask it, whether or not I have been related to something infinite? By *infinite*, of course, we would like to imagine something truly sublime and transcendent with which our deserving life is blessed. But what if, paraphrasing Jung, what crosses my willful path and upsets my views, plans, and intentions and changes the course of my life is in fact an experience of God? And what if this God is really, as he says, reality itself, the reality that I am presented with as the unfolding implacability of my life, just as it comes to me? And what if this all comes in the most humble and innocent and helpless of ways that initially crushes the spirit and sends life reeling?

I am possessed by these questions because, for the past twenty-three years, I have had to turn much of my vital life energy to the care and love of a child who should have grown up playing Little League baseball, should have been fishing in the lakes and streams of his youth, should have gone to university, fallen in love, and set out on his path to seek his life. Instead, because of his catastrophic birth experience, he was not capable of returning to us or reflecting to us in the mirror of his face, body, words, development, or achievement that care and love we showered so hopefully and hopelessly on him. We naturally depend on those reflections and mirrors to reward us as parents, and as humans, so that we can keep relating deeply over the trials and triumphs of the life journey. We need to be restored and refreshed enough at a soul level to go on believing that that journey does in fact lead to a teleology of the wholeness of life as we might understand it. In my case, though, the story being told through the child is that the developmental journey is not in the otherness of the child, but in myself, if I can be successful in retrieving the projections I might try to make him carry for me and focus instead on the phenomenology of the meaning his life carries.

My wife and I had wanted this child and indeed had felt blessed in his growing presence in the womb. But there were warnings from the beginning, coming in dreams and intuitions that something very difficult was approaching. My wife one day was filled with such an overwhelming experience of panic, dread, and horror that we openly discussed whether to continue with the pregnancy, but we were unable to discern if it was a warning or an experience of the archetypal energy and reality of impending motherhood. But at the same time there was also a dream: that we were to follow carefully, exactly, and precisely in the tracks that a deer made in the snow with its antlers in order to find our way successfully, a dream that unbeknownst to us predicted a later, lengthy twenty-year initiation for all three of us as mara'akate, or shamans, in the traditional medicine path of the Huichol people of the mountains of central Mexico. These are the people of the deer who is the creator god, whose heart is the mind of the god and whose tracks lead the people to the sacred plant that grows where the deer touches the Earth, which plant is also the deer's heart, which is the doorway to the mind of the gods, an experience in nature of the Self, a story I'll tell in a bit.

Labor was difficult and very slow and a C-section was called for, which resulted in a seemingly unending series of blunders and errors unfolding in a slow-rolling medical disaster. The child was delivered and given into the hands of the doctor who was to revive and care for him. Already he looked like he had been through a traumatic conflict, blue and battered, as she tried for several minutes to get him to breathe. "I don't think I can save your son," she finally said, so matter of fact, so detached, while she rubbed him and put her fingers down his throat to get him to breathe and moved him about and directed oxygen at him until it ran out, and ran out again, and again. Everything that could be going wrong medically was going wrong now, the minutes going by with no breath, the attempts at revival increasingly frantic. But also going wrong was the sudden destruction of my innocence about the goodness and consistency of life, now in the inadequate hands of a person whose own child had suffered brain damage during its birth and had died in her arms. "I don't think I can save your son," she said again as she tried everything she knew, enlisting my participation to rub the child's back hard with a towel to stimulate him in any way possible and to loudly ask him, entreat him to breathe, to come into the world, to become human and join us. "I don't think I can save your son," she said again as Raef failed to become, failed to be, still alive but failing to live, still blue and beaten up, the many anoxic minutes now accumulating like some deadly, dooming poison. And now, out of this blue otherness of our boy, came the beginning of a long, low, deep, guttural sound, the onset of agonal breathing, the breath that is no breath, the breathing out of the life that can't be. It was an unearthly, unhuman sound, a moan that must have begun in a place so distant and so dark that no being can access it and express it except in that moment when life is slipping away, unattainable, unsalvageable, the distant hoped-for light now dimming as if the life potential in him were breathing out, truly expiring, the spark going out, the agony of not being or becoming expressing itself in a sound so awful that no one should ever have to hear it, so deeply piercing of the membranes of the heart that I cannot ever forget it. And with that sound of Death's breathing I let my beloved child go, seeing him like some meteor that skipped brightly across the atmosphere but failed to penetrate to Earth, and was gone.

At that moment, the doctor casually asked the anesthesiologist if he had any ideas that could help. He came over with an airway and inserted it in Raef's throat and the child immediately took a breath, a full twelve to fourteen minutes after his birth, and pinked up. In that instant, the instant after I had let him go, given him to Death to return back to his world, I made a promise to him from somewhere so deep in me that my life has been lived every day from that place: that I would never abandon him, no matter what, no matter where he led me, no matter what it took, no matter how much damage had been done or what his life would look like. His courage and strength to live and become needed to be honored. Little did I know where this promise would take me. And so began the journey that would take from us all the hope we had poured into an expectation of what life would be, but which, had it never happened, had Raef never been born, would not have allowed me to live my life. Anything I know of any real value I have learned from this hurt child, this little boy, my son.

There is a children's story in which a little bunny wants to run away from his mother, who tells him, "If you run away, I will run after you. For you are my little bunny." "If you run after me," says the bunny, "I will become a trout in a trout stream and I will swim away from you." "If you become a fish in a trout stream, I will become a fisherman and I will fish for you." And so it goes. If the bunny becomes a rock on a mountain, the mother will become a mountain climber and find him, or if he sails away as a boat, the mother will become the wind and blow him back to her, or she will be the gardener who will find him as a flower. Nothing the bunny can change into can get him away from the parent, who promises the child over and over that she will doggedly transform herself into whatever is needed, whatever the situation calls for, to find the child wherever he has gone and wrap him in her love, protection, and steadfastness. The little bunny cannot escape the tie to the parent, no matter how far down a road he goes, or what shape he assumes, or what demands are placed on the parent. She will follow him and wrap him in her parental embrace. Like Psalm 139: "Whither shall I go from thy spirit? or whither shall I flee from thy presence? If I ascend into heaven, thou art there: If I make my bed in hell, behold, thou art there." And then, so beautifully, "If I take the wings of the morning, and dwell in the uttermost parts of the sea, Even there shall thy hand lead me, and thy right hand shall hold me." As the Self is to the ego, so can and must the parent be to the child in the personal realm, especially if the child takes the wings of the morning and dwells in a place that can never be accessed. The child who incarnates in otherness needs to experience that he is known, and knowable, by the parent who has been transformed by the child who experiences such hurt and disability. At the same time, the child is the parent's psychopompic guide to a world never imagined or wanted, but wherein lies his destiny in this lifetime.

When Raef was a year old, I gave some tobacco to a great Lakota medicine man and asked him to pray for Raef during a Yuwipi ceremony he was doing that night. In the middle of the ceremony, when the energy of the singing and drumming was at its height and all manner of things were flying around the room in the total darkness, the medicine man called out to me in English, an unusual occurrence. "Barry," he shouted, "the spirits have a message for you! They say that your boy is a white bird. They say you have hold of one leg, and your wife has hold of the other. Do you know what that means?" As I fumbled for something to say, he shouted again, "The spirits say that you know what that means." And of course, I do now know what that means: that Raef is a pure spirit in an embodied form. But because he was so damaged at birth, he is only partially embodied in the material human form and much more "embodied," if you will, in the spirit world. He has landed in our lives as a human-looking spirit, but from the spirit world's point of view, he is a spirit figure, a white bird in the human world. Right or wrong, we hold on to his legs, each in our own way to keep him here, to love and attend him and get his blessing, as if from that very angel who wrestles with Jacob through that long night. We use all the strength and love we can muster to hold him on the Earth, to hold him in our family and in our lives. He could fly off at any moment, and indeed he nearly has any number of times during many dramatic medical crises. The hold we have had on him is partly desperation, partly hope, partly illusory, but mainly a love, devotion, and dedication that was incomprehensible before that birth/death/birth moment that forged in us a resolve and promise that we have been pledged to keep. He also knows he has permission to fly away if he needs to or if it is time, and we will release him back into his world in a timing we would never understand but would be obliged to accept.

Within months of Raef's birth, I had a dream: I am standing before a tree in a forest, from which is emerging a whitish growth known as a shelf fungus. In the dream I know that this is a very potent medicine. As I contemplate and wonder about this medicine, a strong voice announces, "The boy and the medicine are one!" And the dream ends. At the very outset of my journey with Raef, then, I was told in no uncertain terms that the boy is actually the medicine, presumably the medicine I need to both save and live my life. He is not a problem to be solved, a wound from which to heal, a medical blunder for a lawsuit, an end to the life I thought I was supposed to lead, the sacrifice of pleasure and freedom, or anything else. He is the medicine, my medicine that will heal what ails me, that will bring me into alignment with the Self and what it wants of me, from which I was blindly errant. The dream has echoes of the Grail legend and the philosopher's stone. The boy as the medicine is that creator deer, the medicine deer in whose tracks we must follow completely if we are to live and if, as the Huichol say, we are to find our lives. It is the medicine path that completes us, the deer whose heart we are to ingest so that our eyes can be opened, who goes before and leads us—the boy, the dream medicine, the elixir, the stone, the sacred plant that is also the maize that grows and is eaten for life, the heart and mind of the deer that is the god that is the boy that is the medicine around and around in a circle of imaginal medicine meaning. The dream also says that the medicine does not *come from* nature; it *is* nature. It is the Self as nature, the vegetative aspect of the Self, as Jung says. A radical acceptance of the occurrence of Raef's life and injury is demanded by the dream, just as one would accept the occurrence of a shelf fungus on a tree as completely natural. It is the Self manifesting in and as nature, in and as the world.

By the time Raef was six months old, he had been in an ICU three times, had two life flights to distant hospitals, and had been to the top children's hospital in the country, and we had been told twice by different doctors that they did not think they could save him in a critical moment. He had had life-threatening reactions to every major medication prescribed, and we were finally told by our pediatrician to let him go, that he was an angel and we would be better off to go on with our lives. It was at this point that I muttered that I was tired of people guessing and I wanted someone who could see. Within two weeks of that statement we were on a plane to South America and the Upper Amazon to see a locally well-known Piaroa shaman we had been directed to. When we told our doctor what we were planning, and that I would rather our son die in the rainforest than in any ICU in the country, she said she understood, but she really thought we were going to go in order to let him go. We drove five hundred miles south from Caracas, across the savannah and the flooding Orinoco River on a tiny raft-like ferry, to reach the small village of the Piaroa people on a tributary of the Amazon. The shamans of the region use a powerful plant spirit medicine, called yopo, that is sharply inhaled into the nose through bird bones and sets off an explosion in the brain and mind. The shaman insisted that I use it so I could see what he was doing, ultimately giving me, like Raef, in an exact parallel with his birth/death/birth experience, a complete death journey so strong and so real I was stunned and more than slightly taken aback to wake in my body. The healing work went on all night in the shaman's thatched hut, and in the morning spirit creatures from the time before time, from before creation, entered to drink eagerly a liquid that made the humans in the place throw up violently. For the first of many times we were told in halting Spanish that the boy was OK, that this is how he was supposed to be, that he had come for a purpose and that we needed to adjust to this reality, not to try to fix him, and that we must deal with our own lives.

For the next year and a half, we searched the world, from the Amazonian rainforest to the Canadian woodlands, looking for help from a great variety of spirit healers. Each in turn and in their own way had a very similar message: The boy was OK and had great medicine, but we needed to do our work to allow him to use it. A Chumash shaman in California gave him a medicine blanket he had used for twenty years, saying it was now Raef's. A Zapotec healer in Mexico became his godmother and lifelong champion, once doing spiritual brain surgery on him and sending him home on the plane wrapped in bandages. A Lakota medicine man came to us in tears after a very dramatic healing ceremony and said he couldn't help Raef. When we asked why not, he said that Raef had come and helped him, and that his purity was his medicine power. When a Hopi elder and healer met him, he immediately gave Raef the amber bear he kept in sacred corn pollen in a pouch around his neck, later adopting him and giving him a Hopi name. Often he would call to tell us that Raef had visited him the night before and to tell us the story of what they had done together and what Raef had told him, saying over and over to us that Raef had healed him and had healed thousands of others. A Navajo hand trembler diagnosed him as having a whirlwind illness, presaging his eventual Huichol medicine path of Tamatsi Wawatsari, el Arbol del Viento, the Wind Tree, a very powerful and ancient spirit who manifests as whirlwind and is, among many things, about neurological dynamics, just as the antlers tracks of the deer are about the spiritual and neurological energies of the shaman. An Anishinaabe medicine man in the woodlands of Canada gave him white pine medicine, the true spirit of the forest.

Finally, we met a Huichol shaman we had heard about, a meeting that came through the most sinuous of synchronistic pathways, as destiny often does. I had had a dream perhaps twenty years earlier in which hunter after hunter tries and fails to shoot a deer that was standing still in the forest in front of us. Finally it is my turn, but when I pull the trigger, I purposefully shoot over its head, at which point the deer transforms into a native medicine man who falls to the ground in some sort of heart crisis. I rush to help him, knowing that if I had shot the deer, I would never have realized that the deer was really a native healer, that potential in me to be a traditional healer, whose heart and life I must now save. Now we were approaching a shaman from the Huichol world of the deer, whose heart is the deer and whose medicine power derives from eating the heart of the deer as sacred plant and as the mind of the god. The Huichol shaman took one look at Raef and said he could not see us then, saying that he couldn't help us and to come back in three days, during which time he would fast and pray and dream. When we returned, he asked us forcefully how we had found him. We said something simplistic and he repeated, "No, how did you FIND me?" He had dreamed we would come and had been told that Raef would be his first Wind Tree pilgrim and apprentice, and even he was amazed how it had happened. He explained that he had been told that "they," that spirit-filled Divine realm, could help Raef, but in return they wanted him. This meant that Raef had been called to be a shaman, or mara'akame in the Huichol tradition of this most ancient, powerful, and sacred site, because of his very nature. His story and nature almost completely corresponded with the Huichol myth/story about the Wind Tree Child, who was excluded from his family and village because no one could or would deal with his manifestation as otherness. In his rejection and abandonment he eventually became the Wind Tree in all its healing and transformative power and energy.

I experienced this encounter with the Huichol medicine path as the string that, when I pulled it, moved everything. The archetype of the healer, the promise of life for our child, a physical, psychological, and spiritual undergoing of an ancient tradition that was an embodiment of powerful realities of the psyche and the necessity of an authentic initiation into an ancient, intact medicine path, all spoke deeply to me, as if it were a soul pattern. All three of us were to become pilgrims to sacred sites where dwelt the gods, Raef and I to the Wind Tree in Mexico and my wife to several other sites. The apprenticeships would take six years if all went well before initiation. Each pilgrimage cycle required a period of thirty-five to forty days of fasting and inward turning twice a year, and an intense journey at the limits of endurance and strength up a mountain that in itself is a kakayari, or dwelling place of the gods, there to place offerings and prayers in a most precarious and dangerous manner, to spend the night, still fasting, in wakeful vigil until the blessing came, and then to descend and make our way to the ocean, Grandmother Ocean, Tatei Haramara, to leave final offerings to that unfathomable depth and expanse, that deity from which the gods were born and from which all life springs. Raef, of course, could not and did not go with me in his body, so I carried his sacred bundle with mine to receive the blessings and over the years to activate the contents that would become the implements and instruments of our future healing work.

Each pilgrimage is a ceremonial time that enacts a psychological as well as physical approach to the reality and presence of the Self. A Jungian perspective allows one to see the many parallels with other initiatory ceremonies, alchemical operations, and patterns of the individuation journey. What was so life-giving for me was the opportunity to embody and undergo, within a cultural setting, an authentic indigenous initiation process and to experience with my eyes wide open the confrontations with so many of my psychological issues, the scouring of complexes, the shifting of attitudes, positions, identities, and whatever intellectual knowledge I thought I possessed that was so tested against the absolutes of the archetypal world presenting itself in the imagery and dynamics of a people's religious experience of their gods. Now, twenty-one years later, I still go on pilgrimage to the sacred desert and its plant spirits, the heart of the deer, still learning and dreaming with the medicine that comes through the boy, that is the boy.

At the end of the sixth year there is an initiation, in which, among many events, there is the ritual sacrifice of a bull in the moments just before dawn following an all-night ceremony in the tuki, or god house, in which the shaman has sung the human world and the cosmos into a restored and balanced order. Every apprentice who would cross the threshold to becoming a mara'akame, a healer for his or her people, must kill a bull, by hand, with a knife. It is an acknowledgment that he or she is willing and able to cross back and forth over that threshold of life and death, from one world or dimension to the other, to deal with the blood of the life force of nature that offers itself for this sacrifice and to stand with the archetypal forces who become obliged by the ritual to attend the shaman in his or her life of healing. There is a profound meaning in blood, the vital life essence, the signature of the life force, the contained flowing energy of life itself. No offering to the gods is complete and efficacious without the blood of a deer that is seen and understood to have sacrificed itself for this purpose, and no ceremony like the initiation is complete without the blood of a bull, sacrificed by the initiate, who petitions to enter the community of healers by becoming a familiar of those energies that command life, vitality, power, and wholeness, whose flesh is then also given to the people as nourishment in body and spirit in ways so similar to other more familiar archetypal patterns of eucharistic participation in the ingesting and assimilation of the god.

At the outset of my apprenticeship, I had dreamed of hunting a deer with a snare for a sacrificial offering, in the exact manner of the Huichols. A deer offered itself in the snare, and as it died I felt such grief I wanted to undo it but could not, and ritually, psychologically, should not, since its blood was required to complete my offerings and petitions that would restore the world, and life. Later I dreamed that I was to sacrifice Raef in that same motif of the demand for a life, but when it had gone too far, the same guilt consumed me, but it was too late and I had to go through with it because it was what was called for, for the sake of life. I have to accept, however unwillingly, that Raef, like the deer and the bull, has offered himself to me from the depths of life, from the depths of nature and the Self, so that there can be life, and that his life can be completed through his sacrifice. This is a primordial reality within the psyche. I have undergone by the circumstances of Raef's presence in my life an enactment of the archetype of sacrifice. One could argue persuasively that other religious patterns offer a more redemptive path that does not include such sacrifice, and I would agree, but this was the path that chose me, for better or for worse, and the sacrifice of and for the deer, the sacrifice of and for the bull, and the sacrifice of and for the child is a price for the redemptive understanding and embrace of a meaning that had called me to it, a meaning so distant from consciousness that I have spent twenty years trying to get inside it.

In the biblical story of Abraham's sacrifice of Isaac, Yahweh demands of the father the sacrificial offering of the child he deeply loves, the very symbol of the gift of a new relationship of the Divine with the human world, the Self with the experiencing ego. In his obedience to this Divine demand, the father reaches the penultimate moment of sacrificing his son, who is now bound and on the altar, the fire read-ied to light, the knife raised, consumed by the archetypal energy of this offering. The ram caught in the thicket, the redemptive substitution, represents and signifies the inbreaking into consciousness of a more compassionate god image that no lon-ger demands child sacrifice. If we are in this situation, as modern recipients of the millennia of transformation of the God image, we hope, even expect, the ram to be there. But for me, nearly unimaginably, there is no ram in the thicket. It seems as if the Self is revealing itself in its most primitive aspects, demanding that I participate in the sacrifice of my child, who is offering himself for this very purpose. When there is no ram in the thicket, no substitution, no redemption offered in the outer circumstances, then the deer, the bull, and the child offer themselves up to life, for the sake of life, to be sacrificed for something even greater. My guilt, doubt, and hesi-tation, like in the dreams of the sacrifice of the deer and of Raef, nearly spoiled the completion of the archetypal pattern that will bring into consciousness a meaning that struggles to be made conscious. I must be willing to risk the encounter with the primitive manifestation of the Self in order for this new consciousness to emerge. In such circumstances, we cannot discern what the intention or meaning of the Self is; we can only deal with its phenomenology. We therefore have a choice of how to react and live. We can feel angry, punished, despairing, or philosophical depending on our personality structure, or we can choose to gamble on there being symbolic meaning in the symptom and the event, putting faith in the symbol of the self-sacrificing child that demands our own sacrifice. If I am obedient to the demands of the Self, wher-ever it takes me, if I follow precisely the tracks of the deer and see the events of its manifestation symbolically, then I am in alignment. This process demands a radical acceptance of the just-so-ness of life, which will then reveal the activity of the Self. The proper conscious attitude toward the Self that demands the ego's enactment of its intentions by definition creates sacrifice and the correct sacrificial attitude.

In other words—and this is the heart of the matter—if I accept that Raef, as the shamans all saw, is in this life as he is in order to be able to do his work and be the medicine, I must see his life as a meaningful and purposeful sacrifice. If I do not see and accept that, he has wasted his life on me, and I have wasted his life, as well as my own, in trying not to see in order to keep him alive. If I see and accept him and what he is about, I bring that purpose to consciousness, but in so doing I participate in the sacrifice of the child and, in fact, bring it to completion and fulfill his destiny. The risk is that this move will relax the grip we have had on him as that white bird and he can leave to return to that mystery he came from. Consciousness, then, is the redemptive factor that allows me to see more clearly the nature of the Self as pure, implacable nature, the totality of being that forces and demands a radical acceptance of the way things just are but rewards and redeems from unknowing the hopeful mind that wants to avoid its destiny. There is no bargaining with the indecipherable world of the gods, but one must not avoid the encounter, at the risk of wasting life.

The Divine Child is born alchemically when the concreteness of existence dies, when projections break down, in the defeat of the ego and the resulting experience of death in life. Only then is it possible to transition to another level of awareness. In the midst of putting into words the experience and understanding of Raef's life and my own transformation as a result of his sacrifice and my participation in it, I dreamed that I am assisting at the birth of a beautiful and perfect little brown-haired boy. As his head emerges, still only partially born, I cradle it and speak to him, welcoming him into the world. The dream seems to confirm the work of acceptance and receiving and welcoming the events of life, allowing the Self to be born and enabling the new possibility and potential for life. The emergence of the Divine Child can be the redemption of the wounding and suffering that would otherwise be my lot if I did not gestate and deliver this understanding. My only hope now, and my most fervent prayer, is that I can make my life worthy of Raef's sacrifice.

6

A Compassion-Based
Model of Pregnancy*

INTRODUCTION

Emerging research in Dr. Weinstein's book points out the critical need for a different approach to working with women who are pregnant and their families. Cited research on the impact of stress and trauma to a woman's or girl's biology and the fetal-placental connection demonstrates that a model and an approach must be developed to help a woman during her pregnancy as well as birth and after the birth. These are now moral and civilizational issues that can no longer be ignored for the entire future of the planet is at stake. The most basic missing element is the development of a thorough and unified approach to supporting pregnant females based on the emerging literature of compassion. Without compassion many pregnancies are unsustainable at a biopsychosocial level. Furthermore, the United States is seeing a rise in maternal deaths at birth (World Health Organization et al. 2015) indicating a critical need for a different approach to pregnancy and birth.

PHILOSOPHICAL ORIENTATION

What follows is an analysis of terms and discussion of the four levels of compassion based on a model of pregnancy shown here in figure 6.1. These four levels are:

1. Philosophical orientation
2. Need for compassion
3. Compassion resources
4. Therapeutic processes

---

*This chapter was originally published as "Appendix A: A Compassion-Based Model of Pregnancy," by Michael J. Shea, in *Prenatal Development and Parents' Lived Experiences: How Early Events Shape Our Psychophysiology and Relationships,* by Ann Diamond Weinstein. Copyright © 2016 by Ann Diamond Weinstein. Used by permission of W. W. Norton & Company, Inc.

Each of these categories as the reader can observe is subdivided into three or four subcategories with an analysis of terminology used. This should be considered as an abstract to a much needed treatise yet to be written.

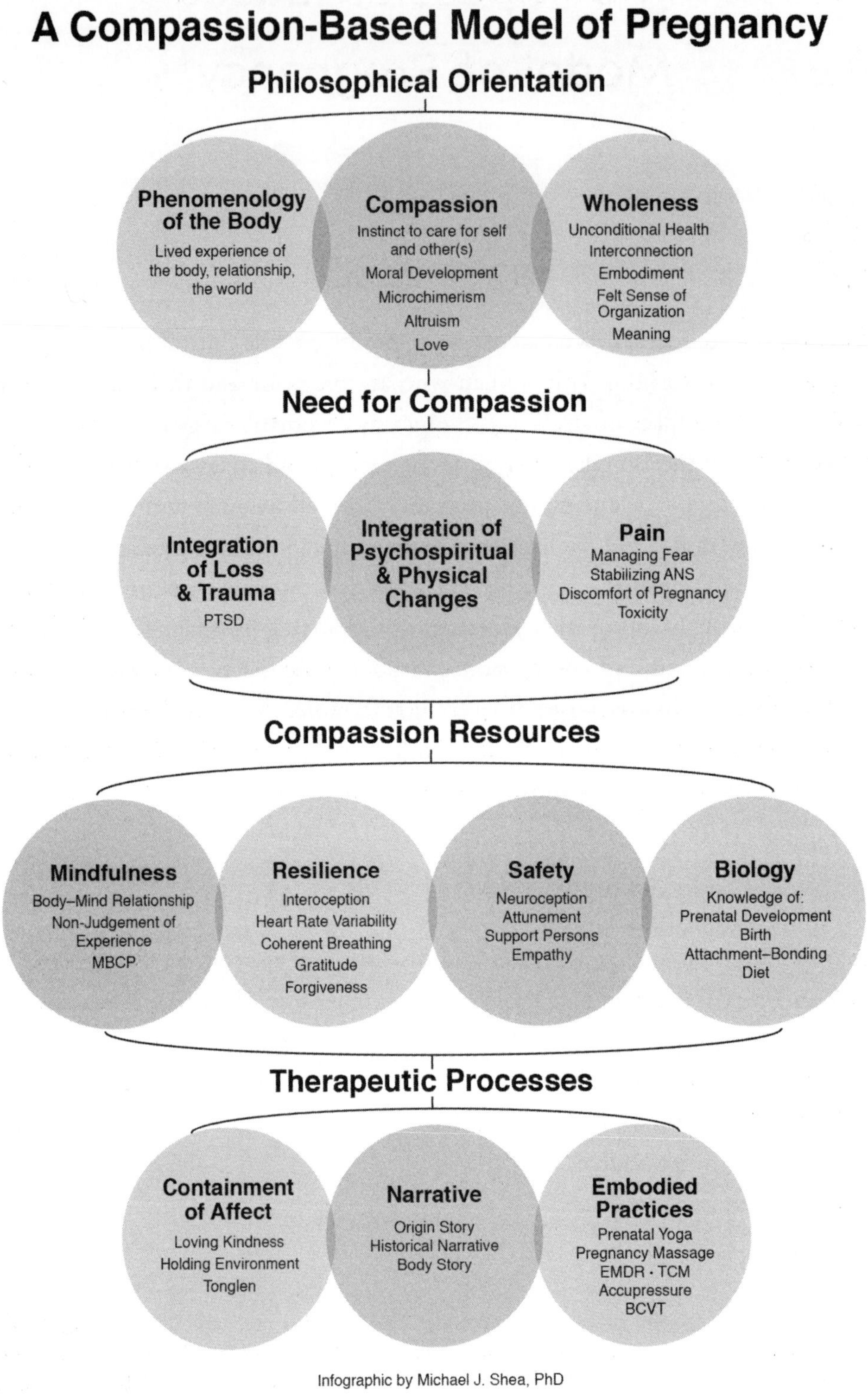

A Compassion-Based Model of Pregnancy

Philosophical Orientation

Phenomenology of the Body

Lived experience of the body, relationship, the world

Compassion

Instinct to care for self and other(s)

Moral Development

Microchimerism

Altruism

Love

Wholeness

Unconditional Health

Interconnection

Embodiment

Felt Sense of Organization

Meaning

Need for Compassion

Integration of Loss & Trauma

PTSD

Integration of Psychospiritual & Physical Changes

Pain

Managing Fear

Stabilizing ANS

Discomfort of Pregnancy

Toxicity

Compassion Resources

Mindfulness

Body–Mind Relationship

Non-Judgement of Experience

MBCP

Resilience

Interoception

Heart Rate Variability

Coherent Breathing

Gratitude

Forgiveness

Safety

Neuroception

Attunement

Support Persons

Empathy

Biology

Knowledge of:

Prenatal Development

Birth

Attachment–Bonding

Diet

Therapeutic Processes

Containment of Affect

Loving Kindness

Holding Environment

Tonglen

Narrative

Origin Story

Historical Narrative

Body Story

Embodied Practices

Prenatal Yoga

Pregnancy Massage

EMDR · TCM

Accupressure

BCVT

Infographic by Michael J. Shea, PhD

Fig. 6.1. A compassion-based model of pregnancy

PHENOMENOLOGY OF THE BODY

Philosophy is about the pursuit of a moral and good life by unifying knowledge rather than the production of academic knowledge. It can be understood as the love of wisdom and more importantly how to achieve that. With the advent of specialization in the twentieth century a loss of a felt sense of wholeness occurred and consequently a loss of the experience of wisdom and compassion in general in exchange for being intelligent and well researched. Thus a starting point to a return to wholeness is a philosophical orientation beginning with *phenomenology of the body*. This philosophical tradition emerged in the early twentieth century in northern Europe as part of a philosophical inquiry into the natural world of the human body. Clearly in reviewing a substantial amount of literature regarding contemporary models of the psychobiology of pregnancy, there is no philosophical orientation or guiding, centering dynamic theory. There is no research that I know of that connects a woman's and girl's body to her mind and emotions as a unified whole during pregnancy. Thus a valid starting point for such an orientation is the female's body itself.

It is through a woman's or girl's biology and her whole body-mind that all experience, perception and growth dynamics occur. Phenomenology of the body holds that the subjective experience of the individual person is of primary importance and a source of meaning. This subjective experience arises first in the body prior to the measurable dimension of nervous system affects and objective science. Phenomenology of the body is usually divided into the lived experience of the body, the lived experience of relationship and finally the lived experience of the world. Lived experience is the unique and individual way in which sensory information interacts with cognition and brings forth individual experience, rather than the other way around in which many people are assumed to have the same experience. Thus the first need in a therapeutic interaction with a pregnant mother is simply to honor her individual body-based experience, which is unique to her. As a rule of thumb in human embryology, all differentiations of structure and function have their own individual timing thus supporting the uniqueness of all pregnancies (Blechschmidt 2012b).

COMPASSION

Compassion is the second philosophical orientation towards what is uplifting, elevating and good. Yet emerging research at The Center for Compassion and Altruistic Research and Education (CCARE) at Stanford University indicates that compassion can be defined as a biological instinct to care for oneself and others (Jinpa 2015). In this way compassion is completely relational and fundamental to being human. This leads to a simple conclusion that it is our collective responsibility as a species to support pregnant mothers and their developing babies as a precious act of compassion. To fulfill this responsibility there is a need for all who provide care to them to hold the heart-felt intention of nurturing the growth and health of the mother-baby dyad and to approach them while embodying a nonjudgmental posture. This includes at a practical level having compassion for one's own self first and then others. Self compassion is the basis of the compassion instinct. Otherwise compassion devolves into narcissism, codependency and burnout (Halifax 2011). Research has clearly shown repeatedly that compassion is an instinct that can even overcome trauma (Valdesolo and DeStano 2011; Hofmann, Grossman, and Hinton 2011).

The new field of Fetal Maternal Microchimerism is a beautiful example of biological instinctual compassion (Boddy et al. 2015; Kallenbach, Johnson, and Bianchi 2011; Mahmood and O'Donoghue, 2014; Rjinink et al. 2015). In what these researchers call a metabolism of cooperation, cells from the developing embryo and fetus enter the mother's bloodstream and gravitate towards her heart, brain, liver and breasts. These cells are now seen to have a healing effect on the mother when she experiences problems in those areas of her body. The fetal cells are known to offer the mother protection from breast cancer and a reduced risk of rheumatoid arthritis. Fetal cells can also alert the immune system of the mother for healing her heart. More than a system of cooperation, it is a system of compassion rooted in the cells of our body. It is an easy step to take, that this innate capacity for compassion could manifest behaviorally, psychologically, and spiritually through the lifespan. Compassion is our pre-existing condition.

Compassion is linked to altruism and moral development. Moral development goes through three stages in which one learns *first* to care for oneself, and second, to care for another person or being (Peterson and Seligman 2004). Taking care of one's self is not associated with self-esteem, self-centeredness or self-gratification. It is associated with self-acceptance, self-tolerance and self-kindness. The *second* phase of moral development includes the numerous helping professions that specialize in caring for others. As an interesting note, when children grow up with pets the tendency to care [for] and consider others is increased throughout the lifespan. The *third* stage of moral development is a sense of care and concern for the entire planet. This is altruism, caring concern for the entire planet and everyone on it. Altruism requires a kind of cultural humility by respecting the enormous diversity of people on the planet and even the uniqueness of each client that comes into the office each day for treatment. Thus humility and respect form the basis of compassion that includes everyone (the whole).

These developmental aspects of compassion are instinctual and as instincts they need to be nurtured to grow and evolve. The contemporary client has too much activation of their survival instinct, which dampens the compassion instinct. This is because the culture has entered the age of fear. This is the next paradigm following the age of trauma we have just passed through in the past hundred years. The natural antidote to fear is safety, and safety is established with the altruistic attitude and embodied presence of compassion. Therapeutically, reducing defensive physiology and survival-oriented mechanisms in a pregnant female is a priority, then instinctual compassion can be fed and nurtured. Once it is fed and nurtured a variety of skillful means based on the awakening of compassion can be applied to help oneself and others.

Ultimately, the skillful means of loving kindness is what is missing in many therapeutic interactions with pregnant females. Skillful means is right action that does not produce harmful side effects. The skillful means of loving kindness is the primary expression and application of compassion. Loving kindness is the instinct to want others to be happy. No matter what profession is involved in helping pregnant moms, they can all use loving kindness as the ground of therapy (Nyima and Schlim 2015). The application of loving kindness is gentleness.

All cultures including our own recognize the vital importance of love, not just as a spiritual feature of life development but as a central organizational living experience in one's heart and social interaction. Some literature points to a relationship between maternal-fetal stress during pregnancy and birth, and aggression and violence later in life (de Mause 1996). One antidote is loving kindness. Even interpersonal boundaries can be set with loving kindness.

WHOLENESS

The third aspect of a philosophical orientation is wholeness. Historically, wholeness became a philosophical orientation in the late [nineteenth] century through the efforts of Goethe (Bortoft 1996). This type of philosophical orientation influenced a generation of medical and scientific researchers early in the twentieth century. For example, in the 1920s and 1930s, research in human embryology included an investigation of the embryo as a whole dynamic being with numerous fields of activity within it (Haraway 2004). So wholeness was investigated as both a biological and functional organizational feature occurring not only in prenatal development but throughout the lifespan. More recently in contemporary literature the terms interconnectedness, unconditional health and inherent completeness have been used as metaphors for wholeness. Health in this context is understood as a unity of mind-body-spirit.

Wholeness as unconditional health is actually the pre-existing condition of the human body and one's total being. Prenatal phenomenology is called morphology, which is the study of how the form of the whole body develops through active shaping processes (Blechschmidt and Gasser 2012; van der Bie 2001). Embedded within prenatal phenomenology are the multi-level ordering principles of an embodied wholeness. These ordering principles operate at the micro level to the macro level and are subsumed at all times by the macro level including the environment of not only the woman's body but the social and environmental context outside of her body. The whole is under constant reorganization via well-defined movements and physical forces that act as the primary influence on the cell nucleus to replicate.

One embryologist, Jaap van der Wal, presented a lecture which I attended where he suggested that the human embryo is 10,000 times more metabolically active proportionally than the adult body. This is how a prenate experiences their body—constant lived experience as growth and development and with a degree of intense activity that is normal. Phenomenology of the body is lived morphology. Thus a phenomenology of the body includes prenatal development and the context of pregnancy—the life of the woman or girl in relationship with others, the world and her body.

Included in more current discussions of the wholeness of the human body and body centered therapies is the term *embodiment*. Embodiment is the experience of *order and organization* in the body. It includes different levels or ways of attending to the body. These levels of conscious attention start with neuroception (Porges 2004), the neurological perception of safety, danger or life threat in a person's internal and external environment. Neuroception is a form of *exteroception*. Exteroception is the way that all the different senses especially vision and hearing continually scan the outside environment in the space around the body. The primary purpose for this is to assess safety and/or detect the presence of danger in the environment. Porges (2004) explains that neuroception is also used to continually scan the body *interoceptively* for pain, fever, and illness within the body.

Proprioception and forms of body movement are both a conscious and unconscious experience of the adult body relating to the space around it. Then comes the basic instinctual urge for pleasure and the avoidance of pain, which is one of the body's most basic sentient biological activities. When the instinct to avoid pain wakes up a variety of physiological responses regarding survival and defensiveness, compassion, pleasure and happiness are buried, or in one apt metaphor being used, they are covered in weeds.

Finally, regarding embodiment the term *body image* is used to describe what we imagine we look like in our minds as informed by early preverbal growth patterns. This includes the way children imitate the posture and mannerisms of their parents thus taking on some lifelong patterns being held in their parent's bodies. Children also use images from movies, for example, to relate to their growing body. It is well documented in the eating disorder literature that adolescent girls who are struggling with an eating disorder are affected by media images of female models and other movie figures who are thin (Roth 1992, 2011). This brings to mind the controversy generated by the appearance several decades ago of a model named Twiggy. The media provides numerous other visual representations of inappropriately thin, svelte females as fragmented body images in teenage magazines such as *Seventeen*.

Men and boys receive the same level of distortion through magazines that focus on body building, guns, violence and so forth. Body image refers to the preverbal internal sense of body wholeness in the first two years after birth. The visual sensory systems are much more active than cognitive systems. Lack of safety preverbally distorts the body image as body resources are fragmented into defensive physiology. This is coupled with the young child imitating their caregiver's body posture and mannerisms all of which adds extra layers onto one's body image and the possible fragmentation of a felt sense of embodied wholeness. This becomes compounded in adolescence as the brain and body undergo another major change process.

Culturally defined images of inappropriate bodies add another layer of fragmentation onto the developing body and being. As a boy, I personally was obsessed with the Frankenstein movies. During my adolescence and early twenties my body image was that of numerous parts coming from other bodies being sewn together without much life moving through it. This generates the need for a unique style and sense of embodiment based on a phenomenology [of] the body and self-compassion. Embodied wholeness must be a goal of all therapy based on a phenomenology of the body, compassion and loving kindness.

THE NEED FOR COMPASSION

The second level of figure 6.1 is called *the need for compassion*. It begins with the integration of loss and trauma. Human beings according to some embryologists experience the highest amount of lost embryos and fetuses of any other species on the planet. Consequently, females are actually experts in death and dying as the majority of women have experienced prenatal loss through miscarriage, abortion or stillbirth. The great tragedy is not the loss itself but the way in which family/social support systems and many professionals dismiss the importance of the loss. This casual dismissal of the loss is a denial of the deep emotional pain that many women experience when losing a child even if it is the size of a lentil as an embryo.

Such minimizing of loss by our culture then impacts the attitude and psychodynamics of the female towards herself and her next pregnancy. This creates a barrier that may inhibit the mother's connection with and attachment to the living being inside her body. In addition, numerous women and girls become pregnant who have pre-existing traumatic stress symptoms or diagnosed posttraumatic stress disorder (PTSD). This may further compromise their ability to relate appropriately to their developing child. This is because the activation of psychophysiological states associated with past traumatic experiences held by a pregnant mother can release stress hormones in her body that may have damaging effects on her unborn child. This is clearly stated by the author of this book [*Prenatal Development and Parents' Lived Experiences*], Dr. Ann Diamond Weinstein.

Pregnancy has the potential to be a very spiritual and joyful time. The creation of a family and caring for children is a vital aspect of human development, culture and society. This period of time is therefore critical to a healthy society. Support for the deep psychospiritual dynamics in a woman's or girl's body that include a deep spiritual relationship with the forces of creation and the urge to become are absolutely necessary. This may mean healing wounds of the past and the present. In addition, the physical changes that a female's body goes through are numerous and affect her all the way from swings in moods and emotions due to a shift in her neuroendocrine system to musculoskeletal discomfort and physical pain. At a base level a pregnant woman's or girl's body and mind and her unborn child need to be supported and cared for with compassion—gentleness and kindness. The act of pregnancy is in itself an act of compassion. It is one of the purest forms of biologically caring for another person. Just consider how seeing a pregnant woman can sometimes center one's attention and open one's heart through simple observation. Anyone working with pregnant females needs to meet the woman with an equal amount of compassion.

PAIN

One of the physical effects of pregnancy and birth is physical pain and discomfort including the fear of physical pain. It is a topic that is not addressed well in the popular or scientific literature. There are phases of pregnancy that can be quite uncomfortable for a woman whether that is morning sickness or low back pain during the second and third trimester. Managing fear, especially in a woman who is pregnant for the first time, is an absolute necessity. Frequently the medical community unconsciously scares a pregnant woman if it is her first pregnancy, especially when she wants to choose a different birth plan or vary from the norm in the hospital where her obstetrician or midwife practices. Therapists must focus on giving pregnant females the gift of non-fright.

Reducing fear and increasing safety comes about in a delicate balance with the sympathetic nervous system and the parasympathetic nervous system via the brain and heart. Any and all therapy for women and girls who are pregnant must have as one of its principal aims the stabilization of the autonomic nervous system. This requires a set of open, compassionate eyes (Cosley et al. 2010).

There is significant literature about the toxicity of the environment and its effect on pregnant women (Paul 2011). This effect comes through the blood and influences the development of the liver and the immune system in the fetus (Paul 2011). Environmental pollution such as secondhand cigarette smoke, automobile exhaust, and other chemicals that may be present in a mother's everyday environment should be avoided as much as is possible.

COMPASSION RESOURCES

The next category in the third row of circles in figure 6.1 is *compassion resources*. Mindfulness is the first level of a compassion-based resource. There is an enormous amount of research literature supporting the efficacy of mindfulness-based meditation practices (see American Mindfulness Research Association website). These meditation practices are used in a wide variety of psychological and behavioral problems. What is mindfulness? Mindfulness is neutral attention to the present moment. Neutral means non-attachment and non-interpretation of experience. The most typical practice of orienting to the present time is attention to one's breathing and heart rate with conscious awareness (cardioception). This can be taught to women without complex trauma. Mindfulness is related to equanimity, a state of mind of peacefulness. These are all subtle emotions that need to be cultivated in order to nourish compassion. They are the fertilizer so to speak of compassion.

It is important to differentiate between what I call corporate mindfulness and traditional mindfulness. Corporate mindfulness is used to help people become more efficient at their work or get them back to work after an absence due to illness or other challenges. It is used by corporations such as Google for their employees to be more efficient. Traditional mindfulness however is aimed at creating a foundation for compassion to become active and grow in a person's life with themselves and others. To be compassionate is to be mindful. Mindfulness is the work of paying attention to right now physically and mentally in order to clearly see the need for compassionate action and the subsequent type of skillful means necessary to be applied in caring for one's self and others. Traditional mindfulness is being implemented more and more in pregnancy and childbirth practices especially in anxiety and pain management.

The Mindfulness-Based Childbirth and Parenting (MBCP) program is an excellent example of the application of traditional mindfulness to helping a woman while she is pregnant and giving birth (Bardacke 2012). Susan Piver (2012) and

Cassandra Vieten (2009) also provide excellent resources for a mindful pregnancy in general. Piver's book even comes with a CD of guided meditations. All these authors suggest loving kindness as the base for all interactions during pregnancy.

Resilience is a key element in managing a contemporary lifestyle. Resilience means consciously being aware of the effect on one's mind and body of challenges and stress and rapidly returning to a steady-state. An excellent practice to develop resilience is called interoception. The first step to become resilient is to be mindful of what is happening in one's body at a sensory level internally. Interoception is the conscious awareness of the internal urges, movements and tonal qualities of the viscera and organ systems deep inside the core of the body. Cardioception is a form of *interoceptive awareness* of the movement and activity of the blood and heart (Couto et al. 2014; Sütterlin et al. 2013). Embodied wholeness and compassion is dependent upon cardioception.

A growing body of research suggests that cardioception can reduce fear and anxiety (Bechera and Naqvi 2004; Craig 2004; Critchley et al. 2004). When this is coupled with the emerging literature on a technique called *coherent breathing,* heart rate variability (HRV) becomes stronger and more robust (McCraty and Shaffer 2015). HRV is a measure of the resilience of the heartbeat and its relationship to the vagus nerve, [which is] responsible for lowering heart rate. Coherent breathing is simply a technique in which one's breathing is slowed down to approximately five cycles per minute. This in turn stabilizes the autonomic nervous system (vagal) connection to the heart in the right atrium. This means that one's heart rate can stabilize much more quickly from a stress or a challenge by slowing breathing or humor (Kok and Fredrickson 2010). Information on coherent breathing is readily available on the internet. It is well established that the mother's heart rate directly influences the heart rate of her baby before birth (Channing et al. 2012). Thus breathing skills to lower the heart rate of the mother will directly affect her baby.

Resilience is also associated with developing a sense of gratitude. Gratitude training is a popular theme promoted by the HeartMath Institute in which an image can be held in one's heart and mind of the person for whom gratitude is felt. There are other ways to sense and feel gratitude such as making a list every night before going to bed of five things to be grateful for during the past day. I feel that forgiveness is a vital element in becoming resilient. All of us have experienced events in our lives that require forgiveness. This includes three levels: forgiving ourselves for past actions done to others, [forgiving ourselves for] past actions done to ourselves [and] forgiving others for past actions done to us. Forgiving others is not about condoning actions that were done but rather simply moving on from those life events. Forgiveness and gratitude are essential building blocks that support an increase in compassion and the capacity for loving kindness to embrace more people.

Safety is a critical element in all therapeutic encounters as well as social life expe-

contact with others. As mentioned above, Stephen Porges explains that we

ion to perceive and evaluate safety, danger or life threat in our environ-

ractions with others. Neuroception is the way in which all humans

sten to the environment and other people to determine if it is safe to

e. This has major implications for therapists in general. Safety is a

ause it initiates the therapeutic process. Therapists need to develop

ment through eye-to-eye contact, facial expressions, hand and arm

movement that expresses loving kindness. Attunement is the qual-

on that is moved between the therapist's mind and body and the client's

and body. The therapist's ability to slow down in the presence of a pregnant mother is one key to generating safety.

There is an event in therapy called the *intersubjective moment* (Beebe et al. 2005; Stern 2004). This intersubjective moment is when the client realizes they are being held in safety and at the same time realizes that the therapist is sensing the client's feeling of safety with the therapist. The intersubjective moment is a two-way street because the therapist must also feel comfortable and safe in the interaction and as that moment occurs, the client will also sense how the therapist feels safe around him or her. Sometimes it is a meeting of the eyes in a clinical interview that generates a feeling of positive embarrassment. This is one possible intersubjective moment.

Pregnancy requires safety at so many different levels. This is why it is important that women and girls who are pregnant have support persons such as midwives and doulas, friends and family to support them in the complex spiritual and psychobiological dynamics unfolding every day during pregnancy. Safety, attunement and support all contain an element of empathy. Mindfulness and resilience also contain an element of empathy. Empathy is the felt sense of feeling what is happening in the other person. All of this contributes to the intersubjective moment and the interconnection of the nervous and vascular systems of two people or what is called a two-person biology, the essence of a compassion-based pregnancy. Mom and baby have their cardiovascular and central nervous systems synchronized. At the same time, in a therapeutic encounter with the pregnant female, the therapist and the mother are synchronizing their cardiovascular and central nervous systems. That is why mindfulness of one's own body is the beginning point of a compassion-based engagement with a pregnant female. The therapist must be aware of his or her own body sensations, thoughts and feelings.

BIOLOGY

Knowledge of the biology of prenatal development is an important compassion resource since compassion is an instinct rooted in our biology. Much is known about the changes that go on in each of the three trimesters in a female's body during pregnancy and a basic understanding of such ought to be known by any therapist working with pregnant moms. This also includes knowledge of the stages of birth, and the attachment and bonding process following birth. These are all complex metabolic and physiological changes that a woman's body undergoes and without such body-based knowledge, therapy runs the risk of becoming disembodied and an intellectual or mental event. This leads to a disconnection from the pregnant female and detracts from the ability to feel safe.

Biological knowledge includes diet and nutrition. A growing body of knowledge supports the need for healthy diet and the potentially devastating effects of eating junk food during pregnancy. Of course it is well known that alcohol, recreational drugs and cigarettes have a very detrimental effect on the developing fetus and it is now well established that a poor diet can thwart growth and development as well.

THERAPEUTIC PROCESSES

Finally the fourth row of circles in figure 6.1 involves a variety of *therapeutic processes*. The first understanding from a therapeutic point of view is the necessity of the containment of affect. Many therapies for adults are oriented around the release and discharge of feelings, emotions and history. However a growing body of research supports the need for what is called *containment*. This is a holding environment that the therapist generates in which the client has the space to self-regulate and become resilient within the context of their own resources.

One fundamental way of generating containment, transformation and self-regulation of thoughts, unwanted sensations and emotions is through the projection of loving kindness from the therapist. Loving kindness is the skillful means I mentioned earlier that is employed with mindfulness which comes from the instinct of compassion. Loving kindness itself is also a subtle emotion and periodically requires a genuine smile to cross the face of the therapist.

Tonglen is the name of a compassion meditation in which the pain and suffering of another person is visualized as a dark color and the therapist is simply breathing that dark color into their body especially the heart interoceptively. This taking in happens for about a minute. Then the therapist projects a sense of well-being and loving kindness towards the client perhaps as a light color. This projecting of well-being also happens for about a minute. In this way the pain and suffering of the client is taken into the heart, brain and mind of the therapist and transformed into its opposite quality of loving kindness, health and well-being. Compassion then is a reciprocal cycle of taking in and giving back out. It begins with one's self and extends to others continually. Scanning the environment with compassion is as strong as scanning the environment for safety.

THE ORIGIN STORY

The personal narrative of a pregnant mother is of vital importance. All cultures have an origin story in which the meaning of life and the consequences of pain and suffering are dealt with and given meaning within the context of that culture. Healing rituals were then constructed to regress a person back through their prenatal time to effect a more permanent healing. In cultural rituals and origin mythologies the way it was "at the beginning" was *perfect undifferentiated wholeness.* The telling of the origin story is the healing event because it awakens the time of perfect wholeness in the present moment (Eliade 1958, 1959, 1960, 1963). This is not so much of a therapeutic process as it is an ancient healing ritual especially among women. It needs to be reawakened. In her book *Talking to Babies,* Szejer (2005) advocates for talking to babies on maternity wards in hospitals. She argues that babies need to hear about the specific conditions into which they are born. They need to hear about the mother and father and even losses that have occurred such as a twin. And these stories need to be told in the presence of the mother and father and preferably by the parents. Through these narratives everyone is helped to "find their place in the altered world created by the birth."

Pregnancy is an excellent example of an origin story at a biopsychosocial level for our postmodern culture. Since most origin mythologies grapple with how a human being is created, the need for an origin story can be done quite simply with a pregnant mom. This may include a historical narrative of the woman's personal history or simply a narrative about the conception and pregnancy along with its progression. The mother can be encouraged to tell this story to her unborn child over and over. Within all of this is a story about the human body. The body narrative *is* the origin story. Most literature on dealing with shock and trauma agrees that at some point the person must be able to tell their story and have it heard and reflected by a compassionate therapist/listener. So with or without a history of trauma, the origin story is of vital importance in a compassion-based model of pregnancy. It can be told in short segments or long epic poems.

There are a number of embodied practices being employed therapeutically with pregnant women and girls. A short list includes prenatal yoga, pregnancy massage, acupuncture, EMDR (Eye Movement Desensitization and Reprocessing), acupressure, Emotional Freedom Technique (EFT) and biodynamic cardiovascular therapy. Biodynamic cardiovascular therapy is a compassion-based process that evolved from the biodynamic craniosacral therapy model. This is specifically the application of the perceptual skills of slowing down and becoming still in relationship to the coupled cardiovascular systems of both the therapist and the client. Biological stillness or quiescence is an essential building block for growth and development through the life span but especially prenatally.

An important element of biodynamic cardiovascular therapy is to nurture and support the relationship between the mother and the growing embryo and fetus inside of her. This is done slowly and by sensing her own heart rate and then sensing the heartbeat of her unborn baby either through simple awareness or by palpating using the mother's hands and fingers to gently palpate the arteries of her baby until a pulse is felt. This is called synchronization and is coupled with coherent breathing, which not only stabilizes the autonomic nervous system of the mother but also that of the baby. It increases HRV in both mother and baby and thus the health outcomes can improve, as well as the possibility of having an easier birth. For mothers who are at risk of becoming activated because of a history of trauma, coherent breathing is the starting and ending point of learning how to connect interoceptively.

Prenatal yoga and pregnancy massage require extensive training and certification. This is also true for acupuncture, a part of TCM (Traditional Chinese Medicine) and EMDR (Eye Movement Desensitization and Reprocessing), which is usually performed by a licensed mental health worker. Acupressure can be performed by a number of health care providers, manual therapists and lay people as well. Regardless of the technique employed in treating a pregnant mom, establishing safety is critical. Treatment involves three steps: establishing safety first, stabilization of the autonomic nervous system and the potential transformation of a woman's experience of her pregnancy. This three-step therapeutic sequence is dependent on compassion. Therapies based on compassion training are showing promise for a wide range of conditions some of which women experience during pregnancy (Jinpa 2015).

The premise of the foregoing discussion is that pregnancy itself is an act of compassion as mentioned. The reader might pause and reflect on this statement upon seeing a pregnant mother. The sight of a woman or girl who is pregnant is capable of generating the felt sense of well-being and happiness in the observer when unobstructed by stress and trauma. Thus, even the image of pregnancy may be healing. It is that embodied image and sensibility of one human being deeply caring for another inside of her that must be restored in our culture.

As a postscript to this chapter, I originally put together a graphic with the various models of pregnancy (see fig. 6.2). I noticed that compassion was not mentioned in any of these models and thus I wrote the appendix to Ann Weinstein's wonderful book. I am blessed to have her contribute chapter 4 to this book.

Contemporary Models of Pregnancy

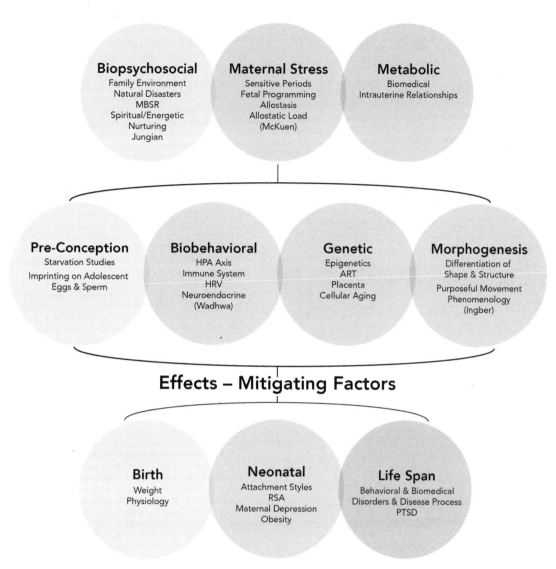

Fig. 6.2. Contemporary models of pregnancy. One of the dominant models of pregnancy is the metabolic model discussed in the next chapter.

7

Vascular Endothelium and the Maternal-Fetal Relationship

MARY MONRO

MARY MONRO has been a practicing osteopath in Great Britain for twenty-five years and teaches post-graduate courses in osteopathy.

> *The unborn child is a feeling, remembering, aware being.*
> THOMAS VERNY AND JOHN KELLY,
> *THE SECRET LIFE OF THE UNBORN CHILD*

The vascular endothelium is the layer of cells lining all the blood vessels throughout the body. It is a critical interface, both between the fluid compartments in the mother (that is, between blood vessels and tissues) and between the mother and baby at the placenta. During pregnancy, 80 to 90 percent of uterine blood flow goes to the placenta, with the remainder going to the myometrium (Wang and Zhao 2010). The vascular endothelium at the placental interface is the fulcrum around which the mother-child relationship (psychoemotional, physiological, transgenerational) is formed. That may seem an exaggeration, but the interaction between mother and child, between the mother's embodied experience and the downstream consequences for her offspring, affects everything from gene expression to temperament and mood. The transmission is mediated at the endothelium, a sensitive, responsive, thinking, feeling, knowing organ.

The vascular endothelium is an intelligent, metabolically active endocrine organ that also forms the blood-brain barrier (Aird 2007; Epstein et al. 1990; Simionescu and Antohe 2006; Ramcharan et al. 2011). In pregnancy, the mother's blood volume nearly doubles and blood flow to the uterus increases four- to fivefold; the uterus receives up to 15 percent of cardiac output at term compared to 3 percent in a non-pregnant woman (Thaler et al. 1990). Consequently, the maternal circulation has to adapt, significantly and quickly, so that the placenta and fetus receive adequate oxygen and nutrients. The modification of the maternal vasculature is facilitated by vascular endothelial growth factor (VEGF), a family of proangiogenic and permeability-moderating factors produced in the endothelium. VEGF also stimulates the release from the endothelium of the powerful vasodilators nitric oxide (NO) and prostacyclin. The distal umbilical cord and placenta have limited innervation and so vascular tone is entirely controlled by endothelial-derived vasodilators and vasoconstrictors (Sobrevia et al. 2016). Vascular tone in turn affects the transfer of nutrients from mother to fetus, so any disturbance to the mechanisms determining tone will result in disturbed nutrient transfer.

As far back as the fourth century BCE, Aristotle asserted that the vascular architecture in the embryo functions as a frame or model that shapes the body structure of the growing organism. Recent research bears this out, with the endothelial cells instructing and regulating organ differentiation and tissue remodeling, from the embryo to postnatal life (Crivellato, Nico, and Ribatti 2007; Ribatti, Tamma, and Annese 2021). Endothelial-derived signals are essential for the normal development of the heart and its electrical system, growth of the liver primordium, pancreatic differentiation and morphogenesis, and the complex structure of the kidneys, the lungs, the musculoskeletal system, and the central, peripheral, and autonomic nervous systems. The intrinsic heterogeneity of the endothelial cells is thought to underpin their ability to influence such a wide range of tissues.

The single layer of cells forming the vascular endothelium is biologically quiescent in health. It becomes activated in response to a variety of factors, mainly driven by oxidative stress (from inflammation) and sheer stress (from increased, decreased, or turbulent blood flow), resulting in adverse outcomes for mother, placenta, and baby and potentially having lifelong consequences for the child. The rest of this chapter looks at these three actors in this drama.

MOTHER

The mother and her social context influence her offspring from before pregnancy, through pregnancy, and throughout the life of her children. If we regard the lives of future generations as important, we have to take steps to support the mental and physical health of potential mothers.

Fetal Programming

A woman considering pregnancy might also consider the potential for her lifestyle to influence the health of her baby. About 10 percent of pregnant women are smokers; 5 to 10 percent drink alcohol. Of the adult female population in the United Kingdom in 2014, 20 percent had a BMI of 30 or greater, qualifying them as obese, while another 31 percent were overweight; in the United States in 2018,

28 percent of adult females were obese and a further 42 percent were overweight (World Obesity Federation n.d.). Such factors can affect every stage of life for a woman's offspring, from the eggs she produces to placental, embryonic, and fetal development to postnatal life and into adulthood. Obesity is a significant public health issue and we must tackle the obesogenic environment (encompassing factors such as poverty, poor-quality housing, ultraprocessed food, sedentary lifestyles, passive travel, and so on) if future generations are to be healthier (Kaczynski et al. 2020; Swinburn et al. 2011).

So called "fetal programming" (a.k.a. the Barker hypothesis) refers to the effect of maternal environmental factors on permanent structural changes in organs and tissues, altered responses to environmental stimuli, and epigenetic changes in the offspring (Smith and Ryckman 2015; Entringer et al. 2018). The developing brain is particularly sensitive to fetal programming effects because the differentiation of major brain structures occurs almost entirely during prenatal life, orchestrated by a cascade of bidirectional interactions occurring between the maternal and fetal compartments and the external environment (Lindsay et al. 2019).

Pre-pregnancy overweight and obesity are linked with gestational diabetes, preeclampsia, recurrent miscarriage, maternal hypertension, pregnancy infections such as Group B strep, premature delivery, C-section delivery, and stillbirth (Leddy, Power, and Schulkin 2008).

Infections, hypertension, preeclampsia, smoking, alcohol abuse, substance abuse, malnutrition, severe type 2 diabetes, and maternal autoimmune disease have all been shown to cause intrauterine growth restriction (IUGR), which can lead to small-for-gestational-age (SGA) babies, who can suffer health consequences into adulthood. Adults who were SGA babies tend to have SGA babies (Kroener, Wang, and Pisarska 2016; Sobrevia et al. 2016). It also appears that assisted reproductive technologies (ART) lead to a higher risk of IUGR and SGA babies, preeclampsia, preterm labor, and C-section delivery, probably due to abnormal implantation and development of the placenta. However, ART also tends to lead to multiple pregnancies and this may explain some of the differences (Da Silva et al. 2020).

All of these complications of pregnancy are thought to be related to endothelial dysfunction. The endothelium is responsible for the vascularization of the placenta and for the production of and sensitivity to substances that transfer between mother and baby. Dysfunction is triggered by inflammation in the maternal vascular system and may be aggravated by a suboptimal placentation process—meaning the mechanism by which the embryonic trophoblast during the second week of development embeds into the maternal uterine wall—affecting the quantity and quality of the connection between mother and child through the pregnancy and having life-long consequences. However, we know that nonplacental organisms also demonstrate transgenerational environmental information flows, so there must be a number of possible mechanisms through which information can be transferred from parent to offspring (Ho and Burggren 2010).

Type 2 Diabetes (T2D) and Gestational Diabetes Mellitus (GDM)

Mothers with high-calorie, highly processed diets produce offspring with adiposity and inflammation that show a higher risk of developing obesity, T2D, and metabolic syndrome in later life (Marshall et al. 2022). The offspring develop endothelial dysfunction and signs of insulin resistance. It appears that in obese mothers elevated levels of cytokines (signaling molecules that mediate and regulate immunity, inflammation, and hematopoiesis), such as leptin (a hormone secreted by adipose tissue that regulates appetite and insulin action), tumor necrosis factor (TNF), and resistin, drive insulin resistance across the placenta and mediate the changes in the developing fetus. Even when the offspring are fed a normal diet postnatally, these changes seem to be irreversible (Archer and McDonald 2017).

Gestational diabetes mellitus (GDM) is defined as novel hyperglycemia in pregnancy. GDM affects about 7 percent of pregnancies worldwide. It increases the risk of obesity, T2D, and metabolic syndrome in the offspring. GDM leads to reduced vasodilation in response to insulin (abnormal insulin signaling affects NO availability in the fetoplacental vasculature and hence vascular tone reactivity). GDM also causes epigenetic changes that lead to a higher risk of cardiovascular disease in the offspring (Smith and Ryckman 2015).

Dyslipidemia (raised blood levels of cholesterol and triglycerides), which is a marker of metabolic syndrome, is associated with GDM and affects fetal vascular endothelium via altered levels of insulin, which is responsible for regulating the transfer of lipids from the maternal to the fetal circulation. Dyslipidemia can result not only in overweight babies but also in neurological disorders and atherosclerosis, indicating the importance of insulin signaling in the transfer of nutrients from mother to baby (Sobrevia et al. 2016; Brennan, Morton, and Davidge 2014).

In T2D and GDM the high levels of sugar and insulin in the maternal blood overactivates the fetal metabolism, resulting in placental hypoxia and increased risk of preeclampsia (Phoswa and Khaliq 2021).

COVID-19 and Pregnancy

COVID-19 infection seems to cause more severe disease and increased likelihood of hospitalization in pregnant women and leads to more complications, such as preeclampsia, premature birth, and stillbirth (Stock et al. 2022), probably as a result of the excessive inflammatory response and its activation of the endothelium. A U.S. study found that pregnant women with COVID-19 were more than twice as likely to deliver prematurely, compared to those recovered from or without infection (Blitz et al. 2021). Vaccination against COVID-19 appears to reduce risk of severe illness and death in pregnant women, with fewer adverse outcomes for the infant (Watanabe et al. 2022).

COVID-19 also disrupts the renin-angiotensin system (RAS) through its use of angiotensin-converting enzyme 2 (ACE2) as a receptor, reducing its bioavailability and interfering with the role of the RAS in placentation and the hemodynamic changes of pregnancy (affecting blood pressure, blood volume, and kidney function). It is thought that both vertical transmission of infection to the placenta and fetus and the depletion of ACE2 may be behind the signs of disease in the neonate (Nobrega Cruz et al. 2021).

Preeclampsia

Preeclampsia, affecting about 5 percent of pregnancies worldwide, is diagnosed as a combination of hypertension with proteinuria after the twentieth week of gestation (Ives et al. 2020). It is a significant contributor to maternal death, stillbirth, preterm delivery, IUGR, and SGA babies (Brennan, Morton, and Davidge 2014); it is responsible for some fifty thousand deaths worldwide every year. Symptoms can involve the lungs, liver, kidneys, heart, and central nervous system. In its most severe form it is known as the HELLP syndrome—the acronym stands for hemolysis, elevated liver enzymes, and low platelets. Risk factors include nulliparity (no previous births), African American race, older age, new partner for a woman who has previously given birth, hypertension, connective tissue disorders, obesity, insulin resistance, and hyperlipidemia. Fetuses exposed to preeclampsia develop elevated cholesterol levels as children and have a higher risk of cardiovascular disease in later life (Andraweera and Lassi 2019). The only effective treatment for pre-eclampsia is delivery of the placenta.

Endothelial dysfunction is central to the development of preeclampsia, although the precise mechanisms involved are not fully understood. It is thought that the embryonic trophoblast invades the uterine spiral arteries only to a shallow depth and that the remodeling of the spiral arteries, to turn them from high-pressure narrow vessels into low-pressure wide vessels, remains incomplete. It is also thought that the invading cytotrophoblast cells fail to transform properly into endothelial cells. These processes are driven by endothelially derived molecules (for example, vascular endothelial cadherin), and in the development of preeclampsia they fail, probably because of maternal inflammation (leading to oxidative stress), infection, and elevated circulating cytokines (which affect both angiogenesis and vasodilation) (Phoswa and Khaliq 2021).

The resulting underperfusion of the placenta leads to a hypoxic state, which in turn causes the release of more inflammatory cytokines and antiangiogenic factors, an elevated immune response, and dyslipidemia. This snowballs into a further inflammatory response and increased oxidative stress, which further activates the endothelium. The result is increased vasoconstriction (as a result of low NO levels), causing increased peripheral resistance and hypertension (Brennan, Morton, and Davidge 2014). However, it is not known which of these processes is the underlying driver and which are consequences (Boeldt and Bird 2017).

Endothelial dysfunction has been shown to be systemic in women with preeclampsia; hence the widespread effects. Endothelial activation is associated with a vasoconstricted environment and reduced responsiveness to vasodilators such as NO. The low level of NO in the system is also thought to adversely affect the level of circulating endothelial progenitor cells (EPCs). In normal pregnancies EPC levels rise through the pregnancy, but they reduce in pregnancies with preeclampsia and remain low postpartum. This is thought to be the root cause of why women who had preeclampsia show long-term elevated cardiovascular risk—they are twice as likely to die of cardiovascular disease as women who did not have preeclampsia (Brennan, Morton, and Davidge 2014).

PLACENTA

In normal pregnancy the embryonic placenta develops from the trophoblast, the outermost layer of cells in the blastocyst. The trophoblast develops into an outer layer, a sort of multinucleate shell called the syncytiotrophoblast, and an inner layer of stem cells, cytotrophoblasts, that form the chorionic villi. The trophoblast is a structural and biochemical barrier, an endocrine organ and driver of angiogenesis. The process of placentation begins with cytotrophoblast cells detaching to invade and remodel the maternal uterine spiral arteries, themselves transforming into endothelial cells. They break down and replace the endothelial lining and the smooth muscle coat, making the arteries larger and of lower pressure, thereby increasing blood flow for gas exchange with the fetal circulation. This low-pressure, high-volume environment facilitates the transfer of nutrients and oxygen from mother to fetus, which happens in stillness (Cowan 2016).

Vasculogenesis (new blood vessel formation) begins at the end of the third week and angiogenesis (additional blood vessel formation) at the end of the fourth week of gestation. The development of the placental vasculature is regulated by Hofbauer cells—macrophages specific to the placenta that also secrete growth factors, such as VEGF, and cytokines such as TNF-α. As in the adult, human placental arterial endothelial cells (HPAECs) are different in structure and function to venous endothelial cells. HPAECs are more responsive to proliferative factors, while venous cells have microvilli and differentiate easily into adipocytes (fat cells) and osteoblasts. This diversity in structure and function is reiterated over and over through life, such that *every endothelial cell is thought to be unique.*

The second half of pregnancy is dominated by placental mass expansion, with endothelial health central to the processes of angiogenesis and vascularization. The placenta and the maternal myometrial spiral arteries have no innervation, enabling the fetus to counter the influence of vasoconstriction driven by the maternal autonomic nervous system (Khong, Tee, and Kelly 1997). Instead, vasomotor tone, and hence fetal blood supply, is maintained by the endothelium. In T2D or metabolic syndrome pregnancies, where insulin resistance and inflammation are present from the start, both the structure and the function of the placenta will be adversely affected.

The placenta is known to produce not only gestational hormones but also almost every known cytokine. These molecules are produced by the vascular endothelium and by the trophoblast. The placenta is also exposed to the regulatory influence of hormones, cytokines, growth factors, and substrates present in both circulations—that is, it is *both source and target* of these chemicals (Murphy et al. 2006). This is the biochemical interface between mother and fetus, meeting like trapeze artists, each time trying to ensure a secure bond in a dynamic, automatically shifting environment.

The placenta has a high level of insulin receptors relative to other tissues, initially in the syncytiotrophoblast (connecting with insulin in the maternal circulation) but toward term mainly in the endothelium (connecting with insulin in the fetal circulation) (Desoye and Hauguel-De Mouzon 2007). Another hormonal shift toward fetal control is via human placental growth hormone, active from fifteen weeks of gestation, which takes over from the maternal pituitary growth hormone to regulate maternal glucose levels to ensure adequate nutrient supply to the fetus. The fetus and the placenta are active partners in the pregnancy, and the quality of the relationship influences lifelong outcomes.

FETUS

As the pregnancy progresses, the fetus takes increasing control, particularly in the third trimester, manipulating the mother's resources and even her behavior (Murphy et al. 2006). The health of the maternal-fetal dyad is inextricably linked, affecting both of their lives for years to come.

The Heart
The fetal heart and placenta develop in tandem. Endocardial endothelial cells derive from the primitive streak and (together with cardiomyocytes) form the heart tube,

septum, valves, and smooth muscle cells through a process called endothelial-to-mesenchyme transition (EndMT). This process is driven by signals from myocardial and endothelial cells (Crivellato, Nico, and Ribatti 2007). These endocardial endothelial cells are larger than most endothelial cells and have microvilli, contributing (along with ridges and furrows in the endocardium) to the large surface area in the heart. They are involved in the contractility, rhythmicity, and growth of the heart and act as a blood sensor. They release large amounts of endothelial nitric oxide synthase (eNOS), which is essential to the health of the blood vessels.

By the end of the first trimester, the placenta and fetal heart are fully formed, and there is a massive increase in blood supply to the fetus and a fall in resistance. The placenta is the largest fetal organ and takes about 40 percent of fetal cardiac output. Abnormalities in the placenta can lead to developmental problems for the heart (and other organs), as is commonly seen with the effects of IUGR. Whether the effects are mediated through reduced transport efficiency, altered endocrine function, or hemodynamic changes in the umbilical circulation is not known (Burton and Jauniaux 2018).

Inflammation

Long-term sequelae of maternal inflammation in the offspring may include cardio-vascular disease, obesity, metabolic syndrome, and neurodevelopmental disorders (Rogers and Velten 2011). Systemic inflammation is associated with oxidative stress, impacting the fetal vasculature and contributing to abnormal fetal brain development (Ginsberg et al. 2017) and diseases of prematurity such as respiratory distress, chronic lung disease, retinopathy of prematurity, necrotizing enterocolitis, and periventricular leukomalacia.

Antioxidant therapies to reduce oxidative stress in neonates have shown mixed results. Vitamins A, C, and E do not consistently improve outcomes and can make things worse. Magnesium sulfate shows promising neuroprotective properties (Ginsberg et al. 2017). Melatonin seems to act as an antioxidant and anti-inflammatory; it is not produced in the term infant until three months of age and is even more deficient in premature infants, especially if there has been neurological insult (Gitto et al. 2009).

The Brain

According to the Centers for Disease Control and Prevention, an increasing proportion of births in the United States are preterm (before thirty-seven weeks, accounting for 10.5 percent of births in 2021) or extremely preterm (before twenty-eight weeks, accounting for 6 percent of those preterm births). The fetal cerebral vasculature in these cases is, by definition, immature and consequently fragile, and although survival rates have increased, the level of neurodevelopmental disability in extremely preterm babies remains high at over 50 percent (Brew, Walker, and Wong 2014).

Arterial development in the brain stem and cerebellum is completed between twenty and twenty-four weeks of gestation, in the basal ganglia and thalamus by twenty-eight weeks, and finally in the cerebral cortex and germinal matrix (an area rich in stem cells under the wing of the lateral ventricles). Vessels penetrate from surface areas to deeper areas, with vasculogenesis and angiogenesis regulated by VEGF, which is deterred in hypoxic conditions.

Brain injury risk factors include the following:

1. The deepest structures are the last to vascularize and the most likely to suffer underperfusion. In the preterm infant, the deep white matter around the ventricles shows lower vascular density than is found in other brain regions, making it more vulnerable to hypoxia, especially from hypotension. The vascular endothelium in the germinal matrix has fewer pericytes and astrocytes supporting it and so is more fragile (and so prone to rupture/bleed with pressure variations) than gray or white matter elsewhere in the brain. Prenatal steroid injections stabilize the germinal matrix vasculature, minimizing the risk of intraventricular hemorrhage.

2. It is known that at birth, cerebral blood flow (CBF) is relatively low and cerebral oxygen extraction (COE) is high, and both of these are exaggerated in preterm infants. However, there is a limit to COE, and this is why preterm infants are given caffeine—it increases the ceiling for COE, minimizing the risk of hypoxic-ischemic injury. Prenatal administration of magnesium sulfate seems to increase CBF, reducing the risk of hypoxic-ischemic white matter injury. Administration of high doses of erythropoietin (EPO) is a potentially promising therapy for brain injury, as it crosses the blood-brain barrier to modulate inflammatory and immune responses, is vasogenic and angiogenic via interaction with VEGF, and helps the brain repair itself (Gonzalez and Ferriero 2009).

3. Another parameter affecting brain perfusion is pressure autoregulation, mediated by endothelial-derived NO, neuronal-derived vasoactive factors, and the autonomic nervous system. Autoregulatory capacity is late developing and so preterm infants cannot regulate cerebral blood pressure adequately, making them vulnerable to hypoxia from hypotension or bleeds.

4. Persistent circulating cytokines in the two-week postnatal period are associated with the development of cerebral palsy in extremely preterm infants, indicating that early postnatal as well as prenatal inflammatory events can influence brain injury (Kuban et al. 2014).

5. The level of oxygen and CO_2 in the blood is also a factor, with preterm infants showing less reactivity to both high and low levels of blood gases. When preterm infants are given oxygen, their CBF falls in response but remains low for several hours after oxygen delivery ceases, potentially dangerously. It is better to give them air rather than oxygen (Brew, Walker, and Wong 2014).

6. Children of overweight and obese mothers have more than a threefold increased risk of cerebral palsy (van der Burg et al. 2016). Maternal inflammation (resulting from, for example, obesity or infection) is known to increase fetal cerebral oxygen consumption and cause fluctuations in cerebral blood flow. Maternal inflammation increases the permeability of the fetal blood-brain barrier (neurovascular unit), leaving the brain vulnerable to the action of cytokines and oxidative stress.

BIRTH

In 2011, researchers from the University of Edinburgh declared: "Human parturition is an inflammatory event" (Golightly, Jabbour, and Norman 2011). It was traditionally thought that the initiation of labor was an endocrine event, driven by hormones such as progesterone (withdrawing its role in the maintenance of pregnancy) and oxytocin (to cause uterine contractions). It is now thought that the immune system is the driving force. Progesterone acts as an anti-inflammatory, and it may be that its role in initiating parturition is that its withdrawal allows the inflammatory state to snowball, triggering labor.

Recent research has found that cell-free fetal DNA (cffDNA) may be responsible for triggering this inflammatory response. CffDNA is shed by the embryo/fetus from five weeks of gestation and enters the maternal circulation via the placenta throughout pregnancy. Toward term, the level of cffDNA increases, peaking just before labor. It provokes a "sterile inflammation" (that is, without infection) response from the mother, causing the release of cytokines and cell adhesion molecules (in the endothelium) that attract leukocytes to the myometrium, cervix, and fetal membranes, causing increased contractility in the myometrium, ripening the cervix, and facilitating membrane rupture (Kazemi et al. 2021).

Corticotropin-releasing hormone (CRH) is a stress hormone normally released through the hypothalamus-pituitary axis. Just before labor, the placenta releases large quantities of CRH, and this has been described as the "placental clock," dictating the duration of gestation. It is thought that the maturing fetal adrenal glands promote placental production of CRH—again, the fetus is in control toward the end of pregnancy. CRH in turn stimulates the release of fetal ACTH (adrenocorticotropic hormone) and surfactant protein A, which help initiate labor (Vrachnis et al. 2012).

Maternal or fetal stress and systemic inflammation (for example, from T2D or COVID) are therefore implicated in premature labor. Recent research on the impact of active COVID infection on pregnant women shows that they are twice as likely to have a premature labor compared to uninfected women or those with past infection (Blitz et al. 2021).

BEYOND BIRTH

Throughout pregnancy, fetal cells cross the placenta into the maternal circulation, where they remain for the rest of the mother's life. Examples of microchimerism—the presence of genetically different cells in the body—these fetal cells are found in a range of maternal tissues/organs, including the brain (Dawe, Tan, and Xiao 2007). They act as stem cells and as part of the immune surveillance system, giving long-term benefit to the mother, protecting against disease and supporting healing (Fjeldstad, Johnsen, and Staff 2020; Vadakke-Madathil and Chaudhry 2021). The phenomenon may be the fetal attempt to protect the mother's health, improving the likelihood that the fetus and then child are well cared for. Perhaps it is an act of love, a gift from the fetus in return for the gift of life.

We are far from fully understanding the intricate dance between a mother and her developing fetus. We do know that as clinicians we can play a part in educating women about the role their health plays in the lives of their children. We can seek to influence the healthiness of the pregnancy and to detect when things might be starting to go wrong. We can support the developing fetus and help them make the best of their environment. Working via the heart and the blood vessels gives us a privileged position from which to support mother and baby at the deepest level.

8

Birth Transitions

MARY MONRO

MARY MONRO has been a practicing osteopath in Great Britain for twenty-five years and teaches post-graduate courses in osteopathy.

> *At our birth, when our umbilical cord is cut abruptly, we are deprived*
> *of our wholeness. From oneness, security and knowing, we enter into*
> *duality, fear and disorientation. This is called the navel wound.*
>
> RADHIKA RAVI RAJAN,
> "OUR NAVEL: THE ROOT OF OUR CONSCIOUSNESS"

When visiting the ancient city of Petra in Jordan, I was intrigued by a sacred carving of an omphalos (see fig. 8.1). The omphalos represents the center of the world, the

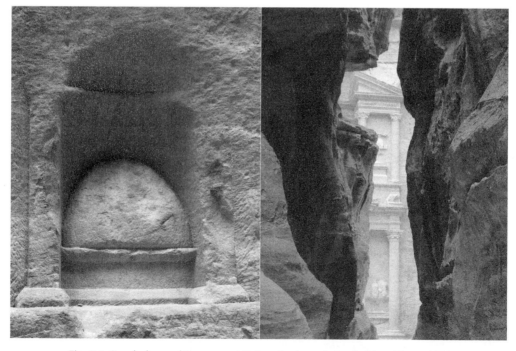

Fig. 8.1. Omphalos and Treasury at Petra, Jordan; photos by Mary Monro 2023

umbilicus, the starting point from which all things emanate, the ever-present origin. The carving is on the wall of the siq, a mile-long, narrow gorge, three hundred feet high, with fleshy sandstone cliffs shaped by water, a birth canal if ever there was one. Despite the fact that I have seen photos of the building many times, as the siq opens out to the famous Treasury, it is as shocking a sight as an infant's first sight of the outside world must be. Amazing, incomprehensible, impressive, overwhelming—no wonder newborns cry! The chief deity represented on the Treasury is Isis, the Mother Goddess. They say the Treasury is a mausoleum. I'm not so sure.

At birth, infants must adapt to an entirely different environment than the one they have grown used to. They must breathe air, make significant adjustments to their circulatory system, consume and digest nutrients, protect themself from pathogens, keep themself warm, and accelerate their neural development. When the cord is cut, they find themself separated, no longer a singular interacting being with their mother; this is the so-called "navel wound." Sometimes they have to recover from a difficult birth that may have left them with physical and emotional injuries. The following sections summarize how these physiological changes are made and what happens when things go wrong.

FETAL CIRCULATION

In utero, the fetus is dependent on their placenta to deliver oxygen and nutrients to their system. The right side of the fetal heart receives both deoxygenated blood from the superior and inferior vena cavae and oxygenated blood from the umbilical vein,

Fetal Circulation

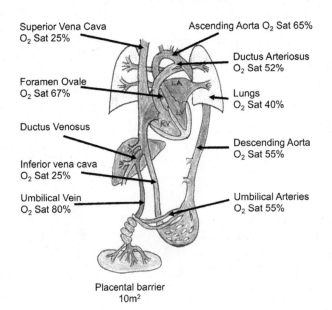

Superior Vena Cava
O_2 Sat 25%

Ascending Aorta O_2 Sat 65%

Ductus Arteriosus
O_2 Sat 52%

Foramen Ovale
O_2 Sat 67%

Lungs
O_2 Sat 40%

Ductus Venosus

Inferior vena cava
O_2 Sat 25%

Descending Aorta
O_2 Sat 55%

Umbilical Vein
O_2 Sat 80%

Umbilical Arteries
O_2 Sat 55%

Placental barrier
$10m^2$

Fig. 8.2. Fetal circulation; image by Mary Monro 2023

which connects to the inferior vena cava at the ductus venosus, bypassing the liver (see fig. 8.2). The blood streams do not mix, due to the greater velocity, viscosity, hemoglobin content, and oxygen concentration in the umbilical blood (Hernandez-Andrade et al. 2014). The oxygenated blood mostly passes from the right atrium to the left atrium via the foramen ovale and then into the systemic circulation (Murphy 2005). The supply of oxygenated blood is delivered preferentially to the vital organs—the brain and the heart (O_2 saturation 65 percent). In hypoxic conditions or acidosis the brain receives a higher proportion of the combined cardiac output (Kiserud 2005). There is very limited blood flow to the lungs, which have high vascular resistance.

PREPARING FOR TAKEOFF

While it may seem that the infant makes a sudden switch at birth and with the clamping of the umbilical cord, in fact the preparations for extrauterine life begin much earlier, at around thirty weeks of gestation. A cortisol surge begins; levels rise from 5 to 10 µg/ml at thirty weeks to 20 µg/ml at thirty-six weeks, 45 µg/ml at term, and 200 µg/ml during labor and immediately postpartum (Hillman, Kallapur, and Jobe 2012). This stimulates the maturation of the heart, lungs, liver, gut, and thyroid. The cortisol surge is accompanied by a catecholamine surge, which raises blood pressure, activates thermogenesis in the brown fat, stimulates the sympathetic nervous system, and begins the adaptation to the use of glucose and fatty acids as substrates for metabolism. There is also a renin-angiotensin system surge, which supports the increase in blood pressure by provoking systemic artery vasoconstriction.

The renin-angiotensin surge is also involved in changes in the pulmonary vasculature, which from thirty weeks shows a higher sensitivity to oxygen levels (Kiserud 2005). Pulmonary blood flow peaks at thirty weeks; the growth of the foramen ovale slows down, the ductus venosus is used less, and blood flow through the liver increases. The production of lung fluid slows down (due to the cortisol and catecholamine surges), and a large pool of surfactant is produced (Hillman, Kallapur, and Jobe 2012).

Normal function of the autonomic nervous system (ANS) is essential to help the fetus navigate the birth transition. The ANS develops asynchronously, with the sympathetic nervous system dominating in the fetal period. Premature babies are thus dependent on the sympathetic nervous system to control heart rate, blood pressure, and vasomotor tone and are less able to cope with changes in external conditions such as oxygen saturation and blood pressure. Steroids given to mothers prior to a premature delivery do help stimulate the sympathetic nervous system, but it is still relatively unresponsive compared to babies delivered at term, particularly in terms of cerebral blood flow autoregulation.

Vagal tone develops late, with a surge between twenty-five and thirty-two weeks and another at thirty-seven to thirty-eight weeks of gestation, generating an increase in heart rate variability (HRV). HRV is a key indicator of health throughout life, part of our resilience and adaptability to an ever-changing environment. Prematurity is associated with low vagal tone, poor HRV, and slowing of ANS development, resulting in poor vagal function into adulthood. This can lead to poor cardiovascular health, mood disorders, and a poor immune response. Abnormal ANS development can also occur as a response to poor maternal physical and mental health (Mulkey and Plessis 2018).

At birth the infant is 80 percent water (allowing increased diffusion rates between compartments) and much of the weight loss in the first few days is water loss. Some 44 percent of a term infant's body weight is extracellular fluid, compared to 20 percent in the adult (Sulemanji and Vakili 2013). In utero, the blood volume is about 10 to 12 percent of body weight, compared to 7 to 8 percent in the adult (Kiserud 2005), partly due to the large blood reservoir in the placenta.

UMBILICAL CORD CLAMPING (UCC)

There has been much research recently into the effects of cord clamping and its timing (which might be characterized as "immediate," "early," "delayed," or, more recently, "optimal"). Between 20 and 35 ml/kg blood is transferred from the placenta to the term infant when UCC is "delayed" by five minutes, with about 50 percent of this being transferred in the first minute (Wu, Azhibekov, and Seri 2016). Delaying UCC by even just one minute has been shown to improve short-term outcomes for premature babies (less sepsis, better blood pressure, less intraventricular hemorrhage, less necrotizing enterocolitis, higher cerebral blood flow, and higher oxygen saturation). It also seems to improve long-term neurodevelopmental outcomes, with superior fine motor and social skills seen in four-year-old children who experienced "optimal" UCC (Andersson et al. 2015; Rabe, Mercer, and Erickson-Owens 2022).

Cutting the cord represents a massive shock to the heart, which, at this stage, has limited resources for coping with sudden change. The placenta provides the left ventricle with its preload in utero, and this is abruptly reduced by 50 percent upon clamping (Wu, Azhibekov, and Seri 2016). It has to be replaced by preload from the pulmonary blood flow, which only begins with the first breath. The afterload on the heart in utero is low and, again, abruptly changes with UCC, as the systemic peripheral resistance suddenly rises with the loss of the placenta. It is much easier for the heart to maintain cardiac output if it has a larger blood volume (from placental transfusion) and the preload and afterload are kept more in balance.

CARDIOVASCULAR SYSTEM

In utero, the heart is constrained by the rather rigid lungs, pericardium, and diaphragm and can increase cardiac output only by increasing heart rate. At birth, cardiac output almost doubles and switches from parallel to series as the pulmonary blood flow opens up in response to the baby's breathing.

The sudden increase in pulmonary blood flow at the first breath increases the pressure in the left atrium, pushing closed the foramen ovale between the atria. The ductus arteriosus, between the pulmonary arteries and the aorta, closes over the first few days. In utero, the ductus arteriosus is kept open by circulating nitric oxide (NO) and prostaglandins (vasodilators) in a hypoxic environment. In the third trimester, the endothelium develops a higher sensitivity to prostaglandin antagonists and to stress and cortisol. At birth, the smooth muscle cells backing the endothelium sense the increase in oxygen level and activate the vasoconstrictive system, in the high-stress, high-cortisol, reduced-pressure environment, to close the ductus arteriosus.

The ductus venosus closes at one to three weeks postpartum, or later in premature babies or those with persistent pulmonary hypertension of the newborn (PPHN). Its closure is triggered by increasing cardiac pressures, falling pressure in the umbilical vein, and reduced endogenous prostaglandins (Poeppelman and Tobias 2018).

Fetal arterial endothelial cells show an unusual phenotype whereby they tend to be endothelin-1 (a vasoconstrictor) dominant and show limited ability to produce or respond to NO (a vasodilator) (Chang, Flavahan, and Flavahan 2016). This seems to be necessary for the development of the vasculature. It changes gradually postnatally to being more NO dominant, but the vasoconstrictive phenotype may contribute to the susceptibility of premature babies to intraventricular hemorrhage and necrotizing enterocolitis, where inappropriate vascular response to stress or injury affects the blood supply to the tissues.

CHRONIC IN UTERO HYPOXIA

Chronic fetal hypoxia can be caused by placental insufficiency, preeclampsia, inflammatory conditions, gestational diabetes mellitus, obesity, and diabetes. All of these conditions set up insulin resistance and an inflammatory response in the fetal circulation. While the fetus is well adapted for a low-oxygen environment and short periods of hypoxia during maternal contractions, in chronic hypoxia it has to redistribute blood preferentially to the vital organs—brain, heart, and adrenal glands—while the gut and lower limbs receive a limited supply, leading to intrauterine growth restriction (IUGR) and small-for-gestational-age (SGA) babies. This in turn leads to asymmetric growth of the body, delayed development of the kidneys and pancreas, and altered development of the heart. Cardiomyocytes suffer from the increased vascular resistance in the systemic circulation, which increases the afterload on the heart and leads to remodeling of the myocardium and great vessels. This may have long-term effects on the person, increasing the risk of cardiovascular, metabolic, and renal disease (Giussani 2016).

KIDNEYS

The placenta does the work of the kidneys in utero, managing fetal fluid-electrolyte homeostasis, acid-base balance, and excretion (Sulemanji and Vakili 2013). Nephrogenesis is complete by thirty-five weeks of gestation, but the glomerular filtration rate (GFR) is low and vascular resistance is high, with these switching at birth with increased blood pressure. GFR increases rapidly in the first two weeks of life but does not reach adult levels until the child is two years old. The renal blood flow expands through the vasodilatory effects of circulating prostaglandins and endothelially derived NO. Premature babies lose more water and sodium in the first days of life than term infants and may need sodium supplementation.

LUNGS

The low-blood-flow, low-oxygen environment of the fetal lungs suppresses the release of and response to vasodilators in the vascular endothelium, though hypoxia in a baby or adult would normally trigger a vasodilatory response. The junctions between endothelial cells are also permeable due to high levels of endothelin-1 (a vasoconstrictor), making for an ineffective barrier (Haworth 2006). Normally the level of endothelin-1 drops dramatically in the first week of life. The high level of oxygen and increased blood flow (and hence sheer stress) to the lungs that are initiated with the first breath stimulate the release of NO and prostaglandins, leading to vasodilation and tighter junctions between the endothelial cells. Breathing also stretches the alveoli and (along with the catecholamine surge) stimulates the production of surfactant in the type II pneumocytes (Hillman, Kallapur, and Jobe 2012).

Breathing itself is stimulated by internal mechanisms, such as the homeostatic oxygen sensing system, comprising O_2 sensors in the carotid bodies and smooth muscle cells in the ductus arteriosus, pulmonary arteries, and fetoplacental arteries (Dunham-Snary et al. 2016), and the hormonal and mechanical triggers that clear the lungs of fluid, and also by external stimuli, such as cold.

Clearance of the lungs is as simple as ABCD (Hooper, Polglase, and Roehr 2015):

A: absorption of fluid into the lymphatics, stimulated by the catecholamine and cortisol surges
B: Blow-drying the lungs, with the inspired air pushing fluid out of the alveoli
C: Clearance into the capillaries and into the wider circulation
D: Direct action of squeeze from the diaphragm and from the mother's contractions causing fluid to exit via the trachea

GUT AND IMMUNE SYSTEM

The gut is both the means by which the infant absorbs nutrients and the principal interface between newly introduced bacteria, including healthy commensals and pathogens, and the infant. In utero, the fetus receives nutrients in the form of glucose via the placenta. As term approaches, glucose is stored as glycogen and fat in anticipation of birth. When the maternal glucose supply is cut off, the cortisol and catecholamine surges regulate plasma glucose and free fatty acids, rather than the usual adult regulators, insulin and glycogen. Premature babies lack both the glycogen stores and the hormonal surges to cope with the loss of maternal glucose and often need glucose infusions (Hillman, Kallapur, and Jobe 2012). The fetal splanchnic circulation is vasoconstricted but develops a greater capacity for vasodilation toward term. Intestinal oxygen uptake and blood flow increase massively at birth to cope with rapid growth of the mucosa and the oxidative demands of digestion (Nair et al. 2015).

There is much debate as to the initiation of the infant microbiome. It has long been argued that the uterus is a sterile environment and that the microbiome is "seeded" by vaginal delivery. More recent research has found some evidence that microbes cross the placenta and that the infant is born with a microbiome. Premature babies have a smaller, less diverse, and less healthy composition to their microbiome compared to term infants. The microbiome is an essential stimulant to the maturation of the gut, the priming of the immune system, and healthy neurodevelopment. As Lee Hill and coauthors say, "Preventing early life dysbiosis may impact future rates of obesity, atopic disease, and neuropsychiatric illness" (Hill et al. 2021). It seems that the principal source of the infant's immunoglobulins (Ig) is the colostrum (first milk), and the microbiome comes from breastfeeding, so maternal health is critical to the development of the infant's microbiome and passive immunity. Mothers with obesity, for instance, suffer dysbiosis (an unhealthy microbiome) and pass this on to their offspring, with long-term effects on their health (Chu et al. 2016).

Breast milk has a dazzling array of characteristics that support the infant's health

(Newburg and Walker 2007; Castanys-Muñoz, Martin, and Vazquez 2016):

- High levels of IgA fight pathogens and inflammation.
- Infant gastric lipases convert milk triglycerides to free fatty acids and mono-glycerides, which are toxic to bacteria.
- The diverse range of human milk oligosaccharides act as prebiotics, contribute to immune function, and support healthy brain development.
- Breast milk accelerates gut barrier maturation.
- Milk proteins (lactoferrin, lysozyme, haptocorrin) are important to immune function, nutrient absorption, and inflammatory response.
- Hormones in milk are immune-protective and anti-inflammatory.
- High levels of leukocytes contribute to the inflammatory response.
- Glycans stimulate the growth of the microbiome and bind to pathogens to neutralize them by preventing them from binding to receptors in the intestinal mucosa.

Formula-fed babies are three to ten times more likely to suffer short-term problems, such as diarrhea. They may also suffer longer-term problems such as inflammatory bowel disorders, allergy, obesity, autoimmune disease, developmental delay, and cancers (Le Huërou-Luron, Blat, and Boudry 2010). In recent years formula milk manufacturers have improved the composition of their products, but it remains difficult to replicate all of the qualities of breast milk with bovine-milk-based formulas.

BRAIN

The brain is treated as a special organ in utero, preferentially receiving the most oxygenated blood via the foramen ovale and the left ventricle. The fetal brain is particularly sensitive to CO_2 levels, and in hypoxic circumstances fetal cerebral blood flow (CBF) can increase from 16 percent of cardiac output to 31 percent (Kiserud 2005). The endothelially derived vascular endothelial growth factor (VEGF) shapes the development of the correct neuronal cyto-architecture as well as blood vessel growth and stability. The endothelium is also responsible for developing the blood-brain barrier and the glucose delivery system (Tata, Ruhrberg, and Fantin 2015). Postnatally, cerebral blood vessel density and volume double from neonate to adult (Brew, Walker, and Wong 2014).

At birth, there is a dramatic drop in CBF accompanied by a sudden rise in O_2 and cerebral oxygen extraction (COE). The pulmonary blood flow preloading, as the lungs start to open with the first breath, is essential for restoring cerebral blood flow. CBF then gradually rises over the first few days of life. For preterm infants, this sudden drop in CBF at birth is difficult to restore, with immature lungs unable to contribute the necessary preload (Polglase et al. 2014). Cerebral vessel autoregulatory capacity develops from superficial to deep, so that the highest risk of injury in premature infants is deep brain (intra/periventricular) hemorrhage, particularly if there is an inflammatory environment (Brew, Walker, and Wong 2014).

NEWBORN FAILURES OF ADAPTATION

The complex physiological changes required for extra-uterine life are not always successfully achieved. Difficulties are often related to prematurity, but the labor and delivery experienced by a term or post-mature infant, or other factors, can also lead to failures of adaptation.

Patent Ductus Arteriosus (PDA)

If the ductus arteriosus fails to close within a few days of birth, it can have a serious impact on the systemic circulation. In the fetus, the ductus arteriosus allows blood from the right ventricle to bypass the lungs and head directly into the aorta. If it fails to close after birth, blood flows back from the aorta into the pulmonary arteries and then delivers excessive blood supply to the lungs, sometimes causing hemorrhage. The increased return from the lungs to the left ventricle can be damaging, but, most importantly, the blood and oxygen delivery to the rest of the body is impaired, with reduced blood flow to the vital organs and systemic hypotension. The drug commonly administered to treat PDA, indomethacin, impairs renal perfusion by acting as a prostaglandin inhibitor (Tóth-Heyn, Drukker, and Guignard 2000).

Persistent Pulmonary Hypertension of the Newborn (PPHN)

PPHN is usually caused by hypoxia and high levels of endothelin-1, accompanied by a low level of NO and poor vascular response to it. Hypoxia can be due to meconium aspiration, poor lung fluid clearance, respiratory distress syndrome, prematurity, or pneumonia. A PDA can also lead to PPHN, as explained above (Lakshminrusimha and Keszler 2015). It is usually treated with NO.

Respiratory Distress Syndrome (RDS)

Multiple pregnancy, prematurity, maternal diabetes, and C-section delivery can lead to damage/immaturity of type II pneumocytes (which then fail to produce surfactant), endothelial damage, and thus RDS, in which the lack of surfactant prevents expansion of the lungs, allows the alveoli to fill with fluid, and thus causes hypoxemia. Approximately 80 percent of neonates born at twenty-six to twenty-eight weeks of gestation develop RDS, whereas less than 50 percent of premature neonates born at thirty to thirty-one weeks of gestation develop the condition. RDS is usually treated with surfactant supplementation and continuous positive airway pressure (CPAP) ventilation. Mechanical ventilation can cause injury, and it is best minimized or avoided using early administration of replacement surfactant therapy, caffeine, and, if necessary, postnatal steroids (Sweet et al. 2019).

Necrotizing Enterocolitis (NEC)

Most commonly seen in premature babies born at thirty-two to thirty-three weeks, coinciding with the highest vasoconstrictor reactivity in the mesenteric arteries (Nair et al. 2015), NEC is related to ischemia, poorly regulated immune response, and excessive inflammatory response in the immature gut. Breast milk is the best treatment, repairing the gut mucosa and providing anti-inflammatory and immune support. Supplementation with l-arginine promotes the production of NO and vasodilation.

Intra/Periventricular Hemorrhage (IVH)

Cerebral blood flow is key to brain health but is not usually measured; instead, systemic blood pressure and oxygen saturation are monitored. CBF is driven by CO_2 levels and moderated by the vascular endothelium, and low CBF is the principal risk factor for IVH and white matter injury. In the presence of chronic hypoxia and inflammation, the brain's capacity for autoregulation is compromised, so a premature baby (with immature autoregulatory capacity) born to an obese or diabetic mother is at relatively high risk of brain injury. This is a public health policy matter requiring review and management of the obesogenic environment (Kaczynski et al. 2020). Neonates who develop IVH in the first week of life show much lower brain oxygenation in the first fifteen minutes after birth than neonates who had no hemorrhage, showing poor responsiveness to changes in systemic oxygenation in the cerebral vascular endothelium (Pichler, Schmölzer, and Urlesberger 2017). For more details on neonatal brain injury and its treatment, see chapter 7.

Head Trauma

The cranial bones are able to mold, bend, and overlap in order to allow the fetus passage through the birth canal. An induced labor that has increased forcefulness of uterine contractions may cause compression of the cranial vault on the base. Prolonged labor, use of forceps or ventouse, the presence of fibroids or a twin, abnormal presentations (face, brow, or asynclitic), and short, sudden deliveries can all leave the cranial and face bones and their protective membranes deformed and shocked (Sergueef 2007). This in turn can lead to irritable, fractious babies, sometimes with feeding difficulties. Neonates have almost no arachnoid villi or granulations and rely on lymphatic drainage of the cerebrospinal fluid (CSF), particularly through the cribriform plate (Papaiconomou et al. 2002; Sakka, Coll, and Chazal 2011; Radoš et al. 2021). Any compression through the anterior part of the head risks disturbance of this delicate mechanism. The change in pressure on delivery, the surge in CSF volume and movement resulting from the restored cerebral blood flow after the first breath (Polglase et al. 2014), and the action of suckling all help restore normal shape and function (Genna and Vallone 2016). Osteopaths with specialist training in child health are well placed to assess and treat babies suffering birth trauma (Frymann 1998; Capobianco 2011; Moeckel and Mitha 2008).

IMPLICATIONS FOR PRACTITIONERS

When asked to assess and treat a newborn infant, we must take into consideration all of the factors that may have affected the mother and the child from the beginning of their story to the present day. The transitional perinatal period is particularly important to understanding maternal and infant health. Be sensitive to the fact that the history may include experiences that were traumatic for mother or child. This is an opportunity for the mother to tell her story, often for the first time, and for the child to have an acknowledgment of their experience. Allow that story to unfold gently.

The following list of questions may be helpful; note that it assumes the child is not under medical care.

- Was the conception natural or assisted?
- How was the pregnancy in terms of maternal mental and physical health? Were there any concerns about the health of the fetus?
- Were there any previous pregnancies? How did they compare and how did they end?
- Did the previous experience of pregnancy or birth affect this pregnancy and delivery?
- How long was the gestation? How long was the baby engaged in the pelvis before delivery?
- Did the mother experience labor or was there an elective cesarean section?
- Did labor begin spontaneously or were any means of induction used?
- Was the latent stage (from the first signs of labor to 3 cm dilation of the cervix) long?
- How long was the first stage (from 3 cm dilation of the cervix to full dilation)? Did the mother receive any drugs to strengthen the contractions or give pain relief?
- How did the baby present—occiput anterior, posterior, face, breech?

- How long was the second stage (delivery)? Were any instruments used to assist delivery? Did the labor end in an emergency cesarean section?
- Did the baby have the cord wrapped around them? An arm up by the head?
- When was the umbilical cord cut?
- How was the first breath? How did the baby look at birth? What were the APGAR scores?
- Did the placenta deliver naturally or with assistance? Did it appear healthy?
- If the baby was born by cesarean section, who looked after the baby while the mother was in recovery?
- When did the baby first feed?
- How long were mother and child kept in the hospital? Were any medical interventions needed?
- Have there been any feeding difficulties? If so, is the difficulty experienced with both breasts or more on one side than the other?
- Does the mother feel adequately supported with feeding?
- Is there any difference in the baby's feeding ability on bottle versus breast?
- Does the baby have any digestive difficulties (trapped wind, vomiting, diarrhea, or constipation)? Is the baby's skin clear?
- How well does the baby sleep? How well does the baby sleep during the day versus the night?
- Does the baby seem unsettled or fractious? Has the baby had any fevers? Any visits to a doctor or the hospital?

We must take care, as practitioners, not to overload infants' busy, fragile, and immature systems. Supporting their health by acknowledging their experience, taking obstacles away, educating their parents, and balancing their autonomic nervous systems may be as much as we need to do. Feeding mechanics and digestive comfort are also important to enable the baby to settle and we have a key role to play here, alongside lactation specialists. It is joyful to witness the entire household relax as the baby transforms from fractiousness to contentment (Carreiro 2003; Moeckel and Mitha 2008; Sergueef 2007; Frymann 1998).

We are a continuum. Just as we reach back to our ancestors for our fundamental values, so we, as guardians of that legacy, must reach ahead to the children—our children and their children. . . . And we do so with a sense of sacredness in that reaching.

PAUL TSONGAS,
ANNOUNCING HIS CAMPAIGN FOR PRESIDENCY,
LOWELL, MASSACHUSETTS, 1991

9

Empty Arms

K. Michelle Doyle

K. Michelle Doyle is both a certified nurse midwife and a certified biodynamic craniosacral therapist. Weaving these two professions together provides Michelle with unending joy.

When first meeting folks and telling them what I do for a living, I invariably hear, "Oh, you are a midwife? That must be the most wonderful job!" It is true, midwifery is a wonderful and wonder-filled profession. But what people rarely consider is how this job is when things are not wonderful. To be a midwife, the name of which translates to "being with woman," means that I enter into intimacy with people in all phases of their reproductive lives. And of course, this includes loss.

The sacred privilege and pain of "being with woman," of midwifing folks through their pregnancy and parenting journey, is especially poignant when there is loss. *Perinatal loss* is a term generally used to cover miscarriage and stillbirth. From my perspective, perinatal loss also includes the desired conceptions that never happened, whether because of medical conditions such as infertility, or social constraints like being single or queer, or just waiting for the right moment that never came. The loss of a beloved child-to-be is an especially intimate journey, a journey that midwives around the world travel every day of every year.

In writing this chapter, I will share my memories of journeying with two clients through perinatal loss. I will also share some suggestions for action that I have found helpful when navigating pregnancy loss. While the events I am about to share really happened, the names of all involved have been changed and the recollections are simply my own. These stories include discussion of fetal anomalies, infant death, and stillbirth. Please take good care of yourself while reading.

In this chapter, I have focused on the parents, especially the mother or birthing person, but many people are affected by perinatal loss: grandparents, aunts, uncles, siblings, nurses, midwives . . . The impact of a perinatal loss ripples outward through friends, family, and even the next generation. Undoubtedly you have been affected by such a loss. Please forgive me for not including your named status in this essay. Please know that I do see you and know you are affected too.

Sunny was pregnant with her first and very much wanted child. Sunny and her husband attended every prenatal appointment together, holding hands, getting teary when hearing the baby's heartbeat for the first time, reveling in all the changes to Sunny's body and their developing babe. They were together for the midpregnancy ultrasound appointment, when they saw their active baby dancing on the screen. They were together minutes later when the room got heavy and quiet: Both the technician and the physician doing the ultrasound realized that this beloved baby had multiple anomalies. For Sunny and her husband, the world stopped even as their baby danced in black and white images.

That ultrasound begat a series of testing—blood tests for possible infection exposure and possible genetic issues, more ultrasounds, a fetal MRI, appointments with specialists out of state (all of New York, where the couple lived, did not have specialists experienced enough to care for this particular pregnancy). That ultrasound and the further testing brought up so many questions that could not be answered. Would this fetus, this little dancing baby, survive until labor began? Would he (a boy!) be able to survive outside Sunny's womb? If he did, would Ezra (he has a name!) live long enough to go home to his beautiful nursery with sunflowers painted on the wall?

At thirty weeks of pregnancy, ten weeks before the due date, Sunny's labor began fast and furious in the middle of the night. Ezra was coming and he was coming soon. The immediate decision for Sunny to make was this: Did she want heroic measures or comfort care? We needed this young woman to decide (while breathing through her contractions): Were we going to do everything medically possible for her baby, or were we going to allow Ezra to be born as peacefully as possible and then held in his mother's arms?

It may seem like doing "everything medically possible" and holding and comforting your newborn could happen simultaneously, but this is rarely the case. From all the prenatal testing, we had learned a lot about Ezra's little body. It appeared very unlikely that he would be able to live for long outside his mother's womb. And now he was arriving ten weeks prematurely, a challenge for any baby. Decisions about heroic care and comfort care included things like staying at the current hospital or traveling by ambulance to the tertiary care center, proceeding with vaginal delivery or doing an emergency cesarean section, planning for Sunny to hold Ezra when he was born or immediately cutting the cord and handing him off to the neonatal care team.

After the first half an hour at the hospital, while options were being discussed and explained, and while she was writhing with contractions, Sunny sat up straight, the room became quiet, and clear as a bell she said, "For my mental health, I need to stay here." At that moment, everyone's attention shifted. Here was a young woman about to meet her baby, on her terms. Sunny then asked for an epidural, stating that she needed to be able to focus on decisions to be made, not on her contractions. Most importantly, she wanted to focus on Ezra.

Acknowledging that I could not give her what she wanted (a planned home birth of a healthy, full-term baby with a long future in front of him), I asked Sunny what she wanted from this birth. Again, her words struck the air like a chime: "I want to hold him." And again, the entire room, all six of us, knew what needed to happen.

Early in the morning, in a peaceful, quiet, and dimly lit room, Ezra slid out of his mother's body, and I lifted him up into her arms. He took one gentle breath as his heart slowed, slowed more, and then simply stopped. (Please, dear reader, take a long, sweet breath on your own.)

Ezra was born into my loving hands and immediately passed into his mother's outstretched arms, where he took his first and only breath. He was then held almost continuously in her arms for the next twenty-four hours. Briefly, he was passed to his father, grandmothers, grandfathers, neonatologist, nurse, and even midwife. Ezra's body was snuggled, treasured, and adored. He was held with love for months after his conception, for moments after his birth, and for a full day after his death.

The perinatal loss journey can begin in many ways. With Ezra, the journey began with the dire findings on the twenty-week ultrasound, deepened with more test results, and then culminated with his birthday being his day of death. Some perinatal loss journeys begin with no warning—a full-term, normal and healthy pregnancy, spontaneous labor, and then somehow no fetal heartbeat heard, the baby gone before birth, before it is even born. Some perinatal loss journeys begin without beginning—no conception, no positive pregnancy test to surprise a partner, no birthday at all.

However the journey begins, a perinatal loss journey always ends with empty arms, arms that ache to hold a beloved child.

Ezra's mother, Sunny, got to hold her child for a day. She felt his weight in her arms and on her chest. Those moments and the memories of them are precious to her. She wrote, "I hardly put him down. It was soothing for my soul." Also, "I held [Ezra] for twenty-four hours straight after he was born. His body and his weight were the only things that calmed me down. It soothed my mama hormones to have him in my arms. I knew his body was just a shell of who he is, but the WEIGHT of him, I craved it, I still crave it."

Sunny has gone on to have another child, a healthy, strong, and feisty baby girl. While Ezra is never far from her mind or heart, her life is full, it is complete. Of course, for some who make the perinatal loss journey, the destination is not one of wholeness. For Sunny, many things supported her healing, a few of which

I will list here. She was treated with dignity and respect while in labor, birthing, and immediately postpartum. Her decisions for her care and the care of her infant were given full authority. Sunny is a woman of faith, and her belief in God, Jesus Christ, and Holy Scripture helped her navigate the stormy days after Ezra's birth and allowed her to treasure the peaceful ones. Having her husband home on paternity leave (yes, his job allowed this even for a demise) was hugely helpful. Having people, family, friends, her midwife, with whom she could share her journey made the loss bearable. In the first week after her baby's birth and his death, she was given a precious gift: a stuffed toy fox that weighed exactly what Ezra had weighed, three pounds and ten ounces.

Death means separation from the embodied being. In perinatal loss, time with the embodied being is either nonexistent (in case of infertility, for example) or fleeting (as in Ezra's story). A friend of mine, Revered Michael Gorchev, says, "Bodies are how we know each other." Without a body to hold, how do you know your beloved child? While terribly simplistic, a touchstone, a necklace, a lock of hair, or a hand-sewn, weighted stuffed fox can help with grieving and remembering.

Sunny's stuffed fox, weighing exactly what her son had weighed, was a small gift of enormous healing power. It meant that Sunny could actually feel his weight in her arms, arms that at least momentarily were not empty. The fox came to her by way of the Jasper Fox Project, a nonprofit organization with the stated goal "to lead parents into the knowledge and salvation of Jesus Christ by placing a Jasper Fox in their arms and walking alongside them through tragic loss." Sunny's fox arrived in a box, lovingly wrapped, and accompanied by a Christian prayer. Holding this cloth fox allowed Sunny and her husband to physically remember their son in a comforting and healing way for days and weeks and months after his death. Now this sweet fox can be hugged by their second child, Ezra's little sister, Molly.

An evangelical Christian nonprofit focused on healing after perinatal loss was a perfect match for Sunny and her husband. It is not a perfect match for all families.

Several months after Ezra was born, I worked with a Jewish woman whose first child, Lenny, was stillborn after a full-term, medically uneventful pregnancy. Like Ezra, this baby was very loved and anticipated; he had a virtual village of friends and family awaiting his arrival. When Lenny arrived earthside stillborn, without warning, his parents were left with aching hearts and empty arms. No air ever entered his lungs. He never felt his mother's kisses on his cheek. She never felt his warm breath on her breast. But she did feel his perfect weight, seven pounds and three-quarter ounce, on her chest and in her arms.

Having seen, with Sunny, what healing could come from a weighted item, I decided to create a simple cloth pillow for Lenny's bereaved mama. I measured the cloth to the same length as baby Lenny, the width to the same as his head circumference, then added an extra 1/2 inch for the seam allowances. This created a simple rectangle. I placed this empty shape on a scale and added enough rice to weigh exactly seven pounds and three-quarter ounce. A few stitches to close the top and the Lenny Pillow was created. I brought this pillow with me to a postpartum home visit and offered it to Lenny's mom. No gift box. No lovely wrapping. No card engraved with scripture or prayers. Just a simple offering of a simple pillow of the perfect weight to remember a perfect and beloved being. Lenny's mama accepted my offering with open arms. That pillow rarely left her side in the early days of loss and then, months later, traveled across the country with her when work obligations resumed. Healing tools can arrive in beautiful gift boxes. They can also arrive in an economy-sized bag of rice.

Being a midwife is hard work; the hours and the physical, intellectual, and emotional demands are relentless. Yet, at its core, being a midwife, "being with woman," is simply about being a compassionate human. Standing next to women and families as they journey through the underworld of perinatal loss is some of the most important work that midwives do.

HEALING TOOLS FOR PERINATAL LOSS

Below are some thoughts on healing tools for perinatal loss that can be utilized by friends, family members, medical providers, and craniosacral therapists. It is my hope that you will find suggestions here that allow you to truly be "with woman," to midwife yourself and your client-friend. It is my hope that you have both the support and the courage needed to stand in compassion even when facing loss.

Attunement
What helps me to stand in the face of unbearable loss, to be truly "with woman" when she has to look straight into the eye of hell? The simple truth is simple: I do the exact same things I do every craniosacral session, which is to attune to myself, my environment, my client, and PR. Through the repeated process of attunement, my attention, the environment, and the folks in it quiet, soften, deepen, and somehow time slows so the most precious moments can become eternities.

Find the Health
Andrew Taylor Still, the father of osteopathy, is credited with saying, "Find the Health. Anyone can find the disease." This charge to find the health has become my sovereign principle. Ezra's little body had so many things that could be labeled as anomalies, yet he had the most perfect fuzzy shoulders and the most precious lips. His day of birth was his day of death, and it was also the day his mother found her

voice. It is the day she and her husband became parents. Health. Find the Health in every client, every environment, and every situation—and work to find the Health in yourself.

Compassion

Merriam-Webster's dictionary defines compassion as the "sympathetic consciousness of others' distress together with a desire to alleviate it," whereas empathy is "being aware of and sharing another person's feelings, experiences, and emotions." Most simply, empathy is feeling what the other feels, and compassion is loving awareness of the other's feeling. I work to stay in compassion and not empathy, especially when supporting folks through loss. I do not find it helpful to feel another's feeling; feeling my own is quite enough. Also, bereaved parents say time and again that no one can know how they feel. Let's not take that from them.

Use Your Voice

Your voice can be a healing tool. Simply saying that you do not know what to say can have a huge impact. Giving voice to your feelings of impotency can actually help. Saying "I have no idea how to help but I want you to know that I am here" can be helpful for a bereaved person to hear. If you know the child's name, say it. Hearing the name of a beloved child may be hard, but parents tell me that never hearing the name is harder. Give a call in a couple days, a week, a month, a year just to say you are thinking of them and remembering their beloved child. Do not worry that you are going to "remind them" of the death—these parents never forget that their baby died.

Make Offerings

An offering is . . . an offering. It is something that you simply offer to another with no expectation that it will be accepted. For families that have experienced perinatal loss, the offer may be as simple as a sympathy card or as involved as a photo album. If you are so moved, make an offering; it might be declined, or it might be perfect. You never know what may be important for these folks on their path to healing.

Here are some suggestions:

- **Time.** Just having someone to spend time with while in the thicket of grief can be helpful. You can offer to hang out, no agenda, just being present.
- **A card.** Yes, a physical card with a real stamp and a bit of ink for your signature. When a baby dies, when a pregnancy is lost, there are precious few things to hold.
- **Mementos.** Most hospitals now have bereavement procedures, which may include mementos like photos, footprints, the child's measurements, and

perhaps a lock of hair or a baby blanket. Volunteers sometimes make baby hats, gowns, or blankets in various sizes appropriate for the gestational age. Occasionally hospitals have a small stuffed animal for parents to take home. One hospital that I am aware of has soft animal forms that can be filled with uncooked rice to match the weight of the infant. Any or all of these things should be presented as offerings, explaining to the family that they are available now or can be held in case they are desired in the future. Of course, the baby's body should not ever be touched or photographed without parental permission.

- **Cleaning services.** If a family has left home suddenly, whether in labor or not, having the place tidied before they return may be appreciated. The usual tidying like dishes, trash, and laundry can be very helpful. Stocking the fridge with a few healthy and easy snacks could also help. Packing up baby's nursery? Maybe. Or maybe not. Newly bereaved parents often have strong feelings about this, so please ask gently first and do not assume that they want everything "out of sight."

- **A call.** Give a call in a couple days, a week, a month, a year. These people will never forget their baby died, and having someone else remember, too, can be healing. Keep your words simple and your ego out of it. ("Hi. I was just thinking of you and Baby Ezra and thought I'd say hello.")

- **A meaningful charm or small stone.** I know a mother who wears a necklace with footprints engraved on a silver heart. It serves as a tangible reminder of the child she never got to take home. There have been times when asked by strangers if she had any children that she answers with the full story. There are also times when she says a simple "no" while rubbing her silver heart.

- **Something to hold in their empty arms.** As discussed above, weighted items may be especially helpful. This can be as elaborate as an item from the Jasper Fox Project or as simple as a beanbag. Even a weighted blanket might be soothing to the grieving folks.

- **Remembrance.** Simply remembering the lost one by saying their name (if there is a name) or sharing any memory can be an offering of compassion. The word *remember* means exactly that: to re-member, to bring back into ourselves. When we say the name or share a brief memory, the little one can be held again for a brief moment.

PART 2

MINDFULNESS AND AWARENESS, EMPATHY AND COMPASSION

10
Beginnings of Healing PTSD
Diné Medicine

I smell your blood
I taste your bullets
I hear your smoke
I see your screams
I touch your mind
All of it
Every moment
Every cell
The hatred of intolerance,
Jihad, fatwah
The folly of aerial bombing
Civilian shields and
Mosques for munitions
Corporate-paid politicians
Moral majority middle America
Hate-spewing social media
Oozes through an open wound
As shrapnel in my psyche
A soldier's stigmata
PTSD

MICHAEL SHEA

On August 19, 2019, the Veteran's Administration (VA) assigned to me a service-related post-traumatic stress disorder (PTSD) disability rating of 100 percent as follows:

We have assigned a 100% evaluation for your post-traumatic stress disorder to include: major depressive disorder, recurrent, severe, with psychotic features, mild alcohol and cannabis use disorder, cocaine use disorder, moderate opioid use disorder (claimed as PTSD to include depression, anxiety attacks, panic attacks, inability to perform activities of daily living, memory loss, mood swings, and disorders of social activities and work) based on:

- Unprovoked irritability with periods of violence
- Suspiciousness
- Depressed mood
- Disturbances of motivation and mood
- Impaired judgment
- Persistent delusions
- Impaired impulse control
- Chronic sleep impairment
- Panic attacks more than once a week
- Obsessional rituals which interfere with routine activities
- Persistent hallucinations
- Difficulty in adapting to stressful circumstances
- Difficulty in adapting to work
- Difficulty in adapting to a work-like setting
- Anxiety
- Occupational and social impairment with occasional decrease in work efficiency and intermittent periods of inability to perform occupational tasks (although generally functioning satisfactorily, with routine behavior, self-care, and conversation normal)
- Difficulty in establishing and maintaining effective work and social relationships

The overall evidentiary record shows that the severity of your disability most closely reapproximates the criteria for a 100% disability evaluation. This is the highest scheduled evaluation allowed under the law for post-traumatic stress disorder.

It would be ten years after discharge in 1973 before I would recognize that I might have a problem as my experience of PTSD continued to incubate, adapt, and manifest in new ways, like a stealthy virus changing to resist a cure. And it would be much longer before PTSD among veterans was recognized by Congress in the 1990s. That was also when I encountered Native American healing and uncovered the depth of my symptoms. I did receive a master's degree in contemplative psychotherapy at Naropa University in 1986, though in the three years I spent there the words *trauma* and *PTSD* were never mentioned.

BEGINNINGS

I met Thunderhorse while I was taking out the garbage one night. He was a Native American roadman who traveled the country offering healings with a medicine wheel. His ancestors were African American slaves and Indigenous Comanche. He was performing his healings in a small apartment next to where I lived. I requested a healing ceremony from him while at the garbage can. I was impressed enough after our first session to ask him the next day to teach me his medicine. I spent a year with him for a brief apprenticeship, which is all he would do with me. I learned all the basics on the proper use of different ritual items such as the drum, the rattle, the feathers, the staff, the eagle bone whistle, the bear skin and buffalo robe, and the medicine wheel in the Comanche warrior tradition. I also learned about Coyote and the Trickster medicine from him. All important lessons. These symbols of healing are external agents to invoke the spirit of the natural world and entrain the patient to an alternative reality consisting of the elements and nature. I learned that these external symbols of healing are powerful and can be internalized by the therapist through the power of perception and visualization. I now use both the external and internal symbols of healing.

This was in the mid-1990s. Thunderhorse said I needed more training. He escorted me and my wife, Cathy, to the Diné reservation in Arizona. The Diné, formerly known as the Navajo, lived in relative squalor. I was shocked at their circumstances: no running water, many homes with only dirt floors, and rampant suicide and alcohol addiction, though there was electricity. The reservation was like a third-world country, and yet the Diné were sublime in their spiritual practice—when not addicted to Westernization. Their origin story tells of the first Diné arising from the earth, and I was about to learn a healing methodology deeply connected to the divine spirit of the earth.*

I was introduced to a shaman by the name of John Nelson and his wife, Ruby (figs. 10.1 and 10.2), along with their whole extended clan. We stayed in their home (fig. 10.3). John told us about his forced education in Christian schools, where students were beaten daily for speaking their own language, which was forbidden. He told us how one of his children had committed suicide in their horse corral, and about many more indignities. John met his wife Ruby when they were both forced to attend the mandated Christian schools for Native American children. John recounted to us the daily physical beatings he received for speaking his language.

With this introduction, my wife Cathy and I began a ten-year apprenticeship with John and his family. In order to receive this learning, we were formally adopted

---

*See chapters 35–36 on the Navajo creation and emergence myth in Shea, M. 2008. *Biodynamic Craniosacral Therapy*, Volume 2. Berkeley: North Atlantic Books.

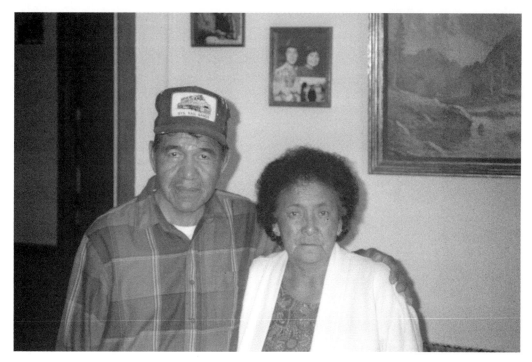

Fig. 10.1. John and Ruby Nelson, our spiritual parents

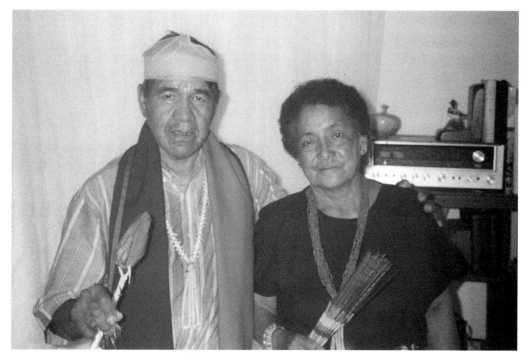

Fig. 10.2. John dressed for ceremony, with Ruby

by John and Ruby as members of their family. Cathy and I referred to them as our parents, and they were our spiritual parents. We were given names. Figure 10.4 shows our baptism and gifting of an eagle feather.

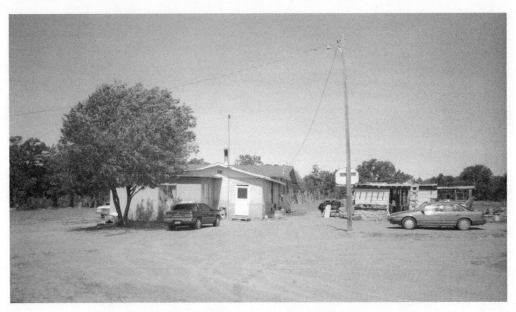

Fig. 10.3. John and Ruby's home on the Diné reservation

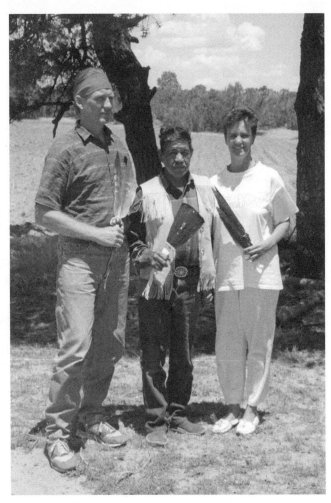

Fig. 10.4. Michael and Cathy being adopted into Diné
family culture of healing

My name is Haskie-yeh-chi'-diiyah, "man going toward something mean and scary without fear." Cathy's name is Yeh'-kas-bah, "woman hunts evil things without fear."

Since the Nelsons' home had no running water, it was quite a chore to prepare meals and clean up. But big meals following ceremony were important. We took it all on. The ceremonies were performed in a traditional hogan, an eight-sided structure (fig. 10.5). The first hogan is said to have been built by the Holy People at creation. The roundness of the hogan is symbolic of the sun, and its door faces east so that the first thing a Diné family sees in the morning is the rising sun, Father Sun, perhaps the most revered of the Diné deities.

When my wife and I began our long apprenticeship with John and his family, we underwent numerous healing ceremonies to learn the structure, prayers, and methods of Diné healing medicine. The first healing ceremony performed on me revealed that I had a significant case of military trauma, now called PTSD. The Diné were very familiar with this condition. Many members of their tribe had served in the military during World War II, Korea, and Vietnam and came home with PTSD. (The Diné were the "code talkers" in World War II. They were the ones who ran the radio communications between the ground base and the flight crews that dropped the atomic bombs on Japan to end the war. The Japanese were not able to break the code of

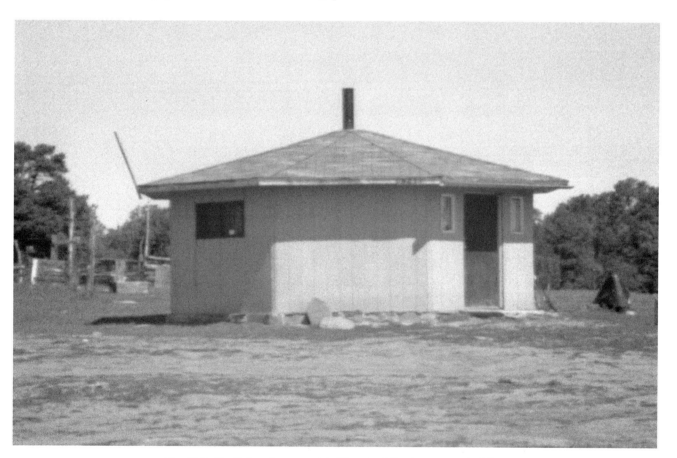

Fig. 10.5. The Nelson hogan, a traditional spiritual ceremony building

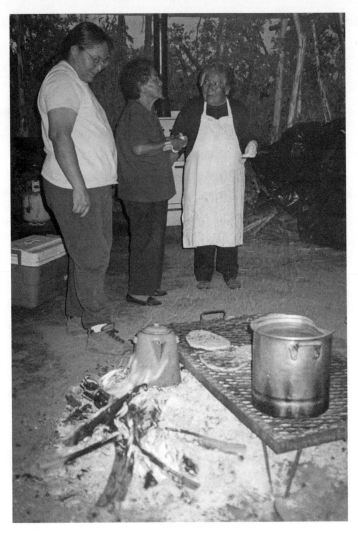

Fig. 10.6. Ruby, Isabel, and a neighbor prepare food to sustain the dancers and leaders of the Squaw Dance ceremony

the Diné language.) The Diné medicine people had designed a new ceremony, called the Squaw Dance,* to perform with the soldiers who were manifesting symptoms of PTSD. And as was the case for all Diné ceremonies, a lot of food was necessary (fig. 10.6). Ultimately, this was the ceremony recommended for me to heal from my military experience.

The Squaw Dance is part of a larger complex ceremony called the Enemy Way. It is a traditional ceremony for countering the harmful effects of ghosts and was chosen by the elders for returning Diné military personnel who suffered the symptoms of PTSD. The Enemy Way ceremony involves song, sandpainting, dance, and

---

*On the reservation the term *Squaw Dance* is not a pejorative or derogatory term. Rather, it derives from the original meaning of "woman" in the Diné language and that of other tribes. The Diné are a matrilineal culture, and all healing comes from the feminine—hence the power of the "woman" in the Squaw Dance.

the powerful mythical figure known as the Monster Slayer. The ceremony lasts for nine days and includes the enactment of a battle. Associated with the Enemy Way is a girl's dance (Squaw Dance), to which young men are invited by marriageable young women. This derives from an aspect of the Monster Slayer myth in which two captive girls are liberated. Thus, the healing is associated with releasing the suppressed feminine. This is a remarkable process to relate with all the unresolved grief for soldiers returning from a killing field.

For the ceremony, the community comes together with several medicine people. It's a multiday, continuous ritual with a lot of singing, chanting, and prayers, which are a main focus of the Diné medicine system. It is a magnificent blessing and a massive community undertaking to observe. The patients, as many as five to ten, are placed in small pens and fed. This time of isolation is important for the healing. They are taken periodically to the center of the field where the ceremony takes place by being sung to and danced to. Their origin story is sung to them to return them to the way the world was at the beginning when the Holy People created humans in wholeness.

The Diné at the height of their culture had the most sophisticated healing ceremonies of all Native American cultures. Part of our apprenticeship was learning a portion of the Blessing Way ritual. In Diné medicine, the Blessing Way is the master ritual from which almost all of the other original 350 diagnostic and healing ceremonies are derived. We learned two parts of the Blessing Way. One was a simplified ceremony in which the patient would lie down over a handwoven rug that Ruby made for Cathy and me. No matter what the patient's condition, there was a sequence of prayers, feathering, and so forth to help remove the affliction from the patient.

The second part was shamanic hand trembling diagnosis. This was John's specialty. The ritual was used both as a diagnostic tool and to elaborate the prescription for the necessary medicine to complete the healing. The ceremony would begin at four or five o'clock in the morning with a huge fire, letting it burn down to hot coals to be used in the hogan. A circular disk of smooth sand was made next to a smoke offering pit (figs. 10.7–10). Smoke offerings were made with ground cedar, and medicine was placed around the floor adjacent to where the patient would lie. John would go through a sequence of prayers and chanting using corn pollen to trace lines of spirit power in the palm of one of his hands. He would then slip into a trance and his hand would dance over the patient, who would be lying to the side of the fire pit. Periodically his hand would pause and draw something on the smooth circle of sand, so that by the end of the ritual a diagnostic sandpainting was created. John would interpret the painting as it was given to him by spirit when he came out of trance.

The key to the ceremony of hand trembling is in the prayer cycle. Since I did not know the language, John had to request permission from the tribal council of the Diné to translate the prayer cycle into English and give me those prayers. The tribal

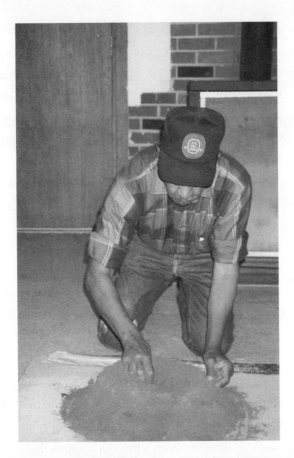

Fig. 10.7. John Nelson preparing the earthen mound for use in the hand trembling ritual in the hogan

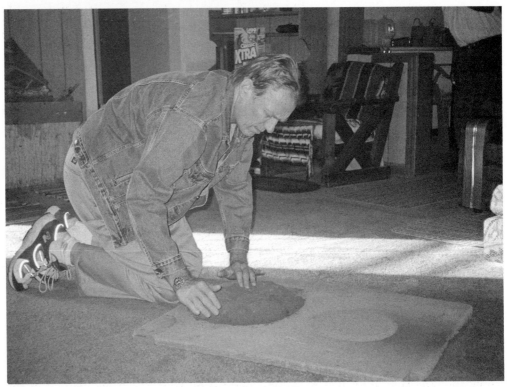

Fig. 10.8. I am learning to prepare the earthen mound for the sandpainting as part of my initiation into being a "hand trembler" in the Diné tradition.

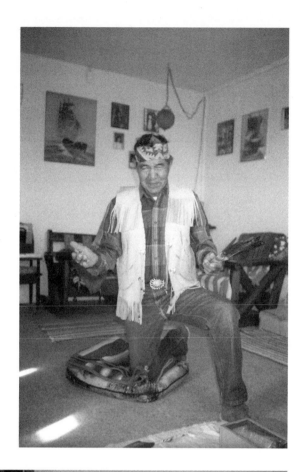

Fig. 10.9. John is now ready to offer prayers and smoke to begin the hand trembling diagnostic and prescription ceremony.

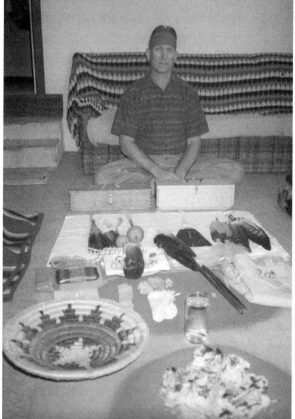

Fig. 10.10. I take my place in the first hand trembling ceremony in which I am the patient.

council voted to give John permission to teach me the English version of the prayers to perform the hand trembling—though not without a lot of dissension among the elders.

THE DIAGNOSIS

In one of the hand trembling rituals in which I was a patient, John drew a large machine gun on the sand disk. Spirit said there was a large gun stuck in my heart and blocking my heart's spiritual energy. I immediately recognized my love of the M60 machine gun (fig. 10.11). When I was in the Army, I loved going to the firing range for marksmanship certification and practicing with all the different weapons I was required to know and teach others to use and to kill with. I especially loved the M60 machine gun. I would get at the end of the firing line so the range officers would allow me to shoot up all the remaining ammunition "John Wayne" style, with the machine gun resting on my hip and firing thousands of rounds of ammunition at targets. It was a huge thrill. The potency of the intoxication with that particular weapon had created a blockage in my heart, which then became linked to the PTSD symptoms.

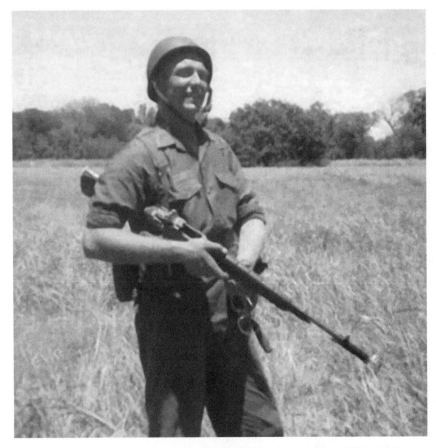

Fig. 10.11. My Army rifle, lodged in my heart while training at Fort Sill in Oklahoma

I grew up with guns and know how to use them. The ceremony revealed to me over time that I was harboring an entire arsenal of guns in my heart. The M60 was just the biggest. In the late 1960s, my father had given me a double-barreled .12-gauge shotgun for bird hunting and a .22-caliber rifle for squirrel hunting, and I trundled them off to college with me, stashing them in my dormitory closet. I had enrolled at Loyola University in New Orleans, and in the craziness that was the 1960s, there was compulsory attendance for all male students to attend not just weekly classes but also weekly military-style parades, with all of us student cadets marching in formation, in uniform, rifles in hand, to the park across from campus. This was the Reserve Officer Training Corps (ROTC) of the Army. The ROTC had their armory in the basement of our dormitory. During my junior year the Army decided to sell off all of its World War II rifles to the ROTC cadets for $20 each. I don't know how many I bought and gifted to friends, but I can say that the men's dormitory was packed and loaded for war.

Of course, that wasn't the end of my long-term love affair with guns. After college, I did seven years of military service in several forms. The weapons training I received was superb. In ROTC we had to take apart and reassemble our rifles every week and memorize the names of the parts of the gun. In the Army, we did the same, but more so. I was first trained as an infantry officer, capable of leading a small group of soldiers to kill other people or in some cases to protect people from being killed by others. I test-fired so many types of guns and weapons of destruction that they are too numerous to name here. I embodied the gun. Part of the embodiment, unfortunately, was in my heart and cardiovascular system.

BEGINNING TO HEAL

PTSD is a multifaceted, developmental, and progressive disorder. Guns and the prevalence of gun violence in America have always been a major trigger for PTSD for veterans, and now for many civilians too. As for myself, I learned that they needed to be removed from my home and my heart. It was a gradual process.

Over the years in which we knew John and Ruby, before they died, we brought numerous people to the reservation for healing ceremony. John was always accurate in his diagnosis, or more accurately, what spirit was revealing to him. The space he offered became a sanctuary of healing and learning, teaching us how to invoke spirit and bless with spirit all who come our way. It is truly the work of the heart to allow spirit a dwelling place in the heart.

I was never able to complete John's prescription for receiving a Squaw Dance for many different reasons. But in 2011 I received the Kalachakra empowerment from His Holiness the Dalai Lama in Washington, D.C., and with that ceremony, the

M60 machine gun was finally removed from my heart. The Kalachakra is one of the more complex cosmologies and explanations of how the universe functions in all of Tibetan Buddhism. As a part of the cosmology, sequential methods are taught to achieve a union of nonduality and relationship with the universe both inside our body and outside. In this way, the sense of separation of me and the world I live in can dissolve into an open awareness that is filled with joy and happiness permeated by a nonthinking mind. And such capacity must be developed with contemplative practices such as meditation described throughout this book.

The arsenal of guns had been blocking the underlying flow of emotions and feelings through my heart and cardiovascular system. With its removal, I could turn my attention to the deeper and more pervasive symptomology of PTSD. I could more deeply explore my anger and rage and learn humility, which has been one of the greatest blessings I've been given as a student of His Holiness. Every session of body work I explore with a client is informed by the prayers of the Diné hand trembling I learned. My hand now trembles as I work on clients, and spirit constantly moves in and through my heart. Everything I teach in the field of the manual therapeutic arts is informed by the potency of invoking the Holy Spirit to fill my heart and hands to infuse the students and their clients with the sacred.

We learned to chant the following prayer to heal PTSD with the help of our spiritual parents, John and Ruby Nelson, on the Diné reservation:

Beauty Way Chant

House made of dawn.
House made of evening light.
House made of the dark cloud.
House made of male rain.
House made of dark mist.
House made of female rain.
House made of pollen.
House made of grasshoppers.

Dark cloud is at the door.
The trail out of it is dark cloud.
The zigzag lightning stands high upon it.
An offering I make.
Restore my feet for me.
Restore my legs for me.
Restore my body for me.

Restore my mind for me.
Restore my voice for me.
This very day take out your spell for me.

Happily I recover.
Happily my interior becomes cool.
Happily I go forth.
My interior feeling cool, may I walk.
No longer sore, may I walk.
Impervious to pain, may I walk.
With lively feeling, may I walk.
As it used to be long ago, may I walk.

Happily may I walk.
Happily, with abundant dark clouds, may I walk.
Happily, with abundant showers, may I walk.
Happily, with abundant plants, may I walk.
Happily, on a trail of pollen, may I walk.
Happily may I walk.
Being as it used to be long ago, may I walk.

May it be beautiful to me.
May it be beautiful behind me.
May it be beautiful below me.
May it be beautiful above me.
May it be beautiful all around me.
In beauty it is finished.
In beauty it is finished.

11

Self-Awareness as a Path to Compassion

To be completely present and open to things as they are, unfabricated reality, this one most precious thing . . . our very life is completely absorbed by the immensity of the immediate. . . . This present moment . . . is a small door that opens onto all of life as it is, an intimate portal that includes the infinite.

JOAN HALIFAX,
BEING MET BY THE REALITY CALLED MU

To care for self and other is a natural biological instinct. It is the basis of compassion. The impulse to care exists on a spectrum from our most basic instinct for self-healing when we are sick all the way to a heartfelt desire to see the world completely free of pain and suffering and the instinct for self-transcendence. Thus, to care is linked to moral development and the altruistic intention for the relief of all pain and suffering. The desire to be free of pain and suffering is the desire to heal, which means to become whole, which means to be connected inside and out with the cosmos. This innate desire for the experience of such freedom includes the necessity to know both at an embodied level and at a wisdom (mind and cognition) level what the causes of pain and suffering are. Mind and body must function together as one unit of function to be free. It is an inside job. It is all about our inner perception.

I was asked recently to be interviewed about alternative approaches to treating cancer. It is only in the past several years that I have begun to counsel cancer patients. I thought about it and concluded that there is only ever really one thing I would say. Every time I talk to a patient who is given the diagnosis of cancer, the fear and terror of death is palpable in their demeanor. My answer is always this: Take your attention and turn it inward, toward spirit located in the body. I am advocating in this book for contemplative practices. When receiving a shock from the diagnosis of a potentially terminal condition, if a person does not know how to turn inward and stabilize by using resiliency skills learned from contemplative practices, it will be a very long and painful road, especially if the patient relies only on traditional forms of cancer treatment such as chemotherapy and so forth. That said, everyone has their own style of suffering, and everyone's decision must be supported. I teach at a European cancer clinic that employs alternative methods such as colon hydrotherapy and hands-on osteopathic treatments. The medical doctors all say that cancer is a disorder of the intestines, and thus to care is to care about real food as a foundation of spiritual health. For me, the inner state of mind, body, and spirit is the next most important after eating real food. Thus, the critical importance of contemplative practices. The healing work we do with biodynamic cardiovascular therapy is a contemplative practice.

Last year my wife was very sick with an intestinal disorder and so we walked to the beach because she wanted to relate to nature. She was unable to determine what remedy to take or use at home. I suggested that while we were at the beach, she lie down on the hot sand and let the animal inside her body tell her what she needed in order to return to normal. After lying on the sand for an hour, she stood up and we went home. She directed herself immediately to the natural remedy of a warm water enema. Within several hours she was free of her physical pain. Our body is capable of informing us how to heal as long as we know how to engage the instinct for self-healing. Sometimes it is sand and water. Sometimes it is prayer and meditation. But our instinct for self-healing may frequently get drowned out in a great sea of advice from others.

At our core, in our organism, we are an animal. The wild animal in us knows how to heal our body, and its raw energy must be tempered with the wisdom of mental peacefulness. The body and mind must work together in order to heal those challenges that derive from an emotional imbalance or strong mental states that cloud judgment. The clarity necessary to navigate contemporary life is easily distorted. Such tempering involves effort and discipline that is not heavy-handed but rather filled with kindness and humility. To care thus includes a whole spectrum of contemplative practices in human development. To care is the basis for all sensation, feelings, and emotions. Even hatred and rage at their core are expressions of caring; hatred, for example, is the caring desire to eradicate evil and all too often is the expression of underlying fear and terror of change.

Humility as a function of caring is birthed from an inner awareness that we can perceive the world only through our own eyes, experiences, and insights. Humility exists on a spectrum from, on one end, being confident to, on the other end, being introspective and contemplative. It involves the constant interchange between inside interoceptive work and outside social interpersonal work. We see in the world that many people hold within them many perspectives encased in a cocoon. And yet these cocoons are transparent and must become porous for humility to birth compassion. Humility requires the inside work of questioning our thoughts and the basic views and assumptions we have of others. It's important to recognize that, being human, we are all lifelong learners. We do not ever have all the knowledge we could possibly need to manage the present moment, let alone our future. Consequently, everyone makes mistakes, and some mistakes are more humbling than others. Which is the point—mistakes are the foundation of humility, not reinforcements for low self-esteem. The task of building a skill set of contemplative practices never ends. We have people close to us who can tell us the truth of how they see us. We can investigate such feedback with humility. Ultimately humility involves wisdom. As Claude Larre and Elisabeth Rochat de la Vallée note in their treatise on the position of the heart in the *Huangdi Neijing Lingshu,* the two-thousand-year-old Chinese classic text of acupuncture, "When the heart is able to take in all that is presented in openness, knowledge is able to become wisdom, the kind of wisdom that is nothing other than to know how to nourish life" (Larre and de la Vallée 2012, 109).

The inability to care generates pain and suffering and is a blockage in the mind-body flow. When the normal flow between body and mind, heaven and Earth, spirit and matter stagnates, it causes a blockage mentally and metabolically, and as my wife frequently proclaims, stagnation requires detoxification and cleansing. We are being polluted constantly in our culture and must develop a cleansing lifestyle. There is an inability to self-regulate and thus transform sensations, feelings, emotions, and cognitive states in the present moment with awareness. Such an inability causes a loss of discernment of knowing what to accept and what to reject in the multitude of daily sensations, thoughts, and choices. By knowing the significance of personal experience through mindfulness and awareness, we can self-regulate with loving kindness and care for our body as a sacred temple.

At a deeper level, this stagnant condition may also be indicative of some form of self-loathing, inner guilt, or a feeling of being a deep mistake of some kind because so many of our daily thoughts are negative. Loss of flexibility in allowing change, of being resilient in the moment, is a degenerative disorder. Thus, a loss of care is also a loss of trust in the most basic human nature of being inherently whole and complete. Interconnected wholeness of outside and inside is the original state.

Contemplative practices, especially mindfulness, compassion, and analytical meditations, are available in abundance in contemporary society. In general, according to research, they do help develop a degree of stability in our personal dance with the inner critic or the inner flaw or the persistent body sensation that nags at one, insisting on anesthetizing it. At the very least our neurosis becomes a little more domesticated and contained. It is repackaged, so to speak, with a prettier bow until we are brave enough to untie the bow and welcome our inner demons. We must make them our friends. Remember that mindfulness meditation in its traditional form arose out of a culture that trusted the basic sanity and healthy nature of the mind-body. Eastern cultures never split mind from body from spirit. In such cultures the mind-body-spirit complex is a unit of wholeness based on the felt sense and perception of the five elements.

Trying to become embodied of spirit and free of mental and emotional conflicts with contemplative practices might only encapsulate the inner flaw and keep it at bay without transforming it. This is called a spiritual bypass. An integrated spirituality includes befriending our innermost demons. We must *be with* the process of self-ownership rather than just talk about it. The core of all human beings that lives in the heart inside the heart is basically and inherently complete, whole, and trustworthy. It is our Buddha nature or Christ consciousness. The core is the spirit of the sacred surrounded by our animal heart that pumps blood. It might help to view our mistakes and challenges—which are natural in life—with humor, which is a demonstration of humility. We can see them as something like the blooper reel of deleted scenes shown at the end of a movie. We seem to be regularly breaking character, in a manner of speaking, and then have to reshoot the scene. Each of us has so many bloopers to look at with humility. This is the humility of awe—when we realize the magnitude of life and recognize that a prime survival tool is humor.

Consequently, to wake up (dare I say, to have faith in) the biological instinct to care means to explore and accept the inner reality of our body-mind-spirit already inherently complete and not flawed in the slightest. That is our spiritual essence and birthright that lives in the heart and moves through our blood under the direction of the sacred heart inside the heart, as it is called in Taoism. We are already complete. The challenges, mistakes, and disorders that we all experience as part of life, with its never-ending mental and emotional hallucinations and other exotic fantasies, are actually the bonus tracks or the director's cut that includes all the deleted scenes in the movie of our life. Everyone has these experiences. No one is exempt. There is no growth without resistance. Our biological origins are defined by resistance to growth, as any embryologist can tell you. Our spiritual maturation includes resistance. And it is usually resistance to change. Consequently, the polarity of hope and fear, problems and their antidotes, is actually held in a preexisting matrix of interconnected completeness and flawlessness.

Though an entire psychological and self-help industry has been created to resolve our flaws or character problems with thousands of antidotes and practices, the rub, so to speak, is that even the flaws in and of themselves must be seen as an expression of wholeness and completeness. In other words, the totality of the human being and all its parts are considered to be equal since its foundation is whole and complete. You cannot fix your brokenness; you can only recognize your preexisting completeness. In other words, focus on what is buried, uncover it, and let it shine through the challenges. Once one part of the body-mind is split off and unintegrated from the whole, our mental-emotional-sensory navigational system is compromised by con-ceptual hallucinations and fantasies that block our knowing of what to accept and what to reject. The flight simulator of our brain cannot possibly integrate all sensory information. The brain makes a best-case simulation of the world, and without a contemplative practice commitment, we crash-land and look for the "black box" of instructions for healing for the rest of our life. That search becomes more and more work, with more and more antidotes (some helpful, some not) applied, from Coca-Cola to OxyContin, physical abuse to emotional abuse, mindfulness meditation to gratitude training.

Nowadays, many mental health and biomedical health conditions are said to be on a spectrum of more to less severity. Thus, the mind-body-spirit is a spectrum of possibilities. Everyone has their own style of suffering and their own style of enlight-enment. But what if it is all just a case of lost heart syndrome? We can return to the metaphor of the Confucian philosopher Mencius, first mentioned in the preface: When our chickens or dogs are lost, we have the good sense to go look for them. When our heart—our understanding of our inherent wholeness—is lost, we do not. Why do we not care enough for our heart to look for its wholeness?

Wisdom is the perception and discernment of our no-flaw essence, and it is the ground of the biological instinct to care. There is a state of mind inwardly that can hold the wholeness of the polarity of growth and resistance and the no-flaw essence together as one thing. This is traditionally called the union of wisdom and compas-sion, but really it is the union of body and mind with the spirit living in the heart. Once the spiritual essence of no flaw is understood as an embodied reality of spiri-tual formation, it can be cultivated and allowed to grow and flourish as the weeds are cleared away. Nurturing wisdom in ourselves enhances the possibility of a great compassion that encompasses all living beings and the wisdom of discrimination to know how to respond with that possibility. This is called unconditional health, from a spiritually embodied point of view. Unconditional health is a synonym for embod-ied wholeness and compassion. It is perceived by the potency of PR increasing at the end of a biodynamic session. This is the human spectrum of wisdom and humility. It is a felt sense. It is consciously discernable. It is innate and instinctual.

The cultivation of caring and the exploration of a constantly evolving embod-ied spirituality is a story, an origin mythology. Classically, an origin story looks at history and the conception of the universe or the human as the starting point of wholeness. However, given the demands of contemporary society and the necessity of healing, we need a different starting point. The starting point is right now. It is the story of nowness, of the present moment as experience continues to unfold seemingly without end.

Many contemporary therapies are designed to evoke and then integrate one's historical narrative, which usually involves one's stress and trauma and the stagnation, as mentioned. This exploration of stagnation goes back many generations. But thanks to molecular biology and epigenetics, an exact starting point for one's historical narrative is actually impossible. The story of stress and trauma is not the authentic story of our being anyway. It is a political-religious overlay justifying wars, slavery, genocide, and all forms of abuse. The trauma narrative needs to be modified and the identification with it suspended. How?

When the story of stress and trauma is being told, it is being held (listened to) by a compassionate therapist in the present moment with care in their heart. Care of the heart begins with conscious interoceptive awareness of the movement and potency of the heartbeat. Care of the heart and listening to the heartbeat is empathy. The present moment, the immediate nowness of the interaction within my embodied spirituality relating to another human being, is the actual living container of a heart-to-heart connection. The present moment is always and immediately inherently complete and whole as a nonreferential awareness. It is the element of space, the perception of dynamic stillness. It is an experience fully integrated with the human body that is breathing and pumping blood in this precise moment of time. Such awareness expresses itself as kindness. *Kindness is caring expressing itself as empathy.* It is an activity born of the present moment and directed toward one's self and another person. Caring expressed as kindness of thought, speech, and touch is the activity of compassion. Compassion, caring, and kindness generate humility and a host of other qualities that support the perception of our heart inside our heart.

Wholeness is described by different metaphors, especially in the biodynamic craniosacral therapy community. Present from the very beginning of our human life and the cosmos, it is currently holding the storyline of stress and trauma better than can be imagined by any comic book superhero. But the accessibility and subsequent exploration of the story of embodied spirituality is made available with the skill of a biodynamic therapist by *listening into the wisdom* of the client with their heart in the present moment.

Listening into the wisdom of the client is a contemplative a practice in which the therapist is oriented to the shape and movement of their own respiratory diaphragm, heart, and cardiovascular system as a whole. Gentle eye contact is made to establish safety. Language is used to establish a reflective, gentle, and genuine connection. This affirms one's own and the other's inherent humanity and spiritual formation. The practitioner attunes to their own body and mind, which stabilizes the therapeutic encounter. The mind of the practitioner reduces its wandering and rests in the movement and activity of their heart.

A biodynamic cardiovascular therapy session begins with the story of nowness. Now is quite simple. The therapist notices any wandering thoughts and returns attention to the shape, power, and potency of their own respiratory diaphragm and heartbeat. The movement of the heartbeat/diaphragm is a rhythmic guide for the therapeutic relationship and itself a contemplative practice to build tranquility and express care. It becomes the metronome of the session and a connection to caring that is metabolized by the client. At some moment the therapist will synchronize with the slow tempo of PR, usually by taking a deep breath.

Biodynamic perception is attuned to slowness and stillness. Thus, the starting point of a biodynamic session is not only a sense of nonreferential awareness (stillness) but also a sense of embodied spirituality (slowness). The starting point is resting in inherent completeness of the heartbeat and breath, slowness, and stillness of the cosmos in which the narrative of stress and trauma is held in a much larger dimension. Now the union of embodied spirituality and compassion can dissipate the past into the simple nowness of open space.

Nowness is the whole of space, the totality of mind, body, and spirit in this very nonconceptual moment. And a daily contemplative practice opens the door to the power of nowness. It is the power of awareness. In this way, the instinct to care wakes up gradually in both the therapist and the client through interpersonal resonance. The end of the session no longer has the goal of establishing embodied wholeness and spirituality, because that is the way a biodynamic session starts. The end of the session is known by clock time and an increase (or not) in the potency of PR. The middle of the session is a perceptual roller coaster of discerning the therapeutic activity of slowness and stillness. The end can go beyond the end of the session. We are giving our clients the gift of our attention. Attention based in the present moment. And the present moment is curative of many ailments. Even physical death is best supported by mindfulness as the basis of caring. By cultivating the ability to stay in the present moment, we are always practicing for our death biodynamically, where slowness and stillness are magnified.

Only one story really gets told in the therapeutic session. It is the story of the therapist. When a client comes in, the client then becomes part of the ongoing narrative in the therapist's body and mind. That is why my friend Sarajo Berman calls biodynamic work "joint practice." At a phenomenological level as a therapist, I can experience only myself, my own body, and my own mind when it is located in my heart. The impressions that my senses give me regarding my client, even in biodynamic practice, are still filtered through a million years of sensory development, cognitive discrimination, and memory within my own body and mind as a therapist. The story of now is the story of embodied spirituality and the story of caring at the most essential level for self and other. This is the story of loving kindness and compassion. It is humbling to sense it as an embodied reality of spirit living in the heart of all beings.

Create Your Own Origin Story

In order to contemplate caring and empathy more fully, I designed a questionnaire to help people develop their own historical narrative and their own origin mythology. Knowing one's own origin is a form of medicine and allows the felt sense of completeness and greater access to nowness.

1. Where did I come from?
This contemplation would include preconception and conception as a transitional state up through the birth process and the first year after birth. Perhaps we are made of stardust and this cosmic perspective can be included.

2. What is an operational definition of Primary Respiration as I perceive it?
Here, we refer to Primary Respiration in its form as the Breath of Life, the so-called animating feature of being human (arriving at conception according to the Bible). Is it neutral or simply an urge to become? Does it have gender? Does it lay down a blueprint for life in the embryo or contain an intention to incarnate as if coming from a divine source into flesh and blood? Consider these two aspects: It is defined by a subtle movement or wind, and its chief sensory property is that it passes through everything.

The human body is also transparent and interconnected to every aspect of the natural world. It can be known at three levels: the intuitive, the instinctual, and the cognitive. To understand Primary Respiration as the Breath of Life is to understand the mystery of a single-celled human being as a whole and becoming a multi-trillion-celled whole. The natural world breathes with the Primary Respiration. The Breath of Life is a light that shines on all appearance before our eyes. Primary Respiration gives form the ability to move. Our search is for its fulcrum, a point of origin if it exists or not. We search for a mystery of beginnings and endings, which means we are on the scent of the sacred. What, where, and how is the source of embodied spirituality? Is it inside or outside the body and heart, or both?

3. Can we accept life as a mystery?
Included in this would be a discussion of the center of the body or what is called the axis mundi in depth psychology. The axis mundi is the center of the universe. It involves the creation energy of sacred space. The axis mundi allows movement from ordinary reality to sacred reality. When you create sacred space, you are sensing your heartbeat and breath and seeing visions guided by Primary Respiration, the Breath of Life and the stillness. It is a big story/space with plot(s), character(s), and setting(s). The notion of the groundswell of Primary Respiration is that, locally, in the human body, it reflexively moves in the water element of the blood from top to bottom and then from bottom

to top of the vascular tree as it fulfills cardiovascular form and function. (This may or may not be important in your own narrative and is an example of a splendid metaphor for creation, but not the only one.) The reflexive movement of Primary Respiration from bottom to top and back again creates the axis mundi for the human body to form around the Breath of Life. This is the creative moment in the Western psyche. Primary Respiration is the quickening of matter through spirit. Other such symbols for the axis mundi are the Tree of Life, the crucifix on which Christ died, and the human heart.

In another powerful metaphor, the shamanic universe consists of three worlds: the upper, the middle, and the lower. The lower world is the world of nature. It is the unconscious. It contains power animals and totems (other power figures). The middle world is the world of humans on the planet Earth. The upper world is the world of the wisdom teachers and spiritual masters. It is the world of death. These three levels stand as a consistent metaphor for the three germ layers of the embryo. What are the relationships of these cosmic stories? What other cultures have similar mythologies? How does Primary Respiration as the Breath of Life bring order to the embryo? What force can be felt or sensed in your own body that is related to the origin of form and function?

It is important to connect with our origins via story and our felt sense of Primary Respiration and to see visions of the Breath of Life. It is a function of normal human growth and development, and all mythologies help us do this. The other and perhaps more important reason creation mythologies do this is to bring meaning to the reality of pain and suffering. Old age, sickness, and death must be seen to have a purpose, as ordained by our cultural concept of the divine, or a culture could not integrate the horror that life presents. Perhaps then life is becoming a mystery as contemporary fixtures of origin are breaking down, much like the Western health care system. Can we accept life as a mystery?

4. Who's in charge?

Who or what is in charge of the world of the sacred? Who or what holds the power? How does the power manifest in the human body, especially the heart? Do the metaphors of Primary Respiration and the Breath of Life work anymore? In the language of embryology, biokinetic and biodynamic forces are in charge. This means biological acausal movement—the movement of the whole. Is it correct to say the fluids are in charge? Or the reciprocal tension between the fluids and membranes throughout the body? Or are the genes in control? Or is it God? Take your pick and choose wisely after deep contemplation.

5. Why is there evil?

There must be an explanation for the faults of the world, whether it's the devil, cancer, senseless killing by senseless people, terrorism, or genocide plaguing the planet.

The contemplation must also include biokinetic forces and environmental influences impacting the egg and sperm transgenerationally, like feast and famine episodes in our lineage. Is there a balance between good and evil, between cancer and health?

6. Who are my people?

Who do I belong with? Who is the *we* of *I*? Who are the genuine people in my tribe? What are the primary relationships of the embryo and fetus that are still accessible in this moment of my life? We know that the growing fetus has cognition via dreams, excellent hearing (especially for classical music), and motor movements while in relationship with the mother and all her relationships. Are we related to just our biological parents or Primary Respiration and the Breath of Life or both?

7. How close should I be to a human?

How close should I be to a man, a woman, or a nonbinary person? This partially depends on one's development of self-regulation and autonomy as well as our social self-regulation capacity. At the same time, mythology is what establishes right relationships between things and people. The embryo is a synthesis of the male and female, not as gender, but as essences from the Breath of Life. We are perpetual embryos at the level of biology. What is the felt sense of your embryo? Have you found your embryo of love?

8. What is the map for human life?

Where am I on the map, and what is my spiritual compass? What time is it in the care of my heart? Where am I on the fate line of my palm? What is the process of my spiritual formation? How does my embryo carry the intention of Primary Respiration and the Breath of Life, my parents, and preceding generations? How does reorientation to slowness and stillness assist the growth and development of *Homo sapiens*? What is the relationship of Primary Respiration and the Breath of Life to patterns of resistance in the body? How do Primary Respiration and the Breath of Life change at birth? How is the map of the sacred changed?

So many questions to contemplate rather than answer.

Intuition is a direct and immediate apprehension of or clarity on a complex situation or set of circumstances. It is intuition that perceives the mythic dimension. Visionary perception takes patience through contemplative practice. To be is to be perceived, to be seen and heard. We exist and give existence by virtue of perception. It is perception that bestows blessing upon the world. Perception brings into being and maintains the being of whatever is perceived. The truth of the imagination is in the invisible dimension of the human heart. Myths have a face found in the heart. It is in the invisible yet perceptual heart that we maintain a contact with the imaginal or the mythic. Perception implies a polarity between that which has manifested and that which has not yet become manifested. Primary Respiration brings the future into the present. From there, we attach values to that which is perceived. Some things are greater, and some things are lesser.

We are constantly living our myth without knowing its roots. The path begins by caring from the heart.

12

Immeasurable Compassion

May I be an isle for those who long for landfall,
And a lamp for those who long for light;
For those who need a resting place, a bed;
For all who need a servant, may I be a slave.

SHANTIDEVA,
EIGHTH-CENTURY BUDDHIST PHILOSOPHER, AS QUOTED IN
A FLASH OF LIGHTNING IN THE DARK OF LIGHT,
BY THE DALAI LAMA

From the very beginning of biodynamic cardiovascular therapy, the emphasis has been on the practice of non-fright. The reduction of fear in the therapeutic relationship is absolutely necessary for compassion to flower and become more manifest. Compassion is the way we are built biologically. And, just as there is a fear center in the brain, it is now known that there are compassion centers in the brain, heart, and gut, which are all associated with mirror neurons.

In the Buddhist tradition, compassion has three basic phases. The first phase is to see and treat all people as being equal. I am the author of a multivolume work titled simply *Biodynamic Craniosacral Therapy*, and the dedication in volume 5 reads, in part, "May all beings be parted of clinging and aversion—[of] feeling close to some and distant from others." As we go about our daily life, it is so important to notice all the tiny and not-so-tiny judgments we have regarding the people we see on the street, in the grocery store, or anywhere else for that matter, and including our family and friends.

The second phase of compassion is to see all people as capable of giving and receiving love and kindness. This means that instead of projecting our own thoughts and feelings onto other people, we begin to see everyone as equal and we start to project thoughts of love and kindness to them. Sometimes it helps during meditation to simply imagine extending love and kindness to everyone on the planet, including animals.

The third basic phase of compassion is the practice called Tonglen. I'm sure many of you are familiar with this meditation, in which you breathe in the negativity of another person and breathe out health and well-being to that person. This makes compassion a deeply personal practice.

All three phases involve the practice of non-fright. When we have less fear, we can develop more compassion. Imagine a garden that has many different types of seeds planted in it. We must stop watering the seeds of fear and start watering the seeds of compassion. Safety and trust must be the foundation of the therapeutic relationship.

In order to experience compassion more deeply, it is important to develop a deeper and more profound view of the way reality exists. The biggest obstacle to seeing the reality of our lives more clearly is mental confusion or what Buddhist teachers call mental complications and afflictions. The contemporary lifestyle, in which we have constant contact with television, news media, advertising, entertainment channels, and social media, involves an unceasing barrage of opinions, beliefs, and ideas about the way the world works. The tidal wave of data is having a clear effect on our biology and state of mind. Research in cognitive neuroscience shows that the brain and soma have no unifying place or point that organizes the sense of self or ego. Researchers say that the brain is essentially like a cocktail party, with many conversations happening at the same time, and that the brain is like a flight simulator, sorting out as best it can the overwhelming amount of sensory data coming in. Such confusion and the resulting hyperreactivity are today the principal obstacles to mental clarity. We have an addiction to being overwhelmed.

Since there is no unifying Self except in the spiritual domain, this lack of existence of a true Self should actually create happiness, tranquility, and peacefulness mentally. However, as human beings, if we are caught in a cycle of confusion, the main struggle is with compulsive behaviors that result from mental confusion. In lectures he gave at Naropa University when I was a student there, psychiatrist Ed Podvoll talked about these habituated and sometimes addictive behaviors that keep cycling through what he called "guilt, repent, rebel." This adds another element to our confusion: emotional problems, or afflictions as they are sometimes called. Emotions are the lubrication of confusion and compulsivity. Physiological reactiveness is rampant in our culture because we live in the age of overstimulation, trauma, and fear. We've suffered a great loss of resilience, meaning the ability to rapidly return to a stable mental and emotional state after a change. The path to such resilience begins in the body with interoceptive awareness. For example, as soon as one's heart rate gets too high (say, above a hundred beats per minute), it should be lowered through whatever reliable and safe behavioral means are possible. This may include medication due to the enormous prevalence of heart disease in our culture. The issue is that most people cannot sense their heartbeat without taking their pulse. The first step in the recovery of our senses is to regularly feel our heartbeat.

Buddhist scriptures point to the need to destroy our fear and anger. I've seen different Buddhist teachers use some interesting images of violence and aggression along these lines. One such teacher said, "All dharmas agree at one point—kill the neurosis." A lama once suggested that we become Buddhist bomb makers and find a way to eradicate our neurosis; indeed, sometimes Buddhist meditation is called a "spiritual atomic bomb." And yes, these are violent metaphors, but they point to the depth of the problem humans are currently in and seemingly always have been. It is not that we need to attack our confusion; instead, we need to learn to hold it and see it clearly with loving kindness. This takes commitment, effort and discipline, which are in short supply in the age of continuous partial attention. Such discipline is the discipline of a warrior of mindfulness who can recognize confusion and cut it or sever it. Contemplative practice is essential to awaken this capacity.

Whether or not one agrees with such imagery, it does point to the enormity of the problem of how to lead an altruistic life in which the welfare of others and the planet becomes as important as the individual. It is through declaring *Enough!* to our own fear and anger that we can be of help to another. There are many ways to work with one's own neurosis. There are certainly gentler ways to do so. Everyone has their own spiritual aptitude. As is said, there are a thousand faces of God. Everyone has their own style of suffering, and the first step is to embrace our totality, including our demons, through contemplative practices. We convert the demons into friends, and this requires the discipline of a warrior. I am of a warrior class because of my ancestry, which includes the Vikings, and my military training as an officer who was on a killing field and sustained a moral injury resulting in complex PTSD. When I sit and meditate, especially when I was learning to first sit and look at my mind, it took a huge amount of discipline to do so. I had to draw upon my roots and training as a warrior to do.

The principal contemplative Buddhist practice is to develop mindfulness and awareness. This is a type of clear seeing of the present moment, of entering non-referential awareness, initially experienced from a witness point of view. Witness awareness avoids attachment; the witness remains mentally calm. Such mindfulness gives us the ability to contemplate and recognize all the different states of mind and emotional ups and downs that are experienced on a moment-to-moment, day-by-day basis. Contemplative practices try to help us get a proper distance from an observer awareness relationship with our inner thoughts and feelings. At the same time, in Buddhism, a process of analytical meditation helps us use our thoughts, feelings, and emotions in a constructive way to discover their inherent emptiness or to simply solve a problem. We must find the steering wheel of our thought stream.

Compassion requires a tremendous work ethic on the part of the individual to get to know themself very thoroughly and very honestly. The first vow in Buddhism, called the refuge vow, is somewhat informal and is more like a unique marriage ceremony in which one promises to marry oneself and get to know oneself. Imagine a spiritual ceremony in which you marry yourself in order to save yourself from a compulsive inner life. Everyone visits hell with their thoughts, feelings, and emotions, and most of us do so on a daily basis. I do.

Compassion is the basis of altruism, the desire to eliminate the pain and suffering of another person and replace it with happiness. That work begins at home, because if you do not have compassion for yourself, you cannot extend compassion to another. (One teacher of mine called it a state of "idiot compassion"; it is sometimes called codependence.)

The central task of altruism is to integrate the personal work of neurosis deconstruction with compassion. In the Buddhist tradition, that work begins with the six paramitas (virtues):

1. Patience
2. Generosity
3. Discipline
4. Meditation
5. Joyful effort
6. Skillful means

They are the behavioral activity of compassion on a daily basis. All of this leads to a greater state of humility and inner peace by making sure that we are regulated by practicing self-care through mindfulness, awareness, and analytical meditation. Gradually, the state of humility and acceptance replaces the state of fear and anger. This style of happiness recognizes the beauty of constant change and the principle of nonduality in which we are all interconnected as one organism. Happiness can also be feelings of gratitude, forgiveness, empathy, and kindness. These are the thoughts to be contemplating during our day.

These teachings from the East are similar to the Seven Gifts of the Holy Spirit in Christianity:

1. Wisdom
2. Understanding
3. Discernment
4. Courage
5. Knowledge
6. Reverence
7. Wonder and awe

Sensuality

The extraordinary problem in spiritual and religious traditions is whether or not sensuality is part of the path. The ability to transform sensuality as part of the path is called Tantra in the East. Tantra derives from a very rich lineage in both the Sanskrit and Tibetan traditions. Basically, nothing is left out of the path to freedom; all aspects of our life are knitted together like a beautiful patchwork quilt.

THE FOUR IMMEASURABLES

The Four Immeasurables, shown in figure 12.1, are a traditional configuration of ancient wisdom regarding the path of mindfulness and compassion. The path can begin anywhere on the map of the heart: in loving kindness, compassion, joy, or equanimity. It is circular; each feeds the others.

Mindfulness gradually develops into a nondualistic awareness of self and other. The practitioner is simply left with the sense of a panoramic awareness or dynamic stillness permeating all perception. The perception of formless openness becomes more pervasive, and the practitioner experiences equanimity—the whole of life in its equalness. Equanimity forms a basis for loving kindness and compassion. The mind, free from fear or anxiety, begins to treat all experiences as equal based on a sense of acceptance in the knowing that life keeps changing and thus there is nothing to hold on to, especially strong emotions and the various storms generated by those emotions and strong mental states. Acceptance transforms into laughter or forgiveness or gratitude.

As figure 12.1 shows, the Four Immeasurables can be enhanced by various factors, such as practices of gratitude and forgiveness, as well as the interoception of our own heartbeat and its potency when we breath consciously (Brown and Gerbarg 2012). The perception of Primary Respiration and stillness is the very basis of all these various states and stages of becoming human and whole.

It is important to mention that resilience is a very important feature of mindfulness and compassion in general. Resilience is the capacity to prepare for, recover from, and adapt in the face of stress, adversity, or challenge in the moment. Metabolic syndromes, a central theme of this book, generate a loss of psychological and metabolic resilience and consequently the need for contemplative (and cooking) skills to recover and restore that resilience. Mindfulness practice and compassion contemplative practices need to be linked to detoxification therapies, dietary strategies, and the rehabilitation of the human body in general.

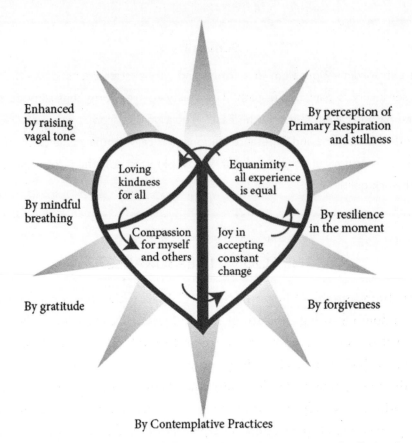

Fig. 12.1. *The Four Immeasurables. Compassion recognizes our personal suffering that we share with everyone. This awakens the instinct to care for self and others. Equanimity is the wisdom of oneness, being impartial. Joy is the wisdom that accomplishes all things. Loving kindness is the perfectly clear reflection of clear light.*

DEVELOPING COMPASSION

The instinct of compassion is the innate biological desire to care for self and others. It is developed with mindfulness, the subject of the next chapter. It consists of how we lead our lives in the world and thus is social, relational, and ethical. Compassion is ignited by mindfulness of our own inner states and the conscious welcoming of our own style of suffering and joy as one interconnected whole. When we accept our own pain and joy and relax into the tenderness of our own beating heart, compassionate action can arise spontaneously from that base of self-knowledge. Happiness or joy for self seeds happiness or joy for the other. In this way, contemplative practices prime the pump of spontaneous compassion.

The *first* step in developing compassion involves interoceptive awareness of the movement of the heart and blood inside the thorax; we call this cardioception. It is a deliberate movement of attention or focused mindfulness of the body in conjunction with awareness of the breath. We bring our conscious awareness to the movement above and below the respiratory diaphragm, down into the abdomen (Calais-Germain 2006). The heart grows and develops in connection with the respiratory diaphragm; they are linked. Research indicates that such awareness of the heart reduces anxiety, fear, and depression and increases empathy and well-being (Craig 2009, 2011; Damasio 1999). With practice, this interoception becomes spontaneous, and the heart-breath becomes home base for investigating the shared world we inhabit.

Second, based on this interoceptive awareness, we can consider being more compassionate toward ourselves. Self-compassion becomes an unbiased acceptance of the whole *me,* which is inherently complete and without flaw or mistake. This is a practice of radical forgiveness of ourselves for all perceived wrongs and mistakes, now and in the past, from little thoughts to big stories to the misuse of the body to uncontrolled emotional episodes. We forgive ourselves for others whom we may have harmed and forgive those who have harmed us.

Third, once we can grasp a picture of our self with compassion, we practice what Pema Chodron (2011) calls "compassionate abiding." This is a quality of resting in our heart with forbearance and patient endurance. Self-compassion is an innate function of being alive that needs nurturing and cultivation through mindfulness practice. It is the ground of a tender heart and the experience of "sadjoy," a type of compassionate emotion that lies just beneath the experience of the totality of our life in the present moment (Desmond 2017).

As an instinct, compassion has a reciprocal movement. The first movement of compassion is to receive. The second is to give. I breathe in the experience of myself, and I exhale well-being to myself. I practice radical self-acceptance and know that all other human beings have a similar experience in which we are all basically good at heart. Gradually, compassion practice generates an awakening in the heart of compassion for others as I become more and more self-regulated and committed to my own self-care and personal spiritual practice.

The Power of Cardioception

Attending to the space around the heart in the trunk and its movement spreading out throughout the body, we become more aware of our living, pulsating experience. This leads to the experience of the potency of the heart, the way it warms the blood and continually creates pressure waves moving throughout the body. Once we can experience the movement, space, and potency of the heart as the movement, space, and potency of the Earth and the ocean, we can learn to feel the radiance of the electromagnetic field via Primary Respiration moving from heart to heart among all mammals.

LISTENING WITH COMPASSION

From the point of view of the therapeutic relationship, we are constantly exchanging elements of our self with the client and vice versa based on the science of empathy. We are essentially a *two-person biology*. This can be brought to consciousness by simply synchronizing with Primary Respiration (PR). The practitioner synchronizes with their own heartbeat as the basis for empathy, the receptive phase of compassion. We feel in our own mind and body what the other person is feeling. When PR changes phase, the practitioner sends out a sense of health and well-being to the other person, toward their heart—the giving phase of compassion. First we receive, then we give. We fill our heart with the universe and radiate it back out through our body and that of the client. This is compassion. Imagine a single beam of sunlight radiating directly from the practitioner's heart to the heart of the client. Imagine visualizing a rainbow radiating from your heart to yourself and the universe.

Listening with compassion can be practiced almost anywhere and anytime, whether with a client, a loved one, a friend, or just someone you've bumped into, say, in an airplane or at the checkout line in the grocery store. I call it everyday compassion practice. It involves conscious movement of attention between the person speaking and yourself, the listener, while paying attention to your own heartbeat and breath. This focus and interoceptive awareness can be very different from the typical person-to-person interaction, in which the mind often wanders and we have little awareness of our own body sensations.

The power of listening with compassion is well supported by the science of interpersonal neurobiology (see Siegel 1999, 2012a, 2012b, and also chapter 14 of this book). Research into intersubjectivity has shown that discrete areas of the brain cause subtle shifts in our body as a response to another person's body movement and vocal tones. In a face-to-face interaction, such a client-therapist session, intersubjectivity means the client *gets* that the therapist, who is listening, is getting who the client is at a deep level. It then becomes reciprocal; each person feels nourished by being listened to and listening with embodied compassion. This is the essence of the neuroception of safety in Porges's polyvagal model of compassion (see page 31). This is when the felt sense of safety arises in the client and Primary Respiration shifts to healing mode in the therapeutic relationship.

Compassion involves a reciprocal movement of the mind, body, heart, and brain receiving from self and others and then giving out to self and others. As a practice, it is based on taking care of one's own needs first (Cosley et al. 2010; Halifax 2011). As a meditation, it can be used to process the difficult feelings and emotions of another person (Hofmann, Grossman, and Hinton 2011). The illness or symptomology of the other person is imagined to be flowing into the body of the listener. It is taken in and processed by the listener's mind and heart, transformed into a sense of well-being, and then projected back out onto the other person in a very slow tempo. For biodynamic practitioners, this connection is literalized as a flow of Primary Respiration moving back and forth from each other's heart.

All human beings have the instinct for compassion—caring for self and others—rooted in their biology. It is one thing that connects all human beings. Compassion is recognizing our interconnectedness.

වෙ

Listening with Wisdom

This listening practice unites the brain and heart through intersubjectivity and compassion. I teach it in the classroom and use it in my daily life. Here, we'll go through the steps as an intentional exercise, but you can practice this sort of listening in any face-to-face conversation.

We work in dyads. Each person should identify their role as the listener or the storyteller.

The storyteller will tell their story and have it listened to with compassion. In the classroom, the time allotted for storytelling is 20 to 30 minutes, and generally I ask students to tell how they got involved in cranial work and what really excites them about this work, whether in their personal life, with clients, or both.

⌣ Eye Contact ∾

The first focus for the person listening to the story is to make periodic eye contact with the storyteller. Comfortable eye-to-eye contact usually lasts for two to four seconds. I ask the listener to make sure that their gaze is soft, yet they are trying to actually look at and see the pupils of the storyteller's eyes, unobtrusively and nonthreateningly, which means with a slight smile or an inner sense of having a dignified posture.

Stylistically, I tend to look at just one eye of the person telling the story. I try to stay with that one eye during the listening, though it is okay to shift and spend time occasionally looking at the other eye of the storyteller. Trying to look at both eyes at the same time is more difficult and not necessary for this practice to ignite compassion.

Eye contact also involves facial expression. One way a person knows we are listening is by our facial expression, which can be a smile or a look of concern and so forth. I encourage the participants to be expressive with their face in a genuine and appropriate manner.

⌣ Interoception ∾

The second focus for the listener is to move some (not all) of their attention to sense the movements of their own heartbeat and respiratory diaphragm. They should feel their inhalation into the belly and their exhalation as the diaphragm lifts. It is important to sense both movements, whether separately or together as one dynamic, because research has shown that the combination of these two movements affords a greater conscious sense of our three-dimensionality and thus more of a felt sense of wholeness in our body while we are listening to another's story. It might feel like just sensing the totality of the space within which these two interconnected movements take place.

∿ Heart-to-Heart Connection ∿

Third, in the cycle of moving attention, the listener periodically shifts a little of their attention to sense Primary Respiration, breathing between their own heart and the heart of the storyteller. Primary Respiration moves with the electromagnetic field of the heart, which is quite strong and extends about fifteen feet out from and around each human heart. As you sit and listen to a story, if you drop your attention to the area of your heart-diaphragm and then extend that attention to the heart area of the storyteller, it is quite possible to sense the push and the pull of the magnetic field breathing in the tempo of Primary Respiration.

There are several locations to place your attention in the heart for the heart-to-heart connection.

- I tend to keep my attention located initially around my sternum, since the heart and diaphragm are just in back of it. Here you can experience the greatest movement of the heart and left ventricle. Posterior to that is where the heart begins to meet other structures like the pericardium and so forth.
- The second location to place attention is in back of the movement where the heart tissue ends as the myocardium meets the dorsal pericardium.
- The third location is the actual space between the myocardium and the dorsal pericardium. Here is a connective tissue bridge that stabilizes the heart in the embryo, and consequently it can be experienced as a suspended fulcrum of stillness, since the pericardium does move in relationship to the heart.
- The fourth location to place attention in the heart is the fascia that anchors the dorsal pericardium with the descending aorta and esophagus.
- The fifth location is a metabolic field between the spine and heart. The neural tube and nervous system grow rapidly in the embryo, while the heart and vascular system grow very slowly. Consequently, there is a fulcrum of stillness directly between the heart and neural tube. It is sensed as a metabolic field where the tensions of fast and slow are neutralized in the stillpoint.
- Gradually, with practice, as the story unfolds and both the storyteller and listener relax into a continuum of deepening connection, the listener might bring

their attention to a sixth location of attention in the back of the body in order to sense the heart as transparent and Primary Respiration breathing through the body, back and forth, in its phases.

Connecting heart-to-heart is only a part of the overall cycle of attention in this practice; it is only one phase of building compassion. Each phase of this practice has a benefit. If it begins to feel like you are juggling too many balls (of attention) in the air, it is sometimes enough to simply imagine or visualize the heart-to-heart connection, resting your attention in the previous phase of the practice.

↺ Reflective Listening ↻

The only other component that gets added to the practice is periodic reflective listening by the listener. This can be as simple as making vocal tones to acknowledge elements of the storyteller's narrative, or repeating words, phrases, and sentences the storyteller has said, or perhaps sharing a brief personal reflection of a similar experience. Any verbalization during the exercise, however, needs to be minimal in order for the listener to stay with the sensation in their body and Primary Respiration moving from heart to heart.

The basic cycle is eye contact, sensing heart-diaphragm movement, and finally, sensing the movement of Primary Respiration in heart-to-heart connection. It is not so much that these are separate activities but rather, after a while, they blend together into a simple but mindful way of being in relationship. It is something like learning musical scales. Gradually, with practice, such compassionate listening becomes spontaneous jazz. This is the continuum of compassion as a jazz ensemble.

I have taught the preceding practice and used it myself now for some time, and it is very exciting to note that many storytellers report after the exercise that they could actually sense the story changing as they told it because they knew they were being listened to with mindfulness and compassion. It is a very powerful way to help clients who hold stress and trauma to organically change their history. Our brains and bodies are designed to change the story of our past in order to integrate it to a more fully functional and meaningful life in the present moment. This is a form of self-healing. We are designed to interpret the past with forgiveness and clarity regarding the importance of life lessons. Sometimes we can accomplish this work by less verbal interaction and more heart sensing to ignite compassion. To wake up the heart is to sense the movement of the heart consciously. Compassion at this level is simple.

13

Mindfulness and Heartfulness

Prior to and during a session of biodynamic cardiovascular therapy, the practitioner establishes and maintains a presence based on mindfulness. From the traditional Buddhist perspective, mindfulness is attention to the present moment of experience without judgment. Many of us are held in bondage to our ordinary wandering mind and its tens of thousands of daily thoughts. This is called "attention capture." For most people, the majority of these thoughts are negative, being caught in the past or future or overwhelmed by the present moment. Mindfulness practice consists of a variety of contemplative skills that nurture freedom from this bondage. As a contemplative and spiritually based manual therapeutic art, biodynamic cardiovascular therapy (BCVT) can help people establish that inner freedom.

Contemplative meditation is a starting point for building mindfulness. For example, mindfulness can be ignited by shamatha (calm abiding) meditation, which can be used to softly attend to an experience in order to remain in the present moment of open awareness without thoughts of aggression or forcefulness. First we learn to make room for our thoughts. Breathing and heart rate are always occurring in the present moment, so they are the most typical objects of attention for shamatha meditation. Gradually, as we come to recognize that our thoughts go away by themselves, with or without noticing the process, maintaining open awareness becomes the object of concentration with mindfulness.

Mindfulness is both an act of noticing when we are being captured by our thoughts and the experience of returning to non-thought, which is awareness without an observer. The non-thought of awareness is the innate ground of our inner perception that lives in the heart, as discussed throughout this book. Mindfulness simply allows awareness to fully manifest in the foreground of our perception. This is the deepest level of the present moment and takes practice to achieve. It is associated with relaxation and freedom from attachment to thoughts, concepts, and emotions. Thoughts go on but in the background.

Contemplative practice, and especially Buddhist meditation, identifies the nature of our thoughts initially as a kind of self-psychotherapy. Shamatha meditation to build mindfulness is a great start because a meditator begins by identifying thoughts of judgment and evaluation. The noticing is powerful information about our inner world. The next step in shamatha is for the meditator to notice two kinds of mental states: speedy, meaning that thoughts are voluminous and rapid, and lethargic, meaning that the mind is lazy and sleepy and cannot easily concentrate. Advanced meditation techniques point to noticing categories of thoughts about the past, future, and present. It is our awareness that notices the activity of our mind. Gradually awareness itself becomes the object of concentration and mindfulness simply becomes watchfulness and finally awakeness—that is, the ease of resting in awareness without an observer. At this point our thoughts are not a problem because there is no mental chasing after them. This is easier said than done. It takes practice.

Altogether, settling and resting the mind in the present moment of awareness without a reference point takes practice in order to identify the four instinctual inner states that serve as foundations for mindfulness. These are the four states of mindfulness and are the essential foundations of understanding and embodying mindfulness. Each state relates to the instinct to remain in the present moment where thoughts might be happening, but they do not capture our attention. These four states are like directions on a compass that create a continuous direct knowledge of the details of interoception of embodied experience. Consider these four states described below as four aspects of our inner life that define a whole universe of space located in the present moment. The inside merges with the outside in a nondualistic state of open awareness.

BODY: THE EARTH

Embodiment is a felt sense or interoceptive awareness of the rhythmic gain and loss of a bodily experience of order and organization. Our experience of our body is like a wave that comes and goes because it includes emotions, moods, and other concepts that are constantly fluctuating throughout the day. Our outer senses seem to compete with our inner interoception. As a side effect of a neutral attention to our breath and heart rate, our mind interprets the body as having pleasure, pain, and neutral sensation. That involves a lot of thoughts. It is here where judgment and interpretation are not necessary—the beginning of mindfulness practice.

The body is the ground of perception because without a body, there is no perception, and therefore all perception comes from a place of basic goodness in the heart, before the many filters of life experience it passes through every day. The five external senses do not need a constant torrent of thoughts interpreting the data, interfering with how the brain functions instinctually. Embodiment is an inner contemplative and spiritual practice centered on the heart. When we feel order in our body, we are open to a larger or deeper whole that could be said to be spiritual. It is earthy, supportive, and clear. At the same time, without negative thoughts, the source is basically good. Even the lack of order is also part of the whole and consequently must also be from a place of goodness. It is simply a process—a wave and then more waves in our body and mind that make our day seem like a roller coaster.

Meditation and BCVT involve practicing a regular body scan from the feet to the top of the head to confirm comfort and ease or to confirm discomfort without judgment. Then the practitioner examines whether they can self-regulate their body with attention on the breath and heart rate or simple awareness. They continually relax into the present moment of experience. This can be done through interoceptive awareness of the core movements in the body, such as those involved in diaphragmatic breathing and the movement of the heartbeat and blood throughout the cardiovascular system.

We inhabit the inner world of the body and its polarity of pain and pleasure, which is constantly switching back and forth in the pendulum of embodied experience. Some days we are in touch with our body, and some days we are long gone from our body. Mindfulness as an instinctual process rides the rhythmic waves of fullness and emptying. Mindfulness is the ship's rudder. Awareness is the ship's keel. Someone must be alert when handling the ship's wheel.

LIFE: TOUCH AND GO

The next area in our inner bodily life to explore with mindfulness is the full spectrum of human feelings and emotions, both positive and negative. The practitioner notices their emotional and mental experience and lets go of the noticing. This fosters a deep insight into impermanence and the constant change process of inner life. Emotions are simply energy and information. Mindfulness allows us to see such energy and information with far more neutrality or equanimity than we usually do. Mindfulness practice involves learning to entirely disengage from, disidentify with, and become nonattached to the experience under review.

Mindfulness neither favors nor opposes inner phenomena such as strong emotions; it does not like or dislike them. All thoughts, feelings, and emotions are welcome, even if they provide discomfort. They are held as part of a larger whole. So many thoughts, feelings, and emotions are happening at once inside of us, all relating to the past or the future. The mindfulness of life touches that experience and then lets it go by returning attention to the present moment of awareness, without a reference point. It is just open space. Letting go means being in that space without further analysis or reinforcement. We are not turning our backs on our experience. We are observing our experience rather than reacting to it. We are calmly abiding. There is absolute peace in the space of the present moment.

EFFORT: INSTINCTUAL RETURN TO BREATHING AND HEART AWARENESS

The ordinary mind consists of thoughts, ideas, concepts, and world views. Typically the initial techniques of mindfulness meditation are designed to reduce the number of thoughts by recognizing them as distracting, entertaining, or compulsive and then returning one's attention to the present moment of breathing, heart rate, and awareness as a priority for developing a calm and peaceful mind. We learn to directly experience the present moment in our body as we attend internally to our breathing and heart rate. Gradually, we learn to turn our external attention to a panoramic awareness of the space or environment around us. Eventually, in therapeutic practice, the present moment of embodied experience and awareness of space merge as a dynamic stillness or void state in which concepts of self and other, of dualistic thinking, are suspended, at least temporarily. In BCVT, the practitioner goes further by applying mindfulness to synchronize with the slower healing tides of Primary Respiration.

With practice, we gradually discover in meditation that the ordinary mind instinctually returns to the present moment by itself. Regular contemplative practice awakens that instinct. There is some effort and discipline involved in taking advantage of the natural flow of instinct to bring a wandering mind back to the mindfulness of breathing, heartbeat, and awareness. It is not heavy-handed discipline. It is the discipline to notice laziness. Sometimes when I sit and meditate my mind starts to whine that I'm too tired or I don't have time for this. I cannot judge those thoughts either.

Once we notice that our mind is captured by wandering thoughts, a spark of mindfulness ignites and we return to the present moment. This is the natural and normal movement of the ordinary mind back to the present moment in which the body and mind are synchronized into an experience of awareness without separation or duality. It can be abrupt, like a sudden change in the course of our thought processes, a strong wind that suddenly blows. The change in course does not define our destination as other thoughts; rather, it presents a return to the open space of the present moment. The ignition of the present moment is the space between the past and the future and is not bound by linear time. It is known by its dynamic stillness and a mind that gradually awakens to the waves of suffering and joy in ourselves and others. This is the innate instinctual mind of compassion. In the present moment is the awakening of preexisting compassion. It is the universe inside us. It is already there. It never left.

MIND: ONE THING AT A TIME

Mindfulness of mind is about contact with our primal life stories, such as those of our family of origin, our career, our life experiences, and so forth. It is our personal narrative, repeated over and over again in our mental life, with all of its plot turns and twists. We must examine whether or not we are resourced by our life stories. How much time do we spend reviewing past experience or anticipating future experience? Do we spend at least an equal amount of time spent in the present moment for balance? Visiting the past can lead to depression. Visiting the future can lead to anxiety. Mindfulness in this way is, again, a type of self-psychotherapy.

A by-product of mindfulness is the ability to discriminate what is healthy or wholesome in these four states and what is unhealthy or unwholesome. We begin to notice how judgment and evaluation about personal experience is not resourcing and thus does not lead to a sense of peacefulness, resilience, and tranquility—that is, to calm abiding. The qualities of calm abiding, such as tranquility, are actually subtle innate. Empathy, kindness, gratitude, and compassion are all subtle emotions. They are like seeds rooted in our biology that need to be watered because the larger stronger emotions have become like weeds and overgrown the garden of our mind. Some of the weeds have deep roots and must be extracted carefully and slowly. The basic technique of mindfulness meditation is to notice and then relax the mind into open awareness, and then any such polarities naturally dissipate. Thoughts are not the enemy and are best left alone.

Mindfulness of mind is about slowing the process of life in order to recognize the potency of the present moment. We can take things one at a time without multitasking and holding on to everything. The present moment is our wireless provider of sanity. The mind operates by looking at one thing at a time, and each thing exhausts itself naturally. In this way, mindfulness becomes spacious and panoramic. This is like watering the other side of the garden, where the seeds of compassion are already growing. In this way, dynamic stillness is not a concept but an actual mind-body experience resulting from regular mindfulness practice. Dynamic stillness is the ground of compassion. Primary Respiration is the movement of compassion.

Calm abiding is the ability to experience both pleasure and pain without clinging to anything, which is a pretty tall order if our mind and emotions are constantly stirred up. We can be aware of what is gratifying and uncomfortable and still abide independently, autonomously, and with self-regulation, without needing things to be other than the way they are in the present moment. The present moment reveals the power of nowness. Inside the universe of the present moment are love and compassion in their totality. Love and compassion softens and warms the space in and around the heart. When we simply bring our attention to the area of the heart, synchronizing our attention with our breath, the potency and radiance of the heart appear. This form of mindfulness can lead to a deeper awareness that ignites heartfulness—that is, compassion.

In closing, I offer a piece I wrote while on a Buddhist retreat called a sesshin. It is about the present moment. It begins with what are called the Eight Negations of Nagarjuna, a second-century Buddhist philosopher.

I prostrate to the Perfect Buddha,
The best of teachers, who taught that
Whatever is dependently arisen is
Unceasing, unborn,
Unannihilated, not permanent,
Not coming, not going,
Without distinction, without identity,
And free from conceptual constructions.

NAGARJUNA
(TRANS. J. L. GARFIELD,
THE FUNDAMENTAL WISDOM OF THE MIDDLE WAY)

I

Yesterday I was so sad I cried
today I laughed so hard I cried
rain does not know happy or sad
rain is
reflecting five colors
a rain of magic
a squall, a gale,
a tropical storm, a hurricane,
all move the rain
yet
no falling
no evaporation
no freezing

II

mind as "stormy weather"
a song
not moving
yet
moving through nothing at all
colored droplets of thoughts
clouds forming

cirrus
cirrocumulus
cumulonimbus
incus (my favorite)
swirling as an artist's palate
Earth's umbrella
nurturing
transforming
each dharma of my neurosis
five colors
making a paraffin self
melting by the heat of mindfulness
a magic rain

III

Cool meets heat
and there is friction
at the edge
becoming
five elements
thunder and lightning ensue
face the wind head on
face the rain head on
the ship has no anchor
in the clouds
guaranteeing a light and sound show
moved by the wind of space
all such dharmas are dreams
recycling the five skandhas
over and over
the elements solidifying a self
the artist's palate
Van Gogh
Manet
Brauner
Klee
Magritte
Kahlo
Picasso

Ah Dali!
It is simply magic rain
thickening the artist's chalk

IV

take shelter in not-knowing
space is freedom
when facing the mind of fear
these heavy dewdrops
were given to an old mule
to write down
may they benefit others
may all beings be safe
may I be safe
may you be safe

MICHAEL J. SHEA

The dharma taught by buddhas
Hinges on two truths:
Partial truths of the world
And truths which are sublime.
Without knowing how they differ,
You cannot know the deep;
Without relying on conventions,
You cannot disclose the sublime;
Without intuiting the sublime,
You cannot experience freedom.

NAGARJUNA
(TRANS. STEPHEN BATCHELOR,
VERSES FROM THE CENTER)

14

Working Heart to Heart, Brain to Brain

If we lack inner freedom, any intense sensory experience can generate strong attachments that entangle us.

MATTHIEU RICARD,
"WORKING WITH DESIRE"

This chapter continues the exploration of the practitioner's perception of mindfulness and compassion in the therapeutic relationship, from the point of view of therapeutic competencies (Siegel 2012) in making a brain-to-brain connection and practical mysticism in making a heart-to-heart connection. Practical mysticism means accessing inner freedom from obsession. It leads to making a heart-to-heart connection with the client and the world that is genuinely responsive rather than reactive. Self-awareness and self-regulation of the practitioner's body and mind are the keys to establishing the inner freedom of a clear and discerning therapeutic resonance. This is gained through consistent reliable contemplative practices. Once the practitioner develops mindfulness of embodiment through the instinct of the four states of mindfulness discussed in the previous chapter (the body as earth, letting go of thoughts, breathing and heart awareness, slow sequencing of mental activity), synchronization with Primary Respiration (PR) can unfold, wherein the practitioner attunes more deeply to the client. It begins with watchfulness.

WATCHFULNESS

Watchfulness is a nonconceptual awareness—an instinctual state of knowing and being—that derives from mindfulness practice and compassion practice. Traditional approaches to craniosacral therapy frequently mention the stillpoint. Biodynamic approaches to craniosacral therapy refer to it as the dynamic stillness. This stillness is rooted in the biology of our body at a cellular level. Its interchange with Primary Respiration merges a sense of spaciousness of the natural world in and around us with being embodied and of the Earth in physical form. The form and the formless merge. Over time, contemplative practice gives us a conscious awareness of this state.

The state of watchfulness is always present but usually buried under thoughts, sensations, emotions, and concepts that form a template for our body and mind—an unnatural condition. The natural state unfolds gradually with contemplative mindfulness practices, such as those outlined in this book, in which mind and body can merge and become one living whole. Watchfulness is available in every second of our life. Typically we experience it in those moments when we space out or briefly glimpse the unity of ourselves with the natural world, but the nonconceptual mind is always available in the present moment. Watchfulness is the pause that refreshes, observing nature without thought. As we take on greater ownership of our own body and our own mind, we gain the insight of compassion, of how oneself and others suffer in the same way. As a species we share the same suffering.

EMPATHY AND SAFETY AS A FUNCTION OF THE SOCIAL NERVOUS SYSTEM

The social nervous system, which governs our relationship with environmental and social cues, consists of elements of the vagus nerve throughout the facial, cranial, neck, thorax, and abdominal structures. This aspect of the nervous system is responsible for interpreting the communication regarding safety and empathy that is constantly being relayed back and forth between two people via eye contact, vocal tone, body movement, and touch. Stephen Porges refers to this evaluation of safety and empathy as neuroception, and it is a function of the limbic system of the brain (Porges 1998, 2001, 2004, 2007, 2011, 2024b). A functioning neuroception system therefore is a prerequisite for compassion. Thus, in the practice of manual therapy in general and biodynamic cardiovascular therapy specifically, the defensive physiology of the therapist and client must be turned off or temporarily suspended for optimal benefit of a session. Mindfulness of the body reduces fear and anxiety and thus helps reduce defensive physiology.

INTERPERSONAL NEUROBIOLOGY

Interpersonal neurobiology (IPNB) can be understood as the cardiovascular and neurological self-regulation of the mind-body in relationship with another person. It has two components: (1) internal or autonomous self-regulation through conscious awareness of the body from the inside, also called bottom-up processing; and (2) self-regulation occurring socially in relationship through the social nervous systems and brains of two people, also called top-down processing. The implication of IPNB is that the therapeutic relationship is a two-person biology. This new scientific reality requires a deeper level of embodied awareness and mindfulness on the part of the practitioner.

KEY COMPETENCIES FOR THE THERAPEUTIC RELATIONSHIP

Below, we'll review the basic knowledge, skills, and abilities that are required for the safe practice of biodynamic and manual therapies. *Biodynamic* in this context refers to the biological wholeness of the human body, one of the core concepts of mindfulness. The intention is to help practitioners embody the individual competencies more holistically and apply them more easily in clinical practice.

The reader might well ask if it is necessary to know and practice each and every one of these skills in every session. These skills take time to develop and gradually become second nature. At first there is a deliberate sense of practice; eventually the practice becomes spontaneous. Some sessions will involve an emphasis on certain skills, while other sessions will focus on different skills. I recommend picking one or two skills that are unfamiliar to the reader and getting to know their meaning and application. If I had to pick a base skill, it would be simple awareness or interoception of the movement of one's heart—cardioception. This is the core of the practice.

Embodied Wholeness

Knowledge: Embodied wholeness is the experience of organization in one's body. The practitioner builds and maintains a therapeutic container based on safety and trust through contemplative practice. This is a holding environment in which normal and natural self-regulation of the body and mind can manifest in the practitioner and the client. It begins with the practitioner sensing their own body-mind. This requires (1) mindfulness, or seeing things from the inside; (2) nowness, the unconditional and total acceptance of one's life; and (3) compassion.

Skills and Abilities: Mindfulness of body begins with correct posture and simple awareness of breathing. Mindfulness of emotions is a nonjudgmental awareness of our current emotional state. Mindfulness of thoughts is awareness of thinking and the natural tendency of the mind and body to synchronize with the present moment. Mindfulness of life stories is about the constant story we tell ourselves about our life, from day to day, week to week, year to year, and so forth. All experience can abide in the space of the present moment.

Self-Regulation

Knowledge: Understand that self-regulation is modulated by two pathways. One pathway is from the body and heart to the brain via sensation and feeling (bottom up), which is slower. It is processed by the right hemisphere of the brain. The second pathway is from the brain to the body via cognition and thinking (top down) in general by the left hemisphere of the brain. Healthy self-regulation of emotional states occurs in the prefrontal cortex in the left hemisphere of the brain. The practitioner needs to affect both pathways in self and other.

Skills and Abilities: Practitioner regularly senses the shape of their own body as one whole continuum of fluid, bone, and membrane with a three-dimensional fluid, wave-like awareness. Practitioner synchronizes with slowness and stillness while orienting to the shape of their body. This generates resonance with the client. Practitioner senses the movement of their heart and breath as a natural place of abiding. The practitioner is aware of the movement of their respiratory diaphragm as a wave, and awareness of the heartbeat to build empathy. This is called cardioception of the heart movement, feeling the space in which it moves, the potency it generates and its radiance spreading through the body.

Relationship

Knowledge: Understand that self-regulation interconnects three elements: attunement, compassion, and intersubjectivity, which are all based on the quality of the practitioner's attention via mindfulness. There are five types of attention in a biodynamic therapy: focused, unfocused, deliberate, spontaneous, and resting or abiding.

Skills and Abilities: Practitioner maintains mindfulness of mental and physical states while in relationship with the client. Practitioner regularly synchronizes with their body, breath, and heart. Practitioner allows their heart to radiate out to the client and back slowly. Practitioner abides in the stillness when perceiving it anywhere.

Attunement

Knowledge: Understand that attunement is the process in which the nervous and cardiovascular systems of the practitioner and client build and maintain a therapeutic container based on safety and trust. This requires neuroception in the brain and cardioception of the heartbeat. Understand that attunement includes the cycling of sensory attention away from the client and back in a slow tempo. At first this is a deliberate movement of attention, and it gradually becomes spontaneous, normal, and natural during a session.

Skills and Abilities: Practitioner is mindful of the slow rhythm of attunement. Attention moves periodically from the practitioner to the horizon and back rhythmically via the third ventricle of the brain.

This develops flexibility in shifting from focused attention to unfocused attention and invites nature into the session. Practitioner is mindful by noticing wandering mental states and emotions and returning to the present moment. Practitioner regularly moves attention back to their heart movement. Practitioner may practice coherent breathing.

Slowness

Knowledge: Understand that under nonstressful conditions, the nervous systems of the client and the practitioner attune on average once per minute. Understand that attunement leads to synchronizing with Primary Respiration and its therapeutic forces.

Skills and Abilities: Practitioner makes soft eye contact when appropriate with the client, especially before and after a session. Practitioner visually scans the surface of the whole body of the client periodically. Practitioner deliberately avoids fast tempos when encountering them in the client or solicits slowness from the client verbally. When stillness permeates the room, the practitioner takes time to abide in it.

Cardioception

Knowledge: Understand that empathy is generated in the brain and heart in order to feel what the client is feeling. It is receptive. Understand that empathy is the foundation of compassion (the biological instinct to care for self and others). It is giving. Understand that the client and the practitioner coregulate each other's nervous and cardiovascular systems through coherence and resonance to generate social coherence (love, happiness, equanimity, kindness) and brain self-regulation. Understand that each person in the therapeutic relationship is affecting the other's nervous and cardiovascular systems equally. Understand that the practitioner's compassion gives the client an experience of being nurtured, loved, and "gotten" (understood). Likewise, the practitioner may feel "gotten" by the client. Understand that empathy and compassion are built through interoceptive awareness of the practitioner's heart and breath, which builds vagal tone. Understand that compassion is the foundation of moral development. Biodynamic therapy facilitates moral development and moral safety.

Skills and Abilities: Practitioner regularly practices cardioception, focusing attention on the movement and activity of the heart and blood. Practitioner pays attention to the heartbeat pulsation spreading out to the hands and three-dimensionally through their body. Practitioner deepens cardioception to include their gut feelings, such as tightening, cramping, queasiness, hunger, need for evacuation of the bowel or bladder, shifts in breathing, streaming, pulsating, undulating, and so on. Practitioner is capable of guiding the client through a body scan. Practitioner notices sensations of heat and warmth in self and client and allows them to permeate the whole body. Practitioner periodically smiles as a type of nonverbal dialogue with the client. Practitioner actively senses their hands as continuous or connected with their heart and that of the client. Practitioner attunes to Primary Respiration in the client's vascular tree.

Loving Kindness

Knowledge: Understand that physical touch when coupled with loving kindness and compassion stimulates the release of the hormone oxytocin, associated with the felt sense of love in both the practitioner and the client.

Skills and Abilities: Practitioner periodically contemplates the flow of loving kindness, equanimity, love, and joy flowing from their heart toward the client or through the hands while in contact with the client. Practitioner contemplates the client's history, sensing their own heart movement while doing an intake or even while in contact with the client.

Mediation of the Autonomic Nervous System

Knowledge: Understand that the client holds stress, trauma, and shock in their body, which is capable of being sensed by the practitioner before, during, and after a session through attunement and resonance with the client. Understand that the client can sense the practitioner's inner state of mind and body, whether consciously or unconsciously. Understand that shock and trauma is mediated in the body by the autonomic nervous system (ANS) and its deeper metabolism.

Understand that at the same time that shock and trauma are held in the body, they are being centered by health, also present in the body. Health is the potency of Primary Respiration. Practitioner synchronizes with the health in every situation with mindfulness of the body, heart, and breath. These are deep innate instinctual resources for healing. Understand that it is important to support a client emotionally but not process the client's emotions.

Skills and Abilities: Practitioner observes signs of the client's ANS seeking allostasis, such as skin color tone, breathing, shaking or trembling, eyes glazing, and so on. Practitioner periodically attends to their own thoughts, feelings, emotions, and sensations while in contact with the client. Practitioner acknowledges the client's ANS activation by verbally soliciting the client's comfort or desire to pause or continue the session or moving their attention out into the natural world and back slowly. Practitioner modulates contact with the client slowly while the ANS is active by slowing down and pausing periodically, waiting for the client to take several breaths. Practitioner brackets or saves personal feelings and emotions that persist in a session for reflection after the client has left the office, with appropriate supervision or therapy.

Healthy Boundaries

Knowledge: Understand that clear verbal communication is an important boundary and facilitates successful therapeutic outcomes. Practitioner maintains clear, responsible, and ethical boundaries with clients.

Skills and Abilities: Practitioner actively acknowledges the client as they speak through soft eye contact, head nodding, sounds of recognition, and/or words of recognition. This includes actively sensing the heart. Practitioner is curious or questioning, but not intrusive if something in the client's story seems to be missing. Practitioner avoids provoking the client's emotions through verbal or manual techniques.

ତତ

Heart-to-Heart Practice

Contemplative practices allow a nonlinear sequencing of living and being in the heart to emerge. This twelve-step process for building a heart-to-heart connection is really a series of simple reminders that incorporate a wide variety of contemplative skills. This process is not limited to the client-therapist relationship; it is the pathway to navigating life.

1. Practice mindfulness of the moment. How am I physically, emotionally, and spiritually organized in this very moment? How do I find the felt sense of my body in this very moment? What is the state of my mind? Am I distracted?

2. Bring attention to the felt sense of breathing. I feel the breath moving down into my abdomen. Am I able to sense how my breathing and Primary Respiration periodically synchronize and ignite wholeness by a spontaneous deep breath?

3. Practice interoception of the heartbeat and its potency. In how large of an area in my body am I able to sense the movement of the heartbeat and its potency? Can the heartbeat in the back of my sternum expand? Can I sense it throughout my body?

4. Inhabit my mind and body as if extending to the horizon with Primary Respiration. Am I able to sense the micromovement flowing from bottom to top, from side to side, undulating in the total volume of blood to the surface of my skin? Can I feel the space around my whole body holding me gently? Can I evenly suspend my attention without overfocusing to the horizon looking

from my third ventricle? Is Primary Respiration moving back and forth from the horizon in the great ocean suspended between me and the client?

5. Make a heart-to-heart connection with PR. I bring my attention to the electromagnetic field of my heart surrounding me and my client. I sense Primary Respiration moving through this shared heart field that connects us. It is a gentle rhythmic, magnetic pull and push of my sternum and pericardium, swinging like a pendulum in the tempo of Primary Respiration. (This is the core perceptual skill in biodynamic cardiovascular therapy.)

6. Ask permission to make contact. Receive permission for hand contact with the client and sense the blood capillaries pulsing under the skin. I contact the whole vascular tree and gradually sense Primary Respiration, first heart to heart and then moving through the vascular tree as a torsioning or lengthening and shortening.

7. Move attention away from the hands. The fulcrum of Primary Respiration automatically shifts between the third ventricle of the brain and the heart. I allow the fulcrum to shift while staying in the tempo of Primary Respiration. I wait until stillness fills the present moment and leaves my perception in the void.

8. Focus on Pericardium 8 in the palm of the hand. I synchronize my hands as Primary Respiration moves from the heart in a spiral out the palms of my hands.

9. Attention is suspended between the horizon in the natural world and the therapist's heart-brain. I gradually synchronize these attentional fulcrums of Primary Respiration into a single continuum from inside out to the horizon and beyond. This includes sensing the stillness moving from the background of my perception to the foreground. I let go of Primary Respiration and relax into the void.

10. Ignite the light in the third ventricle and heart. Is Primary Respiration automatically shifting into colors and forms, into images and shapes made of light? Primary Respiration moves locally in the veins, arteries, heart, lymph, and gut as a wind moving the vascular tree, as a force of nature. Its appearance is colorful.

11. The Void clearly manifests out of the perception of stillness. Dynamic stillness spontaneously manifests from infinite space as infinite space itself. Space is the universe seen and unseen. I completely rest my attention in this awareness, without a fulcrum. I allow the movement of the heart to radiate the stillness as a bright light of the Breath of Life filling my body and extending out into the cosmos.

12. Relax and let go into the Void of stillness. A central stillness spontaneously manifests between the heart and the third ventricle of the brain. I always connect the movement of the heart with the stillness, wherever it is located.

This chapter offers numerous skills that are the foundation of biodynamic cardiovascular therapy. These skills communicate directly to the heart and blood of the practitioner and client. They represent the activity of embodied compassion. Biodynamic practice is nonlinear, however. Our fulcrum of attention is constantly and sometimes automatically shifting. We learn to stabilize our attention with our breath and heartbeat. We learn to automatically shift our attention away from our thoughts. The learning and application of new skills must be done gently and with kindness.

15

What Is Health?

Find the Health, anyone can find disease.
ANDREW TAYLOR STILL, FOUNDER OF OSTEOPATHY,
IN *PHILOSOPHY OF OSTEOPATHY* (2015)

The defining element that differentiates the biomedical paradigm from the biody-namic paradigm is the concept of health. The body is defined in biomedicine as being the structure of health. When something goes wrong with the body, it is considered an unhealthy condition. Much time is devoted to working on the body as the structure of health. In a talk I heard, Robert Lustig, MD said the processed food industry in the United States makes six hundred billion dollars a year in profit and that it costs the health care system a trillion dollars a year to try and fix the negative health outcomes called metabolic syndrome from processed food addiction. The search for the recovery of health is conducted all over its various anatomical systems, right down to the cellular and atomic level. The genes are seen as holding a blueprint for health and disease. And yet it is the processed food industry as I mentioned in my book *The Biodynamics of the Immune System* that is a key problem along with weak government food recommendations that keeps the public unhealthy.

Culturally, the biomedical paradigm results in the drive to manufacture health in the body. Health is interpreted psychosomatically; we are what we think, how we exercise, and certainly these days what we eat. In a word, that is confusing. Our culture prizes a buff, toned body and manipulates the body to achieve a standard of surface health at the local gym. As D. Aldridge (1996) writes in an article on the phenomenon of "becoming" healthy, "Within today's context of cultural insecurity, the body of the person becomes the vehicle for expressing one's beliefs and desires." But this is a half-truth.

In the biodynamic paradigm, the body is the house or container of health, the instinct for self-healing. The body is health's partner. Together, soma (the totality of the organism) and health form a spiritual whole. They intermingle with each other. Health in the biodynamic paradigm is not found in the structures of the human body, nor does it have a genetic code as such. It is a function rather than a structure of the body. It is not an absence of disease; it is an unconditional state. It is found as a process arising around and within the soma, passing through it and sharing the body as a partner in a collaborative event with the totality of our environment. It is the preexisting condition. We feel it in Primary Respiration and dynamic stillness. There is a physiological experience of body, such as the heart pumping. There is the enormity of our invisible metabolism of chemical molecules and cells known by interoceptive awareness. There is a subtle sensory experience moving through the soma and permeating the soma called *Health*.

Iatrogenic Immorality

Theologian and social critic Ivan Illich (1976) wrote that Western medicine is a significant threat to health and well-being physically and emotionally. Illich makes a profound and catastrophic analysis into iatrogenesis, examining how medicine really functions as opposed to the fallacy of healing that has been built around it. His book, *Medical Nemesis: The Expropriation of Health,* speaks of our contemporary society and its addiction to a medical system that is completely draining both its patients and staff of power, money, dignity, and life itself. Since that book's publication, the problem has only escalated with more than 251,000 patients every year in the United States being killed from physician mistakes, and that number is only from 10 percent of medical facilities reporting! Such medical errors are now the third-leading cause of death in the United States (Anderson and Abrahamson 2017). Illich argues that the problem is not with medicine itself but with the medical establishment existing as a pawn of a profit-driven corporate society and government corruption regarding food recommendations. Iatrogenesis will be minimized only if it is understood as but one aspect of the destructive dominance of industry over society and consequently over our bodies. This is a good example of paradoxical counterproductivity driven by profit rather than health, which is now surfacing in all major industrial health-related sectors. Modern medicine deprives the individual of self-determination (agency) in treatment, and unless you have an advocate for your health care decisions close by when entering the system, the chance for an iatrogenic outcome is greatly amplified. The treatment is taken over by a technocratic bureaucracy that tends to declare everyone in need of treatment for a disease rather than for health and insists on a "cookie cutter" treatment based on cohort studies of which many are flawed because of financial bias with the researchers or their journals and then applied to the masses. This is opposed to assisting the patient with self-treatment and awakening their innate instinct for self-healing with empathy and compassion, which is missing. This is grounds for rampant moral distress in the medical system (Rushton 2018). Rushton further uses the terms moral suffering, moral dilemma, unregulated moral outrage, moral sensitivity, moral residue, moral agency, and moral imagination to describe hospital systems. This implies that the medical system is immoral to the core according to both Rushton and Illich. The medical establishment replaces traditional cultural means for understanding pain, suffering, and death with a judgmental artificial intelligence bureaucracy that engages in a failed effort to eliminate pain and prolong life, as I saw so poignantly with my mother and many others. The majority of health care dollars in the United States is spent in the last thirty days of life in an attempt to prevent the inevitability of death—or even after death. When one of my mom's roommates at the nursing home died, the staff came in to do another expensive test on the dead patient. I exclaimed that this person was dead, and the reply was that the test had been ordered, so it would be done, meaning more money extracted from the dead person's insurance or family. This is immoral. The spiritual foundation of Health as a unity of mind, body, and spirit is completely absent.

Before Hippocratic medicine, the practice of medicine and healing was theurgic—disease was seen as divine punishment and healing as divine intervention. Theurgic medicine saw health as a relationship with the things of spirit or the divine will, and illness as a loss of relationship with spirit. While first defined in ancient times, the idea that illness is a loss of relationship with spirit rings true even today. It is the premise of my previous book, *The Biodynamics of the Immune System*, and continues in this book. The patient goes to a healing temple/therapist's office, whereupon the priestess-priest/therapist performs the necessary ritual to invoke the presence of the divine/spiritual/universal. This ignites a spark of the innate self-healing instinct. This vigil might take days, depending on the illness. David K. Reynolds (1982) reports that the fourth and fifth days of "quiet therapies" (Japanese healing regimens, which include Zen meditation) are the most critical. At last, the whisperings of spirit are heard or seen in a vision and the original matrix of Health (with a capital H) is reestablished for the patient. Thus, stillness and silence are a quality ferment for spiritual healing.

Health is carried by chi in Taoist medicine or by the wisdom wind of Primary Respiration that animates the flesh and all the cells of the body in biodynamic practice. It animates the fluid matrix inside and outside the cells. It moves the blood from the heart inside the heart. This Health is the self-healing instinct. Sometimes physical health is referred to as vitality, meaning the capacity to maintain homeostasis in order to function properly. This notion of vitality derives from the science showing that, for example, eating processed food and having a stagnant elimination system (constipation) is a strong predictor of disability in our aging population. Research has shown that having three or less bowel movements per week is a strong risk factor for dementia and Alzheimer's disease. Vitality and homeostasis are manifestations of the instinct for self-preservation, which is itself directly related to the instinct for self-healing, which is Health.

Health is the perception of the animate, the ignition system, and the spirit of all things. It is the original condition, the primal matrix or life-giving force known by different names in different healing traditions. This Health is interconnected with the instinct for self-transcendence, the innate capacity to go beyond the ordinary. This Health is never lost, even with cancer or disease. The body may have a disease, but this does not negate Health and its connection to spirit. Your illness is wasted unless you are transformed by it. The diseased part of the body can be found and even removed by surgery; however, the dis-ease may return. The Health, though, is never lost. It may be asleep, forgotten, or hiding, but it remains present, residing in the heart, waiting for a metamorphosis like a phoenix rising out of the ashes. Everyone has experienced this miracle, either personally or through someone they know. I see it frequently in my clinical practice.

Indeed, Health is difficult to find in a diseased condition of the body and may lose its voice amidst the physiology and metabolism of the disease process. Dr. Jim Jealous, one of my mentors, said that Health is "that which cannot become diseased." During illness, it recedes deep into the instinctual level of body or the mind or both (Kalsched 1996). This Health that I speak of is without observable facts and rationality because of the instinct for self-transcendence that is linked to the instinct for self-healing. It is known and felt as the movement of grace and love. It is a silent partner in the silent communication between the world and the body. It is ineffable. It is found in the perception of stillness and slowness, and thus its connection to Primary Respiration and dynamic stillness. It exists as a function of *not knowing* how to define it. Not knowing is the threshold to perceiving Health because we must pass through a doorway of fear. As John Daido Loori wrote, "We seem to have lost the ability to just be quiet, to simply be present in the stillness that is the foundation of our lives. Yet if we never get in touch with that stillness, we never fully experience our lives" (1996, 5).

The silent communication of Health interacts between the subject (patient) and the guide (therapist). The guide acts as *a finger pointing toward the moon*. The perception of Health dawns in the patient in the fullness of their own time and place, arising as a lucid stillness, in a vision or a deep sensory experience. It is motile and touches the core of the body's fluid essence, the blood. It whispers and hums in the background of stillness. Direct sensory experience and images are emergent properties of Health. There is a sense of *something* that passes through everything, like a warm mist. Dr. Jealous said that the Health is experienced as fire that can consume everything associated with disease.

Stillness is often associated with emptiness. From emptiness, the form of life and

Health arise unique to each human being. Health is in a constant state of becoming new—it is always being reborn. To become new is to accept the constancy of change in every moment. The present moment is constantly shifting and cannot be nailed down. Being present means being present for a newness occurring every moment. We exist in a vast sea of impermanence and thus newness and constant renewal of Health is the most potent spiritual teacher possible. However, the soma experiences only a portion of Health at any given time. The vast amount of Health is withheld from perception as the world is filled with many distractions and information overload. Our brains are easily overwhelmed with sensory information and afflictive emotions. Contemplative practice in slowing down and making time for recovery from information/communication (cultural) overload is needed for Health to become apparent. This is the essence of biodynamic cardiovascular therapy (BCVT). Gradually the body attunes itself to Health, and Health places itself more deeply in the incarnate world of mind, body, and spirit. Health is a conversation of continuous whispering dialogue that unfolds below our ordinary thinking mind. And it offers images of itself that are sacred and can be accessed through contemplative practices.

BCVT is a contemplative practice. A contemplative practice is any act that we regularly enter into with our entire heart-mind essence. It is a comfortable turning inward. It is a way of awakening, deepening, and sustaining a mindful experience of the intrinsic holiness of the present moment. The most important factor is not so much what the practice is, in its form or structure, but rather the extent to which the practice incarnates an utterly genuine and reliable view of awakening inwardly in our perception of self, other, and the cosmos. It leads to total acceptance of the sacred nature of the present moment.

MYSTICISM AND THE CRANIAL CONCEPT

If the recognition by Dr. Andrew Taylor Still of God, as creator of the human body is religious, then the science of osteopathy, in concept, is religious. If the science of osteopathy is religious, then the cranial concept in osteopathy is religious.

W. G. SUTHERLAND, DO (1967)[*]

The cranial concept as developed by Dr. William Garner Sutherland is a mystical exploration into how spirit incarnates into the human heart and how healing occurs as a spiritual function of the human heart. His lifelong investigation of the mechanics of the craniosacral system led him to a direct experience of a divine light in the client

[*]From an untitled talk in 1944 at Des Moines Still College of Osteopathy. In *Contributions of Thought* (Ft. Worth: Sutherland Cranial Teaching Foundation, 101–115).

that he called the Breath of Life from the bible. He observed this divine light healing a client. These aspects of the cranial concept are a mystery. It is said that one can enter a mystery, but one cannot solve a mystery. We have entered the mystery of biodynamic practice. A central feature of biodynamic practice is *not-knowing* and entering the portal of our fear to see it clearly, know it, and befriend it. It is being comfortable in the mystery of transubstantiation, according to Dr. Jealous. Transubstantiation is the act whereby the presence of the divine, the holy spirit, changes itself into the form and functions of the human body. It can be scary to sense our soma as divine. Human beings are created from the food we eat and the air we breathe. Both come from the natural world as the essence of the sacred in giving us our "daily bread." Such metaphorical and real bread (real food) transubstantiates metabolically into blood that carries the virtue of spirit residing in the heart inside the heart to every cell in the body. Breathing energizes the process as the great ocean of chi. The sacred lives in real food and clean air. Our gut becomes the organizer of our creation moment by moment. Our gut builds the blood that spirit moves and fills with virtue. And so we can see why some ministers tell us that processed food is the devil.

BCVT is only partially derived from the cranial concept. It explores on the very practical level of the cardiovascular system how healing occurs in the body with the aid of the presence of the divine in the vascular tree. Ancient sources of animism, in which all of the natural world is medicine, come forward in biodynamic practice. The sacred is recognized by the perception of Primary Respiration and dynamic stillness. BCVT employs skillful palpation to relate to the primal matrix of Health in the body and form a dialogue with this Health via the vascular endothelium. Progressive stages of palpation and perception are used to find the center of Health and its tidal motion underneath all the anatomy, physiology, and distortion that are encountered along the way. As Dr. Jealous said, Health is the potency of Primary Respiration. It is discernable as an endpoint in biodynamic sessions.

THE BREATH OF LIFE

And Lord God formed man of the dust of the ground, and breathed into
his nostrils the breath of life, and man became a living soul.

GENESIS 2:7

Dr. Sutherland said that central to his cranial concept is the Breath of Life—the spiritual blueprint for incarnation. As mentioned he experienced the Breath of Life as a light. The Breath of Life organizes the form of the human body around a spiritual center, the human heart. This relates the natural world of both heaven and Earth to and through the heart and blood. It is a fulcrum of clear light radiating the appearance of the universe in front of our very eyes. The heart inside the heart is the center of this clear light and its radiance. The Breath of Life is synonymous with spirit as used in many other cultural traditions. Indeed one could say in the Christian context that the Breath of Life is the Holy Spirit.

Spirit is an intelligence that is self-existing. It is self-knowing awareness. Its voice is a whisper. It is invisible. It speaks from the blood of the soma by its movement. It animates all the fluids and the blood. Its movement is that of an imprint of a bird in flight. Not a trace is left.

The Breath of Life as Sutherland perceived it is a metaphor for spirit. Spirit includes an expanded experience of the Breath of Life. Spirit is called Health which forms a conjunction and interaction between therapist and client. Both the therapist and client attempt to perceive the field of Health permeating both through perception of the wisdom wind of PR and dynamic stillness. The client is sensing the Health in the therapist as much as the therapist is sensing the Health in the client. The foundation for this perception is safety. Health is mutually searching in each other for a place to *be* in the heart. Both the client and the therapist are on the scent of the sacred. Biodynamic practice is a sacred treasure hunt. The therapist initially is the guide, with their own personal attention directed inward upon their own heart and soma, and then gradually the Health manifests and guides the ignition of self-healing in the client. The therapist can wait, watch, and wonder about the direction of Health and must be patient for the intelligence of Health to manifest its unerring potency in the fullness of its own time.

PERCEPTION

The disease process in biodynamic practice is viewed differently than in biomedicine. It is not an enemy to be conquered. Biodynamically, disease is seen as a series of causes and conditions, such as transgenerational imprints that form a multidimensional persona living in our organism. Disease is a process of outer relationships and inner perception. It is a construction of the mind, the body, and culture (Morris 1998). Culture can be any factor in the past, present, or future that imprints and shapes our body, including processed food and social media. Perception is a processing of exteroception and interoception into meaning, values, and beliefs. Perception is dependent on an ability to be introspective or self-reflective (Wilber 1997). Self-reflection in turn requires the ability to think critically and have room for tension to occur between opposing thoughts, feelings, values, and so on. Contemplative practice is critical to this process.

Health is a reciprocal encounter within my soma between me and a silent partner living in the heart inside the heart. "Health is seen not as the absence of disease, but is a process by which individuals maintain their ability to develop a meaning system that will allow them to function in the face of changes in themselves and their relationships with their environment" (Schlitz, Taylor, and Lewis 1998, 48). This requires acknowledgment and acceptance of life constantly changing. Thus, the present moment becomes the supreme spiritual teacher because we have a choice to accept change or resist change in every moment.

Health involves our ability to synchronize with Primary Respiration and stillness and then expand our perception into the open space of awareness. This allows for what Carl Jung called the *transcendent function* to occur. We are in a constant transition from one spiritual state to another, from one thought to the next, from one emotion to the next. It is the spontaneous and constant arising of the Breath of Life, the personal spirit in us in all of its thousand faces (Kalsched 1996). A wide field of perception that includes the inside and outside allows new possibilities and creativity. A narrow field of perception, attention capture, and continuous partial attention become mentally claustrophobic and is a nutrient field for disease. Such narrow perception invites illness and disconnection from life. It causes a persistent sense of alienation between the body, mind, and environment. We lose our heart.

The Breath of Life is light because of its clarity, the clarity of silence and the awe of perceiving the cosmos. It contains the spark around which the form and function of the body are created. The very nature of the Breath of Life is radiance, clarity, and wisdom. It lives in the heart inside the heart, radiating its rainbow waves of light carried by Primary Respiration. It transforms the blood into a carrier of virtue as the deepest dimension of our fluid body. It carries with it the consciousness of the perfected heart-mind. Sutherland said that it is *unerring*.

ORDINARY MIND

In the practice of BCVT, a client may initially present with "ordinary mind"—busy with the inner perception of mental thoughts, without contemplative peace and quiet. Let us look at this ordinary mind of confusion and the stages of discursive chatter that are perceived constantly during waking reality and biodynamic session work.

Stage 1: Non-dwelling mind. The non-dwelling mind experiences a type of free-floating approach to body/mind synchronization. This may occur in the morning upon waking up, as we are just lying there, with our non-dwelling mind experiencing the fluidity of life. Thoughts come from nowhere and go nowhere. In biodynamic terms this is related to the potency of Primary Respiration, a slow rhythmic enhancement of the self-healing instinct in the body. Potency is self-generated by the perception of a relaxed, non-dwelling mind synchronized with Primary Respiration and dynamic stillness.

Stage 2: Recreational mind. Mind then moves into recreational thinking. We start the day. We mentally review our schedule. We plan. We fill our mind with input. Entertainment is the fundamental occupation of the recreational mind. It seeks to avoid boredom at all costs. Facing boredom, the mind might seize upon one particular thought or feeling and begin to fantasize, often about the past or the future, continuing until some new form of input comes. And then there is the vulgarity and mental pollution of social media and television. I tell students to shut it all down—planning, dreaming, streaming, messaging—a minimum of fifteen minutes before a session begins. A biodynamic session starts early with the contemplation of emptying the mind. And as a session continues we usually bump into recreational mind.

Stage 3: Habitual mind. The recreational mind moves into habitual mind. Thoughts trigger emotions and the building of concepts as though building a house in the sky. Mind begins to fixate on thoughts, emotions, concepts, and states of consciousness that are empty. The more fixated thought processes become, the more the ordinary mind will project a solid reality. This solidness relates directly to the physiology of the body and how thoughts affect the body (Pert 1997). The autonomic nervous system of the body is continually shaped by thoughts, like a puppet on a string. This leads to constant distraction and, in a BCVT session, lack of the sense of safety in the connection between therapist and client. Always the practice is coming back to the moment. Dr. Rollin Becker, one of the great biodynamic osteopathic instructors, said to leave one's ego outside the office. This is easier said than done in contemporary practice.

Stage 4: Obsessive mind. If this habitual mind continues, obsessional thinking is the result. The ordinary obsessional mind may fixate for days on one particular problem or another. Mind is fickle, and it doesn't take much to obsess or, for that matter, to drop the obsession. Sometimes our obsessions dissipate quickly and suddenly, and others do not. Obsessions are a mask for numerous psychological and physical problems and the root for many illnesses. This is the mind of stress and a sympathetically adapted nervous system and a physically unhealthy body. This was one of the great discoveries of Wilhelm Reich (1945): that the body is formed by emotions, which is not the soma. We then carry two bodies: the one of Health and the one that obsesses. And that is a lot of work for the autonomic nervous system.

It is the ordinary mind that recreates, fixates, or obsesses and is related to the cranial rhythmic impulse (CRI) in traditional craniosacral therapy. The CRI is an indication of stress in the body from a mind that is disconnected from body and lacks space. The CRI and other craniosacral rhythms are compensatory to maintain an urban lifestyle. When I did my ten-year apprenticeship on the Diné reservation, as discussed in chapter 10, I put my hands on my teacher and his family members but could not perceive the CRI. In an Earth-based culture like the Diné, it was not present.

The body via the autonomic nervous system is connected to our ordinary mind, and our awareness flickers back and forth between sensations, feelings, and mental events such as thoughts, interpretations, and projections. This movement back and forth between the body and the mind is called *dualistic fixation*. It causes thoughts to be projected as though they were real in order to make them seem solid, and consequently the body becomes solid rather than fluid. In the words of Dr. Jealous, the fluids can lesion. *Lesion* is an osteopathic term describing the situation in which the past is held in the present as something solid and palpable. Dr. Jealous said the fluids turn solid and feel like muscle tissue. Thoughts arouse the autonomic nervous system because ordinary mind is riding the flight simulator of our overloaded brain. That system speeds up and everything around it tightens, especially the endothelium of the vascular tree. It is a form of protection from an enemy that is our own mind and skewed perception. Homeostasis in the body becomes disorganized and vitality diminishes. There is a basic split between who we think we are (ordinary mind) and who we really are (heart). There is constant elaboration with thoughts because of this uncertainty around the flickering back and forth between thoughts and physical sensations from overstimulation of the autonomic nervous system. Then we tend to invest more time to get fixed by the medical system, delaying a much-needed reunion with spirit in the heart inside the heart.

Our ordinary noncontemplative mind tricks us into believing that this trapeze act of swinging precariously back and forth is two separate events without a causal relationship. There is fantasizing. There is indulgence. There is a constant checking in on personal feelings in an attempt to discern good-bad, happy-sad, pain-pleasure. It is because of this preoccupation that chaos and illness are invited in as something solid in our fluid body. There is a loss of relationship to the Earth, to the physical heart of the body, to the environment, and to the preexisting innate unconditional Health. In biodynamic practice, this is the perception of an imbalanced autonomic nervous system due to the rapid movement of mind and body rocking back and forth in an unsettled condition. So many clients I see now are in chronic states of overwhelm; I feel that our work is becoming palliative care.

The autonomic nervous system gets corrupted by excessive mental activity. As noted earlier, we think tens of thousands of thoughts a day, and the majority of them are negative. This creates a significant split between mind, body, and the spirit that lives in the heart. It ultimately creates a dream or an illusion because mind is capricious and fickle. The house is built on shifting sand. First we think of the past, then we think of the future, then we obsess about this moment, then we generate habitual emotions generated by these mental obsessions that are cardiotoxic, such as anger, depression, and anxiety. Thoughts of the past can lead to depression. Thoughts of the future can lead to anxiety. Over time, these interpretations and projections become solid and highly believable. Our bodies and especially our hearts are shaped according to mental states and social situations. This is called psychosomatic body or a somatoform disorder. Psychosomatic body is the home of disease, the complete solidification of mental-emotional states into a coexisting body template up against and preventing change within our real body. This is another body altogether inside each of us. It has its own physiology and anatomy, and it fools us into valuing it as the real thing, the genuine body where Health resides. Our psychosomatic body requires medication and more entertainment from the outside. It prevents us from turning inward toward contemplation and insight gained from contemplative practices.

Disease, then, is self-inflicted at worst and a spiritual maturation at best. It becomes a part of our individual self-expression. Our instincts for self-preservation and self-healing are wounded. Ultimately such disease becomes a defense against the innate ability to create new meaning or discover new possibilities about how to change personal suffering and the suffering of others. Compassion is snuffed out. Biomedicine often becomes a rationalization or a preventive measure against meaning. The patient is prevented from finding personal and universal meaning from their suffering.

UNCONDITIONAL HEALTH

From the spiritual point of view of the Breath of Life, all disease is viewed as an initiatory process. Pain and suffering initiate the wounded into the mystery of self-healing and the darker recesses of healing the heart, literally and spiritually. In other words, with disease, the big picture of the cosmos and its clarity slowly arises from the depths of our inner world at the center of our heart. This is the world of spirit, which constantly seeks a home in our heart inside the heart. The human heart is a complete representation of the visible and invisible spirit world. The union of spirit and mind percolate in the fullness of their own time until the mystery of healing is revealed in the heart.

Unconditional Health is not capable of thinking. It is the absence of thinking altogether. This is the subtle mind of non-thought awareness. Thinking is not necessary; *not-knowing* is. Mind and heart are synchronized with the Breath of Life internally. There is also synchronization with the external environment, which allows the ordinary thinking mind to dissolve out into a wide perceptual field. This connection to expansion and dissolving is facilitated by the therapist paying close attention to interoceptive awareness of their own body, especially their heartbeat and breathing. This builds empathy for self and other. When I feel my heartbeat increase, I can adjust my behavior and thoughts to lower my heart rate. This is great self-care. It helps cultivate a contemplative mind. In biodynamic terms, the synchronizing the fulcrum of heart and mind orients us to the Breath of Life, allowing the light of spirit to reside in the heart inside the heart. It is the animate nature of Health, or the Breath of Life, that links ordinary, contemplative, and wisdom mind together as a unified whole. Ordinary, contemplative, and wisdom mind are neither good nor bad. They are in relationship with each other. It is imperative for biodynamic practitioners to form a relationship with these minds without an allegiance to any. They live in the heart. That is where to place our attention.

In forming a relationship with this big heart-mind, another possibility arises: the perception of the Breath of Life. This awakens the self-transcendent function of the cranial concept. It begins with the therapist rather than the client. As Loori writes, "When the mind is at rest, the body is at rest—respiration, heartbeat, and metabolism slow down. Reaching this still point is not something unusual or esoteric. It is a very important part of being alive and staying awake. All creatures on the earth are capable of manifesting this stillness" (Loori 1996, 6).

The very subtle nature of the Breath of Life is the palpable sense of unconditional Health as a light radiating from our heart. The Breath of Life forms the blueprint and the original matrix of the intention to incarnate—to be. Its basic effects go beyond a sensory level into the imaginal and visionary. The realm of the imaginal requires a shift in perception to the heart inside the heart.

Health, the Breath of Life, and the potency of Primary Respiration are independent of the disease process. Health may hide and spirit may temporarily vacate the heart, but neither is ever lost. By quieting the thinking mind through contemplative practice, we can feel this silent and wordless movement from outside to in and from inside to out, always happening as an improvisational dance. This dance is between the heart, with its blood coursing through the vascular tree, and the breathing landscape that surrounds us and fills the cosmos. Health is a radiant presence known by the perception of Primary Respiration and dynamic stillness. Its originality is in the heart-mind. Health is encountered on the inside as the potency of Primary Respiration communicating and commingling in a dynamic process that constantly draws us into relationship as a type of intercourse between our heart and mind. We encounter this Health outside in nature, in ourselves, and between others as the movement of Primary Respiration and the radiant light of the Breath of Life illuminating all of nature. It is a soft breeze in the treetops on a summer day or the stillness of a frozen lake. It is the horizon beckoning us when we sit at the ocean.

The radiant appearance of the Breath of Life as everything that appears on Earth and in the sky undercuts any opinion or belief system about what Health is or must be. We enter a state of awe. As a culture, our concepts of health have been conditioned by biomedicine to orient around the body. We say things like *My body is healthy* or *My body is unhealthy*, or *I feel more healthy when I take my vitamins* or *I felt awful yesterday but today I am healthier*. We operate under beliefs that *I'm healthy if I meditate every day* or *I'm healthy if I'm working with the Breath of Life*. All of these are conditional points of view. If any of these circumstances change, and they do all day long, then we believe that our health is lost. But Health is unconditional and courageous; it cannot be lost. It must be uncovered by the quality of our attention. The courage of unconditional Health is intrinsic and inherent to being alive. If you have cancer, you are healthy. If you have a mental health disorder, you are healthy. The Breath of Life is neutral. It is pure love and good will. Look at the courage that many clients manifest in the midst of their suffering.

> *On this journey we're moving toward that which is not so certain, that which cannot be tied down, that which is not habitual and fixed. We're moving toward a whole new way of thinking and feeling, a flexible and open way of perceiving reality that is not based on certainty and security. This new way of perceiving is based on connecting with the living energetic quality of ourselves and everything else.*
>
> PEMA CHODRON, "EVERYBODY LOVES SOMETHING"

16

The Mysticism of the
Five Indo-Tibetan Elements

In the center of the heart, the Absolute Body abides naturally as the five
Buddhas endowed with the five Wisdoms and clearly manifesting in an
unceasing mode of luminous visions that are contemplated within the sky.
JEAN-LUC ACHARD, *THE SIX LAMPS*

The five Indo-Tibetan elements—space, wind, fire, water, and earth—are the anatomy and physiology of the universe and the human body from the beginninglessness of time. As conceptual designations for explaining the universe and natural world, the five elements arose out of the animistic healing traditions on the planet hundreds of thousands of years ago. These traditional healing systems contain the oldest medicine in the natural world, and some still survive in their original form. For the Chinese, it was Wu shamanism and Taoism; in India, early Buddhism and Hinduism relied on ayurvedic, Unani, and Siddha medicine dating back to 5000 BCE. When both ayurveda and classical Chinese medicine came to Tibet, they encountered the preexisting shamanic culture of the Bon.

It took thousands of years for these early elemental healing systems to coalesce into the formal pluralistic medical systems of ayurveda, Tibetan medicine, and classical Chinese medicine. These systems of healing derive from a lived experience of the five elements as an integration of spirituality, religion, and medicine. They proclaim a fundamental unity of body-mind-spirit.

Though Western medicine has its roots in the same sort of holistic animistic traditions as these Eastern ones, here body-mind-spirit suffered the trauma of amputation. Spirit was cut off and given to the church; the body was taken by biomedicine. The mind became a function of the devil at the same time in the Christian church because of the intrusiveness of evil thoughts (as they were called). And thus mind became synonymous with discursive thinking. When a contemporary practitioner seeks to work from a unified context of body, mind, and spirit, it requires a contemplative practice for such unity to become clear. In Eastern traditions, the unity of mind, body, and spirit is assumed and built into the educational and medical systems. The body is viewed as consisting of the five elements in the Indo-Tibetan system, which are space, wind, fire, water, and earth. These elements are linked to mind and spirit by association with colors imbued with divine-like sentience. This forms the basis of Eastern cosmology as detailed in my book *The Biodynamics of the Immune System*. The basic principle in these Eastern cosmologies is that the very same molecules that form the elements in our body form the same elements in the universe and thus the human mind, body, and spirit, as well as the idea that all sentient beings are unified from the beginning inside and out. The practical starting point is a contemplative practice that encourages befriending all thoughts without judgment and that builds an optimal relationship with one's body—one that is free of believing completely in debilitating pathological diagnoses. This nurtures a relationship with unconditional health as mentioned in the previous chapter.

It's important at this time in the narrative of Western medicine to reconsider the five elements as the basis of anatomy and physiology of the body-mind-spirit. All five elements are the primary building blocks for a human embryo from the beginning of life. All five exist in an interdependent continuum in the composition of the body and serve as the foundation for the integration of spirit biodynamically.

More important in our contemporary context is our own body sovereignty, meaning "I take responsibility for my body, my mind, and my spirit." It is an oath to take and keep. But how do we reclaim the sovereignty of our body-mind-spirit?

THE ELEMENTS AT THREE LEVELS

The five elements take on a variety of interpretations and levels of understanding depending on our own spiritual aptitude and cultural context. In order to reconsolidate the mind-body-spirit, we must interpret the five elements at three levels:

- the gross (physical) body of anatomy, physiology, and metabolism
- the subtle body of channels, colors, winds, and energies
- the very subtle body of pure light

The Gross Body
The first arena of reconsolidation is associated with the gross or physical body. Here is where the elements have a direct association with those readily found in the world of nature, especially trees, the whole Earth, the seas, and the sky. The elements in this way formed the original medical systems on the planet because these traditions know the relationship of our body to the world of nature. Many forms of shamanic medicine developed an arboreal map of their methodologies because trees were

objects of worship. The roots of the tree symbolized the unseen beings of the earth and water elements. The trunk of the tree symbolized the human-animal domain (comparable to the Garden of Eden), depending on fire for life. The treetop symbolized the heavenly realm of the spirit, or Shen, as it is called in classical Chinese medicine, or the domain of the gods and goddesses, and depended on wind and space. A powerful bird sits on top of the tree, representing the Breath of Life.

In similar fashion, Tibetan Buddhism offers a map of three realms in a broad cosmological sense. The first is form, wherein is found the roots of the trees and all things under the earth. Second is the realm of desire, where visible living beings, such as humans, dwell with the drive (associated with the fire element) to reproduce and its power of sexuality. (*Desire* here simply means more, which most people crave, especially when it means more of that which gives brief feelings of well-being.) Third is the formless realm of heaven and heavenly beings, such as dakinis, angels, Taras, and so forth. The cosmologies around this formless realm of gods and goddesses are elaborate and complex. Such ancient cosmologies can be accessed by prayer and meditation. They can be seen and imagined with certain practices. The visionary is medicine.

In their association with the natural world, especially the roots of trees, the five elements are domains in which categories of sentient beings live. These sentient beings are both seen and unseen, depending on the stories, legends, and myths associated with a particular culture. They can be both benevolent and wrathful. Wrathful means irritable and easily angered but also, and more importantly, protective of certain secrets, so to speak, such as those of the natural world and its healing potential. It requires initiation to learn and practice such secrets.

Think about life in the wild for early humans. For hundreds of thousands of years humans were low on the food chain, prey for the much bigger and powerful predators in the world around them. Early cultures had to figure out the meaning of life in these circumstances. These cultures had ready access to the sacredness of life on Earth and its preciousness. Gradually, those endowed with a greater spiritual aptitude, with a greater ability to see how the divine reveals itself in the natural world, became the priests and priestesses.

In the cosmologies of these spiritual traditions, it's often held that such wrathful beings need to be converted with loving kindness and compassion. Ultimately, they are projections of our own inner being. We all have inner demons. In ancient times, they were given form in images and projected out into the natural world. The natural world is a mirror of our inner perception. It always reflects our state of mind and body back to us.

For example, there were some very large animals, birds, and snakes living close to human settlements that made humans lower on the food chain. Today there are still some big snakes used as a powerful symbol of the Earth and matrilineal cultures. The Florida Everglades, the largest ecosystem in the United States, is home to the Burmese Python, which can grow to thirty feet long and weigh hundreds of pounds. They feast on large animals and are frightening to behold. Humans who live in gated communities to protect themselves from each other in economic oases still find themselves confronted with bull alligators, which eat humans several times a year in Florida. And thus primitive cultures and contemporary humans tend to project their worst states of mind onto the natural world.

At the same time one can imagine the power of seeing a rainbow in ancient times. Even today, the sight of a rainbow causes one to pause and view the majesty of the elements and their five colors. The five colors took on great significance in relation to the five elements. Some ancient peoples most likely worshipped a rainbow and gave it mystical power. Even scientific research now points out the incredible healing power of just walking in nature with unfocused attention and experiencing awe. In Japan it is called "forest bathing." In our deepest instincts we still know both the healing power of the natural world and its frightening power.

The Subtle Body

The second arena for reconsolidation of mind-body-spirit is called the subtle body. It is the spiritually integrated component of the elements in the body, consisting of channels, winds, and subtle energies. The five elements manifest as the five chakras, the five types of wind governing movement in the body, the five wisdoms, and the five colors. This is a whole world of subtlety that can be seen through various meditation practices.

At this level, the five elements take on a spiritual potency that, in both India and Tibet, is designated to be a form of the divine feminine called a dakini. Each of the five dakinis is associated with one of the colors of the rainbow. Though they represent an integrated form of the divine feminine, they can be represented by both male and female deities; they might be considered angels. The dakinis represent the potency of creation associated with sexual desire, playfulness, and its transformation into spiritual energy. Consider that the elements, the lights, and their wisdoms as detailed in my book *The Biodynamics of the Immune System* are in a type of sexual union with each other. Eastern cosmologies understand the power of sexuality and use it as a metaphor for the felt sense of the unity of mind, body, and spirit. In this way the body is viewed as a feminine vessel for the creation of life exactly the way the planet Earth is also such a vessel. In the same way, God is explained as being everything, and everything is God. All together this means that the natural world of both the Earth and of our body is divine and at the very least is sacred as a function of creation itself. The continuity of the sacred bodies of Earth and all sentient beings is the spiritual essence of mind, body, and spirit. How can we see this natural intrinsic divinity? The Buddhist scriptures tell us that in the middle of the brain (third ventricle), a channel branches away from the central channel. Its single column bifurcates and open within the eyes. The gates of this bifurcated channel appear like blossoming mango flowers and are the doorways through which the visions of clear light awareness radiate from the very subtle body (the next level From the cavity (third ventricle) of this channel, the five lights shine like peacock feathers. If we roll up our eyes to the middle of the forehead, the third ventricle gets a mechanical tug, and this ignites the potential for seeing these lights. Such visions can be deliberately generated or given spontaneously when contemplating the list below. My visions as described here occurred in the night while I was also wearing an eye mask.

- The white light appears as a god in union with the goddess of the sky element.
- The yellow light appears as a god in union with the goddess of the earth element.
- The green light appears as a god in union with the goddess of the wind.
- The red light appears as a god in union with the goddess of the fire element.
- The blue light appears as a god in union with the goddess of the water element.

The Very Subtle Body

The very subtle level of the human body is the third arena in which to reconsolidate the mind-body-spirit. The very subtle body of clear light generates the subtle body consisting of the five colors, which become the five elements imbued with the five wisdoms. These aspects of the five elements—colors, goddesses, and wisdoms—manifest as a radiance of the divine essence. It is the divine presence of clear light, of the mind of awareness existing in the formless, invisible void in the center of the human heart. Thus, the heavenly upper shamanic realm is present in the heart of all sentient beings; it comes together with the lower earth-water world of the shamans. The cosmos exists in the center of the heart. The entire universe as a sacred spirit of clear light has a throne room in the human heart.

The heart has a visible and invisible form. The visible form is the gross physical structure. The invisible form is the House of the Lord, the Empress, the Queen. The spiritual journey uncovers this preexisting spiritual essence residing in the heart. This spiritual journey is depicted in the heart meridian in Taoism, and we will examine it in the final chapter of this book.

Sometimes there is no room for spirit to live in the heart and move the blood, infusing it with its virtues. Obsessional thinking, afflictive emotions, cognitive blockages, and unrealistic views of life block the entrance to the heart's throne room of spirit in humans. Such blockages prevent virtue from expressing itself throughout the body as deep Health. The exploration of the five elements within these three arenas of integrated spiritual function is cosmological, physiological, and metabolic in the human body. The contemplative practice is to overcome the duality of inside and outside realities. We need help reconsolidating the five elements, allowing them to become the five spiritual potencies of the dakini goddesses and the five colors radiating the wisdom of clear light through the blood, the body, and the skin. All appearance in the universe originates from a single fulcrum or throne room inside the human heart. Some people call it the fifth chamber of the heart because honeybees have a fifth heart chamber. It is metaphorical. And if grief so enlarges the left ventricle of the heart to experience greater love, then perhaps the left ventricle is the throne room. A heart filled with spirit can radiate the universe and perceive it as a unified whole. Ultimately, all perception in this integrated mind-body-spiritual approach to healing derives exclusively from the inside dimension of the human heart, where spirit mind resides and fuels the body via the blood with radiant virtue. When ordinary mind of constant thinking is diminished, the subtle mind of spirit can manifest in the heart.

Thus, the heart has three dimensions/arenas/realms that include the physical tangible heart, the subtle heart of visionary appearances, and the formless, invisible, yet tangible throne room inside the heart. The five elements are a road map to the heart. This formless heart existing inside as a fulcrum of dynamic radiant stillness is bliss. Bliss is freedom from obsessional thinking, afflicted emotions, cognitive blockages, and unrealistic views. This is peace, happiness, and love.

ⱺⱥ
The Five Elemental Colors
⌁ A Visualization Practice ⌁

This visualization is to be done in the middle of the night when the bedroom is dark. As you lie in bed, visualize each of the five rainbow colors—white, blue, yellow, red, and green—slowly and sequentially arising inside the heart, then radiating through your body, then radiating through the bedroom. Remember that the practice should be done very slowly.

Notice if the bedroom can be filled with the glow of the color. If a radiant glow does not remain in the bedroom, move on to the next color radiating from your heart. Usually one color will remain with its residue lingering, as if it were alive. At some point one of the colors that is glowing in the room will generate the appearance of the Divine Feminine. It may manifest spontaneously, like a mirage. You can also request an appearance and visualize which area of the room she appears in. However she shows up for you, she is imbued with the essence of the universal divine feminine and the originality of the cosmos in its most essential form.

Each of the colors has a different quality. This means that there may be a mind transmission—a conversation happening in your mind with the divine presence. There can be personal instructions given to you and also engagement with her hands and body in relation to your body. Allow her to come alive and then to dissipate on her own terms.

APPARITIONS OF THE TWENTY-ONE TARAS

I experience auditory and visual hallucinations. They are a typical side effect in the PTSD cluster of symptoms. The result of having such hallucinations is a sense of fear and dread; it's like having a nightmare. Through therapy, I came to realize my hallucinations are generated by fear. Fortunately, there are contemplative practices in Tibetan Buddhism to directly work with the reduction of endogenous fear from any source. It is a practice that confronts the fear of death in a very traditional Eastern way. One practice is to meditate in a graveyard, which I did every day for over a year. Another is to visualize your own death, with a mantra practice that goes along with it. After a year of such practice, the auditory and visual hallucinations were transformed into mystical experiences, as follows.

In September 2021, while in Italy on a holiday, I was lying in bed realizing how much fear my body holds. It escalated to a sense of bone chilling immobilizing terror coming from inside myself. I began to sense my heart and breath. Then the colors came spontaneously, and I was visited by a series of Tara goddesses, and the night terror left. I'll describe my experiences here, and you can very easily find more information on the twenty-one Taras online. They are goddesses initiating and healing me.

Blue Tara #7: She Who Conquers

It starts with the Blue Tara #7. Her first appearance in the middle of the night gives me relief from my sense of primordial fear—a deep fear that clearly resides in the marrow of my bones and is ancient beyond any transgenerational family imprint. With the initial contact that unfolded and with the subsequent visits, she immerses her vajra hands into the marrow of my cranial bones and holds my head for me. I feel the support as my entire cranium loses its anatomy and dissolves into the subtle body. (Vajra hands refers to their transparent shimmering brightness of the sacred.)

Gradually the elements as I know them—earth, water, fire, wind, and space—gently dissolve and disappear, leaving simply the outer shell of my body, which is completely transparent and empty of any tangible physical reality yet exists as a subtle human outline. Slowly I am informed with luminosity. The container of my body spontaneously and sequentially manifests five lights: white, blue, yellow, red, and green. They represent the five Buddhist wisdom families that are the origin of the five elements in the Indo-Tibetan system. The lights precede the elements and thus are the intermediate origin of the elements.

The lights appear to be gaseous, like the warp core in a *Star Trek* starship or a lava lamp. With a unified sense of form and emptiness, they seem tangible, with an aliveness, rather than just luminous. In this way they are visibly moving and yet intangible clouds, a beautiful unfolding weather pattern driven by the element of wisdom wind of PR in the empty shell of my body. While the lights are moving inside the frame of my body, they are at the same time luminous and radiating beyond the outer frame of my body. I have no skin but rather an etheric membrane, the thickness of an atom, a translucent luminosity that is just barely perceptual. My mind wanders off, just like in zazen, and I must return to the visualization. I am learning from Blue Tara #7 how first to be empty of anatomy and then gradually to perceive the lived quality and totality of the five lights as the inner subtle reality at the core of my body.

While the inside of my body has dissolved, simultaneously I sense a wholeness, an interconnectedness without structure. My attention is finally directed to my heart. Her last instructions from this first visit are simply to have the five colors radiating from my heart and filling the universe. Thus the protocol is:

1. Sense the living presence of the sacred in the marrow of my cranial bones.
2. Allow the marrow to be clear light.
3. Disappear the anatomical structure of my body from the top down, starting with the brain,
4. Fill the empty container of my body with clouds of the five lights sequentially.
5. Notice the radiance and luminosity of the five lights extending beyond the form.
6. Center attention in the heart. Radiate the colors from that source and fill the universe.

Yellow Tara #3: Lady of Golden Yellow

The next night, Yellow Tara appears. She is the Tara of abundance and a reminder that all manifestation is abundance. She is ocher in color. She begins with her hands immersed in the marrow of my cranial bones. Her lesson this evening is to allow me to see and sense the complete abundance, as if magical, that is our planet, solar system, and universe. I feel an expansiveness and an interconnection to everything.

Green Tara #9: She Who Protects from Fear

The following evening, Green Tara appears. She begins with her hands immersed in the marrow of my cranial bones. She informs me, "You will accomplish your death." A great peace overtakes me and permeates my mind and body.

Red Tara #5: She Who Proclaims the Sound of HUM

The following evening, Red Tara appears. She begins with her hands immersed in the marrow of my cranial bones. Her form dissolves into the central channel of my subtle body. She is the red tigle, the red droplet or vital essence of Ultimate Bodhicitta that will descend into my heart at the moment of my death.

Blue Tara #14: She Who Is Frowning Wrathfully

The next day, I visited Instituto Llama Tsongkapa in Italy. We are given a private showing of the Temple of Chenrezig, a small temple dedicated to the bodhisattva of compassion. His Holiness the Dalai Lama is the reincarnation of Chenrezig. I am given the blessing of the twenty-one Taras to confirm the validity of my nightly visitations from them. I feel their power and majesty. I feel how my heart and body are constructed by them. I am immensely grateful.

That evening, Blue Tara, the Lady of Death, visits me. She instructs me that the void is the starting place for all healing. The void is the absolute ending of the previous universe, from which the wisdom wind containing the seed of karmic residue from the previous universe spontaneously moves to start a new universe. She tells me: Rest in the black form and the black color. Wait for the central channel to clarify the clear light that is the core of the very subtle body. Wait for the spark that is spontaneous, a friction between the power of the wind element and the power of the fire element necessary for ignition. The karmic residue carries the fire of associated realms of unresolved delusions of all sentient beings. There is spontaneous combustion as the elements join into a new form—and thus, a new universe. The five elements arise out of the five lights, which arise out of the clear light. That is the sequence of development.

Red Tara #16: She Who Arises from the HUNG

On a following evening, another Tara appears in her red form. Her instructions help me visualize the channels of the subtle body superimposed within the physical body. I learn how to visualize the color and shape of the central channel, which is blue in relation to anatomical structures. Upon exiting at DU 22, an acupuncture point on the top of the head, the central channel continues through the top of the head so that the eighth chakra above the head is where Vajradhara, the primordial Buddha, is visualized to be in union with a consort. At the appropriate moment that image descends through the funnel and down the central channel into the heart.

Red Tara #13: She Who Blazes Like Fire

On the following evening, a Red Tara appears. She teaches me to disappear and dissolve all the cells in my body except those of the cardiovascular system, including the blood. I am given instructions to form an image of the vascular tree and shown how Shen, the deepest spiritual component of the element of wind, in its most refined spiritual sense, infuses the blood from the back of the heart. This is the highest spiritual essence of the chi.

Slowly she helps me dissolve and melt all the blood in my vascular system into the life channel of the aorta, descending aorta, and abdominal aorta. Then she shows me how the right channel, the red channel of the subtle body, is formed. And then she dissolves the right channel of the subtle body into the red tigle of Bodhicitta that exists above the heart in a central channel. I learn how to purify the right channel of my subtle body.

Next I am given instructions on proper hand placement. The therapist's hands always start in the marrow, the origin. The first focus is on the marrow of the cranial bones, especially the parietal bones. Then the therapist visualizes the disappearance and dissolving of all brain structures. I am given a sequence of contact with the bones, the marrow, the interstitium and capillary beds, and the fascia and lymphatic beds; this is the metabolic evaluation sequence linked to the five elements in Tibetan medicine.

Next she gives instruction on the five lights. The clear light or the white light is specifically pearlescent. It is a bright moon on a cloudless night reflecting on the water. This pearl light dissolves into the left channel with the five skandhas (visual form, sensation-feeling, perceptions, concepts and world views, and consciousnesses). The blue light dissolves into the central channel of the subtle body. The yellow light of complete abundance radiates from the back of the heart. The red light of the future Buddha dissolves into the right channel, also with the skandhas. The green light is the totality of human consciousness existing in the heart at death. It is ejected out the top of the central channel during the Phowa ceremony of meditating on the moment of death into the red Amitabha Buddha of the future sitting above the head in the position of the eighth chakra.

Green Tara #9: She Who Protects from Fear

Green Tara first appears after I arrive home from Italy in late October. She is outside and comes through a wall to the inside of my bedroom and stands right by the side of my bed. She then moves around to the foot of the bed. I am lying on my back. Without any feeling or sense of fear, I invite her to come close. She enters me and I become a luminescent green. The form of my body inside and out is only a luminescent green. Her mind is of complete generosity and wisdom. She is inside me. We are united in the bliss of emptiness. No elements are present, only her luminescent green radiating through my form. She whispers in my ear, "Be confident." This advice occurs the night before I am to have an interview with the dean of the program I am working with regarding critical comments I had made in a group email. The next day, I am able to relay my feedback and rationale with calm and confidence.

Yellow Tara #4: Lady of Complete Victory

On the following evening, Yellow Tara appears. She assists me in visualizing the location of my heart and pericardium, but especially in differentiating the anterior and posterior embryonic fields that develop the heart. With her help, the posterior cardiac fields become a bright yellow. The color appears as a halo in the back of my heart radiating Shen, the highest form of spiritual chi. At times the halo is the dorsal pericardium and then the original dorsal mesocardium of the embryo. And then my heart appears to be the actual head of the Buddha and the yellow dorsal pericardium is the Buddha's halo, the center of which is the fifth thoracic vertebra.

Blue Tara #7: She Who Conquers

It is the middle of the night, around 2 or 3 a.m. This is Blue Tara #7's second visitation with me. I am home in my own bed, lying on my left side. I sense her presence and place my attention on calming my mind. My eyes are closed when she appears. She is very close to my bed. She has a smile and is not only radiating her vajra blue color but also projecting benevolence. All week long I've been in the grip of primordial fear, having been triggered with PTSD in a training the week before. As with previous visits, she reaches out with her hands and embeds them in the marrow of my cranial bones. I see a hint of blue radiating from my cranium. I feel relief from the fear at the core of my overactivated survival instinct. I initiate a conversation of gratitude for her help, and she says, "Of course," and then continues to radiate benevolence through me via her hands and presence. I lose concentration and roll onto my right side. I regain concentration and she is still there and comes into union with me through the back of my body. She completely embeds her presence and her etheric body in my brain and neural tube. I see my entire central nervous system, including the dural covering, cerebrospinal spinal fluid, and bony coverings, all radiating blue. I can feel a deeper relaxation occurring, and it brings a quality of pleasure that is subtle but nonetheless pleasureful. I am in union with her, or more accurately, she is in union with me inside my body.

Now I am given teachings about the five Buddha families, which represent a cycle of psychological states starting with the open awareness of space (Buddha white), the pacifying boundless clear energy of the universe (vajra blue), the expansiveness and enriching energy of the universe (ratna yellow), the separating and magnetizing energy of the decline of the universe (padma red), and the dissolving and destructive energy of the universe (karma green).

I am able to maintain my concentration and invite a teaching from her. What do you want to show me? I see the sagittal plane of my body, and she turns my esophagus the color green, the color of the karma family. Last week the yellow Tara showed me the yellow halo of my dorsal pericardium that is the halo of the Buddha's head that is my heart. My literal heart is actually the head of the Buddha. This time Blue Tara #7 shows me that all the coelomic sacs of the embryo are yellow. The entire pericardium, pleura, and peritoneum are now the color of the ratna family. Then she shows me, starting with my descending aorta, the color red. We slowly go through the entire cardiovascular system, including the heart itself, the descending and abdominal aorta, and the complete capillary system. This is the padma family.

Then I wonder about the Buddha family, associated with a pearlescent white. She starts where she has always begun her teaching with me, and that is in the marrow of my cranium. I see the marrow radiating like a pearl. She then takes me directly to my lower dantian, an ancestral power center below the umbilicus in the abdomen and I see the pearl of my lower dantian beginning to radiate throughout my abdomen and whole body. From there, she guides me through my entire skeletal system, from my cranium down to the bones of my feet, and every bone in my body begins to light up like a radiating moon. I lie there seeing and feeling my body as a field of radiating moonlight. I feel a blessing beyond belief.

We take some time to review the locations of the other colors she has shown to me. We then both agree that this is quite enough transformation to be with for the moment. All fear has disappeared. I am now radiating a rainbow body that simultaneously has a core of moonlight that is all pervasive in the form of my existing body. I am now nothing but a rainbow body with a core of clear light.

I wake up to a newsletter from Khenpo Tsultrim Gyamtso Rinpoche with his quote of the week:

> *No matter what thoughts occur, if good or bad*
> *No matter what feelings are felt, if pleasant or not*
> *Knowing them all to be the clear light mind*
> *Let them be, like an ocean would its waves.*

White Tara #19: She Who Alleviates All Suffering

At night, White Tara appears. As she does with every initiation, she places her hands inside the marrow of my cranial bones. My marrow instantly turns to clear light. This time it is brighter. She then proceeds to place her hands in every single bone of my body. From the cranium, she places her hands in my clavicles and ribs. From there, she places her hands inside both of my hip bones and then each of the vertebra. From there, she goes down through each leg all the way down to the bones of the feet. With each movement, a bright clear light, a pearlescent luminous moon, begins to shine from wherever she had placed her hands. When she finishes, I lie there radiating clear light from my entire skeletal system. She then allows me to see the void at the moment of death as a black space filling the inside of my body, underneath the clear light, so to speak. So I lie there radiating clear light from my skeleton. The rest of my body is nonexistent; I see it with awareness as simply blackness or a darkness without life. The void is the ending of the last universe and the ending of this life when the body dies. This is the essence of origin. I ask her if there is a further teaching associated with this initiation. She says this is the entrance to the bardo. The bardo is the transition that occurs at the moment of death. I lie there in bed contemplating my experience of the clear light and the void of no physical body. I feel totally comfortable and at peace with death. I ask her if there is anything else. She replies, "I think this is quite enough for the moment."

In the morning, while practicing the Kalachakra tantra liturgy during meditation, I visualize Machig Labdron from her tangka directly in front of my meditation cushion. Machig Labdron is the patron saint of Tibetan Buddhism because she is the only person to start her own unique lineage of Tibetan Buddhism associated with severance of all fear by visualizing one's own death. Images of her are painted onto canvases and called tangkas. I visualize her in union with Vajradhara and the two coming together down through the central channel into my heart. From there, I typically visualize the five lights radiating from my heart or through my body. However, this morning clear light begins to shine from inside my heart, radiating outward, filling the whole of the universe. Then each of the remaining five lights spontaneously begins radiating with a brilliant luminosity from my heart.

Machig Labdron

For two evenings in a row Machig Labron appears. On the first evening, she starts just as the Taras do, with her hands in my cranium. Her very essence is pearlescent clear light and I am receiving that transmission from her. All the marrow in my bones gradually lights up as her hands go through each of my bones with clear light. The empowerment I am receiving is on how to achieve what is called the rainbow body. She shows me each of the colors radiating from the clear light in the marrow. I wonder how all five colors can manifest at once. She has me rest in the water element of my Hara, or abdomen, in order to contemplate this visualization. I feel the rhythmic movement of my fluid body centered in the lower dantian.

On the second evening, we go through the same process and she gives me the instructions for looking in the biosphere that surrounds the human body like a cloud, a warm wet field of moisture that can refract the five colors like a rainbow and manifests the appearance of the rainbow body. She had given me a glimpse of that on the first evening, and on this second evening it becomes clearer that all five colors are being refracted through Zone B. I am given only a brief glimpse. I come back to the fluid body in the lower dantian, feeling the rhythmic waves of motion inside the body. They are colorless, a darkness or blackness, yet moving.

I question the difference between the five lights manifesting from the heart and the lights manifesting from the marrow through Zone B. I question the difference between the Five Buddha Families and the five colors, if there is such a difference.

I am directed to the upper dantian of the third ventricle of the brain in order to see and sense my rainbow body. It starts with sensing the pearl, the moon of clear light, coming from the lower dantian. Then I move to sensing the heart, the middle dantian, and the five lights of the Five Buddha Families manifesting sequentially from the heart. Then I am sensing the upper dantian as a sphere of water. Rolling the eyes up to the middle of the forehead places a slight tug on the optic chiasm and stimulates the upper dantian. It is from this place that the field of vision expands to include Zone B and the ability to see the prism effect of the clear light radiating through the warm wet fluid cloud of Zone B surrounding the body. It is here, after aligning the lower and middle dantian, that I am given a glimpse of the rainbow body in Zone B.

Green Tara

She appears for three consecutive evenings. Each evening is about allowing her green radiance to permeate me. As with all the Taras, she begins by sinking her hands into my cranium. On the final night, she stands at the foot of the bed and begins to move toward me, coming to lie down on top of me. At first I experience fear, but then I receive a transmission to let go of my fear, and her body completely permeates and is absorbed into me and my subtle body.

ⵯ

Meditation on the Five Elements

This contemplative visualization and breathing practice uses the five Indo-Tibetan elements (space, wind, fire, water, earth) inherent within the element of space to purify the gross elements inside the body with color (Norbu 1999). This leads to the possibility of recognizing clear light in the deepest void space of the heart within the heart. When the elements are coupled with their origin in the element of space—earth space, water space, fire space, wind space, and the space of space—the visualization is like seeing a morning mist entering and leaving your body.

1. Begin by visualizing yourself inhaling clean, clear, fresh yellow earth air/space. Allow this yellow earth air/space to come in through the nose, into the lungs, down into the belly, and then through the entire body. Upon exhalation, visualize

the exiting breath as a smoky or grayish color, which is a sign of the cleansing and detoxification process going on within the subtle body inside. Repeat three to five times.

2. Visualize yourself inhaling clean, clear white water space. Allow this white water space to come in through the nose, into the lungs, and then permeate the entire cardiovascular system as it merges with all the blood in the body. Imagine turning the color of blood to white. Upon exhalation, visualize a hazy grayish color like a mist leaving your nostrils. Repeat three to five times.

3. Visualize yourself inhaling clean, clear red fire space. Allow this red fire space to come in through the nose, into the lungs, and then fill the heart, where the deepest essence of the fire element and its sacredness is located. From there, this red color descends into the abdomen, surrounding the liver, kidneys, stomach, spleen, and intestines. Allow the exhalation to be simple; visualizing it having a smoky color will enhance the purification process. Repeat three to five times.

4. Visualize yourself inhaling clean, clear green wind space. This time, imagine you are inhaling this clear green wind space from above your body, down through the top of your head and down the central channel of your body, which is located between your spine and descending aorta. Allow this wind to permeate the whole body and, like a mist in the early morning, dissipating out every pore of the skin. Upon exhalation, visualize a smoky, hazy grayish color exiting your nostrils. Repeat three to five times.

5. Finally, visualize yourself inhaling the beautiful, clear deep blue space of space. This time, imagine you are inhaling this beautiful blue color through the front sternum of the body and directly into the heart. It leaves a dark blue shimmering radiance in the heart inside the heart. This dark blue begins to glow and radiate a powerful light extending in all directions. With each exhalation, dullness and lethargy leave the body as a smoky gray color passing out through the sternum. Repeat three to five times.

As you become more familiar with this visualization, you can deepen the practice to allow all the colors to rest in the heart. Allow the heart to become each of the five colors associated with the five elements.

If the practice seems too complicated, simply breathe in each color and transform your heart into that color for three to five cycles of breathing.

Sometimes visualizing the hazy grayish waste product can be challenging. If that is the case, use each exhalation as a vent for any negative thoughts; just allow the negative thoughts to exit your body through your nose. They exit while riding the wind of exhalation. How easy it is.

I leave you with my interpretation of a Buddhist poem.

It's All Basically Good*

Illness and its painfulness have neither cause nor origin.
Relax into it, fresh and uncontrived,
Revealing an essence way beyond all speech and thought.
Don't shun them; pain and illness are basically good.

Just as conception, birth, old age, and death
Have no beginning and never end,
Nothing exists without everything else.
Here today, gone tomorrow. It's all good.

The confusion that's occurring is negative forces at work.
But it's your own mind of awareness, simple, unborn, unceasing.
Without anxiety or even worrying at all,
Don't shun them; demons and gods are basically good.

Emotions are islands in the stream.
The stream goes around them;
A body is perturbed by them and fixates.
You are free to choose which style; both are basically good.

When the agony of illness strikes your body systems,
Don't grasp at stopping it; don't get angry when it won't improve.
Such adversities have the flavor of bliss that's free of the contagion's blight.
These emotional extremes are not to be shunned; they're basically good.

Sensation is the voice of the body, ebbing and flowing.
Breathing flows on, out and back.
The whole world stops in between.
Stop and go, out and back, what's the difference?

---

*Based on "Eight Cases of Basic Goodness Not to Be Shunned," by Gyalwa Gotsangpa (thirteenth century CE); original translation and arrangement by Jim Scott (1997), under the guidance of Khenpo Tsultrim Gyamtso Rinpoche.

All the joy and the pain we go through, all our highs and lows,
When seen through, have no substance; they are our friends.
Don't try to stop pain; don't try to be happy; be free of all hope and fear.
Intense dissatisfaction is not to be shunned; it's basically good.

Empathy and compassion make the world go around.
So do anger and rage, not to mention sex.
The embryo creates temporary boundaries necessary for growing.
Adults needlessly defend the boundaries. Both styles are basically good.

And though this whole life is frequently plagued by the torments of falling ill,
Don't think that's bad; don't plan to get around it.
Avoidance will become your badge, your proof of suffering.
Yet your suffering's not to be shunned; it's basically good.

Enemies, naysayers, and obstructionists abound.
Resistance happens; make space for nature to twist and turn.
Pause, don't move, become the center of a friendly world.
Only offer your heart; take it out of your body and give it away.

There's a Hindu story about Krishna that I like in which Krishna says, "Whoever wishes to follow the spiritual path, I will give them the tools to follow the spiritual path, and whoever wishes to not follow the spiritual path, I will give them the tools to not follow the spiritual path." Now we are finished with part 2. In part 3, we will explore embodiment through interoceptive awareness, and I will present important suggestions for reframing PTSD and trauma.

PART 3

INSTINCTS, METABOLISM, AND EMBODIMENT

17

Embodied Evolution

The different stages in evolution are each characterized by the appearance of a new structural principle. The new design enables the species to expand its habitat and to multiply, often at the expense of the original species. The new development is not reversible.

ULRICH DREWS, *COLOR ATLAS OF EMBRYOLOGY, 134.*

I ask myself: Can I know my body as an evolutionary organism made of stardust? This chapter and several that follow explore the life-giving and life-sustaining properties of the human body in perpetual evolution. Scientists have deduced that sponges were the first lineage to separate from all the other animals. These results suggest that our ancestors were simple creatures like sponges, feeding by filtering tiny particles from the water—an early map of the function of the human gut. Though 750 million years have elapsed since our evolutionary split, sponges have changed relatively little since then, so they provide a window into our past. Now we are very different from sponges, but at some point in the past we did share a common ancestor (Feuda et al. 2017).

OUR INSTINCTUAL NATURE

Since the beginning of cosmological time, when the first organisms appeared on Earth, life on this planet has relied on three primary instincts: to be nurtured (self-preservation), to detoxify (self-healing), and to grow (self-transcendence). They are a part of the underlying drive that makes us human and the core of origination that we share with all sentient beings, to some degree. Some say that this instinctual nature started four billion years ago with acellular organisms, of which there are many in residence in our body.

All organisms, no matter how primitive or complex, operate with the pleasure-pain principle at the core of our instincts: We move toward that which is nourishing and away from that which is irritating. We move toward that which feeds us, from food to love to spirituality with the seen and unseen world, and away from that which does not nourish or is fearful. And though this innate capacity driving our organism can be damaged, it can also be repaired or reinvigorated.

Comparative embryology teaches us that the human embryo shares a structural similarity in its stages of development with the earliest organisms on the planet. As sentient beings, we need to rekindle our innate capacity to naturally relate with the unseen world, which is both microscopic and ancient. This relationship with the whole of our environment internally and externally has been present from the very beginnings of life on our planet. Imagine being present for such creation. It was divine and still is.

Self-Preservation: Evolution of the Nervous System

The instinct for self-preservation is primary in the human organism, having helped our earliest ancestors survive by learning, through trial and error over a long period of time, what to accept and what to reject. After all, even that which seems to nourish can prove false. Eventually, our instinct for self-preservation transitioned to the physical structure of a nervous system. Some say this happened just 500 million years ago—a relatively short leap back in our evolution.

The first step toward any nervous system was the creation of an organizing midline, called the notochord, which eventually evolved into our spine and specifically the nucleus pulposus of the intervertebral discs. This slowed the organism down, which could be dangerous, but it allowed for greater nutrient density to be ingested from the environment. When the filtration net of the organism stiffens it slows down the flow through of nutrient. When nutrient can stay longer, a greater breakdown of the nutrient can occur extracting more nutrient and causing greater growth. In this way nutrient density requires specialization for digestion, assimilation, and elimination vital to human instincts. Though not without risks, and needing evolutionary time to solve problems via the genetic mutation pathway, the organizing midline proved a great long-term strategy. Stephen Porges (2023) discusses this in detail in his elaboration of polyvagal theory.

It wasn't until the lamprey eel came along around 450 million years ago that we could get a sense of the next step in the evolution toward a mammalian nervous system. This eel has a much better integrated neural circuit, allowing it to immediately assess pleasure versus pain, along with a greater ability to move, especially in an aquatic environment. That circuit evolved into the reticular formation of the anterior brain stem and spinal cord. In this way, the organism could use its more sophisticated proprioception to move toward that which was nourishing and then use all available proprioception and motor skills to move away from that which was irritating or non-nourishing.

Then came the triune brain. In the slow evolutionary development from the reticular formation, we gained the brain stem for differentiated defensive and aggressive maneuvers for self-preservation and self-healing. Then came the midbrain for differentiating emotional responsiveness for a better chance at longevity and raising children. Finally came the cortex or frontal lobes, the newest part, serving as the executive control center. The nervous system then needed hundreds and hundreds of thousands of years for that development to have an innate capacity to downregulate emotions and maintain inner and outer social harmony.

Self-Transcendence: God

The instinct for self-transcendence, also derived from the originality of pleasure and pain, involves the parietal lobe of the cortex, which is vital for sensory perception and integration, including the management of taste, hearing, sight, touch, and smell. It is home to the brain's primary somatic sensory cortex, a region in which the brain interprets input from other areas of the body.

Activity in the left inferior part of the parietal cortex, an area of the brain involved in awareness of self and others, as well as attention processing, seems to be a common element among individuals who have experienced a variety of spiritual experiences, according to some studies (Hardy 1979). I saw on the cover of a Time magazine some years ago the discovery of a "God module" in the human brain that derives from the fact that epileptic seizures in the left temporal lobe are associated with ecstatic feelings sometimes described as an experience of the presence of God. If a seizure creates a spiritual fulcrum, then shock and trauma have the same potential. The point is that prayers and contemplative practices affect the same area of the brain across religious platforms.

Homo sapiens and related species, such as the Neanderthal, about one hundred thousand to two hundred thousand years ago, had burial rituals that most anthropologists agree represent a differentiated spiritual or self-transcendent instinct of the *Homo sapiens* lineage. But if mammals evolved three hundred million years ago, then how is it possible that self-transcendence started only later with the development of the frontal lobes of the brain? This instinct—to move toward that which is fulfilling and to honor those with whom we are connected, even a bacteria—must have been present since the beginning of our planet. The nature of loss has been present from the very beginning. All living organisms on planet Earth since the very beginning were and are sentient in some form, and they would have this potential for self-transcendence. In this way, all sentient organisms know the whole. Each human cell also knows the whole of all the cells in the body. This is human biology. That's divine!

Self-Healing: Repair

Much of what we do with our contemporary clients who are metabolically challenged (including 93 percent of Americans) is palliative. Repair and restoration are a big job for the body's metabolism, especially when political, corporate, and medical systems are broken. It is coupled with the continual degradation of anatomy, physiology, and metabolism from processed food and reactive emotions, causing some scientists to state that important parts of our microbiome (think beginning of time on the planet) are becoming extinct, making our intestinal milieu uninhabitable. This leads to multiple organ failure, heart disease, dementia, many psychological problems, and death. We live in the microbial world. They do not live in our world. They outnumber us at a cellular level in the human body.

Biodynamic work potentiates a spiritual fulcrum. Synchronizing our perception with Primary Respiration (PR) and the stillness is the context of the whole. We exist in this ocean of perception at the elemental level cosmologically. This biodynamic spiritual fulcrum enhances and supports the self-transcendent instinct of all beings, including humans. However, as one of my teachers told me, "Not all clients want to see God." And that's okay. PR does the choosing of where to go and what to treat rather than the therapist. The first development of biodynamic treatment is to engage the self-healing instinct of the body. A Neutral takes place as the central (brain) and cardiovascular systems of the client and therapist synchronize to establish mutual safety. The Neutral is the autonomic nervous system of the client reducing its defensive physiology just enough to shift towards self-healing. From there, PR chooses whether to engage the instinct for self-preservation and metabolic dysfunction or the instinct for self-transcendence for spiritual support. How wonderful that all three instincts are engaged biodynamically! Sometimes all three instincts are being enhanced and supported. As therapists we do not have to know how to or even try to direct PR. It's enough to know that holding presence with the exchange of PR and the stillness as a balanced interchange of a single wholeness, a vast ocean of possibility, allows our ancient instincts to ignite and express coherence. Our instincts know how to automatically shift for optimal benefit to our body, mind, and spirit. We are touching much more than a nervous system in biodynamic practice. We are always touching the beginninglessness of time. That beginninglessness is always available in the present moment.

EPIGENETICS

The microbiome is intimately related to the function of our epigenetics. The epigenome is a sleeve that surrounds the DNA in what is called a methylation zone. It controls what aspect of our DNA is expressed. Epigenetics can be seen as sheet music, needing a well-calibrated, well-tuned orchestra for proper expression. But all the orchestra's instruments are provided by the last meal we ate. The orchestra starts playing the sheet music (the epigenome) with the instruments they were just provided. If we ate ultraprocessed carbohydrates with all sorts of chemical additives, including added sugar (a dose-dependent chemical toxin), the sound is horrible and off-key because the genes that are expressed are not those that are needed for proper metabolic digestion, absorption, and elimination. Thus metabolic syndrome begins to gestate.

We all inherit a particular set of sheet music from the beginning of time. We have DNA for type 2 diabetes (hyperinsulinemia), obesity arising from starvation studies in our ancestors, cancer (gene mutations, the majority of which are caused by a poor diet and wrecked intestines), and more. Whichever form of disease is prevalent in your parents' lineages lives on in you only as a potential. And then there are dementia and Alzheimer's, in which brain cells are constipated from ultraprocessed food. Some authors call such memory disorders type 3 diabetes.

The epithelium that lines the gut is an endocrine organ and immune system modulator; it controls gut permeability, identifies threats, and coregulates the metabolism required for homeostasis in the body. The ingestion of ultraprocessed food is so devastating to the gut endothelium that complex inflammatory processes continually recapitulate and spread to the endothelium of the cardiovascular system. The microbiome in the gut degrades, and our indigenous connection to our planetary origin erodes. The breakdown of the epithelium is then mitigated by the endothelium of the vascular tree, liver, spleen, and heart. Epigenetically, the endothelium can change its cellular shape and function from quiescent to hyperactive to interrupt blood flow. This means that systemic endothelial inflammation greatly interferes with the proper exchange of nutrients. (So, in a biodynamic session, when we palpate the artery, the most important metabolic part of the human endocrine system that we can touch is the endothelium. And it is covered with fascia, muscle fibers, and houses blood flow. These are the three basic levels of artery palpation, as we'll cover in chapter 24.)

The liver is a major player in the conversion of our food into energy for the mitochondria. These ancient nonhuman organs in every cell produce the energy we need to live; they lie at the core of our instinct for self-preservation. Once the barrier is breached in the epithelial lining of the intestines, the liver must work overtime to deal with excessive levels of irregular, undigestible molecules (hyperinsulinemia). It turns many of them into fat cells, which are inflammatory cells. Obesity is a visual example of the inflammatory process, expanding the size of the human body. And since the inflammatory process originates in the gut, we have to look at other factors, such as the client's trauma history and so forth, and the other comorbid impacts on the gut. Everyone has their own unique epigenetic sheet music, and the physiological orchestra needs the right instruments to play a melodious tune for metabolic health. Every client is unique and individual in their instinctual unfolding if they choose to shift from palliative care to self-healing care. And that is the third instinct, the instinct for self-healing, the starting point of a biodynamic session.

When we eat processed food and ignite inflammation, the brain starts to lose optimal function. There is so much continual daytime sensory information, and the brain is like a flight simulator that pilots use when they're practicing flying on the ground. With dementia and Alzheimer's, the flight simulator is in really bad condition from a plane crash. Yet it is still giving a signal because we are not dead yet, and the black box from the crash went to the bottom of the ocean and it's going to take some work to recover it. The recovery and restoration of the human intestinal system requires diligence, support, and a change in lifestyle. Ultimately water and fasting are the best medicine. The next level of medicine is already in your backyard or close to where you live. Every plant in the area where you live can be medicine. The instinct for self-healing involves relating with the unseen world as all our original ancestors did through recorded time. When we eat real food, as endocrinologist Robert Lustig calls it (2022), we form a relationship with the innate sentience of plants and animals, just as our indigenous ancestors did. Self-preservation becomes tempered with self-transcendence and self-healing. This is the starting point to repair our relationship with our origin and the unseen. It is deep. It is old. And it is inside us already as the microbiome.

LIFE FORCES

Everything we eat gets broken down to a molecular level through numerous pathways to support the instinctual processes of self-preservation, self-healing, and self-transcendence. This all occurs in a microbial milieu supported by the blood, an aspect of our fluid body in biodynamic practice. There are also physical forces at play, embodied metaphors for our vitality because they move our vitality. The wind element, Primary Respiration, the Breath of Life, the Tide, the long tide, the primary respiratory impulse, chi—these are all descriptions of the wide variety of life forces. Biodynamic practitioners are fond of comparing to ancient slime molds made of protoplasm. They move the protein building blocks from the genes to the extracellular space, and without them, we would all be dead. They drive metabolism. They power the blood.

The delivery system for nutrients throughout the body is first and foremost the cardiovascular system. And there is a lot of molecular and cellular traffic in the cardiovascular system. It contains hundreds of different cells, a unique microbiome, and precious oxygen, glucose, and ketones, the fundamental triad of fuel for the human organism's instinctual needs. And the brain prefers ketones to glucose.

As noted earlier, the endothelium is an endocrine organ and an immune system modulator. It is highly receptive and protective at the immune level. With inflammatory processes coming from the gut endothelium, the immune system floods the bloodstream. The endothelium has a limited repertoire of protection for itself; its only recourse is to stiffen, just like a muscle does when injured. Its cells lose their quiescence and become hyperactive, causing leakage of different-size molecules, which further pressures the immune system. When under stress, the immune system at that level of the endothelium will shut off nitric oxide (NO), which is the sympathetic vasodilator of the artery. This is the metabolism of the sympathetic nervous system. The artery is traumatized metabolically via the sympathetic nervous system. The artery has stretch receptors, as it needs to expand to meet the demands of its endpoint organ sites, and when it loses that ability to dilate and can only contract, its blood flow becomes erratic. Blood flow, which is spiral in nature, becomes staccato and stutters constantly, which causes a significant interruption in the whole-body energy metabolism and (over time) increases in blood pressure, kidney problems, and so forth. Inflammation in this way can gestate metabolic syndrome.

QUIESCENCE

What is common to all three primary instincts is that they serve the requirement for periods of quiescence for proper metabolic functioning. This quiescence is known by many names—the Neutral, the stillpoint, the gap, the pause, and other metaphors that indicate a period of stillness and silence. It is extremely valuable in relationship to the instinct of self-healing but for the other instincts as well. At the molecular level, scaled across the universe, all molecules are related to each other in their function of transmutation—everything is constantly becoming something else. Molecular transmutation is the very core of our biochemical metabolic processes, which are driven by the self-preservation instinct. In the transmutation from one molecule to another, there is a stillpoint—a moment of quiescence, of stopping, of neutrality. We must pause and intersperse periods of quiescence for biology to function well. It is safe to assume that such quiescence has been with us since the very beginning of the smallest biological organisms. And thus dynamic stillness is the essence of instinctual transmutation, then and now.

META-ORGANIZATION OF
THE AUTONOMIC NERVOUS SYSTEM

The self-preservation instinct is built on conscious interoceptive awareness. Interoception, the felt sense of the body's internal physiological-metabolic states, underpins homeostatic reflexes (both visceral-somato and somato-visceral), motivational states (especially hunger), and sensations (contributing to a wide spectrum of emotional experiences from joy to grief). The continuous nature of interoceptive processing, coupled to the instinctual behavior of self-preservation, is implicated in the neurobiological construction of the sense of self. Moreover, interoceptive mechanisms appear central to somatic disorders of brain-body interactions that involve the autonomic nervous system (ANS), including functional digestive and elimination disorders, chronic pain and trauma, and comorbid conditions, particularly metabolic syndrome (Bonaz et al. 2021).

The meta-organization of the ANS integrates exteroception, interoception, and proprioception. More importantly, meta-organization of the ANS is based on the primary instinct for self-preservation. The self-preservation instinct is specifically defined as gathering food for the primary energy needs of cellular mitochondria in the body, including the brain. This includes metabolic processing of food in the gut and distribution to the brain and body. These metabolic processes, typically referred to as anabolism and catabolism, are linked to the instinctual physiological allostatic responsiveness of the brain needing to predict what the nutritional needs are and how to get them. Then the body's homeostatic ANS reflexes operate relatively autonomously to deliver the goods, so to speak, and remove the waste products. It is a big dance requiring a good orchestra. Allostatic responses in the brain and homeostatic reflexes in the body need to be accurate and reliable since the self-preservation instinct is the oldest human instinct, with the ANS and endocrine system being the main drivers of both the neurological and organismic aspects of interoceptive awareness.

Interoceptive awareness of the gut and pelvis is the attentional priority regarding the procurement of food and the elimination of waste products to continually fulfill this primary evolutionary instinct. Awareness of the body's interoceptive systems, such as hunger and satiety, is critical, as are urination and defecation. Such awareness is coregulated by the endocrine system. The enormity of the ANS reflexes associated with these key interoceptive systems, especially those regulated by the vagus nerve, provides a wealth of conscious sensory information for determining interoceptive reliability and state of internal safety.

Interoception in general is related to proprioception, sometimes called kinesthesia. When the brain says eat, the body must move to the source of food, such as the kitchen or, as is all too often, the drive-through window at a fast food restaurant. Proprioception is the ability to sense stimuli arising within the body regarding position, motion, and equilibrium. All soft tissue, muscles, and fascia in the body are connected through proprioception. Its center of organization lies in the abdomen, where we also find, in Eastern systems, the Hara, the lower dantian, and source chi.

The primary interoceptive system linked with the self-preservation instinct is fear. It is integrated with the neurobiology of interoception and the acquisition of social safety from exteroception. Exteroception is defined as any form of sensation that results from stimuli located outside the body and is detected by exteroceptors, which include taste, vision, hearing, touch, or pressure. This includes our ordinary thinking mind trying to figure out the data coming from our external environment. The central autonomic network, where all this information comes together, has its main hub in the brain at the insular cortex. This area of the brain is the first embryonic fold of the cortex, beginning at six weeks after fertilization. It is partnered with the amygdala embryonically. The amygdala forms the core of a neural system for processing fearful and threatening stimuli, including detection of threat and activation of appropriate behaviors in response to such stimuli. It develops directly adjacent to the insula, and no doubt the two regions share many cells embryonically. The ventral vagus is also on that circuit.

If the insular cortex is the distribution center for the engine of interoception, then the amygdala is the transmission driving the fear car. The dorsal vagus is the gas, sending fearful information to the brain in terms of inflammatory processes in the gut. It is the fear of not having enough food or not being able to use it and assimilate it, even in people who are obese. (In the same way, the intestines are the distribution center or engine of the body's homeostasis and metabolic safety, and the heart is the transmission or driver of an interoception of spiritual safety and confidence.) Fear resulting from a concussion or trauma can also dramatically interfere with interoceptive systems of the gut and physiological responsiveness of the brain. The barrier function of the intestines is diminished in trauma, causing "leaky gut," and the vagus nerve then signals a state of metabolic fear interoceptively, alerting the brain to complex inflammatory processes and altered immune-endocrine function. These vagal signals go to the brain for allostatic processing, which ramps up anti-inflammatory signaling for self-healing of the whole body.

All humans are warriors. We train in the fear of death continually. Our body is biologically programmed to die at a cellular and metabolic level. The food we eat is already either dead or dying (and ultraprocessed food is ultra-dead food). Urination and defecation are training in the release of decomposing waste from the body. As much as we gather in for self-preservation, we are equally bound to letting go.

Death is a composting necessary to bring forth new life. Life requires death, universally, biologically, and even within our gut. When the microbiome is disrupted, its ability to participate in the life-death cycle is disrupted. The result is dysbiosis. Dysbiosis is the hallmark of a disintegrating microbiome and the cause of many psychological problems because our fear of dying is an innate part of our interoception of an unsafe metabolism. Under the trauma of inflammation and a radically altered microbiome, our gut becomes a wild predator, destroying our body and brain. To self-liberate the fear arising from the gut requires, to start, substantial repair of the intestines, liver, heart, and brain. There is no mental health without gut health. There is no heart health without gut health.

The martial arts are also known as the Way of Death. Training in defending ourselves from predators, both animal and human, involves training in killing. To know how to kill requires the readiness to die at any moment. And to be ready to die at any moment requires the capacity to self-regulate innate fear and terror through contemplative practices because these art forms target the brain areas that regulate fear and prepare the body proprioceptively to take appropriate action and resist unreliable action. If you want to know how to die at any moment, begin to get in touch interoceptively with your immune system, the somatic executioner specialist. Eighty percent of the immune system forms part of the lining of the intestines. Start there because killing our thoughts, concepts, and unrealistic views as mentioned at the beginning of this book ignites healing.

Our three primary instincts of self-preservation, self-healing, and self-transcendence, in turn associated with real food, real healing, and real meaning, must be nourished by the integration of interoception, exteroception, and proprioception or else our life withers on the vine. This is embodiment of safety. We attempt to domesticate death by avoidance of our innate metabolic fear and terror until it is too late for many people. Why wait? "The kingdom is now or never," as Thich Nhat Hahn (2018) said.

18

The Metabolic Functions of Human Instincts

I now intend to integrate a metabolic-instinctual understanding of the processes involved in human trauma, whether recent trauma or trauma developed through the life span. I do not consider this offering to be an antidote or a solution. Perhaps it is a resource for relating to our deepest sense of self—the heart inside the heart. It includes a continuation of my story of the spiritual and therapeutic discoveries I made as I worked to save my own life after having been on the killing field in the military and suffering from PTSD. It is intended to help the reader consider what they might need to accomplish in the spiritual and metabolic realms to save their own lives. It is not a list of therapeutic suggestions, although it undoubtedly contains some lifesaving treasures.

I discovered a healing principle that PTSD forms its own identity over time, regardless of therapeutic input. The identity deepens over time because it is self-reinforcing in the same way as all of our other identities in our career, family, and religion of origin. I constantly recruit all aspects of my historical body-mind to reinforce a protective barrier, commonly called avoidance by my therapists. My military identity was shaped by the Vietnam War, seven years of officer training to lead a group of soldiers to kill others, and my experience of a terrorist bombing attack. This includes the subsequent cultural denial of the impact of such moral violations; after my discharge from the Army in 1973, I came home to rampant anti-war fever. While in uniform I was spit on, and while driving my car I had paint thrown on it. I went underground and hid for many years.

Some but not all of the therapies I've tried:

Massage therapy (and its infinite variations)	Group therapy
Gestalt therapy	Marriage counseling
Sensory awareness	Continuum
Feldenkrais	Laughing yoga
Rolfing	Hatha yoga
Contemplative psychotherapy	Kundalini yoga

Mindfulness meditation   Somatic experiencing
Craniosacral therapy   Prolonged exposure therapy
Somato-emotional release   Jungian analysis
Cognitive processing therapy   Alexander technique

Some of these therapies were temporarily helpful and others were downright retraumatizing. The word *reliable* is used to navigate inappropriate reactions versus appropriate responses from the literature on instincts. For example, a walk on the beach is seemingly more reliable than getting drunk. But maybe not. What is reliable today might not be reliable tomorrow. Being with embodied trauma is a lifetime adventure as it constantly seeks to reinforce its identity physiologically and metabolically. Visually this can be seen in Victor Brauner's surrealistic painting *Consciousness of Shock*. It is a constantly shifting neurological and somatic landscape as I learned in every decade of my life.

Over time, I discovered that metabolic-instinctual explorations are important but often missing in contemporary forms of trauma therapy. Most important are the three foundational instincts described in the preceding chapter: self-healing, self-preservation, and self-transcendence. Now we will explore these instincts more deeply. What follows can simply be considered a menu, a buffet of sorts, from my fifty years of learning to inhabit my experience and explore its identity from the contemplative state of deeper awareness that has no observer. I found that contemplative skills are absolutely essential for navigating this landscape. Now I would like to offer the reader some detail regarding the most ancient three instincts of *Homo sapiens*. I separate them below yet they are all intertwined with each other as the reader will see.

INSTINCT FOR SELF-HEALING

When we cut our finger, we trust that the bleeding will stop eventually. The blood will coagulate; a scab will form and gradually fall off. Time heals most wounds. It is this way with all of human physiology and metabolism. Self-healing is built into our body and mind. And there are many varieties of the self-healing instinct. Trauma dissipates across all systems of the body, with each having their own place and timing for healing throughout the life span. These physiological systems are regulated by the cellular metabolism of anabolism (break down nutrients; build up energy and tissue) and catabolism (break down nutrients; remove waste from the process). In classical Chinese medicine, trauma is said to gradually dissipate like a mist, emerging from the center of our bodies and passing out through the pores of our skin and other elimination channels.

Positive Factors

These factors ignite the possibility for self-healing. There is only self-healing, and therapeutically the ground for such in the body and mind can be supported by BCVT. Yet, it is each individual that must follow through on that ignition especially behaviorally.

Detoxification

The instinct for self-healing depends upon reliable behaviors to function properly. I heard in a podcast that one out of six deaths on the planet right now is from pollution—pollution that we eat, breathe, and have placed in our body medically, dentally, or otherwise. Lifestyles must now be oriented to regular cleansing and detoxification. I feel that, proportionally, detoxification is the priority. The term "detox lifestyle" in contemporary literature summarizes the shift necessary to manage both our minds and our bodies. My detox lifestyle includes (but is not limited to) doing liver cleanses, taking enemas, and having regular colon hydrotherapy as well as doing meditation retreats. I also love to sweat and work outdoors in my mango grove constantly; the work gives me states of non-thought and is a deep contemplative practice for me. Of course, I do have measured indulgences since I am not an impeccable yogi.

Attunement with Natural World

Large amounts of research show that self-healing depends upon a connection with the animate world. This is on a spectrum from what is called forest bathing in Japan all the way to the ingestion of psychedelic substances (plant spirit medicine) therapeutically or recreationally. When no therapy was available to me in the military or following discharge, I experimented with LSD and other natural and synthetic psychedelics. They exposed me to the sentient nature of the natural world and larger environment. The natural world and everything that is alive is sentient, and when we cut ourselves off from that intelligence, disease follows in the body and mind. This is the most ancient wisdom for self-healing.

Igniting Interoception

Embodiment entails coming to our senses, literally. Our senses have been captured and held hostage externally by media of all forms and internally by our mind of thoughts, ideas, and concepts. Contemplative neuroscience suggests that we tune in to our senses without judgment and interpretation, starting on the meditation cushion and then throughout our day. It is critical to regain the trust of our body. Our body must regain its trust of our awareness for reliable behaviors. We let our body know that we trust it to reciprocate.

Each of our five exteroceptive senses activates different physiological and metabolic components within anabolism and catabolism. The five senses are also linked to interoceptive awareness of heartbeat, hunger, satiety, elimination, and much more. This is where physiology meets metabolism and where the brain's interpretation of the environment and physiological predictions for behavior meets the inner organism of interoception (Weng et al. 2021, Quigley et al. 2021, Chen et al. 2021).

Nutrition is coregulated by the instincts for self-preservation, self-healing, and self-transcendence. Nutritional balance requires a deep relationship with heaven and the Earth and how we ingest the Earth with our metabolism. And we must constantly navigate many refinements, adaptations, and addictions because metabolism is a continual process and a balancing act between input and output 24/7. Nutritional balance requires a deep respect for trial and error. Our bodies can be forgiving when we maintain the intention of eating real food and allowing our channels of elimination to remain functional. This requires maintenance of interoceptive awareness.

Self-Compassion

Self-compassion is the inner world of trusting and caring for our body, mind, and spirit. All of us have a metabolism of autonomy that must be nurtured and supported at the metabolic level. It is equally as important as our metabolism of social connectedness. It is critical to understand that out autonomy comes first, and thus self-compassion is vital. We live in a world of trauma, and we are the trauma species. We all have it! Yet no matter what the trauma is, it contains a potential and is embedded or linked with our spiritual formation over our life span through what Carl Jung called liminal space. Liminal space is where we find the potential for all experience to be sacred and thus compassionate as I did.

Some of us have heinous trauma to work through, and finding its sacred nature might not happen in this lifetime. I have worked with both adults and children who were tortured and know this type of trauma well. "I'll work on it later" is a familiar refrain from clients, but we can only kick the can down the block for so long, as developmentally the window for self-healing narrows while the window for spiritual formation also narrows. Many folks are hoping for a deathbed conversion to the sacred. That is risky business. We are accomplices in our own suffering through avoidance of the natural world and avoiding the spiritual depth of the present moment. And we all go through the doorway of the fear of change.

Elimination

To trust our senses, we need to open our elimination channels, especially that of the large intestine. Enemas are an essential part of our medicine bag. Yet humans are experts at abusing things, even enemas. Our body needs to trust us to make wise choices to withdraw and take care of ourselves, following the elusive yet obvious need for self-compassion. It is nonetheless difficult for most folks caught in the spin of Red Bull and Starbucks, of Facebook and Instagram. We learn self-care over time through trial and error, through mistakes and a constantly changing landscape, mentally and emotionally. It is exhausting to begin to care for our self because it requires time for our body and mind to trust our innate awareness. We can ignore our exhaustion for a long time, but eventually, inevitably, we crash.

Our metabolism depends on anabolism, the buildup of tissues in the world's biggest construction site: our body, with its thousands of major and minor construction pathways. Then there is catabolism, the removal of waste products, which are constantly being sloughed off by the entire cellular metabolism of the body, with major and minor pathways to get it all out of the body. It is a lot of work and requires a lot of help to repair these channels and to detoxify the body on a regular basis. The amount of pollution you are exposed to, regardless of how clean your diet is or how much exercise you get, is staggering.

From moment to moment, day to day, week to week, month to month, and year to year, our metabolism is constantly shifting to maintain metabolic and nutritional balance. Knowledge of the four basic nutrients the human body requires—proteins, fat, simple carbohydrates, and micronutrients—is essential. Obtaining all of them means eating approximately thirty different fruits and vegetables every week. When I first heard that I was overwhelmed, but gradually I have worked up to thirty different types of fruit and vegetables, including herbs, spices, and seaweed. It is about real food. And capacity for overwhelm largely depends on (but is not limited to) stress levels, exercise, the climate you live in, the availability of fresh local food, and your transgenerational family history. Our autonomous experience of the world requires a unique approach to everyone's self-healing needs.

Following detoxification, the next step in self-healing is to balance the gut microbiome. This happens through eating naturally probiotic fermented foods and prebiotic foods rather than downing probiotic pills—which are a waste of time since they are freeze-dried. When the gut microbiome is restored, then finally the gut's epithelium, the lining of our intestines, can go through its healing process to rebuild its proper barrier function and stop "leaky gut." Everyone needs to start exploring indicator diets such as acid-alkaline, blood type, low fat/high carb, keto, and so forth. Our nutritional needs change from decade to decade from the moment of conception. I do not know of anyone in my fifty years of experience who can sustain a long term mono diet even if considered healthy. If you are eating a lot of processed foods, the body becomes acidic and begins to rob the bones and tissues of its calcium to buffer the acidity. That leads to a host of other metabolic problems.

Negative Factors

Spectrum in the context of the three instincts refers to escalating or deescalating degrees of intensity and experience. So, at the other end of the spectrum of the self-healing instinct are the following considerations.

Pervasive Trauma

The media-driven world provides constant images and sounds of trauma. So do family systems, community systems, and common daily activities like driving. I notice my aggressive tendencies more when I'm driving than in any other activity. If I hadn't noticed this tendency, I probably would have lost my driver's license many years ago. I practice driving now as a contemplative practice.

Homo sapiens has always been at war. Stop the war internally first. To change the world, we must change ourselves internally. After 9/11, I remember hearing Peter Levine, the founder of the trauma resolution therapy Somatic Experiencing, say that the most important way we could care for ourselves and heal ourselves is to simply feel our heartbeat consciously. This practice—cardioception—is the essence of interoceptive awareness. When I feel that my heartbeat is elevated, I know I must immediately change the behaviors of my outer and inner life.

Systemic Inflammation

Systemic inflammation starts in the gut with a diet that includes ultraprocessed foods, added sugars, preservatives, and other things that kill the gut microbiome. This cascade of gut disintegration interferes with the senses and thwarts interoceptive awareness, while the resulting inflammation dysregulates the heart and the autonomic nervous system (ANS) via the endothelium.

Ultraprocessed food is engineered to be addictive; it uses the same metabolic pathways as cocaine and opioids. It causes our bodies to gradually become uninhabitable, non-safety zones, and untrustworthy. Our trust then frequently gets projected upon medical professionals, who are also prone to make debilitating mistakes and tend to fit us into treatment boxes of their norm, not ours. This is food trauma, or inflammation trauma.

Self-healing is rooted in our body's metabolism. But our inner garden is overrun with weeds. And not just the gut but also, especially, the mind, the domain of self-transcendence. This is really a call for retaking sovereignty over our body. It is time to individually recall the dignity and preciousness of human life.

Evolutionary Imprinting

Imprinting is a way in which a trait or characteristic of an organism builds an instinct. From the moment of the appearance of the first life forms on Earth, the imprinting of pleasure and pain, nurturing and non-nurturing, formed the core of our instincts. This is where our ancestry transitioned from the origin of the universe into a more solid form and continues to transition between being formless (the mind) and forming (the body) in the present. Imprinting then becomes like the age circles in the diameter of an old tree that show what the tree experienced at a given period of time in its life. One of the oldest parts of the mammalian nervous system is the reticular formation. It predates the vagus nerve (though not really by much). The reticular formation functions like an unconscious first responder; it receives input from the enteric nervous system (ENS) and responds even before the brain gets to elaborate on the input. The ENS spreads out its input to the spinal cord three to five segments which is much broader than input from the musculoskeletal system into the spinal cord. The processing goes from the spinal cord posteriorly towards the reticular formation for the initial evaluation of pleasure meaning go toward that which you're in relationship with for nurturing and care. And the reverse, to move away from non-nurturing. It is a very primitive reflex and discussed in chapter 20 in more detail.

This gut level information has a conscious sensory knowing called interoception related to hunger, thirst, pooping, and peeing; all are integrated with desire and the orgasm reflex. One way to understand this is through a joke about three engineers arguing about what type of engineer God would be. The mechanical engineer says the exquisite movement of our body is an art form only God could have created. The electrical engineer says the vast connections of everything that happens in the body through the electrical system of the central nervous system proves that God is an electrical engineer. The civil engineer says only a genius God would know to place a sewer line in the middle of a recreational area. Metabolic circuits driven by the hormones of interoceptive awareness always involve pleasure and pain circuits.

Insecure and Disorganized Attachments

Babies develop their sympathetic nervous system (SNS) through attachment with a caregiver. The prime function of the SNS in that phase of attachment with a caregiver is to experience joy (love) throughout the soma. This is through social affiliative behaviors and touch. At the same time, the baby's parasympathetic nervous system (PNS) develops withdrawal behaviors for self-soothing with pleasure. However, sometimes babies are born into families that are emotionally unhealthy, insecure, or at worst forming disorganized attachments. When a baby's attachment is insecure or disorganized, which happens in upwards of 70 percent of the Westernized human population according to a lecture I heard by Allan Schore, the baby's SNS and PNS must manage varying degrees of fear in a very immature brain. The fear processing center of the brain is the amygdala, and it is the most metabolically active part of a baby's brain in the first several months after birth. Insecure attachment experiences alter the development of reliable interoceptive bodily awareness. It activates defensive allostatic physiological states in the autonomic nervous system (ANS). If the attachment breach is not repaired, it may thwart development of the entire ANS, both physiologically and metabolically. This leads to metabolic syndrome. The lived interoceptive experience of safety may be dysregulated, especially at the core of the body, including the pelvis, gut, and heart.

The SNS at a metabolic level regulates vasoconstriction and vasodilation of the artery. Vasodilation can be compromised even from prenatal stress and trauma. Consequently, heart disease starts during pregnancy and in childhood.

As mentioned, a baby needs time alone to experience autonomy periodically and develop interoceptive awareness as pleasure rather than pain. This allows the PNS to experience happiness coupled with somatic explorations including self-soothing, which is the self-preservation imperative to explore the inner world and to suck, swallow, and breath, mimicking the SNS behavior of breastfeeding. If this capacity is thwarted, then the default state of the PNS becomes dissociation and numbing as a form of self-soothing and unreliable adaptation.

This original design function of the ANS for joy and happiness as well as the spectrum of its default modes related to overwhelming stress create what is called a "setpoint for stimulation." Every human has a unique ANS setpoint for stimulation, determined by transgenerational imprinting and embryonic development of the ANS. Setpoints involve a variety of allostatic physiological responses and somatic metabolic reflexes. They can be seen as automatically shifting fulcrums, especially with PTSD, in which the buffering, stabilizing capacities of the ANS are broken. Today's setpoint for calm is tomorrow's setpoint for overwhelm. If we focus on the metabolism of accumulation and dissipation at the neurological exteroceptive and somatic interoceptive levels, then in some ways, trauma reactivity is like the game show *Wheel of Fortune*. We spin the wheel repeatedly every day, not really knowing where it will stop or if the stopping point will be a winner or loser in terms of whether the trauma symptoms will overwhelm the interoceptive systems in the body and brain. Consequently, self-love is a prerequisite for self-healing. And that is related to self-care. It is about turning the focus inwardly and contemplatively.

Developmental Features of PTSD

Post-traumatic stress disorder is perhaps the most common and pervasive diagnosis for human beings; we are the trauma species. PTSD changes and transmutes its symptomology as we progress through the different stages of our life. For example, upon reaching our sixties, we begin to do a life review and thus come into constant contact with earlier traumas. When I was in my sixties, I reexperienced every concussion I had ever had, from playing contact sports to accidents. I had already received many years of craniosacral therapy and its biodynamic sister, and I had to start all over again. There was a much deeper fulcrum that needed to dissipate.

During each developmental phase of life, therapy and resourcing must also change and evolve to support the instinct for self-healing. Some of the therapies I experienced opened aspects of my being. For example, gestalt therapy showed me my emotional body. I cried for over a year in every session for the first time in my life. My emotional body was ignited, and some therapists insisted on repeating the crying and wailing in each session, which was nonsense and retraumatizing. Contemplative psychotherapy showed me the nature of my mind and its seeming chaos. It also showed me how much anger I held and importantly gave me a glimpse of consciously recognizing for the first time my symptoms of PTSD, such as avoiding the post office when walking to work or being startled when approached from behind by a friend or lover. This first awakening to the symptoms I experience took place a decade after the initial event in the Army. And even then, I did not consciously link them to the event. I just noticed this peculiar behavior and wondered, *Why?* The instinct for self-healing I came to recognize as always functioning even at an unconscious level. My inner being had constant courage to face every subsequent event in my life.

INSTINCT FOR SELF-PRESERVATION

The instinct for self-preservation, a.k.a. the survival instinct, tells us to move toward that which nourishes and move away from that which irritates. As above, it began with the earliest organisms after the Earth was formed some five billion years ago.

Positive Factors

These factors support a clear and conscious sense of the instinct for self-preservation. I start with interoception again, as this is the key to embodied spirituality and survival.

Interoceptive Awareness

The gut comes first in the evolution of body systems. The cells destined to be the viscera differentiate first in the human embryo. They begin to function before their definitive structure appears. They serve as a manifestation of the instinct for self-preservation, which depends on the development of reliable behaviors associated with hunger, satiety, and elimination.

Humans, like all mammals, must seek out food, avoid pain, and immobilize to eliminate. But other mammals have a specialization for survival that develops at the end of the embryonic period, such as exaggerated teeth, claws, snouts, or speed for chasing down prey. We humans are different; we are perpetual embryos, always maintaining the potential of becoming something new and being able to adapt to changing circumstances.

To accomplish the demands of survival, humans rely on an exquisite conscious awareness of our internal organ signaling. We must be able to feel our heartbeat (cardioception) and the sensations of hunger, satiety, and elimination (visceroception). This is a beautiful and necessary sensibility to cultivate over the life span. However, in contemporary society, the gut has become a garbage dump for toxic corporate pseudo-food, causing a host of problems, including chronic visceral pain and disintegration, metabolic syndrome, heart disease, and dementia. The disruption means that interoceptive awareness no longer functions naturally. We do not know when to eat, what to eat, when we are finished eating, and when to use the toilet. Our heart is lost, and we don't have the sense any longer of where and how to look for it.

Self-Regulation

Self-regulation relies on the development of a felt sense of safety over the life span. There is external safety, registered unconsciously via neuroception, as detailed in the polyvagal model of Stephen Porges (2024b) and there is internal safety, registered consciously via interoceptive awareness in the sanctuary model of Sandra Bloom (2013).

To secure fuel to feed the mitochondria of every cell in our body for vitality and energy, it is important to experience embodied safety. Much of the food we eat these days is not safe, meaning that rather than nurturing us, it causes inflammatory trauma that interferes with all levels and types of safety. In contrast, eating real food that fulfills our nutritional requirements creates embodied safety and manifests the deepest level of the instinct for self-preservation.

Intermittent Fasting

Humans have always been subjected to periods of famine followed by periods of feasting. Our metabolisms adapted to this dynamic. The problem today is that for many of us, a constant nonstop feast is available 24/7. Some of us face poverty, and thus famine is also present in our culture. However, whether in feast or famine, the majority of Westernized people are malnourished because they rely on a diet of processed food.

Linked to self-healing, self-preservation requires real food, as noted above. At the same time, the body also requires periods of "famine," meaning in this case fasting, to trigger autophagy, the cannibalistic behavior of our cells to consume waste products and make them easier to excrete. Autophagy occurs in each cell of our body, managing the waste products from energy metabolism, specifically from the mitochondria, a nonhuman ancestor running our cellular metabolism and creating the energy we need to live and love. This takes time and is greatly interfered with by overeating and snacking frequently, especially late at night. Fasting in this way contributes to purification of the body, which improves metabolic and spiritual health.

The United States had famous fasting farms, as they were called, until the 1970s, when they were all put out of business by big medicine. Only in Europe can someone still go to medically supervised fasting clinics, such as the famous Buchinger Wilhelmi Clinic. We must learn the science of not eating for regular periods of time—that is, intermittent fasting (IF) or time-restricted eating (TRE). This begins with a minimum of twelve to sixteen hours between the last meal eaten in the evening and the first one the following day. This supports deep metabolic elimination of waste products.

For me, there was a point after several prolonged fasts where an emotional switch happened. I felt like I finally had regained the control of my body that morbid obesity had robbed me of. My body and I were one organism that I now had sovereignty over, and no one could ever take it away. It was an ignition of somatic sovereignty.

The Kitchen as the Center of Compassion

So many people do not cook. So many people do not know how to cook. So many people do not like to cook. My mother-in-law raised ten children and hated cooking. So many people eat regular meals from a drive-through window at a fast-food joint. The reasons for that are manifold, but I'll just say: The current politics of food science and government dietary recommendations are genocidal.

We must relearn how to trust our body and for it to trust the decisions we make about what we put into it. This takes time and a shift in our priorities and values based on repairing interoception, which requires detoxification, repair of the gut microbiome, and repair of the intestinal epithelium. Start in the kitchen with what I like to call the seven phases of real food: planning, gathering, prepping, cooking, praying, eating, and cleaning up. The kitchen is not only the new ER but the center of compassion in any household. It is the hearth. The place where fire ignites the food being cooked with the potential for love, infusing every aspect of the process right down to scrubbing the kitchen floor. When the kitchen is a sanctuary of mindfulness, the beauty of our attention penetrates the food we are prepared. Compassion begins in the kitchen. Healing begins in the kitchen.

Negative Factors

At the other end of the spectrum of our survival instinct we find the following.

Metabolic Syndrome: Cellular Starvation

To review, the results of the ultraprocessed food diet and the addiction to sugar drives a variety of disorders, especially obesity, type 2 diabetes, most cancers, memory disorders, and on and on. This is called metabolic syndrome, as mentioned. The cells of our body are being starved for correct molecules from real food and become toxic from an overload of waste products and the inability to free the metabolic channels for elimination. We are literally starving ourselves with junk food. This includes food trauma, organ failure, cellular starvation, and sepsis (dying from being overwhelmed with inflammation).

Inflammation: Epithelial-Endothelial Dysregulation-Dysbiosis

To review, the breakdown caused by ultraprocessed food begins in the epithelial lining of the intestines and its milieu of the microbiome and immune system. This leads to "leaky gut" in which the barrier function of the epithelium of the gut disintegrates. This causes "leaky everything everywhere" from metabolic syndrome. Inflammation and the breakdown of the barrier function of both the epithelium and endothelium are the source of a majority of ills, including even mental illness, which is linked to dysbiosis, the degradation and species extinction of gut microbiome.

Over 80 percent of our innate immune system is integrated within the gut microbiome, ENS, and dorsal vagus nerve. A breach of the barrier of the epithelial lining upregulates the immune system and generates an inflammatory response that is then mediated by the vasculature adjacent to the epithelial lining, which all goes first to the liver. The endothelium is the master coregulator of homeostasis in the body and lines the entire cardiovascular system, where the blood flows. It is an endocrine organ and loses its function for properly sharing nutrients and oxygen and transporting self-healing molecules across its barrier. This whole process is mediated by the gut microbiome, and it changes its makeup and loses its integrity. All systems of the body have their own unique microbiome. And they all talk to one another. This is the deeper metabolic nature of trauma that must be addressed in trauma resolution therapy.

Epigenetics

The microbiome is linked to the function of our epigenetics, and consequently pathways of inflammation are related to our unique epigenetics. When we eat ultraprocessed, preservative-laden, sugar-rich corporate food, our body expresses different genes than those that are needed for proper metabolic digestion, absorption, and elimination. The DNA being expressed is damaged, genomic instability ensues, and thus metabolic syndrome begins to gestate, with its exact manifestation dependent on our family ancestry of disease and suffering.

Violence

When I was studying to become a Buddhist chaplain, my biggest spiritual challenge was the very first precept in Zen Buddhism. My cohort was asked to contemplate the following statement: The support of all life involves the taking of life. I had been on a killing field, as it's called in the military, and could not even begin to comprehend such a statement at that moment. Yet since then, I've learned that for me simply to eat every day, all manner of vegetation and animals must be killed. Even vegetarianism involves killing. We are not only the trauma species; we are the violence species. And we have the capacity to transcend these base functions of our instincts. Certainly, killing other human beings is not the foreground of our instinct for self-preservation. The consequences psychologically and spiritually for killing or maiming another human being are devastating. This is why I work with other veterans. There are no easy answers. This is only a contemplation and not an exercise in virtue or morality signaling.

As a side note, because I was so reactive when asked to contemplate the above Zen precept, it ultimately led to my dismissal from the chaplaincy training. I wrote the following poem, called "Another Homeless Vet," to commemorate my dismissal.

Another homeless Vet
kicked into the street
home away from home
sleeping on cardboard under a bridge
begging for food without a bowl
wearing rags and fingerless gloves
I wear the Tathagata's teachings
alone at last, away from the dogma
pushing my old shopping cart
full of Heart Treasures
begging at stop signs in the pouring rain
a quarter here, a dollar there
enough for a needle and a Bud Light
to patch up the hole in my ancient, twisted Karma
what more can a Vet ask for?
Just another kick into the dark end of freedom
A Zen Peacekeeper
On the streets for fifty years
Homeless at last

Cardiotoxicity

In *The Mass Psychology of Fascism*, Wilhelm Reich (1980) said that there are three levels of human relationship: the superficial social engagement level, the deeper level of rage and hatred that we all experience in its various guises, and the lifetime of work to get to the deeper level of transforming hatred into love. I find it better to say that hatred can come into balance with love, as hatred in contemplative psychotherapy is also related to the discernment of evil. Reich is saying that as a species we have the innate capacity to overcome the animal side of our instincts. After all, we are animals.

We live in a world that is stuck in its fascination of shock and terror, even at the therapeutic level. The instinct for self-preservation is related to these states because hunger becomes a longing, and the longing has the potential to become an ideation, for good or not. As a species, we migrate with our social groups to seek better opportunities because we long to have food readily available for ourself and other, and that is linked to a longing to be free of political oppression and racism in all of its forms.

Reich also said that it is not in the best interest of political systems to give their population freedom of embodiment. Indeed, today we eat the worst kind of junk food that is medically sanctioned by governments, especially in the United States. The junk food industry makes $600 million in profits every year, and it costs $1 trillion for the medical system to try to fix it with pills and stomach stapling. When we establish sovereignty with our body, when we know how our body as a spiritual temple functions, we also withdraw from mainstream culture by necessity. We escape the political, medical, and corporate iatrogenesis of kill-for-profit. And with the instinct for self-transcendence, we eliminate the need to blame anyone once we establish somatic sovereignty.

INSTINCT FOR SELF-TRANSCENDENCE

The maturation of body and mind and their spiritual healing come together with the instinct for self-transcendence. This instinct requires a turn inward away from the external senses and thus BCVT is a contemplative practice that awakens the instinct for self-transcendence.

Positive Factors
These factors are the sparks that ignite self-transcendence. It is said that the ground for our spiritual heart is full of weeds, and we must weed the garden of our heart and free it from emotional toxins and unrealistic concepts and notions of how life functions. We must find our heart at the literal level of self-healing physically, and we must find our spiritual heart whose form is beauty and wisdom itself.

Spiritual Formation
The contemplative arts are a wide variety of body-mind practices. I have been a licensed massage therapist in the state of Florida since 1976. I had planned to become

an attorney, as I come from a family of attorneys, but the terrorist bombing attack in Germany in 1972 gave me a U-turn into my future. It wasn't until I was doing a lot of professional massage in Miami that I came to the realization that I didn't like people. That was my first conscious clue that something was amiss in my compassion ethic as a newly trained fresh-out-of-school healer, though I did not connect it to a symptom of PTSD. Eventually I moved into the field of pediatrics, and I worked with infants and children with mild, moderate, and severe developmental disabilities for more than forty years; they taught me great compassion, as I detailed in chapter 2.

In 2022, when I was undergoing prolonged exposure therapy through the U.S. Department of Veterans Affairs (VA), I had to recount the story of the terrorist bombing more than a hundred times. During one of those times, as I was recounting/reexperiencing the peak moment of lifting a decapitated body into an ambulance, the memory of the liminal space of the sacred and spiritual essence of compassion came back to me. It was a vivid reminder of the potential for trauma to be a portal to compassion. I did not know that then in 1972, yet my body and mind instinctively and immediately moved in the direction of compassion. I knew my life ended and I needed to heal my body. That was the ignition. I know that now that such compassion was sparked around the fiftieth anniversary of the bombing attack. It needed a long time to gestate.

Some of the manual therapeutic arts are contemplative and valuable in the exploration of trauma. Some are not. Babette Rothschild, a well-published author in the field of trauma resolution, once told me personally that she does not refer clients for manual therapy because "you people have no boundaries." This means many of my tribe have not done their own inner work. And it is not only about a lack of inner work. It is about the continual reinvention and proliferation of release-based cathartic therapies, which have the greatest potential to retraumatize a client. It can be so damaging. Containment of affect is a more appropriate model from the field of affective neuroscience and interpersonal neurobiology. Containment entails creating a safe space through a variety of perceptual processes that can be considered contemplative in their application, such as mindfulness.

A Note on Cathartic Therapies

The only literature that supports release-based cathartic therapies is the spiritual literature regarding the healing practices in some religious congregations around the world. While their relevance was impactful in the 1950s and '60s, their intention was to crack open the hard shell of the post–World War II body. With the advent of the pandemic of metabolic syndrome, the hard shell in the body has already broken down. Release-based cathartic therapy is old stuff and very unreliable. "Seek not, forbid not" is the best advice I've ever heard regarding processing a client's emotions. It is not possible to know what the deep core of a client's problems are. As biodynamic therapists, we can create a holding environment for containment and transmutation of the client's inner existential complex with the perception of PR and dynamic stillness.

Contemplation is an attempt to decrease the externalization and projection of our discomfort onto others and to turn our attention inward to explore a highly personal and awkward landscape of our body and mind. It begins with a thorough investigation of one's heart on its full spectrum from physical to the spiritual. There is a heart inside the heart where the spirit lives. Contemplative art forms span from formal classes to making a garden in your backyard. As is said in Buddhist meditation, anything can be the object of meditation. That is why at the beginning of many meditation practices the breath is the object to stabilize a busy mind. And yet 25 percent of meditation practices can trigger adverse reactions. Like many lifestyle interventions, contemplative practices are a trial-and-error proposition, which is a recurring theme in the journey to recovering body sovereignty. I tell my meditation students that the moment their heart accelerates, they should get up and leave the meditation room.

Nonduality refers to the cultivation of a meditative awareness that already exists in us. Such awareness is also called self-knowing awareness, nonreferential awareness, or awareness without observer. This deep awareness is already present in our heart inside our heart and leads to deeper states of wholeness and interconnectedness with self, other, and the universe. These are the deeper levels of mind in which we can see through the perception of subject and object and the machinery that creates subject and object as separate and solid. This is innate. This is the preexisting condition. In Christianity, it is the idea that God is everything. The world can fill us with awe when we recognize it. It's not about eliminating thoughts and emotions. That ticker tape will always be running more or less at the bottom of our mental television screen. It's about letting those thoughts be. It's about recognizing the nondual awareness already inside us, which has no reference point such as the breath or our thoughts. Yet it is readily present and available as we go through our day and naturally experience gaps in our thoughts and emotions. It is about the stillpoint.

As Shakespeare said, "Get thee to a nunnery," and in my case, I began to learn Buddhist meditation shortly after arriving in Boulder, Colorado, around 1980. From the moment of receiving my first instruction, I felt immediately at home on the meditation cushion. I felt awe at the vastness of being introduced to my mind. I had tried transcendental meditation, kundalini yoga, and other techniques, but unsuccessfully, as they bored me to death. And then I began to watch the Coney Island of my mind with simple shamatha (calm abiding) practice. I discovered my mind was and still is a roller coaster, and I can now insert space and intervene in most states of mind. Sometimes I am lucky with my awareness intervention, and sometimes not. I hold the nature of my mind with a sense of awe and deep respect. This awe makes me humble.

Creating Sanctuary

Dr. Sandra Bloom's sanctuary model (2013), designed to help organizations establish safe space for working with clients who've experienced trauma, names four levels of safety: psychological, social, moral, and cultural (Bloom 2013). The safety of neuroception, which we might call social safety, is also a central component in Stephen Porges's polyvagal theory (2024b) and for other authors in the trauma resolution community. These manifestations of safety increase our embodied and conscious awareness by reducing fear. *Sanctuary* implies sacredness, and indeed, the safer we feel, the greater the accessibility of self-transcendence.

In my multivagal model, detailed in my book *The Biodynamics of the Immune System,* I adapted Bloom's four levels of safety as social (neuroceptive) safety, compassion (emotional safety), embodiment (metabolic) safety, and moral safety. Once we travel below the brain and heart, we arrive in the gut and pelvis. This level of embodied safety is the deepest from an evolutionary point of view. Self-healing and self-preservation are linked to self-transcendence not only through the brain and heart but also through the gut and pelvis. Some people start their journey to safety through the brain and some start their journey through the heart. I started my journey to safety through my gut and pelvis with its elimination channels. Where does a client's journey to safety begin? And how do these four areas lend themselves to a single state of embodied self-transcendent safety?

Spiritual Maturation

To uncover the innate sanctuary of the heart inside the heart, our mind of hatred and separation must begin to be held in loving kindness, as we are told by our spiritual leaders. I mentioned earlier the work of Wilhelm Reich in this regard. We develop awareness that is nonjudgmental and much vaster than the hatred itself. This requires constant contemplative practice. It is daily work. It is a lifetime of work.

As part of my own therapy, I underwent cognitive processing therapy (CPT), an evidence-based trauma resolution therapy. I had developed a lot of avoidant mental habits that included hyperreactivity to various stimuli, leading to anger and periodic rage. As they say in AA, I had a lot of stinkin' thinkin'. I then underwent prolonged exposure therapy (PET), in which I repeatedly told the story of being on a killing field, as mentioned. I now hold the symptoms of PTSD with much greater compassion. Compassion is a state of mind that makes it utterly unbearable for us to see the suffering of others sentient beings. The way to develop this is through seeing our own suffering (first). When we become conscious of our own suffering, we have a spontaneous wish to be free from it (self-compassion). If we are able to extend that feeling to all other beings, through realizing the common instinctive desire we all have to avoid and overcome suffering, then we arrive at that state of mind called great compassion. So, to develop compassion is to become so impartial that it can include all sentient beings within its embrace, whether friend or foe. This begins with cognitive empathy, through which we put aside all judgment of another person and feel into their thinking and conceptualization with equanimity.

Spiritual Authority

Trauma has the potential to lead us to spiritual maturation and deepen our empathy for self and others. Over time spiritual maturity becomes a type of spiritual authority in which there is no longer any need for ministers, priests, chaplains, and so forth. Each of us has the capacity for direct experience of the sacred, no matter what our tradition, religion, or preferences. This is awe. Even an atheist has direct experience of the sacred when we define it as that which brings meaning to our life. As His Holiness the Dalai Lama has said many times, there are more than a thousand spiritual aptitudes.

As mentioned in my Introduction, biodynamic cardiovascular therapy was founded in the osteopathic community by a group of Christian mystics under the rubric of the rule of the artery. My career is now a ministry of laying on of hands using my hands to bless my clients. The terminology used in biodynamic practice lends itself to mysticism and the awe of direct experience of the sacred in a multifaith context. This is the reality of the contemporary client that is unable to make the changes necessary to heal their metabolic syndrome. Biodynamic work becomes a unique form of palliative care in which we make our offering and give our blessing for its potential to Ignite the client in their self-transcendence.

Incorporation of the Unseen

Unseen refers to the unseen sentience of every living being. All living, sentient beings have Buddha nature or Christ consciousness. Another way of saying this is that God is everything, as mentioned earlier.

As noted earlier, animism-shamanism is the original medical system on the planet. In the East, the ancient animistic-shamanistic traditions have as their basis the construction of physical reality being composed of the five elements, as described in chapter 16. Each of the elements is a unique domain in which sentient beings other than those that we can see, such as plants and animals, some animistic-shamanic traditions, and especially Tibetan medicine, refer to what are called provocation disorders. A provocation disorder is diagnosed as an unseen entity from one of the elemental domains interfering with a person's body and mind. This is seen in Western religious traditions in terms of devils and demons taking over the mind and requiring exorcism rites. The idea of the unseen provocation is important when it comes to relating with trauma. It requires that biodynamic therapists think outside the box when we observe a client who "seems to be possessed." We have all had experiences with such clients. Many trauma patients seem to be possessed, which to me is a spiritual process. A short visit to any VA hospital will give you this view rather quickly. Spiritual authority is a power to remove so-called entities that seem to be in possession of a client's well-being. Living from a sacred place in the heart inside the heart can change a curse to a blessing with a thought or a beam of light, just as Jesus did. And there are many spiritual reinforcements, deities, and avatars to help relieve anyone of their illness. All wrathful entities can be converted with loving kindness. I am not suggesting that biodynamic practice is an exorcism rite. I am advocating for expanding the depth of our heart to include the living sacred spirit that lives there an opportunity to manifest its unerring potency in healing the world.

Reverence for Death

Everyone and everything everywhere dies. Embrace your inner corpse. See the discussion of this concept in chapter 3.

The Sacred Heart

The heartbeat is the new church. It is a potential that is ignited via contemplative practices.

The simplest instruction for life is to become able to feel our heartbeat without taking our pulse. Research is clear that the capacity to sense our heartbeat generates empathy, specifically emotional empathy.

The moment we feel our heartbeat is elevated, it is the signal to expand our awareness to the whole and practice resilience in getting the heartbeat back to its natural rhythm (seventy or less beats per minute). This includes knowing and sensing through interoceptive awareness the potency of the ANS in its innervation of pulmonary circulation in the trunk of the body.

At the same time that we can sense our heartbeat, we can experience the felt sense of potency in the area all around the cardiac and pulmonary plexuses on the inferior border of the aorta. The strength of that potency is sometimes deceiving, as it may feel as if a powerful heartbeat is more rapid than it actually is. This is when it's important to take your pulse at the radial or carotid arteries and confirm the difference between a strong but regulated heartbeat and a strong potency radiating throughout the trunk and beyond from pulmonary circulation. Once these first two perceptions are established with interoceptive awareness, we can synchronize with the subtlety of PR originating from its fulcrum at the posterior heart fields (dorsal myocardium and pericardium).

In a therapeutic session, that same emanation from the client's heart fields extends beyond the body into all surrounding sentient beings. The client-therapist relationship becomes a unified heart of potential love. This makes Primary Respiration (PR) the movement of love itself, as many clients have described to me. There is a stillpoint in the heart inside the heart that generates the radiance of PR. Find the stillness.

Negative Factors

At the other end of the spiritual spectrum we find the following.

Spiritual Disease

The shamanic diagnosis of spiritual disease is the gradual alienation of ourselves from the natural world, and then an alienation from our society and community, and then an alienation from our own body, and finally an alienation from our own mind of awareness, openness, and clarity. In this view, the natural world is the world of the divine. It is the sacred in all of its appearances. When spiritual disease is the diagnosis (and I argue all contemporary physical and psychological disease is spiritual) it means that the antidote is supporting the instinct for self-transcendence in all its contemplative forms especially biodynamic cardiovascular therapy.

Spiritual narcissism is a form of spiritual disease. It entails an overidentification with one's role as a healer, a light worker, or whatever term we use for the identity we have taken on our career path. It is an inflation of identity that blocks the living reality of the shared pain and suffering on the planet. It is an identity crisis and overidentification.

The term *spiritual bypass* frequently describes clients who use meditation and other contemplative practices to avoid their emotional problems. It can be a difficult diagnosis to make; everyone is doing the best they can with what they have in the present moment. And yes, it looks really strange sometimes. As one of my professors once said, "We need to learn to treat strangeness with respect." Not-knowing is the first principle of healing in the Zen tradition. As therapists, we first confront our inner fear of not really knowing what the client needs. This fear is the threshold of a door we sit at until the compassionate response naturally arises. We must do as Dr. Jealous instructed: "Wait, watch, and wonder."

Addiction to Digital Propaganda

Digital propaganda and our culture's obsession with social media is the true scourge and pandemic of our time. We all know it, we all talk about it, we all see it in our children and our friends and throughout our communities and at every restaurant. It is the new addiction brought to us by corporate and political greed. We see it everywhere around us. Even when we are driving—last year alone in the state of Florida, eighty-seven thousand accidents were recorded as the result of distracted driving from a driver being on a cell phone.

My wife and I make agreements to have weekly TFDs: technology-free days. Try it.

Lost Heart Sickness

When we don't recognize the need for stability of mind, with space between thoughts and a practice of open awareness, emotions can run wild. This generates overconceptualization. Conceptions can build a sense of false security, create projections of rage and hatred, and distort our view of reality. We are all human, and human emotions are unavoidable, but we can learn to recognize them and befriend them with a greater allegiance to open awareness. Lama Tsultrim Allione (2008) refers to it as "feeding your demons."

The worst form of duality is an emotional and conceptual state of affliction that becomes an entrenched view of life or belief system. It fosters systemic anger, rage, and hatred. We now navigate a culture of conspiracy theories, and we are an accomplice until we move our mind and body away, and this means turning the mirror on ourselves. We must turn inward and weed the garden. It is time to become the host of our experience, rather than a guest. This was my main takeaway from cognitive processing therapy. As I detailed earlier, I was capable of very intense world views directly linked to my military experience. Each one of those worldviews had to be examined and gradually deconstructed. Such a deconstruction is necessary for our innate empathy and compassion to manifest. We do not have to heal the world we see through the media; we really only have to heal ourselves and care for those around us. I've learned to "stop helping other people," as Anne Lamott said in her 2017 TED Talk. I can sit with my clients and relate with them heart to heart. I can offer a blessing with my hands or a prayer with my words. I can call in the Holy Spirit. Can I ever really know the depth of their suffering and how their deep inner spiritual formation is organized? No. But I can say that I don't know to a client and also let them know I am here for them. I can sit in the awe of not-knowing as a radiant light.

Death Phobia

We fear change and impermanence. This is the core. Change is constant, and such impermanence is a doorway to the reality of our physical death. Without acknowledging and accepting the permanence of change, mentally, emotionally, and physically, we become death phobic and at death we are unprepared, leaving while regretful, anxious, short of breath, and in physical pain. Resilience is required to recognize the nature of constant change in our life. We must learn to recognize our reactivity to change and disengage as quickly as possible. Then, as death approaches, the other possibility is self-transcendence, which can happen without regret, anxiety, shortness of breath, pain, or fear.

Humans have abdicated their innate sovereignty of their body by being careless and irresponsible. This is called ignorance in Buddhism fueled by negative karma. It is an abdication of agency for our own body-mind-spirit and an abandonment of our instincts.

Our instincts contain an innate intelligence for self-healing, survival, and spiritual formation. The work is turning on the light inside the heart inside our heart before trying to help someone else ignite their missing pilot light. As is said, there are a thousand faces of God, and this indicates numerous doorways to integrating our trauma every moment of our lives. We can restore our sense of awe with this mystery called life.

19

PTSD

An Evolutionary View

This chapter begins to explore the evolution and metabolism of trauma more deeply. I start with my hypothesis that post-traumatic stress disorder (PTSD) is the evolutionary side effect of natural dissociation. The original organisms on the planet were dissociated by their nature and gradually associated to higher levels of complexity while keeping their core of dissociation. Our most basic default state of being is therefore dissociation. I call this *original dissociation*. It all began with these five factors:

- Immobility to increase metabolism
- Very low levels of oxygen metabolism (anoxia, similar to fetal development)
- Inefficiency at sustained growth or development due to hostile environments
- A complete trial-and-error method of living with limited filtration of experience
- The ever-present reality of death

This may sound like the present moment on our planet, but in times of planetary stress, we naturally return to our most original metabolism. Our origin is dissociation. In this *natural originality*, we are always in the present moment metabolically, as it really all began with the interaction of the tiniest molecules and elements from the periodic chart, which are still active in our body. This full spectrum of dissociation is the natural state inherent in any expression of PTSD. In *Living in the Borderland*, Jerome Bernstein writes:

> In the case of individuals who encounter . . . trauma . . . , they too have come into the world with their "origins story" in place at birth. However, the impact of their traumatic experience(s) overlays a new and powerfully charged story—a trauma story—which, because of its impact on the self, takes on numinosity *as if* it were their "origins story." . . . [It] tends to leave the individual cut off from his pretrauma "origins story" with which he came into the world *as if it never had existed.* (Bernstein 2006, 146–47)

THE VAGAL CONNECTION

I learned of Stephen Porges and his work back in the early 1980s. I had just begun my study and practice of Rolfing, and he was on the research committee for the Rolf Institute. But it was not until I opened the science section of the *New York Times* one Tuesday in 1990 that I could see his brilliance and the unveiling of his polyvagal model at that time. As a practitioner and teacher of craniosacral therapy, especially the way it was handed down through the osteopathic community in the past century, I already had a deep knowledge and interest in the autonomic nervous system (ANS). It became embedded within the osteopathic model of the cranial concept starting at the turn of the last century. The polyvagal model is primarily a model of metabolic and physiological safety. Its relevance to the therapeutic community is very important because it is the felt sense of safety that Ignites the instinct for self-healing. It is palpable and observable by a therapist with discerning eyes, mind, and hands.

When my career practicing Rolfing was over, it was because I had blown a disc in my neck from years of sleeping on my stomach and overnight I lost my ability to do Rolfing. I transitioned to working with craniosacral therapy and eventually a biodynamic approach, wherein I integrated contemplative psychotherapy. Out of a deep need to understand my own emerging dilemma with PTSD, I earned a doctorate in somatic psychology in 1995. Then I became an academic embryologist and taught courses on pre- and perinatal psychology and somatic psychology in doctoral programs at the Santa Barbara Graduate Institute. I also taught embryonic morphology and its phenomenology. I studied the evolutionary development of the body systems and in particular the developmental sequence of:

- gut *first*
- heart *second*
- brain *third*

The dorsal vagus is a large nerve that runs down along the front of the spine and through all core viscera starting from in back of the ears all the way to the large intestine and hypogastric plexuses in the lower abdomen and pelvis. It is considered to be the oldest part of the polyvagal system. It is the evolutionary default system in terms of our metabolic and physiological responses to traumatic shock, especially including the gut and heart. The connection of the dorsal vagus to the gut is now a major player in our understanding of metabolic syndrome and gut-related pathophysiologies (Porges 2024a). Vagal tone and vagal resources are important regulators of heart rate variability (HRV). Importantly, there is a relationship between the heart's metabolic function and those people who have adverse reactions to common vagal tone practices, especially breathing techniques. The problem is sourced in the metabolism of the human gut. I propose that the dorsal vagus is the co-regulator of the contemporary orientation of pathological unhealthy dissociation. And at the same time, it is the manager of all visceral metabolic functions. I am making the case that understanding the organismic and instinctual levels of human evolution, as described in the preceding two chapters, is necessary to consider dissociation as a natural phenomenon.

FIVE STAGES OF MORPHOLOGY

We can explore the natural phenomenon of organismic dissociation as an evolution through five stages of active shaping (morphology). This includes metabolic changes for increased longevity, which require growth resistance. Growth and development in the human embryo is a constant flow against different scales of resistance. Resistance induces growth and development in all domains of life, especially in the activity of the three primary instincts as presented in chapter 18. Resistance is a requirement for longevity.

Step 1: Resistance, Passivity, Transparency

I love snorkeling. Florida has the only underwater state park in the continental United States. It is just an hour and a half south of my home. It is called John Pennekamp Coral Reef State Park, and here all the varieties of sea sponges are available to watch in their undulating dance with the currents and tides of the Atlantic Ocean. If these beautiful organisms are our ancient sisters, as discussed in chapter 18, it is easy to see their originality of resistance, passivity, and transparency underwater. They become resistant to large movement because they grow into the floor of the ocean. Their connection to the Earth binds them in form and function just as it binds us in form and function through our feet (for an excellent discussion of this, see David Abram's *Becoming Animal: An Earthly Cosmology*). This resistance is really the first consideration for stabilizing the ANS of a client, as many trauma specialists have pointed out. With my own PTSD, I feel the cascade of sensations and debilitating thoughts and then the urge to resist. It is the urge to resist in my body and mind that keeps me alive, while other veterans have lost their urge to resist and give in to despair and sometimes suicide. In my therapy at the VA, I was able to make a distinction between my unnecessary resistance to change and that which was necessary from being overwhelmed originally while in a terrorist bombing attack. I learned the need to transmute my form of resistance, which involved bouts of paranoia, nightmares, panic, and anxiety, to a process of recognizing the resistance and relaxing.

On the ocean floor, we can see how resistance allows the sea sponges to be passive, subject to the whims of the water they live in. Resistance is not about the ANS, it is about rooting to the Earth, allowing our senses to expand and our attention to confer with nature rather than other humans. It is about slowing down and being still so our molecules can transmute.

Nature is not like a Disney movie. Though it is full of dangers, it is not intentionally malevolent. Nature is not out to get you. The shore birds where I live continually pluck fish out of the water. They aren't malicious; they simply want to eat. I watch this dance of instant death every time I sit on the beach.

Passivity is vital to healing, whether that's a good night's sleep or withdrawing from culture and society by being nonattached. By being passive, sea sponges have a gesture of being carefree and aloof. They're just hanging out! Passivity can also be associated with relaxation, though in recent years it has become negatively associated with psychology. Nevertheless, passivity is the organismic urge that supports dissociation in its most organic form. This urge to simply be takes the form of a deep longing that is instinctual and the core of self-healing. In his poem "For Longing," John O'Donohue (2008) writes, "May you have the wisdom to enter generously into your own unease, to discover the new direction your longing wants you to take." This longing is known by interoceptive awareness. Schleip (2014) describes interoception as the felt sense of urges coming from the viscera. The conscious awareness of a visceral urge coming from the core of our body is sometimes described as a fire in the belly. A fire in the belly in this context is not the inflammatory processes raging in people's viscera; rather, it is the longing for safety and freedom from, for example, the oppression of food trauma and the pornography of social media addiction. Whether the urge is to eat, stop eating, urinate, defecate, or fall in love when the heart is throbbing, the felt sense of inner urges and being reliably responsive to them is critical. This is deeper than the sensory awareness of exteroception, aches and pains in the musculoskeletal system, and the proprioception bias that is prevalent in today's therapy culture.

Returning to our sea sponges, we see that these beautiful sea creatures are also transparent. Ocean flow moves through a porous mesh-like network that provides both resistance from strong currents and also the capacity to gather nutrition as particles adhere to the inner surface, much like food passing through human intestines makes contact with the inside mesh of the epithelium. This transparency and flow through is vital to all organisms. It is also the hallmark of the first stage of human heart development, in which the heart looks much like a sea sponge finger fan. The heart and our most distant human ancestors begin with a boundary-less capacity to survive and at the same time be nourished through those molecules that adhere to the surface.

The latest research on PTSD and its metabolism indicates that during a traumatic shock, such as a concussion, the epithelium of our gut, a single-celled lining from the mouth to the anus, becomes more transparent and the gaps between the cells widen. Through the necessity of opening our metabolic boundaries for survival, traumatic shock awakens our originality of resistance, passivity, and transparency. Our body insists on managing inner physical metabolic safety first. This is an indication that healing the lining of our gut and its microbiome should be the highest and deepest priority for survival, healing, and transcendence. Interoceptive awareness is critical to this repair.

When Leaky Gut Persists

Trauma can break the barrier function of the epithelium. When the trauma is long-term or unaddressed, it can lead to the condition commonly called "leaky gut." The primary cause of leaky gut is the trauma induced by overeating processed foods and added sugars. The modern diet carries other dangers as well. For example, excessive dietary fructose, such as from high-fructose corn syrup and its derivatives, stimulates cravings, impulsivity, risk-taking, and aggression and increases the risk for ADHD, bipolar disease, and aggressive behavior. Moreover, salty food and high-glycemic carbohydrates are converted into fructose and then glucose during metabolism, leading to hyperinsulinemia, heart disease, and obesity, just for starters. These are evolutionary responses to the highly processed food that people ingest daily. As a culture, we are constantly in feast mode and have forgotten famine mode, the skill of not eating.

I've given these details elsewhere in this book. I acknowledge that I am repeating some information. I want you, the reader, to consider that you are listening to a song, and while there is a familiar refrain in each chapter, there are new lyrics that correspond to the refrain. I want you, the reader, to be crystal clear on how to save your life.

Step 2: Separation of Inside from Outside

Early tubular sea sponge organisms in the Precambrian period (450 million years ago) had to become less flexible and less mobile for more efficient collection of nutrients in the template of the primitive tubular gut. The structure of the notochord (our original skeleton) appeared as a cylinder or rod to rigidify and make the internal organism better fed through less movement and stillness for increased nutrient absorption. But this increase in immobility created more vulnerability. This is the original double bind. The organism dissociates itself (separating inside from outside) with its new immobility but must change its shaping and movement (morphology) to survive. This is the original evolutionary engine of natural dissociation. It built the potency for longevity, immobility, and separating inside from outside while undergoing a shape changing that took millions of years to accomplish and then adapt.

The notochord appears three weeks after fertilization in the human embryo. It gradually disintegrates and becomes part of the nucleus pulposus of the intervertebral discs. It is also instrumental in the human embryo for generating a short period of axial resistance in growth and development through immobilizing the center of the embryo. It does this through tension, with each end being pulled in opposite directions. It is not inert or lifeless. Scanning electron microscopy shows the embryonic notochord as a wiggling snake. Thus, our earliest instincts are linked to our mobility (morphology) as well as behavior (nutrient metabolism). And even the human embryo recapitulates this originality with a dynamic stillness in the arising notochord at the center while accelerating growth movement in the periphery. The heart needs the stillness; the brain needs the speed. The double bind of stillness-movement is the core feature of this organic developmental dissociation.

It all begins with millions and millions of years of trial and error for selecting what comes in, processing it, recycling some of it to extract molecular nutrients, and disposing of what is not necessary, toxic, or organic waste. Everything gets used, so any excrement is compost for other organisms locally. It is the same today as it was hundreds of millions of years ago. We are set up to manage waste but not the volume of toxic pollution our bodies are asked to hold now. The immune system is overwhelmed, and a simple virus can take the body into a spiral of decline and death from a weak and polluted immune system. I am clear as I treat the contemporary client that by the '90s the client's nervous systems had exceeded their design capacity. In the following decade I noticed that my client's intestines were beyond capacity as well as their cardiovascular systems and finally the immune system. We are not designed for the amount of pollution we ingest daily at every level of our sensorium. And we may not recognize it until it too late, because metabolic syndromes may take many years to gestate before manifesting symptoms.

Step 3: Take In and Move Out

With a greater capacity to gather nutrients and initiate novel movement patterns for survival, the next evolutionary step from the gut as a filter was followed by the enteric nervous system (ENS) to process and move (propel) nutrients through the organism as efficiently as possible, along with the capacity to assimilate a large amount of potential nutrients and to discard or recycle what was not used or potentially harmful. These were the first two steps, according to some evolutionary biologists. Once again, this makes the gut the original initial structure of the human body to develop. This originality is also seen in human embryonic development, as the stem cells of the gut are the first to appear at the end of the first week post-fertilization.

The engine powering the body from the gut and its septic systems *must get built first* throughout the entire evolution of the pre- and postmodern human body. We must first learn to dissociate from noxious substances entering our body constantly. Thus, the evolution of PTSD as it relates to dissociation has been organized metabolically in the gut from the beginning of time. PTSD is a metabolic instinctual condition that is natural and is expressed on a spectrum of evolutionary possibilities. This means that our body is constantly repurposing older evolutionary structures and functions including PTSD symptoms.

Gut efficiency for processing input exists on a spectrum from rapid to slow. For example, I process caffeine slowly. One cup of coffee takes me thirty-six hours to process, while other people can drink ten cups of coffee in a day and sleep well at night. Metabolic cycles of anabolism (building up the body from carbohydrates, proteins, fats, and micronutrients) and catabolism (removing the waste products) have their own unique timeline for each of us. There are many redundant metabolic systems supporting anabolism and catabolism in order to be most efficient at balancing these processes in the event of a breakdown at any level of metabolism. However, chronic or repeated stress and trauma shut down numerous metabolic pathways. Trauma further interferes with the dynamic morphology of the organism and its critical movement patterns that support the metabolic pathways and cycling of anabolism-catabolism. Their cycling must be in a stable relationship or stagnation and toxicity build up and interfere with growth and development in all phases of life.

Step 4: Attraction to Pleasure, Repulsion from Pain

The fourth phase of evolutionary organismic development, from a metabolic basis, involves making physical distinctions between pleasure and pain. In chapter 18, I discussed the reticular formation of the spinal cord and brain stem, which evolved from approximately 540 million years ago to 485 million years ago in the Cambrian period. Some have said that the reticular formation was the original functioning structure upon which a human nervous system was initially designed, after the notochord. This theory comes from fossil studies of the lamprey eel from the Cambrian period. The notion here is that before there was much of a body per se, there was an original sensory organ interconnected to the whole organism that stimulated the organism to move closer to pleasant stimuli and farther away from noxious stimuli. Thus, movement becomes vital.

It makes perfect sense that, after the first three metabolically inspired morphological developments, the body learns what to accept and what to reject as an organism. The simple distinctions of pleasure and pain evolved. Imagine if these original metabolic and morphological functions are disabled in some way. Certain death for many primitive organisms; certain PTSD for some developing humans.

It is important to note that the impulse to separate from a source of pain, internally or externally, is a fundamental aspect of the contemporary pathologizing of dissociation. As humans, we are designed to be repulsed by pain and overwhelm. This quality of repulsion moves us away from the center of a toxicity, such as some contemporary social discourse, and if it does not, then emotional afflictions and conceptual confusion reign. With contemplative practice, such organic repulsion causes us to go deeper inside to seek solace. Or we might long to go outside and further into nature, which is now supported as a healing practice by so much literature (see for example, *Your Brain on Nature* by Eva Selhub and Alan Logan). Our aboriginal ancestors already had a much closer interrelationship with nature. Many ancestral groups considered nature to be a direct representation of the divine. Consequently, the people who moved farthest away from their own culture into the wilderness became the healers, the shamans, the cave-dwelling gurus, the ascetics, and so forth. Illich (1976, 130) says that "all traditional cultures derive their hygienic function from this ability to equip the individual with the means for making pain tolerable, sickness or impairment understandable, and the shadow of death meaningful." This occurs through the absolute support of the natural world. That possibility is now extremely difficult because of the pandemic of metabolic syndrome and the abdication of responsibility for our own body, turning it over to biomedicine, Big Pharma, and tribalism. This creates a metabolic and morphological double bind that requires a lot of help to resolve.

Early in my career, when I was practicing Rolfing, I saw that many clients were able to move out of toxic relationships or toxic careers when their body had the felt sense of safety and realignment. I learned the importance of body work. Subsequently I learned to contemplate my mental resistance without judgment through meditation and other therapeutic means. This was vital to ignite the potency of repulsion in order to separate from pain and suffering and to understand it, as Illich says.

Having dismissed and pathologized the potency of repulsion, we face the implosion of aberrant mind-body patterns culminating in the pandemic of metabolic syndrome. Our metabolic body becomes the new demon because spirit is flushed from the heart and blood with the systemic toxicity from inflammation. This leads to a painful death, usually in an ICU with multiple organ failure and sepsis.

It is my contention that pathologizing dissociation is a great aberration and morally distressing activity because it suppresses the natural repulsion to get away from culture and society and wake up and reclaim the health and healing intrinsic in the human body from beginningless time. Yes, we have an obligation to help our clients become stable and to assist them in their urge to withdraw from the center of a toxic culture. Such trauma work is a civilizational challenge. The trauma resolution community is simply a part of the biomedicine bandwagon celebrating pathology and maintaining the right medication so that people can return to work and produce more widgets, never living in the heart inside the heart. And yes, some of these therapies seek to stabilize the client, which is important, but stabilization needs to be coupled to transmutation into a new purpose. Complex PTSD is now considered a moral injury resulting from a moral violation. The main effect of a moral injury is an impaired ability to distinguish right from wrong. Moral injury goes beyond our limited understanding of the ANS. Metabolic syndrome is a civilizational issue and is caused by the moral violation of food trauma, its government and corporate sanctioning, and constant polarization from social media. One-third of Americans do not know how to cook and rely on corporate fast food and the television on how to feel about life.

The magnitude of PTSD in our culture right now has created a classification of personality that Joseph Bernstein calls the "borderland personality." His chilling perspective is that fragmentation is no longer a pathology even though it causes an untold amount of suffering. Rather, the borderland personality has embodied the deep split and separation from nature created by the history of our culture's alienation from the natural world. The new character structure is attempting to reconsolidate the split of body, mind, nature, and spirit, especially holding the enormity of the split from nature. "Ultimately," he writes, "the abhorrence of nature as *the* enemy became a characteristic of the western ego and of western culture itself, resulting in what I have come to call a 'fragmentation complex'" (Bernstein 2006, 36). He says that this leaves one with a feeling of self-disintegration from powerful irrational forces that cannot be explained. It is a feeling of "abject terror." This is a state even more frightening than a physical threat to one's life.

Step 5: Pressure Regulation

The fifth instinctual development has to do with oxygen and the integration of the pulmonary circulatory system and heart with the lungs. This capacity developed when our ancestors first crawled out of the ocean and onto land. These early organisms were equipped with gill arches that filter oxygen from water, but more oxygen was necessary to power locomotion on land, which meant more power, which required more energy from oxygen. Thus, the five lobes of the lungs and the four chambers of the heart developed to process much of the greater oxygen needs.

The oxygen molecule can be disrupted through stress, and thus oxidative stress from food trauma becomes a disruptor to the metabolic function of the body's oxygen processing capacity. Since we are practically talking about natural biological breathing in the present time, the consequence of food trauma is a pandemic of anoxia in most everyone.

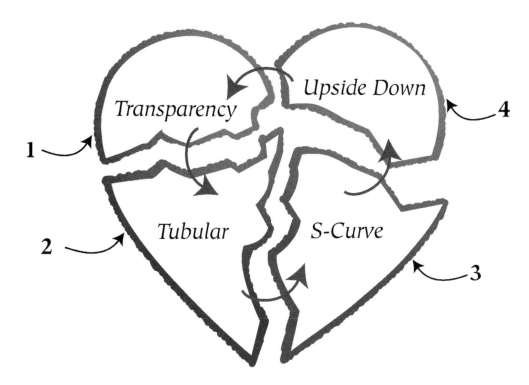

Fig. 19.1. The embryonic development of the human heart

1. A plexiform heart (*first phase*). Cardiogenic cells form in clusters. They are transparent, and water flows through this porous network of mesodermal cells.

2. A tubular heart (*second phase*). Whereas the heart tube of fish grows into a two-chambered heart, humans grow four chambers from their original tube. The heart at this point is completely upside down, with the atria at the bottom of the tube and the ventricles at the top.

3. An S-shaped tube (*third phase*). When the tube starts to curve, the inside lining of cells get squeezed and become quiescent, which means dynamically still. This induces growth of the four chambers.

4. Turning upside down into separate chambers (*fourth phase*). Initially the chambers start to dilate and balloon. First the left ventricle balloons, followed by the right atria Then the cushions and valves separating the chambers develop.

Such organization and morphology allow the generation of complexity, developmental robustness, and evolutionary flexibility or evolvability (see fig. 19.1). The human heart never stops growing and evolving (for an excellent treatment of this subject, see Margaret Kirby's *Cardiac Development*). This is because the inside of the embryonic heart has poor circulation and must repurpose and recycle myocardial cells that are dying for the overall construction project before blood can begin to flow through the chambers. And since there is a bypass valve from the lungs to the right atria in utero, there is no blood coming from the lungs into the heart.

The four-chambered heart at one level is a type of pressure pump, and although the "pump model" of the human heart has grown out of favor (except if you are a heart surgeon), the point of this chapter is the need for interoceptive awareness of pressure differentials in the center of the human body. Furst (2020) calls the heart an "organ of impedance," meaning an organ of slowness, which is the embryonic model. In biodynamic morphology, the heart grows slowly and the nervous system grows quickly. The fulcrum where these opposing forces meet is posterior to the dorsal pericardium, adjacent to the neural tube. Interoceptive awareness is conscious awareness of the signals from the body's organs. Simply sensing one's heartbeat in the middle of the chest builds empathy and is a critical biofeedback barometer of internal states.

The gut does not operate with the same type of pressure that the heart and lungs do. Thus, interoceptive awareness of the urge to urinate or defecate has a different felt sense that many people ignore. And while blood pressure is a major marker of heart health, so are healthy bowel movements. Three or fewer bowel movements a week is a risk factor for Alzheimer's. This central body pressure system is most easily modified by our breathing, vagal stimulation, and vagal maneuvers, all covered in detail in my book *The Biodynamics of the Immune System*. In the last part of this book, many hands-on skills will be shown to help the heart and gut.

Both pressure and reciprocal reflexive breathing are an originality that far predates neurological reflexes as we know them today. These dynamics are also seen immediately after human conception. All adult function in the human is pre-exercised in the human embryo; the first week after fertilization is one of immense pressure inside the young embryo, and the pre-exercising of reciprocal breathing can be observed in the fertilized egg. Conscious attention to our heartbeat and breathing that inflates the transversus abdominis muscle covering the abdominal cavity is critical for central pressure regulation since the lungs have negative pressure and the abdomen has positive pressure. All central pressures must maintain balance. The transversus abdominis muscle interdigitates with the respiratory diaphragm. It expands the abdomen during inhalation and the abdomen relaxes back during exhalation. It synchronizes the respiratory and pelvic diaphragms. It balances central pressure.

With stress and trauma, our central body pressure of the heart and lungs (pulmonary circulation) can easily become disturbed, which is a dissociation from its original nature rather than a pathological artifact. The double bind of a dysfunctional blood pressure–lung breathing process is very painful, and ERs are full of such "old" problems: asthma, COPD, heart disease, apnea, and types of atrial fibrillation.

MYSTERY AND MEANING

With these five primary metabolic functions of anabolism (building/nurturing) and catabolism (waste removal/recycling) and interrelated shaping morphology of biokinetics and biodynamics, the foundation for an original instinctual metabolic PTSD is demonstrated. In other words, PTSD has been here from the beginning of life on the planet as we know it. It cannot be otherwise. Our bodies have preexisting ways of dissipating trauma metabolically. Biodynamic cardiovascular therapy assists these original instincts into something discernible by allowing the body to be in an evolutionary cycle and to support the repurposing of older structures and functions.

I am always amazed that anthropologists constantly find artifacts in more and more ancient burial sites indicating the nascent development of a transcendent spiritual function. Primitive people sat around a fire gazing at it and could experience a stillpoint integrated with the natural world and a resetting of their neurological reflexes at an unconscious level. They collectively entered a state of awe and wonder. This is also a normal natural state of dissociation from the ordinary world. They could more easily access their original dissociation for resistance through binding to the Earth and transformation through right-brain activation, the Zen center of our brain as it is called via fire gazing. I know this state as I have gazed at many fires for long hours in Native American healing ceremonies. The effect of a natural dissociation from ordinary senses comes from the fire imbued with sentient qualities by original peoples, and the stillpoint gave birth to the self-transcendent instinct of mystery (awe at wholeness) and meaning (of pain and suffering).

Competing instincts oriented toward our animal nature and toward our human nature created a huge double bind for survival. A double bind is built into our original metabolism, as described above. All double binds have a metabolic component, as does dissociation. Choices are created by such binds. And clearly there would be a spiritual aptitude identifying one's location on the spectrum of dissociation and to what degree dissociation is experienced within the mystery of wholeness to debilitation. Enter the complex world of neurobiology, the contemporary basis of a scientific aptitude for growth and development. Yet the heart is known by all cultures in the East as the center of spiritual growth and development. Is the doorway through the double bind as simple as being aware of one's heartbeat?

The Double Bind of Migration

Yet another organic double bind in terms of evolutionary development can be seen in the human pattern of migration. Humans, from prehistoric to present times, migrate, usually because they need to move away from noxious stimuli like wild animals, violent neighbors, and food insecurity. A dear friend of mine has volunteered in refugee camps all over the Middle East and Europe, including more recently in Ukraine, for more than forty years. Her stories about these camps reveal them as an unfolding tragedy in many cases. There are no easy solutions to these civilizational issues. All people have a right to healthy food, shelter, and clothing—and the right to worship spiritually.

The double bind of migration is that sometimes humans need to move to find safety and food, and yet also humans need a stable settlement, especially for child development. At this time on our planet the United Nations reports that there are more than sixty million people in refugee camps worldwide, more than at any other time in human history. We simply must appreciate the fact that human beings are repulsed by fascism and seek to become stable. We can turn to Wilhelm Reich's third layer of character structure, balancing out hatred with love. Consciously relating with one's experience of trauma is associated with overcoming fascism inside and outside, as described by Reich (1980).

THE EVOLUTIONARY CORE OF PTSD: A REVIEW

When we look at these five core evolutionary (organismic) developments of the various systems of the human body, the core of PTSD is as follows.

1. Resistance, passivity, and transparency. Our boundarylessness becomes an organic double bind (being rooted in the Earth also creates vulnerability as an adaptive response).
2. Separation of inside from outside. Immobility and shape changing as the basis of growth and development becomes an organic double bind (I become immobile from my fear, and I must immobilize to have a bowel movement, urinate, or make love with my wife). Which immobilization is which when I am under stress?
3. Take in and move out. The innate capacity to know what to accept and what to reject is disrupted. It becomes an organic double bind when a moral violation creates a moral injury, weakening one's ability to differentiate right from wrong.
4. Attraction to pleasure, repulsion from pain. The issue of pain and pleasure is hugely disrupted and magnified given the complexity of the human organism now as opposed to in ancient times. Ignorance was indeed bliss for paleolithic people. We have another organic double bind when pain and pleasure both become triggers and the ANS periodically reverses sensory systems at random as a regular side effect of complex PTSD.
5. Pressure regulation. The heart and lungs, the centers of the brain that coregulate and monitor oxygen saturation, and movement of the respiratory dia-

phragm into the abdomen are compromised because of oxidative stress from food trauma. Another organic double bind is conscious awareness of an elevated heart rate (tachycardia) and shortness of breath. These are my constant companions.

So, my new definition of PTSD is based on these five stages. PTSD is an original, metabolic, and instinctual process from an evolutionary-organismic point of view. It predates neurological models by millions and millions of years. The neurological safety reflexes originating in the brain stem undoubtedly codeveloped with emotional regulation in the limbic system for socialization until finally humans could settle for longer periods of time and develop moral reflexes cortically. Metabolism and morphology preceded neurological reflexes by a long shot. This is a possible direction for post-trauma health.

Those with complex PTSD, such as myself, are experts in the felt sense metabolism of dissociation. Many diagnosed with PTSD live with it, and it is the constant new normal. We here in Western civilization are the only ones that pathologize dissociation. Yet extrasensory information, the principal side effect of contemporary PTSD, gives access to intimate complex knowledge of life and death, the natural world, other species, and other humans. And yet such information is pathologized. It is also damned uncomfortable having PTSD without some form of anesthesia—legal, illegal, spiritual, or rational. Dissociation is the natural ground of becoming a healer to oneself and others if that is one's aptitude for self-regulation in the midst of these deep organismic and instinctual double binds. As Yogi Berra once said, "If you see a fork in the road, take it." I drive on the road of an ancient double bind, an endless fork in the road.

The rates of depression and anxiety keep increasing, and pharmaceuticals are not effective. I have tried so many therapies, and while some provide relief for longer periods than others, the healing work continues to be trial and error. What works today might not work tomorrow. There is no universal antidote except the longing to be free of the worst of the symptoms. This longing keeps me going. Consequently, it is not possible to make a recommendation to the reader for help except to stop the food trauma. Stay in the longing for that which naturally is reliable and nurturing.

TRAUMA REVISED

The stages of human development have been well defined by many experts, with, of course, Jean Piaget being one of the more notable. Trauma is complex because you never really get over it; it can never be erased from your memory bank, neurologically or somatically. One of the problems with trauma resolution therapies is that some methods are used like cookie cutters—one size fits all. Depending on where someone is in their life development, a cookie-cutter therapy might help, or it might not, or it might retraumatize a person.

As Robert Thurman, emeritus professor at Columbia University, said in a lecture,* "Homo sapiens is the trauma species." That is our distinct specialty as human beings, and at the other end of the spectrum is love. All clients fall somewhere on that spectrum, with their own unique symptoms. Consequently, every single biodynamic session requires something new on the part of the therapist. And unless the therapist is doing their own work to spiritually mature, the client may experience negative side effects. Some might not manifest for a while. The healing process is timeless. It is timeless up to and including our death.

I use contemplative practices to maintain stability of my mind and body and to develop awe. Human instincts are powerful beyond belief; they run our entire biochemistry and metabolism. We must come into relationship with our instincts and our soma consciously and slowly over time. This can be very painful—thus the prevalence of spa therapies, relaxation therapies, and the contemplative arts. Ultimately, the realized intention of the life process is to recognize with mindfulness when our attention is captured and relax into open awareness. And it's virtually impossible to simply tell someone to relax and have them do it. To recognize and relax is also preparation for death. Trauma implants an unconscious phobia around death, which we can experience as a felt sense of terror. There is no off switch regarding human instincts, and it is critical to know when our metabolism switches into detoxification mode so we can learn to let go of that which is dead and dying inside of us, including our terror.

The uniqueness of each client and the necessity for a new composition and a new relationship with each session is the essence of biodynamic practice. There needs to be a deeper knowing about the instincts, biochemistry, and metabolism of what keeps trauma in place, like processed food and the pornography of social media. The medical community seems to be especially clueless in this regard. The trauma resolution community needs a metabolic understanding of trauma and to differentiate developmental periods of the life span as they relate to PTSD. Every decade of life changes the matrix of trauma such that what worked last year might no longer be relevant this year.

There is no lasting stability for any human being. Instead, we must learn to embrace and accept constant change. I can now accept the frequency of my episodes of anxiety or deeper fear and terror states. With contemplative practices, I can transmute terror into a spiritual essence in the heart inside my heart. I believe the entire trauma

---

*The lecture, entitled "Wisdom is Bliss" with Professor Robert Thurman and Dr. Nida Chenagtsang, was held on February 18, 2022, in Los Angeles at Pure Land Farms.

resolution fantasy needs a dramatic metabolic revision. We cannot go on supporting the capitalist system we function in geopolitically. It is time to move attention away from the corporate center of our planet to heal rather than trying to get back to work in a dysfunctional job. I'm trying to get better at leading my life, which is the developmental demand through each stage, because it only gets more existentially complex the older I get. And I'm at an age (seventy-five at the time of this writing) where I contemplate the nature of my own death and dying every single day. This is not an obsession or suicidal ideation but rather a natural instinct manifesting as daily thoughts and wonderment about a natural death, if I should be so lucky. In the samurai tradition, this was called the Way of Dying. A warrior's most basic intention is to keep death always in mind, day and night. When death is kept continually in mind, "both loyalty and filial piety are realized, myriad evils and disasters are avoided, you are without illness and mishap, and you live out a long life. In addition, even your character will be improved. Such are the benefits of this act" (Wilson 2015, 81).

Most people aren't ready to die. That means all of us have to start preparing now. Anxiety, shortness of breath, and pain are the big three symptoms while in the dying process, not to mention the level of regret that many people have in the dying process. Yet it is possible to die wise, as Stephen Jenkinson says in his book by that title. Spiritual traditions describe an almost blissful process of death and dying if one is well prepared mentally and emotionally.

Many trauma resolution therapies have failed to help American veterans with PTSD. I would love to see some long-term follow-up studies to prove me wrong. I've done several years of evidence-based therapies at my local VA hospital. It is the biggest form of group therapy I've ever experienced. Just walking into the clinic allows one to encounter hundreds of veterans missing various parts of their bodies and minds. The level of kindness by the staff at the hospital is extraordinary. The whole of my therapeutic experience at the VA, even with individual therapy, was within the context of being in a larger group in which everyone, including the therapists and vets, has the same intention: to help heal each other. Many of us have experienced extraordinary horror. As a species, we are not designed for killing each other (Grossman 2009). Somehow we can kill animals and plants to eat, but when it comes to killing another human being, our instincts repulse and the side effects are devastating as mentioned previously. And that's a whole other topic because the killing of each other hasn't ever stopped since the beginning of time.

The point is that trauma resolution therapies in the public domain are largely ineffective for veterans and many other folks. When I hear an expert throw out the line "I worked at the VA," it simply means that veterans are lab rats for every conceivable therapy available, including even psychedelic-assisted therapy. A therapist with even just one or two years of internship at the VA earns a merit badge with the right to say "I worked with veterans." It is meaningless without context. I'm a very willing lab rat. I also enjoy my life and can manage these powers of anxiety and fear. I practice the Way of Dying daily. Not all vets and other folks dealing with trauma are so lucky. The trauma resolution community has deficiencies in not knowing the metabolism of trauma. It is time to go back to a metabolic drawing board for helping human beings with a history of trauma. We must appreciate how it develops and morphs over each decade in our life. We must know how to treat it metabolically.

Bayo Akomolafe (2017) talks about trauma not as what happens to the body, but rather as the body in its constant external world-shaping, internal form-taking capacity, and overreactivity. Trauma is how modern bodies are manufactured, especially by hospital births and the abysmal rate of maternal and infant mortality in the United States. Wars have not stopped. Gun violence has not stopped. The fundamentalism of the mainstream discourse on trauma and its history as a clinical concept began with Pierre Janet's famous work in the late 1800s on hysteria in women. The diagnosis of hysteria completely covered up the reality of pervasive sexual abuse. Then as now, psychological wounds are concealed by the politics that sponsors them. Today, that means putting trauma survivors back to work in the corporate production model of finance and work ethic, with mindfulness and self-care used for anesthesia.

Trauma is the contemporary grammar of loss and the vocabulary of embodied sorrow. That loss is never given a funeral; its grief is never able to be resolved, especially for veterans. Unresolved grief is passed on and rarely integrated. We must be cognizant of the danger posed by healing paradigms that are dedicated exclusively to recovery but initiated by corporate greed or religious fervor. The body speaks metabolically; we must only learn to listen consciously to our gut and heart.

20

Interoceptive Awareness of
the Gut and Pelvis

WITH CATHY SHEA

CATHY SHEA is licensed in massage and colon hydrotherapy in Florida since 1992. She also holds full certification in Swiss Biological Medicine from Thomas Rau, MD.

The preceding chapters have introduced the reader to importance of interoception. To briefly review, this complex sensory system in the body is based on the instinct for self-preservation and energy needs. The driver of interoceptive awareness is the metabolic need to eat and eliminate. The critical implication is that interoceptive awareness means being consciously sensing signals from the body and interpreting them correctly regarding getting food in, digesting, absorbing, and removing waste products expeditiously. This is the cosignaling dynamic of the endocrine system. When we feel hungry, it is a hormone telling us that. Such perception of the body requires a great deal of mental, emotional, and somatic clarity. This clarity is primarily derived from eating real, whole food and regular elimination of waste and toxins via the sweat, urine, and feces. That is the source of deep metabolic energy, and it powers every single cell in the human body to sustain all the hard work it's doing and to discharge its waste products routinely and efficiently with optimal conditions.

ALLOSTASIS AND HOMEOSTASIS

The brain generates a massive set of physiological responses to meet its energy needs to maintain allostasis and achieve stability. This includes instructions to the body to meet those needs. It turns out that the body has its own independent system of homeostatic reflexes to manage its energy needs. These unique metabolic pathways are functionally separate from the brain's; they include the gut's enteric nervous system (ENS) and others, such as the autonomic nervous system (ANS). The body's system of homeostasis becomes a form of interoceptive awareness when we consciously perceive the activity of the ANS and endocrine systems. So basically, the body has double duty. It must produce high-level fuel for the brain, and I do mean high-level fuel, primarily from ketones and minimal glucose. It must also produce fuel for its own musculoskeletal system, which is a dynamic energy consumer, especially for mobility, such as foraging and migrating to get proper nutrition, in order to fulfill its primary instinctual drive for self-preservation. This is primal and primitive.

THE VAGUS NERVE: GUT–BRAIN HIGHWAY

The vagus nerve is a major player in interoceptive awareness, as is the entire ANS, including the parasympathetic nervous system (PNS) and the sympathetic nervous system (SNS), as previously discussed. The vagus nerve is the majority of the PNS. The vagus has two parts. As discussed in the previous chapter it has a dorsal part going down toward the pelvis. It has a ventral part that goes as far as the heart and keeps the heart toned to a heartbeat around 70 BPM. Please see *The Biodynamics of the Immune System* for a through description of the vagus. It contains most of the sensory information coming from the gut to the heart and brain. It's a sophisticated feedback system and superhighway in the middle of the body. The brain uses the constant flow of sensory information being delivered by the vagus nerve to coordinate allostatic responses in the body, predicting metabolic needs and then directing impulses for physiological balance.

THE INSULA

The main processor of interoception neurologically is the insular cortex, also called the insula. The insula needs a strong connection to the prefrontal cortex, and hopefully enough of the prefrontal cortex is wired in after birth to make appropriate and wise decisions about reliable physiological responses. As discussed in *Biodynamic Craniosacral Therapy* Volumes 1–5, the majority of infant–caregiver attachments do not end up with the prefrontal cortex being optimally wired for optimal life span growth and development.

The brain stem and the amygdala are other major players. Evolutionarily, they precede the insula and also the hypothalamus and frontal cortex. The brain stem, of course, houses both parts of the vagus nerve, the old primitive part that extends to the gut and the new one that determines social safety. The amygdala is a significant processing center for emotions, especially fear. It is linked to other areas of the brain regarding memories, learning, and the senses and thus interoceptive awareness.

As humans develop, the insula is the highly coordinated complex part of our cortex. The insula is called the *first fold* in embryology. It is the first level organizing the growth and development of the entire cortex in general and starts developing between six and seven weeks after fertilization. The neural tube closes at that time, and the top of the neural tube becomes the third ventricle of the brain. According to Dr. James Jealous, all structure and function in the head and neck arise from the third ventricle. It is a fluid bubble folding and lengthening into discrete geographic regions of the brain, preceding definitive structures.

Hunger and Satiety

Hunger shows itself so differently with all of us. For example, I rarely feel the signal of hunger in my stomach. Sleepy, dopey, loopy, hangry, cranky, impatient, thirsty, blurry, achy, hot, cold . . . these are some of the body signals that I get when I'm hungry. The most common awareness for me is loss of concentration. I also noticed that my vision begins to blur. Sometimes I find myself rushing to get things done and then realize I'm doing it because I need real food.

In our culture, with its abundance of processed, sugary, salty, fried, preservative-filled food, the hunger signal is often obscured and clear interoceptive awareness for reliable allostatic responses in the brain is clouded. The same can be said for satiety signals. We simply cannot tell when we need sustenance, what will satisfy us, and when our metabolic needs have been satisfied.

There is also a hunger for meaning, a hunger for joy, a hunger for peace, and a hunger for love and happiness. So, we're left with a question: What reliably satisfies our body, mind, and spirit?

THE GUT TUBE

The oldest structures and functions of the body are in the gut tube. It is almost thirty feet from mouth to anus in the adult human (see fig. 20.1). That's where it started nearly a billion years ago and that's where it ends in the human today. Data from the dorsal vagus below the diaphragm is spread throughout the gut. All visceral and all metabolic functions in the gut are innervated by the dorsal vagus. It manages and relays information to the heart and brain regarding every level, physiologically and metabolically, of digestion, absorption, transport, and elimination in the abdominopelvic region.

A lot of decisions are made by the ANS about the distribution of what's going to the brain and what's going to the body. The PNS is sending information via the vagus up the center of the body, and the SNS is sending data to the spinal cord and

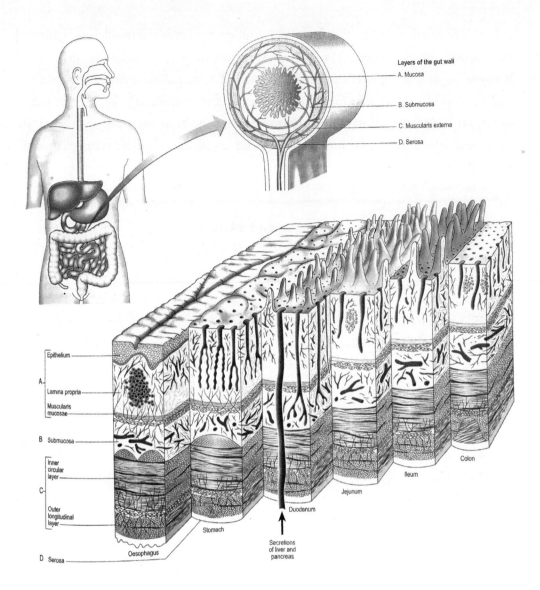

Fig. 20.1. The general arrangement of the alimentary canal, showing the layers of the gut wall

up. Eighty percent of the information flow is up from the gut brain to the head brain, with 20 percent of the flow coming down to the gut via the vagus nerve.

As mentioned in the previous chapters, the ancient reticular formation in the spinal cord evaluates irritation, pain, or any non-nurturing quality that causes the organism to retreat, withdraw, or move away from the irritant. The reticular formation is the organismic immediate unconscious response. The insular cortex is the body's evaluator and predictor, but compared to the reticular formation, its reaction can be delayed or, due to maladaption, inappropriate signaling, and so the reticular formation is an important coregulator of response.

In either case of moving toward or away from that which we are in immediate relationship with, the circuit of insular cortex–vagus–enteric nervous system–reticular formation regulates a vast amount of physiology and metabolism in the body and informs our interoceptive awareness via three pathways. The first pathway starts in the gut and the pelvis and goes up to the brain through the heart, which is the vagal pathway in the anterior or central body cavity. Second the neural tube pathway to the brain with the reticular formation is the posterior pathway, with the ENS being connected both to the vagal system anteriorly and to the reticular formation area of the spinal cord posteriorly. The third pathway of interoception is humeral (endocrine). The endocrine system signals the gut-heart-brain axis through the cardiovascular system and blood. Biodynamic cardiovascular therapy and NeuroVascular Colon Hydrotherapy engages with these three pathways.

PELVIC INTEROCEPTION

Somatic awareness of the functions of the pelvis are vital to human health and well-being. The urination reflex, the defecation reflex, and the flatulence reflex are coregulated through the sacral outflow of the PNS. That PNS outflow is synchronized with the pudendal nerve and pudendal plexus. The pudendal nerve innervates the clitoris and vulva in a woman and the head and shaft of the penis in a man, so that the reproduction reflex is potentized with pleasure anatomically. All the nerve fibers for urination, defecation, and the orgasm reflex share the same dorsal vagus connection with the sacral outflow of the PNS. They are all integrated via the sacral outflow of the PNS, where complex synapses occur with the posterior vagus at the inferior hypogastric plexus and the anterior vagus at Cannon's point, close to the splenic flexure of the large intestine. These nerve fibers all require conscious interoceptive awareness for proper functioning. Always remember that interoceptive awareness arose from evolution as an effect of the instinct for self-preservation, the so-called survival instinct. This is about food and hunger and reproduction, as discussed in chapters 17, 18, and 19. Protocols for these areas of the abdomen and pelvis are taught in part 4 of this book.

The core metabolic instinct of self-preservation is about meeting immediate energy needs: procurement of real food and pure water and regular elimination via the bladder and large intestine. The bladder and large intestine must be evacuated whenever they send the signal to do so. Everyone needs training to consciously discern these signals and respond appropriately as soon as they become aware of the urge. Everyone who has had food poisoning knows the sensation of urgency. I recently had a bout of food poisoning and felt like I lived on the toilet for two days. It triggered memories of past food poisonings, binge eating, and my history of morbid obesity. The gut clearly holds memories of the past. But when we are not ill, the wave may not be as strong; the sensations may fade as we age, requiring more attention to the body's subtle signals; the brain may be overwhelmed with exteroceptive information coming from our five senses, so that it ignores what is needed interoceptively. Yet any delay in answering the call to these homeostatic reflexes create stress in the PNS, and consequently the SNS gets involved at the level of the cardiovascular system, opening the door to the potential loss of vasodilation regulated by the SNS of the endothelium. In other words, when we ignore or don't hear the signals to use the bathroom, our body tightens all the way to the blood vessels themselves in order shut down the signal to eliminate. We primarily teach people how to listen to their body.

ENTERIC NERVOUS SYSTEM

Gut pain is also a local feedback loop in the layers of the enteric nervous system (ENS) embedded within the gut tube. The ENS was originally considered a component of the ANS, but research has shown it to be so independent that the ENS is now considered its own organ system. In his book about the ENS, titled *The Second Brain* (1998), Dr. Michael Gershon notes that it has more neurons than the brain and spinal cord combined and produces over 90 percent of serotonin. The embryology is important because the ENS derives from neural crest vagal cells in the cervical region of the embryo. These cells move down the center of the embryo along the canalization zone that's going to become the gut tube of the endoderm. They are squeezed down morphologically like a tube of toothpaste from the top of the neural tube down the center of the fluid body of the embryo. The vagal neural crest cells being moved down into the gut tube terminate at Cannon's point, which is two-thirds of the way over to the splenic flexure on the transverse colon. The stomach attaches to Cannon's point via the mesentery. This is where a specialized fascial connection of the mesentery called the transverse mesocolon at the bottom of the stomach attaches to the transverse colon. This area gets stretched with overeating and creates a skew in the signaling for satiety. It also promotes a prolapse condition and the potential for the transverse colon to drop down and press on the bladder and reproductive organs. Many reproductive challenges are related to digestive dysfunction, particularly overeating, which also leads to obesity and puts additional stress on this area of the gut.

The remainder of the ENS from Cannon's point to the anus is built from cells coming from the pelvic floor, the adrenal-gonadal-mesonephros area of the embryo, which ends up becoming the sacral outflow of the PNS. This point is also where the vascular supply of the large intestine changes from the superior mesenteric artery-vein to the inferior mesenteric artery-vein. The importance of Cannon's point to the structure and function of the entire gut cannot be stressed enough; gently touching this area upon awakening in the morning to stimulate peristalsis is helpful as part of gut self-care. We teach this to our therapists and clients.

At the same time in the embryonic development, sympathetic nerves are exiting the thoracic and lumbar spinal cord. These nerves form ganglia and plexuses from back to front in the embryo. In the adult they are in front of the spine, interacting with the descending/abdominal aorta. Ganglia and plexuses are miniature brains capable of receiving sensory information and sending out a motor response, called a visceral-somatic or somatic-visceral reflex, locally and/or globally. These are the primary homeostatic reflexes in the body mainly regulating blood flow.

The sympathetic nervous system and the parasympathetic vagus (the two parts of the ANS) come together in front of the descending aorta and abdominal aorta. They are sometimes called the aortic plexuses because of their coregulation of the arteries. The ganglia and plexuses are an integrated ANS circuit. This means that the plexuses are an integrated system of both PNS/vagal data and SNS data. There is a constant flow of metabolic dorsal vagal information from every organ going into the abdominal aortic plexus and all ANS plexuses in front of the entire spine. It's very complex circuitry and informs sensations.

GUT PAIN

The sensation of gut pain is usually caused by emotional reactions, excessive gas from poor food combining, or inflammation from food sensitivities/allergies and ultraprocessed food. It can vary from mild to moderate to strong. It is likely that flatulence is a specific reflex because the urge to pass gas is very relieving when it happens without interference or embarrassment. The anal sphincter is the most sophisticated muscle in the body because it must differentiate between solid, liquid, and gas. Flatulence moving through the large intestine can stretch the tube housing the ENS and trigger its pain receptors, which go to the ANS plexuses and then to the spinal cord. ENS pain from inflammatory processes associated with small intestine leaky gut syndrome is a major stressor for the vascular and nervous systems because it goes not only to the spinal cord but also through the center of the body with the vagus. Allostatic responses in the brain can be severe because of the immune-endocrine input from pain interoception. The complex inflammatory conditions caused by ultra processed food can greatly enhance this pain cycle and lead to brain alterations that, in turn, manifest in metabolic syndrome that affects the entire body.

The ENS sends pain signals through the sympathetic ganglia back to the spinal cord. It's not a strong signal, but if it's constantly flooding the cord with pain, the homogeneous neuronal pool will light up. Then it can become a systemic problem because areas of the body that are already inflamed or in pain receive a boost in reflex signals and local pain increases. This means that other than the brain and heart, where the data are headed, ENS pain can register anywhere in the body (visceral-somato reflex pattern) as it stimulates the spinal cord and all nerve pathways somatically. It also explains how a low back issue may result in gut upset (somato-visceral reflex pattern).

There is no way of knowing where that information will go to enhance a potential subclinical condition underneath conscious awareness and then bring it up to the level of interoceptive awareness. Remember that all this somatic reflex information must be filtered by the heart and then the brain, which is also receiving input simultaneously from the vagus nerve and the endocrine and immune systems via the blood.

CARDIOVASCULAR SYSTEM

The cardiovascular system is the significant link between the body's two instinctual metabolic consumers: the brain and the body. Interoceptive awareness includes the need to develop an exquisite conscious sensitivity to the cardiovascular system. That starts with cardioception: being able to sense your own heartbeat without having to physically take your pulse or use a digital heart monitoring app. Try mentally counting seventy heartbeats. Then look at the sweep second hand of your watch (or have your digital watch show a countdown minute timer) and repeat the counting to seventy again. Verify if your pre-watch perception was accurate even without the timer. This is a practice of interoceptively knowing the tempo of our heart. Practice sensing your heartbeat until the mental counting and watch counting match regularly. Seventy beats per minute is considered the gold standard for a resting heart rate. The more precise you are, the better. Cardioception is the foundation of interoceptive awareness, and this signals the empathy path in the brain.

Local, global, and neurological decisions are being made by the metabolism within the cardiovascular system itself. It is the driver for all the energy that needs to be transported to every cell in the brain and body, especially the endothelium. Knowledge of how much nutrition goes where moment by moment is discerned by the endothelium and the end organ it is serving. Knowledge of global immune system needs regarding inflammation are also coregulated by the endothelium. Consequently, the function of the endothelium is cosmic. The decisions about how much oxygen, micronutrients, ketones, and glucose are triggered by the molecular communication between the artery, the heart and brain, and the end organ. I am frequently asked about the venous system, and we cannot forget about its importance. Yes, the veins play a significant role embryonically when all vascular structures led to the embryonic heart, especially the umbilical and subclavian veins. The endothelium and wall structure of adult veins, however, are different and have more of an association with thermal regulation of the body than does the artery itself. The heart works harder to circulate heat in the blood. This important metabolic capacity of the heart and veins can be compromised in metabolic syndrome, especially in the gut where dysfunction originates.

BREATHING

All the activity in the abdomen and pelvis requires a mechanical churning motion. The respiratory diaphragm expands the abdomen during inhalation, and then during exhalation there's a relaxation at the level of the pelvic diaphragm. Breathing includes interoceptive awareness of how the respiratory diaphragm and pelvic diaphragm are synchronized in their motion during inhalation and exhalation.

The movement of the respiratory diaphragm also stretches the dorsal vagus and the pericardium and keeps them physiologically toned because of the enormity of the flow of neurotransmitters and other signaling molecules within the ANS central highway of the body. Consequently, the breath will also tone the ENS so that its function of creating peristalsis is supported because the dorsal vagus also helps with the wavelike neurological activity in the gut tube. This amazing symphony of activity informs our nutrient absorption primarily in the small intestine. This segment of our gut tube houses the lymphatic tissue known as Peyer's Patches that inform 70–80 percent of our innate immune activity. There are critical signaling molecules from the Peyers' Patches that are essential for the acquired immune system.

Proper abdominal breathing also stimulates the necessary relaxation response to facilitate ease in swallowing and the transport of gas and feces through the large intestine."

All of this interoceptive awareness is to know the oldest and deepest instinctual capacity of the human body: the elimination and reproductive reflexes. Listen to your body as it nurtures and heals itself.

21

Ignition, Midline,
and Spiritual Aptitude

Now, being grounded in interoceptive awareness and the state of mind for compassion to manifest, we move into biodynamic cardiovascular therapy (BCVT) practice and perception.

IGNITION

My mentor, Dr. Jim Jealous, taught a five-step perceptual process that he called Ignition. It was Dr. Sutherland, however, who first coined that term in the 1930s based on the vocabulary being used for automobiles. Dr. Jealous associated Ignition with the fire element and its potency. I am offering an interpretation and update of the Ignition process based on the therapist's potential spiritual aptitudes and the core biodynamic perceptions of Primary Respiration (PR) and dynamic stillness. I make this offering to the reader through the lens of the Indo-Tibetan system of elements (space, wind, fire, water, earth). This offering is based on the great metabolic illness now being expressed in most of our clients. This is my interpretation of Ignition

1. Spark

The first step in the five-step process is spark. Spark is the initial perception of friction created by the element of fire and the element of wind in their very deep and broad relationship inside and outside the body. The spark is like rubbing two sticks together on a rock, the element of earth, yet more subtle. In the perceptual process, the spark is the first moment of awareness that generates the pervasive felt sense of the element of fire in the body, which is warmth. Dr. Jealous said that sweating and getting hot in a biodynamic session is the essence of a biodynamic process. I say it is sorrow and compassion waking up. It is a deep expression of the metabolism of the body, fueled by an evolutionary relationship of embodiment with the sun over many millions of years. The friction is constant because of the need for warmth linked to the instinct for self-preservation. This includes the growing, cooking, and eating of real food, the critical fuel that the viscera must break down and assimilate for cellular mitochondrial function. Because of the temperatures in the body's core, the food we eat continues to be cooked and processed inside us, especially by the stomach and small intestine. Fire is the essence of metabolism and the deepest expression of the heart inside the heart. Consequently, a lot of heat is needed, and in the Indo-Tibetan medical system, the fulcrums for the fire element are the heart, liver, kidneys, eyes, and skin, including their associated arteries. Fire is balanced by water and the blood is the element of water. BCVT focuses on this vital relationship. The spark is always at the change of phase of PR.

Regarding palpation, the spark needs space between the hands and the skin. A spark in electricity must jump in between a gap between objects—in this case, the skin of the client and the therapist's hands. Consequently, Zone B, or what Dr. Becker called the biosphere, is of critical importance. This is the space immediately around the body, extending fifteen inches or more from the skin. When we make physical contact, our hands begin to conduct heat through the clothing or skin of the client. We are always literally "in touch" with the heat. Sometimes we can feel beads of sweat trickling down our spine, under our armpits, or down the brow of our face. Sometimes our clients remark that our hands are on fire. Just as skin-to-skin contact helps a baby thermally regulate, so too the client-therapist relationship is an interpersonal thermal regulation system. Consider the possibility that the client had difficulty thermally regulating as an infant and that capacity may be in the process of restoration simply from our palpation. Sweat linked to thermal regulation comes from the blood. The heart brings excess heat in the body to the surface via the vascular tree. Thus, Zone B has humidity linked to the evaporation of water filled with different metabolites coming from the blood. Zone B is part of the vascular system. It contains a mix of a variety of metabolites and microbiota from the exhalation of the breath as well as infrared heat and electrically charged water.

We make minimal contact with the client's skin or clothing to allow the spark, the first moment of recognizing fire, to ignite in the protocols taught in this book. The skin has differential rates of heat escaping from it as well as thermal spikes like a flame that can repel the therapist's hand(s). Our hands can function like a sensitive spring, always ready to be repelled from the client's body. The spark can be a sudden deep breath or loud noise.

2. Ignition

With ignition, the fire starts, just as the car starts when you turn on its ignition. The engine in the core of the body vibrates. As a child, I tried to burn down our neighbor's garage when I first learned to play with matches. I learned the power of fire early. These remaining four steps are about one thing: the potency.

According to some anthropologists, fire came about 800,000 years ago in our evolution. What a miracle it must have been to our ancestors. It was given godlike status. We learn to heat the body or insulate it from the cold outside. We learn physiologically to keep the core of our body warm, which is regulated by the hypothalamus in the brain. The kidneys and liver do major metabolic work that is fueled by fire and need proper care and maintenance through drainage therapies, intermittent fasting, liver flushes, and so forth to keep the waste removal channels open. The heart produces vast amounts of heat, which is mediated by the pericardium and channels of heart meridian. There is a heart inside the physical heart, and the fire of compassion is damaged in this inner heart. The stove in the gut—our digestive fire—has been damaged as well. We must have the courage to claim our fire, our will to claim dominion over our body and begin healing it. All these metaphors revolve around fire. What gets ignited is self-healing and deeper refinement of the instinct for self-preservation. And all of that is directly linked to an awakening of the instinct for self-transcendence and the fire of love. This is the potency.

3. Permeation

This is the third step in Dr. Jealous's Ignition sequence. *Permeation* describes the penetration through a solid, such as a membrane, at the molecular level. In Taoism, permeation is imaged as a colorful mist arising in the core of the body from the various viscera and moving up, down, and out of the body. Permeation delivers the smallest of molecules to the whole of the body. The water molecule is the smallest molecule in the body and can pass through any structure in the body. This phenomenon was first described by Erich Blechschmidt (2012a) in his embryological studies.

At this stage of Ignition, heat begins to permeate like a mist, supporting every cell in the human body and its proper functioning. The fluid body, a term coined by Dr. Jealous indicating the total fluid and water content of the body at this level, is the blood and interstitium. In biorheology (the study of the flow properties of biological fluids), fascia is considered a super-cool fluid or gelled water, which is the original embryonic matrix around which all the organs develop. The water matrix of the fascia holds the blueprint for structure, function, and metabolism. The fascia likes heat and can stretch better. It likes hot yoga. The mist, the fluid fascia, and the blood are all aspects of permeation and with our palpation can feel like a bed of plankton under our hands, expanding and contracting. Primary Respiration (PR) in its expansion phase carries the mist that fills the body. It exits the skin and fills the universe. The practice is to allow our body to become transparent to the tide of PR, following the evolutionary urge to embody transparency, as discussed in chapter 19.

Permeation is a very creative and spiritual aspect of Ignition because it is associated with the spreading of love from the heart inside the heart. Imagine love being a mist of bright light generated by the heart and capable of spreading everywhere in the universe. The divine lives in our heart if we allow it, and we can allow it to radiate everywhere. This is the Breath of Life, according to Dr. Sutherland. This is potency.

4. Stillpoint

Step four is a stillpoint. The stillpoint relates to biological quiescence, which is an essential component of cellular development and the function of the endothelium. As mentioned earlier, the endothelium is a single layer of cells that are, in a healthy organism, biologically quiescent. Yet today these quiescent vascular cells are in deep trouble, especially regarding the new information on the glycocalyx covering of the endothelium. The glycocalyx is a thin gel-like layer of proteins covering the lumen surface of the endothelium. It maintains vascular homeostasis by changing shape depending on which organ and capillaries it is related to. Individual cell membranes metabolically need to be repaired, as do the physiological systems that are connected to them. It starts with repairing the epithelium of the gut. This is spiritual practice; it is caring for the temple of the Holy Spirit. The stillpoint as a state of quiescence is how body systems function optimally. At the same time, millions upon millions of cells are dying in our body every second. In a way, we are relating to our inner corpse through the stillpoint of metabolic death. This stillpoint allows the proper drainage of dead and dying cells along with a wide variety of waste products from our metabolism to process and dissipate. Without the stillpoint, even the blood has difficulty functioning since the inner core of blood flow is a dynamic stillness.

In biodynamic practice, we know and experience different levels of stillness. Dr. Jealous called the deepest level of stillness the void. I define the void as the absolute ending of the previous universe or the absolute ending of the previous concept, thought, emotion, or feeling I just had. The void is the restart button. The void is where we reboot a spontaneous Ignition of form and function. It is one of the great gifts of biodynamic practice that a client can experience this level of void in relationship with our perceptual process of the interchange between PR and stillness. It is the home of creation and originality. Thus, the spark of creation ignites the human being as well as the universe. We are truly palpating the potency of the cosmos.

5. Breath of Life

From the void state, we can observe step five, in which the self-knowing intelligence of PR, as the wisdom wind, moves in the body and chooses its fulcrum for healing in that moment. Its menu contains the three instincts of self-healing, self-preservation, and self-transcendence. Dr. Sutherland transformed the whole cranial concept when he had this experience for the first time in his career in 1948. It was the birth of the biodynamic approach. That is also when the first schism developed in his followers as Dr. Sutherland dropped into a very mystical understanding and used Christian metaphors to describe the sacredness of what he was experiencing. Others maintained a secular-mechanical view. His spiritual experience was elegant and beautiful, and it offers the same for us. And for him, the Breath of Life was a light in the subtle field of his perception at the age of seventy-five. I will be seventy-five years old in the year of this writing and have fully entered the domain of spiritual maturation.

BIODYNAMIC SPIRITUAL APTITUDES

The Buddhist mystical path looks at three practitioner aptitudes for self-transcendence, or spiritual aptitudes. Which of these three is the gate, portal, or perceptual preference for you, the reader, to access the biodynamic therapeutic process?

The First Spiritual Aptitude: Perception of Stillness

The first aptitude is the perception of stillness. Some meditators can stop their thoughts from moving for many hours at a time and it's quite a blissful state. I've touched the edge of that with meditation in various retreats, all while sequestered in a monastic setting. So, in this sense stillness is an awareness of the distraction of inner noise, emotional amplitude, and the volume of our thought stream, which rapidly can build concepts or unrealistic views of life. As is said, neurotics build castles in the sky; psychotics live in them. Stillness is easy to recognize because it is associated with the element of space, which is everything and everywhere. It is preexisting. You do need a little training on how to quiet your mind by placing attention on your posture, your midline, your breath, and your heartbeat. These are doorways to stillness. Leave your thoughts alone and they will dissipate on their own. Biodynamic practice is really an inner yoga of the perception of stillness, slowness, and light.

The Second Spiritual Aptitude: Perception of Primary Respiration

As is said in Genesis, "God formed the man from the dust of the ground and breathed into his nostrils the Breath of Life, and the man became a living being." Thus, step five of the ignition process is perceiving the Breath of Life, using Sutherland's biblical metaphor for Primary Respiration (PR). And perceiving the movement of PR is the second spiritual aptitude. I know many students, including myself, who love hanging out in PR. It moves everything, absolutely everything—every thought, every molecule, every photon, everything! PR moves between the third ventricle of the brain and the horizon of the planet and between all hearts. It moves our whole ancestry through the umbilicus for nine months (that is a teaching I received from Dr. Jealous). It's connected to very deep neurological reflexes, called the head righting reflexes (HRR). Among other characteristics, the HRR mean that when the cranium is balanced on the atlas, the eyes can rest attention on the line of the horizon. PR moves between the third ventricle and the horizon when the HRR are stable. In biodynamic practice, meditation postures are used to facilitate correct HRR to access PR. I practice this regularly, especially when I go to the beach. If you have access to a broad view of the horizon in the natural world, it is spectacular. One of Dr. Jealous's favorite books is *The Heart of the Hunter*, by Laurens van der Post (1980), in which van der Post said that the Kalahari Kung people of Africa could see PR moving back and forth from the horizon. What a gift to be guided on the planet with this capacity to see the movement of the Holy Spirit.

The Third Spiritual Aptitude: Perception of Appearance

And now we arrive at the third aptitude, which is the visualization of appearance. When we allow our minds to continually name and conceptualize the world around us from the data we receive from our sense organs, it's like constipation for the mind (Suzuki Roshi once said that zazen meditation was like toilet paper for the mind). Appearance involves the five elements and their colors. Before the elements appeared, there were the colors of the rainbow, and before that the Breath of Life. So, appearance means the shape, form, and sound of what is being perceived by our sense organs without mental labeling. We must relearn how to sit with or walk in the awe of the natural world and its myriad appearances. The emotion of awe is the feeling we get in the presence of something profound and vast that transcends our current understanding of the world. Just sitting at the beach allows my mind to stop thinking and digest the majesty in front of me and all around me. Being with a newborn baby fills me with awe. Awe is the basis of visualization of the five colors of the rainbow and other combinations of colors. Awe promotes self-healing while we treat the client biodynamically. Such awe is a side effect of awareness. Visualizing awesome beauty is considered medicine in Eastern traditions. Learning appropriate visualizations and recognizing their spontaneity, as Dr. Sutherland did, replaces a lot of mental chatter and interfaces with the body's metabolism to restore well-being.

It takes practice to see the Breath of Life as Dr. Sutherland did. Part 4 of this book will take the reader through a series of visualization practices for biodynamic cardiovascular therapy sessions. This aptitude is already present in biodynamic practitioners and needs to be balanced with the aptitudes of perceiving stillness and PR.

The Second Pair of Hands

The other practice associated with the Breath of Life is the second pair of hands. It refers to the idea that you can invite the sacred into the room in whatever shape and form is beneficial, benevolent, and not fearful to you or the client. You will learn to visualize a divine essence of the universe preexisting inside your heart. It is the place of the heart inside the heart. From that place of void, the universe is created and filled with love, and it, she, or he lives in your heart. Even the client is a creation of our heart. This is the Ignition of great compassion.

MEANING AND MIDLINE

In the summer of 2022, the U.S. space agency NASA released the first images from the new James Webb Space Telescope showing images of distant galaxies believed to be five to ten billion years old. At the same time, the U.S. Supreme Court took away a woman's right to an abortion, placing the human embryo front and center in the consciousness of humanity, not just U.S. citizens. These political and scientific investigations of our origins bring about a deep contemplation of not only our values but how to make meaning out of suffering. These explorations of origins have been embedded within the instincts of our organism since the beginning of time. They indicate a great revival in cosmology and embryology in contemporary society, which is beautiful and unfortunately unconscious regarding the deeper meaning associated with healing. The Webb telescope images are incredible, and images in embryology books fill me with awe. The images alone can be curative or healing to our unconscious need for meaning-making. Meaning takes place in the presence of awe. Step into your awe.

Relatively recently in our human history, religions formed to explain and mediate suffering. Before that, traditional cultures faced the same challenges as ours. *Every culture old and new must face the reality of pain and suffering of its members, try to explain it to the satisfaction of its members, and create healing rituals to link the origin story with healing pain and suffering.* Prior to the advent of modern religions, traditional peoples embodied their origin story of how life was at the beginning of the universe or the beginning of the embryonic period, when the sacred formed humans in a state of original wholeness. This is still true in many parts of the world now. Such embodied spirituality is based on a deep relationship with the natural world as being sacred and living much more closely to the sacredness of nature. We are designed to participate with nature in awe of its divinity, rather than dominate it and extract its resources for sale. Biodynamic practice touches both the embryo and the cosmos.

Origin stories old and new are not without drama. It does not seem to be easy generating a universe. The Book of Genesis is one of many examples of such drama. Some origin stories in oral traditions are memorized and sung to a stricken patient as a way of the community participating as a whole in the ritual of healing. It provides a sense of right placement in the universe and thus deeper meaning for people's suffering. As described in chapter 10, I apprenticed on the Diné reservation some years ago, and occasionally many community members stood outside the hogan (healing space) and sang the entire Diné origin story while the ceremony inside enacted that same origin story much more rigorously with the patient. Some traditional cultures constructed monuments representing the origin story and placed them in the center of their villages in order to have a constant recognition-orientation to origin and its potency for healing. To lose one's orientation to origin creates chaos in the culture.

Romans knew this quite well, and when they conquered a culture, they would remove the various symbolic representations, such as sculptures, obelisks, and other symbols of that culture's origin story, and bring them back to Rome. Then the Roman origin story would be imposed upon the culture as a form of enslavement. I once taught a biodynamic craniosacral therapy foundation training outside Rome. As a final project for graduation, one of the students photographed each of the statues and obelisks scattered around Rome from conquered cultures and then detailed where they came from and the stories they told of origin. Some of these cultures have begun the process of reclaiming these monuments back to their original location.

There is another common element to these monuments and sculptures symbolizing origination. Midline is a term commonly used in biodynamic practice. It most often is related to embryology and its organizational function, called axial symmetry. In this way a midline provides optimal organization to the whole in growth and development. When observing a contemporary construction site, very large, tall booms or cranes fill the sky around the site as they provide the organizational materials for construction of the foundation of the building, just as an embryo does with several of its structures. The same argument is made for cultural midlines that organize the spiritual function of a culture, such as a cross in Christianity or the name of God in Islam. Many cultural midlines are phallic in appearance. For example, among the Native American cultures (Haida) of the Pacific Northwest, the totem pole is a huge representation of the origin story and is traditionally found in the center of their villages. These poles frequently feature a bird on top, representing the Breath of Life. In fact, some traditional cultures use the term "breath of life" to designate origin. In a similar vein, for a hundred years now, we have glorious drawings and photographs of human embryos with exquisite detail and long narratives about growth and development from a single cell to a human being. Thus, the origin story, whether it be of the universe or the embryo, depending on the culture, is often represented on a symbolic midline. The origin narrative is critical psychologically and spiritually to derive meaning and purpose for pain and suffering. Cultures must be able to orient to a midline of meaning and the meaning of the midline.

Once a narrative of origin is established, whether cosmologically or embryologically (or both), a culture then develops rituals and ceremonies to connect its people, especially those who are stricken with disease and illness, back to the origin story. A necessary embodied spiritual bridge is made between the origin story and the healing rituals for meaning to be remembered. Trust, devotion, and faith in the sacred meaning of origin become key features of healing through an origin story. Without such a bridge to the meaning of life, a culture becomes easily conquered by its people's fears and those imposed upon them through violence and war. In this way, a culture's medical system, which was originally animistic-shamanic, was connected to the origin story. Treatment would then involve awakening a person's instinctual knowing of how to heal their body with the help of a reliable healer connected to the natural world who knew how to reconnect the stricken patient back to their origin. Then it would be up to the patient to integrate the experience. In other words, the healing of suffering or the mitigation of its effects was linked to an agreed-upon cultural midline, a cosmological or embryological narrative. As the Romans found out, it is easy to defeat a culture when the symbolic narrative of origination is obliterated or removed. It is a primary human instinct to make meaning from one's suffering by exploring the source of the universe. When that is not possible, chaos and illness are the result.

Today in the Western world, it appears that the only remaining cultural midline is the bank. I remember hearing Joseph Campbell lecture on this. He said that in the nineteenth century, the central structure in every town was the church. Then it was the factory and finally the bank. It is all about money in the West; it's about who has the most and can protect it with legal teams. And we wonder why mental health is failing in the West, especially among young people. Our culture is full of chaos and illness, and money is a powerful midline. The drive-through windows and smart phones play a part in this chaos, further killing our capacity for awe and wonder. These are the new false gods.

The beauty of Eastern medical systems, whether they be ayurveda, Tibetan medicine, classical Chinese medicine (which is linked to Taoism), or some other traditional healing system still existent, is that their methods maintain a link to the cosmological origin narrative. Many young people in these cultures still learn that the composition of the universe is the same as that of the human body and consists of five elements. All things are constructed of the five elements in Eastern healing systems. This is because the origin stories are clear that the five sacred elements were present at the beginning of the universe and are also present at the conception of the human embryo. Please see my previous book *The Biodynamics of the Immune System* for a primer on cosmology

Part of the healing enacted through biodynamic therapy is returning our midline to the heart inside the heart. As I said in chapter 18, the heartbeat is the new church. The center of the universe is the heart inside the heart seen as a clear light. Dr. Sutherland (1967) literally saw this and called it the Breath of Life. He mentions it seventeen times in his writings. Andrew Taylor Still, the nineteenth-century founder of osteopathy, said that "the rule of the artery is supreme," which lends itself to the Tree of Life in the Book of Genesis being associated with the vascular tree in the Kabbalah. The Kabbalah is the mystical school of Judaism and must be appreciated because of its premise that the complexity of origin narratives are beyond comprehension—and certainly beyond the scientific mind dominating Western culture. Photographs and drawings of origin are meaningless without the context of their deeper connection to the sacred. "Mystical" does not mean supernatural or anti-science. Rather, it is about having direct phenomenological (felt lived experience) of the sacred rather than cognitive intellectual understanding. As is said, "You can enter a mystery, but you cannot solve it." We can ask: What is the source of PR and the stillness? But we cannot know their source except to say they were present at the origin of the universe and the embryo. They are always present now in their original form in biodynamic practice. When I once asked Jaap van der Wal, professor of embryology at the University of Maastricht, what the source of movement is in the embryo, he replied, "There is only movement in the embryo, no source."

In this way, biodynamic practice already has integrated elements of a Western and Eastern cosmological narrative. The midline is, of course, fundamental to biodynamic practice. The biodynamic midline is a transient and local embryonic feature of the human body and necessary for healing in the ritual we call biodynamics. There is no structural midline in the embryo organizing growth and development. The only such midline is a fulcrum centered in the heart. However, the biodynamic midline is internally located in the heart inside the heart, and when blended with a cosmological perspective, it becomes extended externally all the way out to the edge of the universe and back to our heart.

The Breath of Life lives in the heart inside the heart and radiates all appearance in the universe. How can we help the contemporary client make meaning of their suffering, which is so prevalent now? First, we must develop the skill to help the client orient to the center of their heart, which extends to the center of the universe, and symbolically this means the void before there was a universe. This begins with synchronizing with PR and the stillness, the yin and yang of the Breath of Life and the first appearance of the universe, the light inside the dark void. The practical skills associated with a cosmological orientation in biodynamic practice are visualization techniques. They are based on the knowledge of the five elements in the Indo-Tibetan tradition as well as the Sino-Tibetan tradition.

Orientation to the Breath of Life as a light in the heart inside the heart allows the emergence of a preexisting spiritual aptitude to integrate into biodynamic practice. The starting point is always the embryo and its fluid body, while the vascular system lends itself to a connection to the cosmos. Making meaning of the midline now includes perception of the structure and function (the psychology and spirituality associated with the cosmological origin) of the whole universe, of which we are not separate from but included within. We are transparent to the whole and can perceive this through our hands, our brain, and especially our heart with the perception of the wisdom wind of Primary Respiration and awareness of the spaciousness of dynamic stillness. Our perception expands to include a larger interconnected whole through spacious awareness at the core of dynamic stillness in the heart inside the heart. This is the midline, according to Dr. Jealous.

Many origin stories describe a fulcrum or point of originality, as seen especially in the growth and development of the human embryo or the event called the Big Bang in astrogeophysics. For example, in classical Chinese medicine, the points ST 25 (Tianshu) and ST 23 (Taiyi), which are lateral of the umbilicus, and REN 3 (Zhongzi), which is superior to the pubic bone, are named after pole stars, meaning the stars that appear to align with the Earth's axis of rotation. In Chinese medicine, this abdominal region is seen as a microcosmic reflection of the center of the universe. The umbilicus is seen as a symbolic fulcrum of the origin of the universe. Thus the Taoist vision is that the microcosmic (metabolic) universe in the body is a mirror of the universe itself. As biodynamic practitioners we must explore these original fulcrums of the umbilicus and the heart as deeply as we investigate the neurological system and its housing of bones and membranes (the earth element) and fluids (the water element). Then a subtle central channel between the gut, the heart, and the brain can be properly reestablished in relation with the elements of the fluid body, the potency of the fire element, PR as the wind element and, dynamic stillness as the element of space. In this way, when we come into relationship with a client biodynamically, not only do we touch the origin forces still present from their perpetual embryo, but we can and must also touch the entire universe with our hands, heart, and mind, visualizing the origin as color for healing the contemporary client. Such color is alive and moving with the wind and space through the vascular tree as the Tree of Life containing all aspects of the sacred.

It also means that we can begin to expand our perception of PR from a heart-to-heart connection with a client into a heart-to-heart connection with the universe. We can develop a felt sense of PR interacting with the client's pain and suffering using color and the light of the Breath of Life. We can dilate our perception of the client's heart center to include the entire universe as a dynamic stillness, the element of space, the so-called origin in some Eastern origin stories. We can expand our perception of the fluid body to be transparent with the entire universe beyond the horizon of this planet without fear. We stay with our heartbeat and the colors associated with origin. Thus, the universe as we perceive it becomes a coloring book in clinical biodynamic practice. Each of the elements has its own color. It is a rainbow radiating from your heart. Thus, the perception of PR and stillness includes not only a felt sense but also the appearance of a living breathing color pattern of beauty and grace. We can know the efficacy of this emerging adjunct to biodynamic treatment only by feeling the universe in and around the client who lies on our table. It starts heart to heart with PR.

Allow your sessions to be a mystery that unfolds moment by moment. Stay grounded in the earth element of your physicality and weightedness. Feel your heartbeat everywhere. Dissolve into spacious awareness transmuted into a vision of great love and compassion. This is the deepest aspect of heart Ignition.

THE LIFE SPAN DEVELOPMENT OF THE CARDIOVASCULAR SYSTEM

Art by Friedrich Wolf
Vascular maps by permission
from Elsevier Publishing

It is my great joy to introduce you to twenty-four images drawn by Friedrich Wolf of the embryology of the human heart. We have been working on this project for more than a decade, and it has now come to fruition with this section.

The second half of this section (plates 26–35) contains important vascular anatomy images that are also referenced throughout the book. These plates are reproduced courtesy of Elsevier Publishing.

All the images in this color insert should be contemplated, studied, and embodied. The heart is a profound organ, both physically and spiritually. I believe the reader can see where spirit lives in the heart and flows through the body by seeing and understanding these images.

Starting with the embryo, then the adult, and finally ending up with the Sacred Heart of Jesus, the reader can tour their own inner being, like touring a labyrinth visually to find the center. I was raised Catholic and have training as a multifaith chaplain, so I contemplate aspects of the life of Jesus and other religious figures, especially Buddha. This particular image of Jesus in plate 36 appeared to me while receiving a Sufi healing session on my heart.

I invite the reader to contemplate all of the images contained here one by one while remaining centered in the awareness of your heartbeat. The intention is to find your heart.

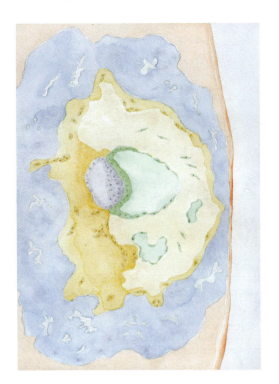

Plate 1. *Overview of second week postfertilization: The placenta begins to form pockets of still fluid called lacunae (a type of lagoon). The embryo is now surrounded by stillness. The green is the future gut, and the blue-violet the future nervous system. You can see the maternal lacunae in white located in the surrounding placenta, drawn in blue. The lacunae will be filled with blood soon.*

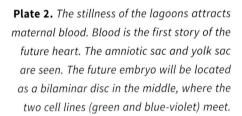

Plate 2. *The stillness of the lagoons attracts maternal blood. Blood is the first story of the future heart. The amniotic sac and yolk sac are seen. The future embryo will be located as a bilaminar disc in the middle, where the two cell lines (green and blue-violet) meet.*

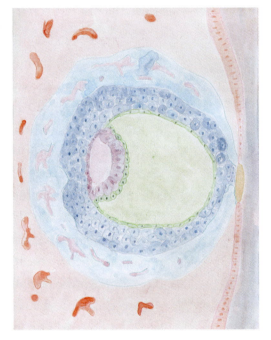

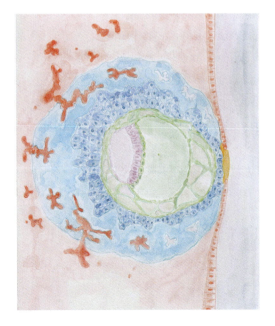

Plate 3. *Mother's blood arrives into the stillness. Blood vessels begin to form in the early placenta, with nutrients diffusing through the cell wall to feed the embryo. The green honeycomb becomes early embryonic blood. A blood-to-blood connection is formed outside the embryo. Blood and its vessels form outside the embryo, in the periphery, first.*

Plate 4. *The midline location of the umbilicus is determined. Toward the end of the second week, the chorionic cavity forms (see plates 1–3) and the connective tissue in the early blood begins to form a connecting stalk attached to the amniotic sac (the future third ventricle) of the embryo.*

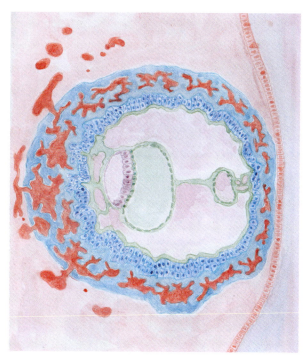

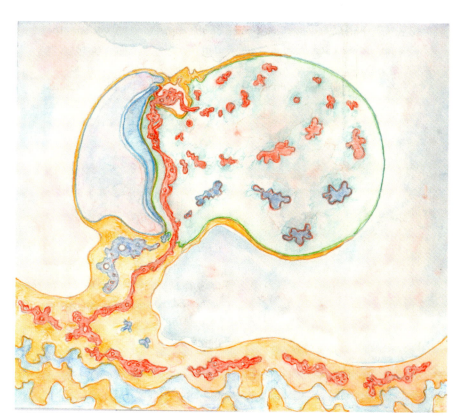

Plate 5. *Overview at twenty-two to twenty-four days: Extra-embryonic angioblast islands are sprouting on the outside of the yolk sac. A primitive arterial vascular system develops. Chorionic blood islands (in the chorionic wall near the connective stalk) and an incomplete umbilical artery and veins are seen.*

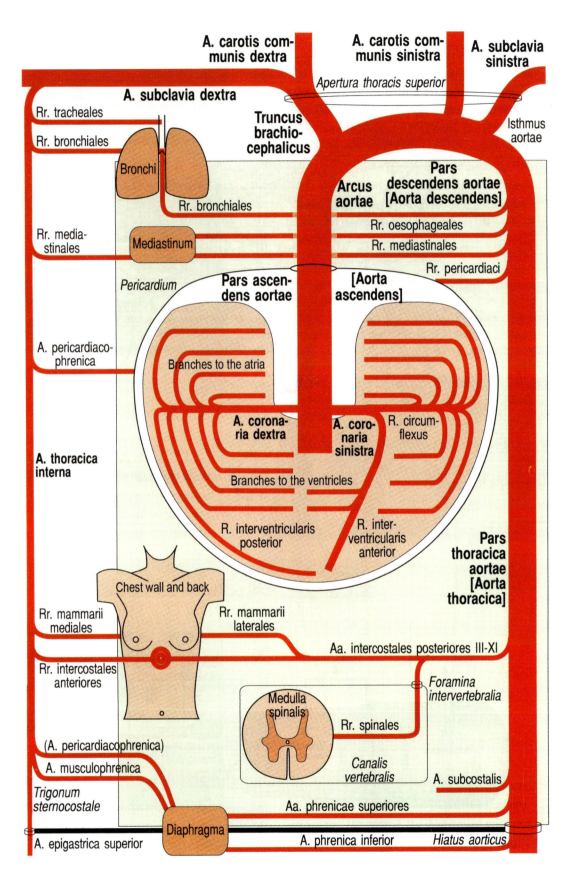

A. carotis com-munis dextra

A. carotis com-munis sinistra

A. subclavia sinistra

Apertura thoracis superior

A. subclavia dextra

Rr. tracheales

Rr. bronchiales

Bronchi

Truncus brachio-cephalicus

Isthmus aortae

Rr. bronchiales

Arcus aortae

Pars descendens aortae [Aorta descendens]

Rr. media-stinales

Mediastinum

Rr. oesophageales

Rr. mediastinales

Rr. pericardiaci

Pericardium

Pars ascen-dens aortae

[Aorta ascendens]

A. pericardiaco-phrenica

Branches to the atria

A. corona-ria dextra

A. coro-naria sinistra

R. circum-flexus

A. thoracica interna

Branches to the ventricles

R. interventricularis posterior

R. inter-ventricularis anterior

Pars thoracica aortae [Aorta thoracica]

Chest wall and back

Rr. mammarii mediales

Rr. mammarii laterales

Aa. intercostales posteriores III-XI

Rr. intercostales anteriores

Foramina intervertebralia

Medulla spinalis

Rr. spinales

(A. pericardiacophrenica)

A. musculophrenica

Canalis vertebralis

A. subcostalis

Trigonum sternocostale

Aa. phrenicae superiores

Diaphragma

A. epigastrica superior

A. phrenica inferior

Hiatus aorticus

Plate 26. *Coronary arteries and chest aorta*

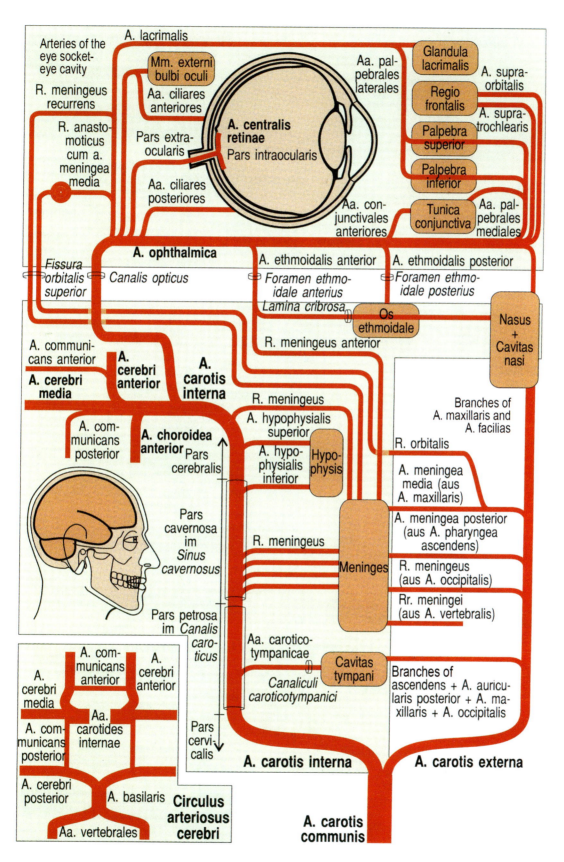

Plate 27. *A. carotis interna*

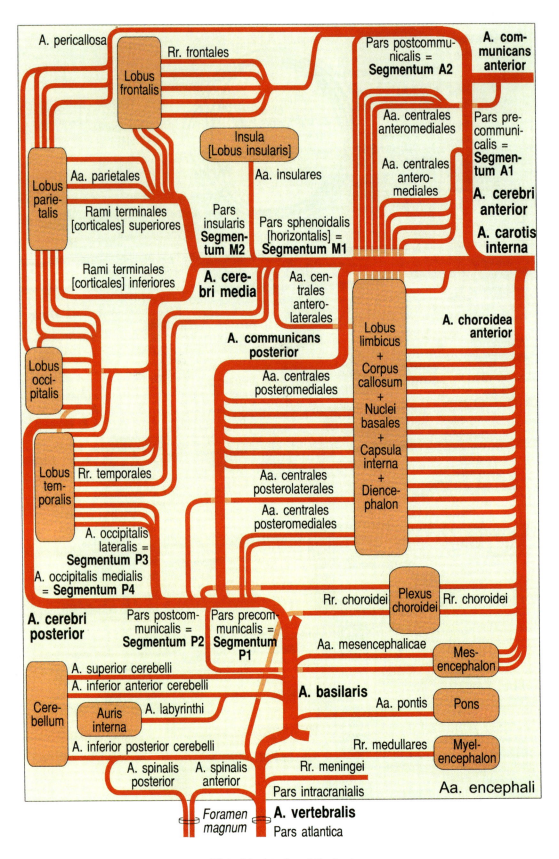

Plate 28. *Arteries of the brain*

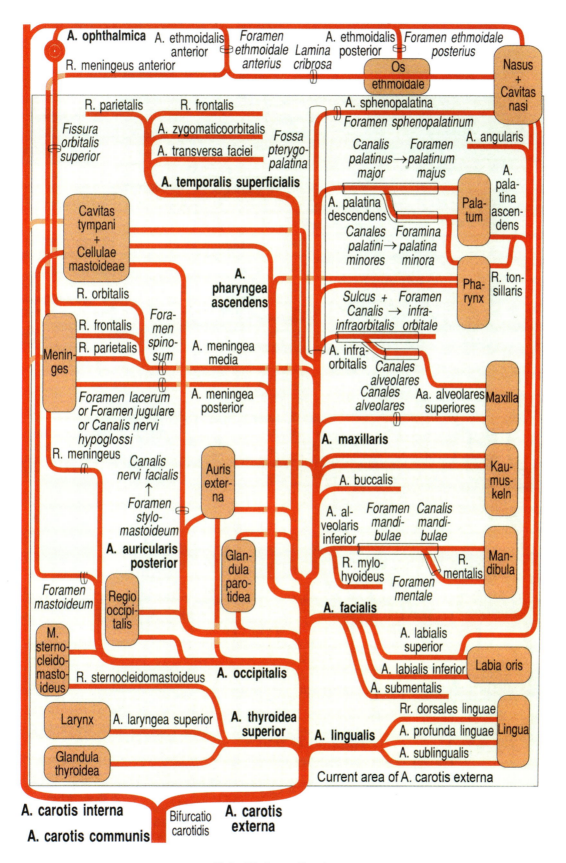

Plate 29. *A. carotis externa*

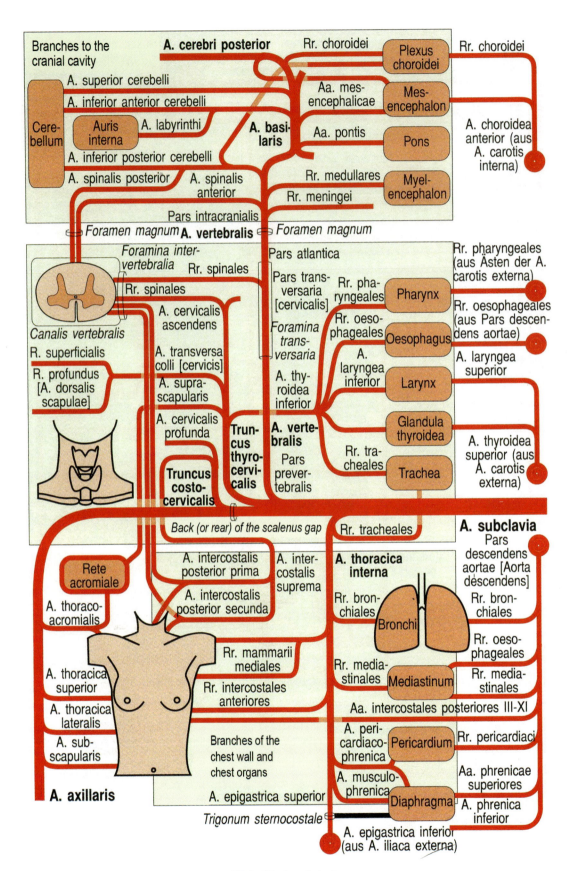

Plate 30. *A. subclavia*

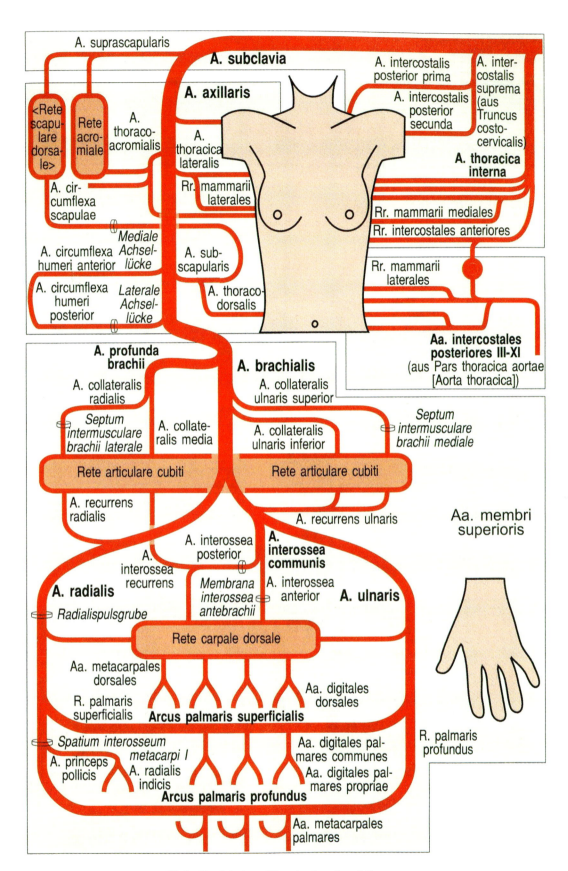

Plate 31. *Arteries of the chest wall and the arm*

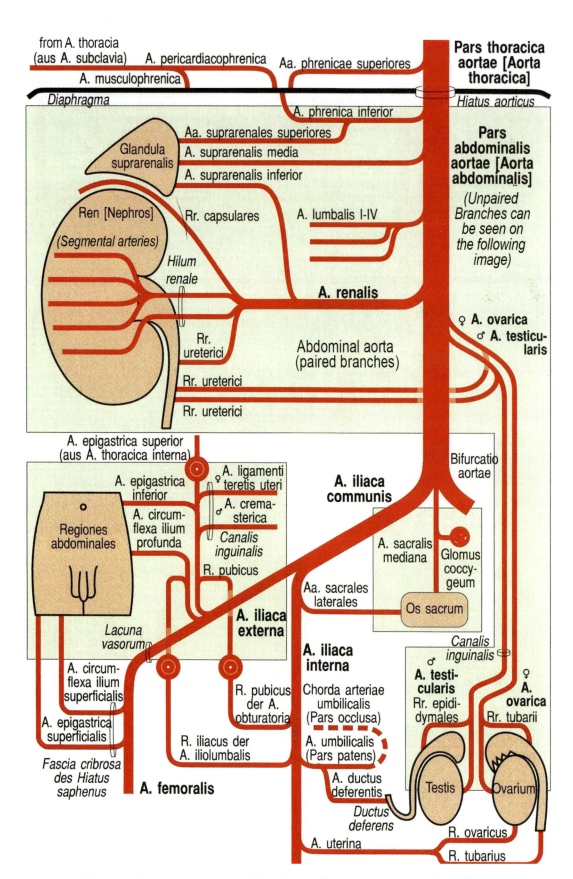

Plate 32. *Abdominal aorta (paired branches), A. iliaca externa, A. sacralis mediana*

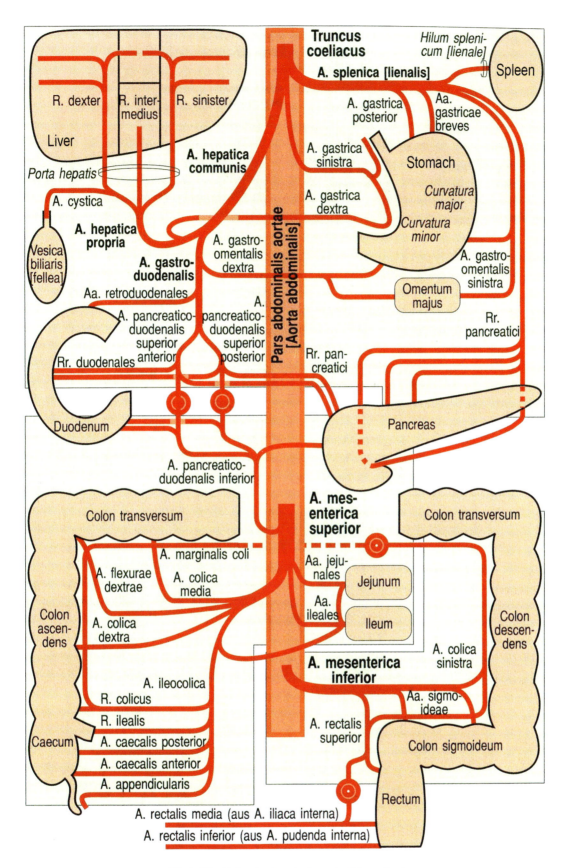

Plate 33. *Abdominal aorta (unpaired branches)*

Hepar: *the Greek word for the liver. In antiquity, hepar was originally connected to the concept of pleasure, showing that in ancient times the liver was considered the seat of the soul and human feelings.*

Gaster: *a synonym for the stomach, meaning (from the old German) "full of guests."*

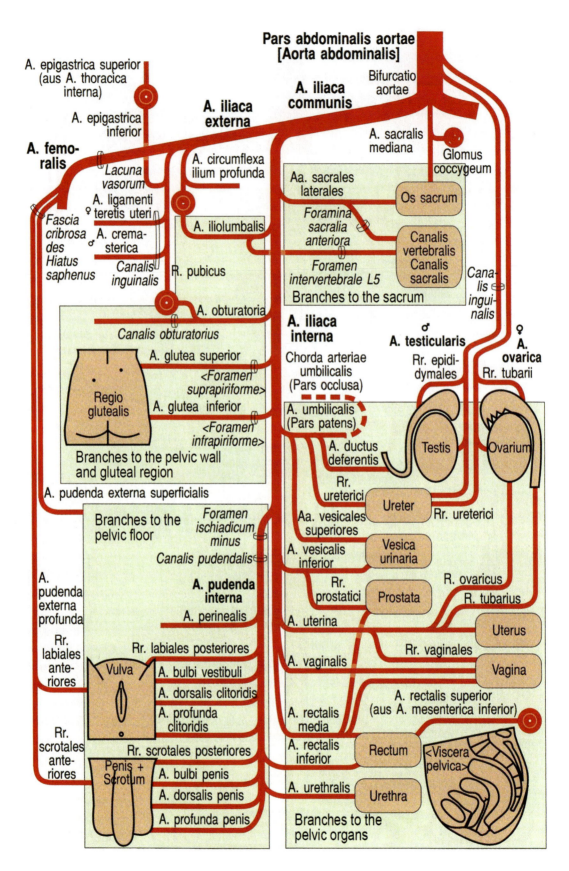

Plate 34. *A. iliaca interna*

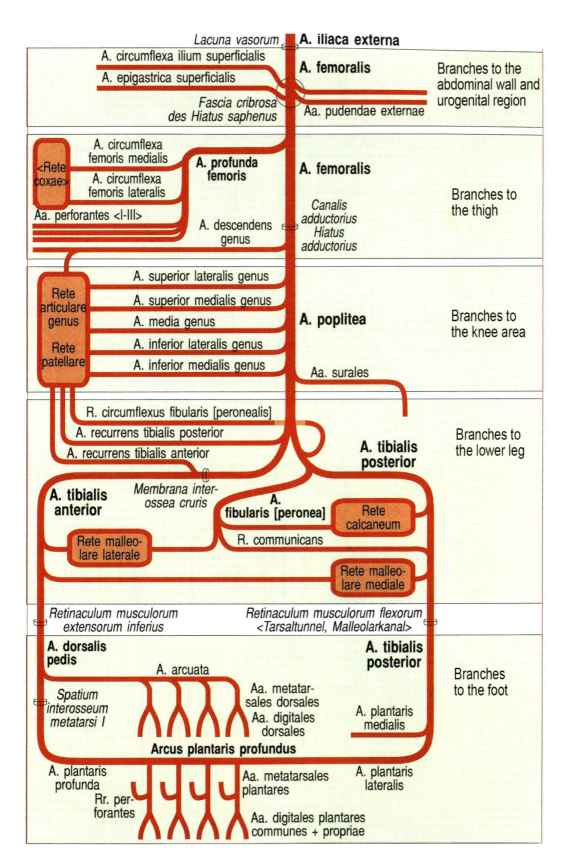

Lacuna vasorum · **A. iliaca externa**

A. circumflexa ilium superficialis
A. epigastrica superficialis

A. femoralis

Branches to the
abdominal wall and
urogenital region

Fascia cribrosa
des Hiatus saphenus
Aa. pudendae externae

<Rete coxae>

A. circumflexa
femoris medialis

A. circumflexa
femoris lateralis

**A. profunda
femoris**

A. femoralis

Aa. perforantes <I-III>

A. descendens
genus

Canalis
adductorius
Hiatus
adductorius

Branches to
the thigh

Rete
articulare
genus

Rete
patellare

A. superior lateralis genus
A. superior medialis genus
A. media genus
A. inferior lateralis genus
A. inferior medialis genus

A. poplitea

Branches to
the knee area

Aa. surales

R. circumflexus fibularis [peronealis]
A. recurrens tibialis posterior
A. recurrens tibialis anterior

**A. tibialis
posterior**

Branches to
the lower leg

**A. tibialis
anterior**

Membrana inter-
ossea cruris

**A.
fibularis [peronea]**

Rete
calcaneum

Rete malleo-
lare laterale

R. communicans

Rete malleo-
lare mediale

Retinaculum musculorum
extensorum inferius

Retinaculum musculorum flexorum
<Tarsaltunnel, Malleolarkanal>

**A. dorsalis
pedis**

A. arcuata

**A. tibialis
posterior**

Spatium
interosseum
metatarsi I

Aa. metatar-
sales dorsales
Aa. digitales
dorsales

A. plantaris
medialis

Branches
to the foot

Arcus plantaris profundus

A. plantaris
profunda

Rr. per-
forantes

Aa. metatarsales
plantares

A. plantaris
lateralis

Aa. digitales plantares
communes + propriae

Plate 35. A. femoralis

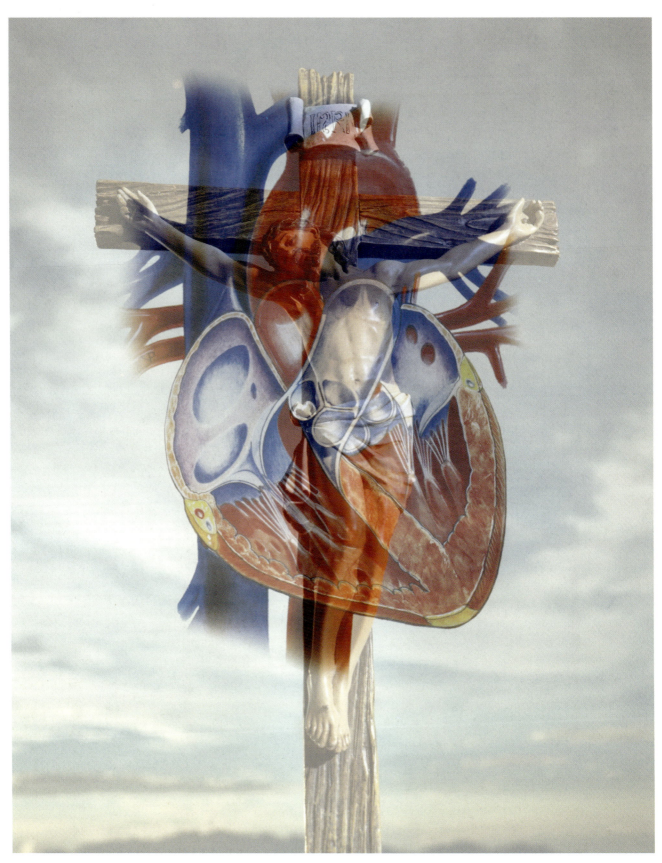

Plate 36. *Sacred Heart of Love. A vision given to Michael J. Shea*

22

The Embodiment of
Primary Respiration and the
Five Elements

Biodynamic practice is a study of the embodied perception of Primary Respiration (PR) and the five elements. In this chapter, we will establish an entrance point to sacred space, the ground of perceiving such slowness and stillness, by elaborating a set of principles for that perception and embodiment. I rediscover these principles every time I am with a client or even while waiting in line in the grocery store. Each session is a personal discovery of the stages to perceiving PR; it unfolds differently in every moment because every moment is impermanent. There is a moment of awe when PR becomes free to move in the body and mind of the practitioner, without restriction. In every moment the past is gone and the future has not yet arisen

DEFINING EMBODIMENT

The transition from exteroception, interoception, mindfulness, and compassion to embodiment necessitates a different perceptual tone. Our teachers have lent us their perceptual terminology, especially Dr. W. G. Sutherland and Dr. Jim Jealous. It is not so easy to give words to the embodied experience of PR and the elements, but we need a starting point!

The embodied perception of PR, as I use the term, is the felt sense of order and organization in the body and mind. Order and organization is episodic on a daily and lifelong basis. It comes and goes, waxing and waning like the moon and the ocean tide. We are linked to a much larger intelligence in the natural world that permeates our body and is our body. To become embodied is to experience the internal vascular pulsations and breath in their shifting locations and their unique ever-changing rhythms. It is through the perception of PR that order and organization become embodied. Everyone has their own unique experience of the natural world inside and outside the body. Like an embryo, we are constantly informing and outforming with a multitude of sense perceptions and trillions of metabolic processes occurring right now, in the moment, mixing us together with the outside world. It is said in Buddhist Tantra: "As without, so within." Every molecule must become still for transformation and without a calm mind such embodiment is lost.

Wholeness

Embodiment implies wholeness, wherein the parts are viewed not as separate but as one. Wholeness is our aliveness. Dr. Jim Jealous would say, "Wholeness is the smallest subdivision of life." To embody wholeness is to have a felt sense of the heart, mind, and body being synchronized. Conscious awareness automatically shifts between being in the mind with its cognitions, in the senses monitoring the external environment, and in the internal body with its interoceptive awareness. You could say that we have an ordinary mind sense (thoughts, cognitions, and emotions) and a body sense (interoceptive awareness). Typically, we have too much mind sense and not enough body sense. Embodiment of wholeness is an automatic constantly shifting fulcrum. It can be buoyant and dense, earthy and airy, fluid and fixed, hot and cold, vulnerable and courageous. It seems like it is always shifting. This is the embodiment of aliveness of change and impermanence.

Again, as embodied beings we are constantly informing and outforming with the senses and with our mind. "There is a tide in the affairs of men," as Shakespeare wrote. These phases of our bodily tides are experienced timelessly, through the seconds, the years, and the whole life span. Embodiment is developmental because of its changeability over time. We do not achieve embodiment like we might finally reach a plateau. It is a continuous gathering and sorting, a type of ongoing integration of the total features of our body's experience of vitality and aliveness mixed with the awe of the natural world.

Integration allows for different qualities to become embodied—for example, what we accept and what we reject, both biologically, psychologically, and spiritually. We embody dietary choices, attitudes, and emotions. Our embodiment shifts over time with a constant loss and gain of somatic experience, like putting on a pair of shoes to see if they fit or trying on a shirt that didn't fit originally but fits now. Order and organization depend on how we set the sails on our ship to catch the wind of PR. It is a slowing and becoming mindful of which way the wind is moving. We occasionally pause, hold the mast of the ship as Odysseus did. As Louisa May Alcott said in *Little Women*, "I'm not afraid of storms, for I'm learning how to sail my ship."

The somatic experience of embodiment is an ebb and flow of both exteroceptive awareness and interoceptive awareness. Our sensory systems perceive the density of the inside of the body and the environment outside on a living, moving continuum of interconnection. To embody a sense of buoyancy and transparency within this continuum might take some contemplative practice (there are many contemplative methods from which to choose). When we experience the interconnected whole of our universe internally with watchfulness and gradually over time with PR, then its natural order and organization becomes embodied. This is the birthplace of appropriate compassion.

Synchronization

Synchronizing is a term used in biodynamic osteopathy to mean bringing our perception to the spiritual aspects and embodiment of Primary Respiration and stillness. I once wrote a poem attempting to explain how the five elements from Eastern medical systems integrate with biodynamic practice. As it turns out, the poem is about synchronization. We can train our attention to include simultaneous processes.

> *There is no spiritual order without dynamic stillness.*
> *There is no movement in the universe without Primary Respiration.*
> *There is no heart without fire.*
> *There is no blood without water.*
> *There is no food without earth.*

PRIMARY RESPIRATION (PR)

Principle: Embodiment of PR is a multidimensional experience. Practicing that embodiment begins with the following basic understandings:

- Embodiment is based upon each individual's unique experience of their body-mind-spirit continuum as a personal spiritual maturation. Everyone has a differential spiritual maturation trajectory.
- PR is the constant automatic fluctuation, the coalescing and dissolution of the total substance of the inner and outer space of the body in a slow tempo.
- PR is the interconnecting movement of wholeness, which extends beyond the horizon but also governs the metabolism of the body. It is potent. It is vital. It is life.
- PR has multiple levels and dimensions occurring simultaneously.
- Biodynamics begins as a training in the embodiment and perception of PR one layer at a time.
- Synchronizing with PR happens both two-dimensionally and three-dimensionally. One possibility is sensing two-dimensionally out the front or back of the body to the horizon. Then the practitioner waits for PR to reveal its three-dimensionality. This awareness of PR automatically shifts its fulcrum from the third ventricle of the brain to the heart inside the heart.

Rates and States of PR

Principle: PR has three types of rates and states in clinical practice.

1. **Reciprocal or biphasic.** Reciprocal or biphasic direction PR states are variable; they are usually perceived starting at around six cycles per ten minutes (two fifty-second phases per cycle) up to twenty-minute cycles and more. Different teachers give different names to longer rates. It is more desirable to have students name their own experience.

2. **Uniphasic (one direction only).** Here PR is in a constant rhythmic, balanced interchange with the intermittent perception of stillness (a pause) expanding in all directions three-dimensionally. A simultaneous two-way direction or phase is also possible, with PR going in one direction in an artery and the opposite way in a vein, and both being centered by stillness in the middle of blood flow. PR does not stop but rather fades to the background of perception for the dynamic stillness to come forward. Thus, at this level PR and stillness are the same thing, just two sides of one coin. Perceptual nonduality is innate.

3. **Nonphasic.** These nondual unpolarized states of PR are without any reference or fulcrum for source or origin. They are associated with the feeling, sense, perception, or subtle emotion of loving kindness, compassion, joy, and equanimity. These are called the Four Immeasurables in Buddhism.

The Four Immeasurables

May all beings enjoy happiness and the root of happiness.
May they be free from suffering and the root of suffering.
May they not be separated from the great happiness devoid of suffering.
May they dwell in the great equanimity free from passion, aggression,
*   and ignorance.*

Mystical Nature of PR

Principle: PR has no beginning point, source, or cause, nor any end point, nor any anchor in time. This is its mystical character.

It is a waste of time to look for the cause of PR. There is only movement and stillness. Trusting the Tide, as Dr. Becker said, includes the capacity to perceive the tide of PR and its various currents. We are being moved by the tide rather than the practitioner observing the tide from the shoreline. This is the essence of embodiment. We must learn how to sail our ship and become biodynamic navigators.

Ultimately PR is about healing since it is timeless. The therapeutic process during a session is time dependent only because we make appointments and give sessions based on clock time. A practitioner cannot know the timing of the client's healing process. It may take forever. It may happen overnight or not at all. Who knows?

MINDFULNESS

Principle: PR is not given automatically in a biodynamic session. It is uncovered by the quality of the practitioner's attention.

Synchronizing includes the embodiment of the practitioner. It begins with the earth element, the starting point of exploration. It requires mindfulness of how the body-mind is constantly automatically shifting. The practitioner synchronizes with their own state of mind, body, and emotions at the beginning, middle, and end of a session without judgment. This is the core of compassion: to care for oneself and to be friends with the totality of oneself. This requires contemplative practice.

Mindfulness is a state of mind free of judgment and interpretation. Synchronizing at this level involves the recognition of one's attention being captured and the conscious automatic shift back to the element of space and stillness, like a gentle wind of PR. It is spontaneous awareness. It begins in the tempo of PR and then time dilates and loses relevance in a session as the timeless dimension of PR and stillness is entered. The timeless dimension is the void, according to Dr. Jealous.

The body-mind instinctually synchronizes frequently with mindfulness. The practitioner becomes conscious of what is happening in their body-mind. When the mind is distracted or wandering, mindfulness notices the distraction and resynchronizes attention on the unity of the body and mind. Mindfulness is a spark or sudden experience of returning home to embodiment. Mindfulness is the basis of synchronizing with PR. The instinct of mindfulness is extinguished in many clients; the practitioner's attention is a spark to ignite mindfulness in the client.

Principle: PR cannot be sensed with the ordinary mind. It can be known by mindfulness of the body and sensing our innate neurological orientation to the horizon.

Contemplating the nature of one's mind and its tendency to wander and get distracted by emotions and story lines about life is important. It is our unavoidable human condition. It's natural to return one's attention to the body of sensations, where PR lives internally and externally. PR moves all thoughts and emotions in its function of the wind element, and the ordinary mind cannot know the therapeutic intention of PR. The organism of the body and its instinctual metabolism can. It is a different tempo that is interconnected to all things, not just the movement of thoughts and emotions. The brain is not the source of our connection to the world but a necessary component of that connection. The heart is the universal connection to all; it is our deepest spiritual essence.

BREATHING

Principle: Synchronizing with PR occurs with biological anatomical breathing.

PR is already synchronized with the breath of air. We are constantly being synchronized with the wind element. Periodically take a deep breath to synchronize with PR when it changes phases. This practice starts deliberately and eventually becomes spontaneous. A phase change is also known by a change of thought or a sound or a light entering our perception. Everyone must become a conscious master of their own breath. PR is breathing us and regulating the movement of our respiratory diaphragm with help from the brain.

Gradually this process leads to synchronizing directly with PR. This involves linking the start of an inhalation with the change of phase of PR. It's about a deep full breath sensed from the central tendon of the diaphragm, the bottom lobes of the lungs, and a sense of filling and emptying the whole space inside the abdomen. The transversus abdominus muscle interdigitates with the respiratory diaphragm. Consider the skin as the diaphragm of PR. There is a gap at the end of an exhalation. Without changing the breath, get to know this gap and the diaphragm of the skin simultaneously. The change of phase of breathing, usually with the initiation of inhalation, synchronizes with the change of phase of PR, usually with its expansion phase. And sometimes it is the opposite. All directions are happening simultaneously, and the great learning is to allow our perception to synchronize with its slow motion and then to notice its power for Ignition.

THE FLUID BODY

The fluid body is the most mystical aspect of biodynamic cardiovascular therapy. The fluid body is composed mainly of the water element and the earth element. In Taoism, the water element is the source or origin of the universe, which is the equivalent of the element of space in Tibetan medicine.

Blood is considered to be the essence of the water element inside the body. One of the main reasons for this is that water makes up 70 percent of the blood. The vascular system is responsible for managing the distribution of the fire element through the whole body, and that happens via the blood. When heat is shunted to the skin, the blood secretes water that we call sweat. This generates a cloud that is charged electrically and ionically around the body. This is Zone B or Dr. Becker's biosphere, and it contains earth elements, bacteria, and fungi, making up a microbiome of the fluid body that is an extension of the vascular tree. It is exactly the same as cloud formations in the sky of the natural world. In this way, the fluid body includes the total contents of Zone B and is the Tree of Life, as it is known in the Kabbalah.

Regarding synchronization with the fluid body, there are five principles to explore.

Principle: The fluid body can be sensed as "one drop" shaping itself three-dimensionally, either purposefully or playfully. The fluid body expresses heat and electrical potency. The body is about 92 percent water and generates heat and electricity. Jump in and feel this potency.

Biological water has longitudinal, lateral, and transparent movement along, toward, and through every tissue in the body. These are the three laws of fluids, according to Erich Blechschmidt (2012a). Its potency moves the blood (and of course PR moves the blood). Thus, the fluid body has its own natural intelligence, a potency existing before the nervous system, cognition, and emotions arise in development. It expresses originality.

Principle: The fluid body is known by flow, a micromovement associated with a felt sense of currents, waves, eddies, and stillness. Recent research on the interstitium of the extracellular fluid environment indicates a global communications network in the fluid body. Many metaphors for the embodiment of the fluid body are possible. I like seaweed for a spine and jellyfish for the diaphragms. Be your own aquarium.

Principle: The fluid body expresses buoyancy in its constant shaping process. The lift of the fluid body counteracts the pull of gravity. Such a lift in no way is dissociating. The body acts as a coral reef to maintain the proper density for embodiment. Buoyancy is somatic freedom.

The fluid body is continuous with the natural world. Therefore, the fluid body is the natural world inside the body. If a client's capacity to have their fluid body transition from inside to outside the body is compromised, then the client's capacity to relate with the totality of the natural world is compromised. We are only partially bound by the skin. Clinically, practitioners integrate the inside of the fluid body, under the skin, with its outside, in the biosphere of the body. Its capacity to transition (via conduction, evaporation, and so forth) from inside to outside is compromised in most clients. Thus the skin plays a vital role in the continuity of the fluid body.

Principle: The fluid body is a completely receptive vehicle. This is a law of nature. Allow the stress in the client's fluid body to completely dissipate in your own fluid body. It will naturally settle itself in a short time. It is essential in biodynamic practice for the practitioner to be completely receptive at all times when with a client. We are already naturally giving all the time. It is not reciprocal, although it seems that way. Both activities occur simultaneously.

Principle: The fluid body operates at the level of body metabolism. The core of human metabolism depends on the water molecule to function properly. Consequently, biodynamic practice functions to support and shift toward health the body's metabolism. The fluid body is a principle focus of healing in a biodynamic session. The potency of the fluid body is called the fluid drive. The fluid drive is a quality of the nature of water itself. It is related to but different from the potency of PR (see page 283).

Regulation theory from the field of affective neuroscience teaches us that we self-regulate both when connected to another sentient being and when managing the need for autonomy. The cycle of attunement (see page 275) establishes balance in both forms of self-regulation. This helps dissipate stress held in the fluid body organically and is a step in turning off defensive physiology in the client so a Neutral can manifest.

THE NEUTRAL

Principle: In a therapeutic setting, synchronization with the Neutral occurs first in the practitioner and then in the client. "The therapeutic process does not begin until the will of the patient [meaning the autonomic nervous system] yields to the will of Primary Respiration," as Dr. Becker used to say. This happens in the Neutral, or the stillpoint, the space in which the natural instinct of self-healing is remembered by the body's metabolism and ignited by PR.

The Neutral depends on the interpersonal neurobiology (IPNB) principle that the client-practitioner relationship is a two-person biology, as discussed in chapter 14. This is based on interpersonal central, autonomic, and cardiovascular systems. Both the client and practitioner are automatically synchronized and interconnected with each other at these three basic physiological and metabolic levels.

The Neutral is achieved by the cycle of attunement (COA), detailed in the next section. Its establishment is linked to the client's sense of safety and the quality of the therapist's attention. Healing requires safety. The COA establishes and maintains social safety via the social engagement system, according to Porges (2023). Compassion safety or spiritual safety is established through the heart-to-heart connection with PR, and inner metabolic safety is established through PR moving through the umbilical fulcrum (see page 278) . All three states of safety must be synchronized to facilitate optimal self-healing, which increases embodiment. When these three states of safety are synchronized, there is moral safety. Moral safety is lacking in today's culture.

When we achieve the Neutral, the defensive physiology of the client dissipates without overactivation of the autonomic nervous system (ANS). It is a law of nature in classical Chinese medicine. Severe trauma does present challenges for achieving a practitioner-client Neutral. The ANS must be stable before it can recover its original functions of the Four Immeasurables (loving kindness, compassion, joy, and equanimity) with the help of PR. Stress and trauma cause the ANS to live in its default state of defensive physiology and fear. Even if a Neutral is not perceived, PR is increasing the potency of the instinct for self-transcendence in the client. PR chooses the instinct it wants to relate with. It is out of our hands, so to speak.

The Neutral is a two-way street. The practitioner achieves one in themselves through contemplative practice, and then the client can find it in the practitioner and have a reference point for safety, even if only for the short term during a session. A client might need to experience the Neutral over and over again before they can trust it and embody it.

Practice with PR homogenizes the three primary instincts of self-healing, self-preservation, and self-transcendence. It does not know them as separate. The Neutral might simply be perceived as a stillpoint in the homogenizing process. The Neutral has many ways of manifesting in a session. Synchronizing with PR and stillness provides guidance in recognizing a Neutral when it appears in the natural world, as birdsong, for example, or an open thought-free state of mind, however temporary that might be.

In the Neutral, the therapeutic direction of PR may be observed to automatically shift in its function. The Neutral is interwoven with the many faces of PR. The language is not as important as the practitioner's individual perception and felt sense. The Neutral is a state in which transmutation is potentiated. As a potential, it is a doorway of perception. The Neutral is frequently sensed as a stillpoint.

CYCLE OF ATTUNEMENT

In a therapeutic session, the practitioner establishes the ground of compassion by first attuning to themselves as a spiritual being. This is always the first synchronization in biodynamic practice; it allows us to acknowledge the biodynamic process with awe. Having laid the foundation for compassion, the practitioner then synchronizes with the natural world and then, to allow the heart-to-heart connection, to the client.

The cycle of attunement (COA) refers to the manner in which the practitioner deliberately and then spontaneously shifts their attention (attunement) between self, nature, and the client in the tempo of PR. This mimics the prenatal and neonatal development of the ANS in which approach behaviors increase sympathetic tone and withdrawal behaviors increase parasympathetic tone. This rhythm of approach-withdraw needs to remain in an optimal window of tolerance for the developing brain to experience joy and happiness and thus the need for the buffering activity of stillness and PR.

The COA is the basic unit of work in a biodynamic session and in life. Such work implies the need for effort at evenly suspending one's attention throughout inner and outer space while staying grounded and connected to the Earth.

Attunement to Oneself: Establishing the Ground of Compassion

Embodiment from the attunement point of view involves interoception, exteroception, and awareness of the five elements. Interoception includes conscious awareness of the heart, stomach, and intestines in their function of emotions, hunger, satiety, and elimination. This inner awareness blends with the exteroception of our five senses in the natural world. The effort requires settling and slowing, recognizing and relaxing. The fulcrum of attention automatically shifts between the elements of wind, earth, water, fire, and space in the body of the practitioner and in the natural world surrounding the practitioner.

Principle: Physical comfort and ease of breath are a priority for attunement and to avoid transmitting discomfort to the client in a biodynamic session.

Physical discomfort interferes with the accurate perception of PR. This makes it vitally necessary to use supports and props for the arms and hands, pelvis, and legs. We can think of our physical positioning in a session as a creative set of yoga asanas. "The posture itself is enlightenment," as Suzuki Roshi (2011) said. With that in mind, keep the following guidelines in mind:

- Your knees should stay below the plane of pelvis.
- Visualize your diaphragms like jellyfish; make sure they are aligned, open, and free to automatically shift.
- Keep your mouth slightly open to mix inner space with outer space. Breathe through your nose.
- Keep your eyes open. Periodically look down for humility, to the horizon for compassion, and slightly above the horizon for wisdom. These are the three planes of vision for inviting PR into your perception.
- Stay mindful of the breath between the respiratory diaphragm and abdomen.
- Stay mindful of the heartbeat and its potency.
- Stay mindful of the fluid body around the skin, in the biosphere.

Principle: Every hand position and contact with the client can be considered a mudra eliciting sacred space. Biodynamic therapy is a ministry of laying on of hands. We use our hands to evoke self-transcendence.

Principle: The perception of PR is Ignited by the Cycle of Attunement. There are many starting points for the perception of PR. The three exercises below offer guidelines for working with three embryonic fulcrums that readily engage with PR: the third ventricle, heart, and umbilicus. They are presynchronized with PR and activated by the quality of the practitioner's attention.

෨෨
Horizon Therapy

↩ Perceiving PR through the Fulcrum of the Third Ventricle (Space) ↝

Explore this practice when a view of nature is available. If the outdoors is not available, an image of nature hanging on the wall or even a houseplant will do.

1. Close your eyes and place your attention on the space between your eyes and the occiput.

2. Roll your eyes up to the middle of your forehead, hold briefly (for several seconds), and then release the eyes. Repeat several times. This movement of the eyes tugs on the anterior third ventricle of the brain.

3. With your eyes open, look to the horizon with the gaze of compassion. Sense PR moving back and forth between the third ventricle and the horizon. It is a subtle tide melting the brain and eyes and dissipating them to the horizon, and then PR changes phase and the eyes and brain reassemble. Be filled with awe.

4. Periodically resynchronize with the breath.

Practice horizon therapy whenever possible, if only for a breath or two. Stand at a window and let your attention go. It will come back in a minute or so.

෨෨
Fire as Light

↩ Perceiving PR from the Heart inside the Heart ↝

1. Sense your heartbeat. Differentiate the stillness in the back of the heart from the movement in front, next to the sternum. Gradually allow the pulsation of the heart to expand and include the whole body. The dynamic stillness in the back of the heart becomes unified with the perception of the movement of the heart in front.

2. Sense the potency of the heart as the sum of all autonomic input to the heart. The heartbeat is not the potency but part of the potency. This potency is the electrical grid of the heart's conduction system.

3. Sense PR moving from your heart and intermingling with PR from the client's heart. PR travels in the electromagnetic field (ECM) of the heart, which extends approximately fifteen feet around the body. The fulcrum for PR is in the stillpoint

in the back of the heart known as the infinity point. From this fulcrum, all hearts are interconnected. We are constantly in an interconnected heart field. The entire universe is an interconnected heart field.

The ECM conducts information from heart to heart just as PR does, with waves within waves, or frequencies within frequencies. It is usually a communication of deep safety and coherence. This generates empathy and compassion via emotional safety.

4. Sense the transparency of the heart. PR moves through without stopping. This is the original function of the embryonic heart. When sitting or standing outside, you can sense the wind moving through you as well as around you, wrapping you like a baby with its gentleness. These are not separate functions; they occur simultaneously.

Practice these four stages of perceiving PR from the heart inside the heart to develop extrasensory perception of the originality of the embryonic heart and to activate universal love. Exploring your perception of PR from heart to heart is the treatment. It is enough until PR decides to shift its fulcrum.

___

On Grief

The heart is related to the emotional safety of not only bliss, pleasure, and joy but also grief. Grief causes the left ventricle of the heart to expand. It mixes with transgenerational sorrow and expands the field of love.

___

ඊඞ
Fire of Earth
⌁ Perceiving PR from Three Levels of the Umbilical Fulcrum ⁓

The gut and consequently the umbilicus is the true metabolic center of the body. This fulcrum must be explored thoroughly, and contact with the abdomen is a recommended part of every biodynamic session.

The abdomen (and its viscera) is the location of inner metabolic safety. It holds the fire of the earth element. Such safety is compromised by metabolic syndromes (which are associated with eating ultraprocessed food), most prescription and over-the-counter medications, and added sugar of any kind in the diet. This compromised safety is directly associated with states of inflammation initiated in the gut that become systemic via the endothelium of the entire cardiovascular system.

There are three levels of umbilicus clinically.

1. The first level is the prenatal biological connection to our mother. Even after our birth, this umbilical cord is always connected to us, energetically and emotionally. It is always there, breathing with PR. In a session, the hands and arms of the practitioner become an umbilical cord—the vein and artery. The two-person biology of the therapeutic relationship is similar in this way to pregnancy.

   To connect with this first level of the umbilicus, practice belly breathing to deepen this knowing internally. Sense the umbilicus moving out and back with each breath. This is embryonic breathing in Taoism.

2. The second level of the umbilicus is our connection to the Great Mother of planet Earth.

   To connect with this second level of the umbilicus, sit under a tree for ten to twenty minutes. Then stand up and place your umbilicus directly against the tree to sense PR moving back and forth between your umbilicus and the tree. Another option is to simply visualize an umbilical cord between your umbilicus and your favorite place in nature. Sense PR moving back and forth.

3. The third level is the divine feminine umbilicus. She is the center of the universe. All life, all creation, flows through this point in Taoism. Joseph Campbell called it the World Navel. Become familiar with the Taoist principles of Chi Nei Tsang (refer to the books by Mantak Chia) and Tuina massage and the traditional Chinese medicine principles of the Hara and dantian. These ancient systems recognize the navel as the center of the universe.

   To connect with this third level of the umbilicus, begin by forgiving your parents and honoring your ancestors. Then reconnect to the Earth from the perception of being part of the Earth rather than simply being on the planet. Finally, build your own origin story of creation, life, death, and beyond (see the exercise on page 135). It all comes through the umbilicus to the heart and then the brain in the embryo.

The Body as the Second Placenta

The body is the second placenta, according to A. T. Still. This is clear metabolically, with abdominal visceral fat in obesity. For self-healing, the body seeks an origin point in the embryo from such a similarity in form and function. And thus obesity tales on the healing potential of a placenta that ultimately must be discarded. Spiritually, the placenta is an organ of great compassion, sacrificing itself after birth. The biodynamic cardiovascular therapist becomes like a placenta and gives their heart to each client and becomes transparent to the Tide of PR. In this way, the body is always a metaphorical second placenta.

Attunement to the Natural World

Attunement to the natural world is a process of unifying the natural world of our inner space with that of the space outside our body. It is a metaphor for the fluid body, as mentioned earlier in this chapter.

Principle: The natural world is presynchronized with PR and its potency. The natural world constantly invites us to synchronize with her.

Whenever possible, make an umbilical connection with nature, as described above.

In a session, explore all the exteroceptive and interoceptive senses to relate with the natural world, especially feeling (kinesthesia), hearing, smell, taste (gather saliva in your mouth and swallow periodically), and sight. Automatically shift between that exteroception and interoceptive awareness of your inner natural world.

Allow the natural world to participate in the session. This is indicated by the natural world synchronizing your attention with the change of phase of PR through birdsong, a sunbeam, a breath of wind, and so forth. Even street noise that is seemingly a distraction is synchronizing. The primary function of the elements of space and wind is the conduction of sound. All sound is sacred (unless, of course, local ordinances ban it).

Principle: Any aspect of nature can bring one's attention back to the present moment for synchronizing with PR. Sparks of Ignition are everywhere, not just in the practitioner and client.

As noted, biodynamic sessions employ all the senses, inside and out, for synchronizing with PR. Train by meditating outside in nature. The Buddha and Jesus did not have covered arenas in which to instruct their followers. PR invites the whole sensorium to synchronize with it.

Attunement to the Client:
Establishing the Heart-to-Heart Connection

Synchronizing with the client occurs through the five elements in their manifestation of density, flow, movement, space, and heat. Every practitioner has different training and different palpation skills, and therefore, each practitioner is unique in their approach to watching the priorities of PR unfold in a session and in life. Own this work. Each biodynamic practitioner has their own unique gift.

Practitioner Tip

Remember: Track PR in yourself first. Then move to attune with the flow of PR in your client and establish a heart-to-heart connection.

Principle: All senses, including the mind sense, are involved in contacting the client. Suspend the mental labeling of objects and sensations. One's mind must be calm for the hands to synchronize with the natural wisdom of PR.

Contemplating the client's pain and suffering is important. Compassion then is bearing witness from the heart inside the heart, which is capable of expanding infinitely. Then the practitioner can make a nonverbal wish that the client's pain and suffering be eliminated, using the biodynamic mantra of the Four Immeasurables (see page 270).

Principle: The practitioner's hands are afferent, or inward seeking. Yet they remain at the surface of the client's fluid body until the impulse arises to explore the three springs, as they are called. At the basic level they are the tissue (outer layer of skin), fluid (the inner layer of the endothelium), and energy (the dynamic stillness in the center of blood flow). The three springs will change depending on the location of the client's symptoms and the embryology associated with those symptoms and the Health. During palpation, the hands are not static or inert; they pause and listen frequently.

Bring attention to the hands when invited by the client's potency of PR and their breath. Wait for a signal to be given by the client rather than letting the mind energize the hands. The practitioner's willpower and desire to add force must be suspended. The intention is to Ignite the client's instinct for self-healing, not to direct it.

Principle: A biodynamic session has three overlapping phases:

1. The cycle of attunement associated with the perception of a Neutral
2. The Ignition of a therapeutic or healing process (therapeutic processes are time dependent; spiritual healing processes are timeless and transparent)
3. The endpoint, when the potency of PR increases (or when the client's clock time is finished and the next client is in the waiting room)

Note that the client's Neutral does not usually happen immediately or in every session. The key is for the therapist to achieve a Neutral in themselves first.

Principle: The cycle of attunement is partially based on the infant-mother attachment that establishes stability in the ANS. Such stability is the basis for states of stress to transform into joy or at least stability and resilience after a therapeutic Neutral occurs.

Sympathetic nervous system (SNS) tone rises with approach behaviors, and parasympathetic nervous system (PNS) tone rises with withdrawal behaviors. This rhythm creates the felt sense of safety (or lack of safety) and, depending on the infant's family circumstances, exists on a spectrum of normal and joyful to stressful and traumatic. The cycle of attunement is paced with the rhythm of PR to repair early attachment complications (as one of numerous possibilities not under the control of the practitioner). Consider such repair as a normal side effect rather than the intention of a session.

THE THREE DIRECTIONS OF PR

Synchronizing occurs with the three cardinal directions of PR:

1. **Outside in.** The initial perception is typically that PR is coming inward from the horizon, intersecting with any or all the embryonic fulcrums of the body.
2. **Inside out.** With deepening perception PR can be felt to originate inside the body, usually from the heart inside the heart or any embryonic fulcrum, and from there move outward.
3. **Transparency.** This is the experience of no source, origination, or cause of PR. It is in a nonphasic state and moves through the body unrestrictedly.

The cycle of the three directions is happening in you, the client, the natural world, or all three. A typical session will demonstrate the entire cycle. Just remember that it is a nonlinear process.

This is not a belief system or dogma about a source or cause of PR but rather an open ended perceptual clinical process in the moment. It is an exploration of mindfulness becoming watchfulness and compassion as the foundation for the embodiment of self-transcendence, self-healing, and self-preservation.

THE POTENCY OF PR

Synchronization occurs with the *potency* of PR, which exists on a spectrum of sweet to strong, liquid to firm, sad to joyful, hot to cold, and so forth. There are many currents in the ocean. It is an expression of all the elements in every manifestation—internal, external, and cosmic. Remember the potency also expresses heat and fire.

Principle: The elements are spiritually sentient, expressing the cosmic dance of life. They express the vitality and aliveness of the body in their spiritual function. The spiritual essence of PR strengthens as a session unfolds. It may initiate visionary and mystical experiences of light and the appearance of the sacred.

Principle: At death, the potency of PR is very sweet and gentle. It merges back into its universal expression of infinite expansion.

Principle: Some biodynamic sessions end like death; the potency of PR dissipates and merges with the greater tide of PR. It is very transparent. Other sessions end with a stronger potency. Still other sessions end in the potency of dynamic stillness.

Principle: Train by sensing the potency of PR in the natural world. The potency of PR is known in many ways through all the senses. Relax and open the senses. Train by noticing the impermanence of all things big and small. Change is constant.

IGNITION (WIND AND FIRE)

Synchronizing occurs with numerous types of Ignition processes. Ignition is on a spectrum from combustion (emotional release) to initiation (spiritual revelation) experiences. It is a metaphor for the self-directed therapeutic activity of PR. It directly involves the elements of wind and fire.

Traditional biodynamic approaches to Ignition consists of four types: conception, heart, birth, and death. Every change of phase of PR is a conception Ignition. Every heartbeat is a heart Ignition. Every inbreath is a birth Ignition, and every outbreath is a death Ignition. Keep it simple. These four types are automatic shifting fulcrums of attention.

Principle: PR undergoes changes of phase. Ignition usually happens in a change of phase. The change of phase is one important entrance to the therapeutic activity of PR.

Rest your attention in PR's change of phase when your fluid body, the natural world, and the client's body synchronize with its potency. This does not mean to focus or concentrate but rather to relax into open awareness, in which your attention is evenly suspended to infinity.

Practitioner Tip

Avoid the trap of trying to perceive the entire cycle of PR like a dog chasing its tail. It dances with everything, especially stillness. It fades to the background and then comes into the foreground in a constant exchange with stillness.

Principle: The potency of PR is the fire element. It is associated with the activity of the Holy Spirit. When I asked Dr. Jealous the meaning of conception Ignition, he said only one word: annunciation. The iconography of the Annunciation of Mary shows the Holy Spirit as a white dove radiating Mary and impregnating her with the son of God. This is the fire power of the sacred and the divine. It moves itself under its own power (potency). This potency radiates from the heart inside the heart. Such potency is directly associated with the vitality or life force of the body.

Principle: The potency of PR upon Ignition spreads or automatically shifts in multiple planes or areas inside the practitioner, client, or natural world or all three.

The potency is the current(s) within the tide of PR. Spend time in the ocean to become familiar with its currents and thus the tide of PR. Special snorkeling equipment is not necessary. This is perceptual practice.

Principle: Upon Ignition PR has its own timing. A change of phase can be longer than a quick spark or sometimes nonexistent. The subtle wisdom wind of PR continually surprises and dances with all appearance.

Principle: All perception of PR is nonlinear and noncognitive. Ignition processes manifest in a triad of hot to cool, slow to fast, and mundane to spiritual. Thus, Ignition can also be an initiation of the instinct for self-transcendence with a strong spiritual fulcrum. How often have we heard a client say they felt the movement of grace in the session?

The potency contained in the wisdom wind (PR) is the Four Immeasurables within the instinct for self-transcendence. It maintains the stability and continuity of a spiritual Ignition process. We are only ever in a continual process of spiritual formation and spiritual maturation in our relationship with life and death in every moment. Ignition is the harbinger of change, both big and small. We must learn to accept change and to forgive with such powerful potency. Have no regrets at death.

RESTING IN A DYNAMIC STILLNESS (VOID SPACE)

Synchronization occurs when we rest attention in a dynamic stillness. There is a dynamic stillness in the midst of motion and reactivity that is free of intention, direction, and time. It is a complete allowing of what is from moment to moment. At some point in the Ignition process or the Neutral, a pause occurs, a type of panoramic opening of space that requires no tracking or work to perceive. It simply arises as a conscious awareness, and we discover that it is here all the time in our heart inside our heart. Dynamic stillness is a metaphor for many perceptions, especially awareness. Awareness is knowledge of the natural state of the body and mind independent of thoughts, concepts, or scientific intelligence. It is not a "presence" but the actual direct empirical knowing of a sacred dimension that discerns itself directly as it is. It is self-knowing wisdom without a reference point.

We observe it and then dissolve the observer through contemplative practice and principles.

Principle: All that is necessary in the stillness is to rest, abide, dissolve, melt, and connect with the pulsation of one's heart. It is the pulsation of the universe.

Our ordinary mind jumps to examine such emptiness, yet it is not necessary or possible to figure it out on the spot. It is break time from one's ordinary perception. Biodynamic practice involves extra-ordinary perception. The essence of synchronizing is a type of shamanic perception; it is crucial to but not limited to biodynamic practice. It is a natural state of awe. Relaxing one's attention into a panoramic awareness is key. One no longer waits; one is abiding and resting without analyzing in the stillness.

Principle: Stillness is associated with the element of space.

Space in this case is the intangible spiritual domain in which visions of the natural state appear. Their appearance manifests the spiritual activity of the wind element. It is a colorful form of space. Access to such visualizations depends on the practitioner's capacity for the spiritual aptitude of perceiving appearance. Remember that this is just one of three spiritual aptitudes (perception of stillness, of PR, and of appearance). These three spiritual aptitudes are not a hierarchy; they are equal developmental phases of biodynamic cardiovascular therapy.

Principle: The stillness of Ignition is a reorientation to conception, in which the spiritual potency of PR and the dynamic stillness direct molecular transmutation to become renewed in an original wholeness. We are actually in a constant state of conception Ignition, a form of embodiment that flows and changes constantly during all phases of life from a spiritual point of view. This is the present moment.

Principle: The midline is the dynamic stillness that automatically shifts from inside the body to outside and back.

The midline is a metaphor for the felt sense of the embodiment of order and organization of the totality of body-mind-spirit centered in the heart inside the heart. Ignition processes are said to place a client back on their midline, which is the heart inside the heart, the true center of the universe. Thus there is only one Ignition in life and death: that of the heart.

Principle: There is no growth and development without biological quiescence (dynamic stillness).

The biological organization of the heart specifically and the growth and development of the body in general is always in reference to biological stillness. All molecules must pass through a stillpoint for transmutation as mentioned.

Principle: The dynamic stillness is a multidimensional experience of an embodied heart. The heart develops around a hub of quiescent cells, as described below. The movement of the physical heart is held in the womb of stillness in back of the heart and the quiescence of its inner endothelium as a single unified experience. The heart expands and contracts from its own quiescence. This is the Breath of Life radiating from the heart inside the heart.

Principle: PR and stillness are one thing, one living self-knowing whole. This whole book is talking about one thing with a thousand different faces.

Principle: Embodied stillness is the preexisting condition of the Health.

Categories of Biological Stillness

Dynamic stillness is integrally linked to our biology. To be more specific, dynamic stillness has three roots of embodiment: embryonic fluid fields, growth resistance, and cell biology.

Embryonic Fluid Fields

Lacunae. The lacunae (lagoons) are pockets of still fluid surrounding the embryo in the structure of the pre-placenta in the second week of development. Their function of stillness is to invite the maternal blood vessels into the pre-placenta and form a connection for the embryo to be nourished. (See plates 1–4 in the color insert.)

Somites. These blocks of cells are seen next to the neural tube starting in the fourth week of development. Each somite initially contains a center of still fluid, a lacunae (lagoon). This stillness invites the blood vessels to grow toward the neural tube and thus begin connecting and nurturing the central nervous system.

Notochord canal. It begins to develop anteriorly of the neural tube around the same time as the somites. It begins as a tube of dynamically still fluid. Its cellular structure retains that stillness all through the life span as an orientation for the central nervous system.

Venous system. The venous system carries 70 percent of the blood in the body. The veins are like lakes or ponds of almost still fluid, moving with the tidal movement of the heart, diaphragm, and body movement in general.

Growth Resistance

In general, metabolic fields (the biokinetic activity of cells coalescing to create structure in the embryo) create resistance to each other, some more so than others. This is because they each have their own unique position, shape, and prestructuring dynamic. The interfaces between the metabolic fields have varying degrees of biological stillness and pulling apart, especially between the heart and brain/neural tube. The universe consists of these metabolic fields, pulling us, contracting us, and so forth. They are universal cosmic fields of creation.

Cell Biology

Wedge-shaped epithelium. When the heart begins to go through its looping phase, the inside hub of the loop becomes pointed or narrow and the outside of the cells becomes wedge-shaped or broader. The inner narrow end of the cells become metabolically less active and thus dynamically still. Stillness forms the core of the heart in this way and induces the growth of the cushions and valves between the chambers of the heart as well as the endothelium of the inner structure of the chambers of the heart. (See plate 14 in the color insert.)

Quiescent cells. This is a category of cells that are metabolically less active and thus dynamically still. These cells are seen in the phases of blood development prenatally and are critically important in the endothelium of the arteries in the adult body, among other structures. Inflammatory processes rooted in the intestines can cause these cells to lose their dynamic stillness and become hyperactive, which is a marker for metabolic syndrome and disease.

Senescent cells. When cells of this type are dying in the embryo, they give off a growth factor that provides nourishment to the surrounding cells. Thus a cell that is dying in the embryo and dynamically still can produce factors for growth and development in the surrounding environment. In the adult, however, these same cells signal the immune system to generate an inflammatory response. (Note that senescent cells are differentiated from apoptotic cells, which have programmed death and give off no growth factors in their death.)

THE EMBODIED COMPASSION OF PR

Synchronizing occurs with the three compassionate intentions of PR, as detailed in Tibetan medicine. These intentions may be observed to automatically shift during a Neutral, during a change of phase of PR, or at any time during the cycle of attunement and the Ignition process.

1. **Create:** The activity of constant renewal, constant spiritual heart Ignition whose fulcrum is the present moment. The change of phase of PR is a dilation of the present moment, which has no past and no future. It reminds me of an expression of the Navy Seals: "Slow is smooth and smooth is fast."
2. **Repair:** PR is self-directing, following its own priorities for engaging the instinct for self-healing. This is known only by observation, just as Sutherland discovered in 1948, when he started the biodynamic model, upon observing PR shift to repair mode.
3. **Maintain:** PR has a constant interconnection to the whole. It establishes the baseline for all metabolic and physiological function inside the body and out.

These intentions unfold from compassion, one of the wisdom aspects of PR. Compassion is the ability to feel the pain that we share with others. It is established in the heart-to-heart connection, which is Ignited by the therapist sensing their heartbeat.

Principle: Compassion requires humility. Bowing one's head during a session is important. When appropriate, make a nonverbal aspiration for the client to be completely free of pain and suffering while sensing your heartbeat.

Principle: The present moment is the supreme spiritual teacher, no past, no future.

THE FIVE GATES AND FIVE ELEMENTS OF PR

This discussion of the five gates (which are organizing fulcrums for PR in the body based on the five vayus in ayurvedic medicine) and five elements is based on an understanding of the animism-shamanism integrated in Tibetan medicine. Shamanism in this sense means the practice of harmonizing the relationship between the individual and the environment through working with the five gates and five elements inside and outside the body. The intention is to Ignite the felt sense of embodiment as an interconnected whole with the environment.

Synchronizing occurs through the five gates of PR in the body with the five

Indo-Tibetan elements (earth, water, fire, wind, space). In ayurvedic medicine the gates are called the vayus; in biodynamic practice, we might call them fulcrums. PR (or chi, prana, or wind, depending on one's orientation) enters the body synchronized with the breath of air. It separates into five gates (fulcrums) to govern the form and function of the human body.

Element	Gate/Fulcrum	Aspect of the Body
Earth	Throat	Tissue
Water	Kidneys/bladder	Blood
Fire	Superior mesenteric-renal arteries	Metabolism
Wind	Heart	Breath
Space	Top of the cranium	Mind

All five elements, however, are simultaneously moved by the element of the wind. Some say that wind is the horse upon which each element is mounted (so, yes, there is wind mounted on the wind). From a shamanic point of view, then, naturally PR is an aspect of the wind element and consequently a critical spiritual aptitude. PR is the wisdom wind.

Principle: The five internal gates (fulcrums) of PR govern all structure and function in the human body.

These gates (fulcrums) and the aspect of wind/PR associated with them are as follows.

Life-Sustaining Wind: The Wind of Space

The wind of space emanates from the top of the cranium. This is an important level of wind that governs all the others. It is where the highest spiritual expression of wind and space enter the body vertically.

The cranium relates to the element of space. Space in this sense is synonymous with dynamic stillness. Whenever a practitioner is working around the cranium, the dynamic stillness permeates the room and total environment. Therefore, the element of space is always associated with the perception of dynamic stillness.

All-Pervasive Wind: The Wind of Wind

The wind of wind emanates from the heart horizontally. Thus, the all-pervasive wind moves the blood and the virtues of the sacred circulate everywhere in the body.

Upward-Rising Wind: The Wind of Earth

The wind of earth emanates from the throat. The cycle of attunement to the natural world with the third ventricle (linked to the central and autonomic nervous systems) connects to the element earth. Any contact around the head and neck of a client needs to be grounded in a perception of the earth element and its density.

Breathing activates the element of wind. Feel yourself breathing from inside the breath rather than from outside at the surface of mind and thoughts.

Downward Voiding Wind: The Wind of Water

The wind of water emanates from the kidneys-bladder. Wait in the fluid body of micromovement and dissipation for PR to enter as if it were a royal guest. The fluid body is the element of water and the blood, longitudinal, lateral, spiral, and playful. This is the metabolism of flow.

Once the fluid body moves with PR, Health becomes available. All the elements move under the power of PR. Everything in the universe that moves does so with the power of PR.

Digestive Metabolic Wind: The Wind of Fire

The wind of fire emanates from the superior mesenteric artery, which feeds most of the intestines. It governs the metabolism of the body and the formation of blood.

Eat real food! Cease eating ultraprocessed food and any food with added sugar. Sugar is a chronic dose-dependent toxin. It poisons the blood.

Intermittently fast, not eating for twelve to fifteen hours between the end of the evening meal and the beginning of breakfast at a minimum. (Thus, the meaning of *break-fast*.) That is a good start unless you are medically compromised such as with hypoglycemia. It promotes inner safety and decreases many metabolic problems by nudging the metabolism of the body toward catabolism, opening the cellular drainage pathways.

Belly breathing activates the fire element located in the gut. Feel the umbilicus move out and back. The umbilicus is our connection to a universal origin entering our body horizontally. It is a key point in biodynamic practice.

THE THREE LEVELS OF PR FUNCTION

Synchronizing occurs with the three levels of PR function. These functions may occur after a Neutral or during an Ignition process.

1. Gross: Guiding the constant structuring and functioning of the human body.
2. Subtle: The movement of cognition, emotions, and self-awareness through the five chakras (crown, throat, heart, belly, and sexual) and three channels (one

central and two lateral). The yoga of breath, the yoga of body, and the yoga of meditation are helpful in purifying these channels. The color of PR in the central channel is aquamarine blue.

3. Wisdom: The movement of loving kindness and compassion emanating from the heart inside the heart is the virtue of the life-sustaining wind. PR at this level transforms emotional energy into wisdom energy. Wisdom PR is the self-existing energy behind the nonduality and felt sense of an interconnection to all life. One could say that it is the energy of enlightenment, or the essence of the Breath of Life.

Principle: Everything in the universe is moved by the wisdom aspect of PR.

Principle: The biodynamic universe described above is all happening simultaneously. As the elements form a body and a universe, they are also dissolving a body and a universe at the same time. Biodynamics is a training in the perception of the whole of life and synchronizing with the layers necessary for Health to manifest. As my wife Cathy always says, "Slowly is holy." Jim Jealous always said: "wait, watch and wonder."

Final principle: "Be still, and know that I am God," meaning Divine Pure Awareness (Psalm 46:10, often quoted by Sutherland and Becker).

May these random thoughts of mine reverse confusion rather than cause confusion in the biodynamic community of practitioners and teachers that I love and respect. May these ramblings of mine be a cause for compassion to flourish everywhere and bring peace to those who are not at peace. May these many thoughts be a cause for kindness to be felt everywhere and in every body. May our ministry of laying on of hands shower blessings continually with the grace of Primary Respiration. May we trust the Tide.

The Buddha did his enlightenment; you must do yours.

You are the host of your mind and emotions, not the guest.
Know the difference.

There is only one koan—You.
Zen Master Ikkyu (2000)

RECOMMENDED READING

The following books are very important to my understanding of healing from an Eastern perspective. I had the great privilege of studying with brilliant Tibetan physicians. These books and their authors informed this chapter and the maturation of my spiritual journey to a great extent.

The Ambrosia Heart Tantra, a fourth-century Sanskrit text, annotated by Dr. Yeshi Dhonden, trans. Jhampa Kelsang (Library of Tibetan Works and Archives, 1977).

Biokinetics and Biodynamics of Human Differentiation: Principles and Applications by E. Blechschmidt and R. F. Gasser (North Atlantic Books, 2012).

Chi Nei Tsang: Internal Organ Chi Massage by Mantak and Maneewan Chia (Healing Tao, 1990).

Crow with No Mouth by Ikkyu; versions by Stephen Berg. (Copper Canyon Press, 1989; originally written in the fifteenth century).

Death, Intermediate State and Rebirth in Tibetan Buddhism by Lati Rinbochay and Jeffrey Hopkins (Snow Lion Publications, 1979; orig. written in the eighteenth century).

A Flash of Lightning in the Dark of the Night: A Guide to a Boddhisattva's Way of Life by the Dalai Lama (Shambhala, 1994).

The Fourth Phase of Water: Beyond Solid, Liquid, and Vapor by Gerald H. Pollack (Ebner & Sons Publishers, 2013).

A Guide to a Bodhisattva's Way of Life by Shantideva; trans. Stephen Batchelor (Library of Tibetan Works and Archives, 1979; orig. written in the eighth century) *(There are many translations of this book. This is my favorite.).*

Healing from Within with Chi Nei Tsang by Giles Marin (North Atlantic Books, 1999).

Healing with Form, Energy and Light: The Five Elements in Tibetan Shamanism, Tantra, and Dzochen by Tenzin Wangyal Rinpoche (Snow Lion Publications, 2002).

Health through Balance: An Introduction to Tibetan Medicine by Dr. Yeshi Dhonden, trans. Jeffrey Hopkins (Snow Lion Publications, 1986).

Medicine Buddha Teachings by Khechen Thrangu Rinpoche (Snow Lion Publications, 2004).

"Neuroception: A Subconscious System for Detecting Threats and Safety" by S. W. Porges, *Zero to Three* 24, no. 5 (2004): 19–24.

The Places That Scare You by Pema Chodron (Shambhala Publications, Inc., 2002).

"The Polyvagal Theory: Phylogenetic Substrates of a Social Nervous System" by S. W. Porges, *International Journal of Psychophysiology* 42, no. 2 (2001): 123–46.

"The Science of Respiration and the Doctrine of the Bodily Winds in Ancient India" by Kenneth G. Zysk, *Journal of the American Oriental Society* 113, no. 2 (1993): 198–213.

The Spiritual Medicine of Tibet: Heal Your Spirit, Heal Yourself by Dr. Peme Dorjee with Janet Jones and Terence Moore (Watkins Publishing, 2005).

Tibetan Medical Paintings: Illustrations to the Blue Beryl treatise of Sangye Gyamtso (1653–1705), volume 2: *Text* by Yuri Parfionovitch, Gyurme Dorje, and Fernand Meyer (Harry N. Abrams, Inc, 1992).

"Tibetan 'Wind' and 'Wind' Illnesses: Towards a Multicultural Approach to Health and Illness" by Ronit Yoeli-Tlalimy, *Studies in History and Philosophy of Biological and Biomedical Sciences* 41, no. 4 (2010): 318–24.

The Tibetan Yoga of Breath: Breathing Practices for Healing the Body and Cultivating Wisdom by Anyen Rinpoche and Allison Choying Zangmo (Shambhala Publications, Inc., 2013).

Treasury of Knowledge, Book 1: *Myriad Worlds* by Jamgon Kongtrul (Snow Lion Publications, 2003; originally written in the nineteenth century).

Zen Mind, Beginner's Mind by Shunryu Suzuki (Weatherhill, 1970).

PART 4

A MINISTRY OF LAYING ON
OF HANDS

*Patients with serious heart conditions should receive medical clearance
to have biodynamic cardiovascular therapy sessions.*

23

Perception and Palpation in Biodynamic Cardiovascular Therapy

Spirit is given. It is not produced by our attention. It is uncovered.

JOHN TARRANT,
THE LIGHT INSIDE THE DARK

Our teachers tell us there are deeper levels of Primary Respiration (PR) and the stillness. There are, as I outlined in the previous chapter. The tide of PR exists superficially with its rate of six cycles every ten minutes. In practice, it gradually becomes timeless. Gradually, it reveals to us its beauty, wisdom, and grace. Some practitioners and clients experience its love, as did Dr. Fulford (2002).

It is similar with the stillness. There is a stillness in back of our heart that generates a potency that moves the blood and expresses love. The stillness deepens into a void that can fill all of space in our perception. The stillness is the midline. It is deep pervasive peace. William Garner Sutherland developed his cranial concept with these insights, which he attributed to Judeo-Christian cosmology. He called the unexplainable and experiences of a bright light with his clients the Breath of Life. The contemporary client needs to be held in a therapeutic container that has deeper levels of instinctual perception available in the practitioner. This chapter explores three levels of perception found in Eastern cosmologies that complement Dr. Sutherland's insights. I describe progressive stages of perception, from superficial to deep, associated with cosmology. These stages describe a possibility and potency in each biodynamic session.

THE BREATH OF LIFE

The Breath of Life is the unmodified precision of the mysterious wisdom of the whole universe as it's expressing itself in that particular form.

JIM JEALOUS,
PERSONAL COMMUNICATION WITH THE AUTHOR

Dr. Sutherland wrote extensively about the Breath of Life, including his spontaneous visualization of it. Based on those writings and the work of Drs. Becker and Jealous, I derive three levels of meaning for the Breath of Life:

1. The first meaning is the metaphor of light, liquid light, the light coming from a lighthouse beacon.
2. The second meaning is movement associated with potency and ignition of the breath of air. As Sutherland said, it is the Breath of Life, not the breath of air. It ignites breathing by its potency, as can be observed in the cerebrospinal fluid. Such ignition includes the entire physiology and metabolism of the human body. We become animated by the Breath of Life, and physical movement is initiated and directed by PR.
3. The third meaning revolves around Sutherland's use of the term *intelligence*. Over his life span, Sutherland could sense a deeper intelligence in the Breath of Life. Probably because he was a devoted Christian in the lineage of the founder of osteopathy, A. T. Still, he came to equate the intelligence of the Breath of Life with the sacred and its God-like nature manifesting in the human body.

Sutherland stated, you could consider the cranial concept to be religious in nature. I interpret that to mean spiritual in nature, with a direct connection to the sacred, regardless of which tradition and religion you might have grown up with (or without). The Breath of Life evokes a deeper inner development of one's heart as the spiritual center of love, beyond space and time. This spiritual intelligence equates to the awareness spoken of in Eastern traditions, which I will speak to shortly.

PERCEPTION

Perception is composed of subject, object, and the organismic machinery connecting the two. The interoception literature describes neurological perception as being similar to that of a flight simulator used by pilots to practice flying. Our brain is simply making predictions based on enormous amounts of sensory input about what's needed physiologically in the body to manage its energy and safety needs. We must really learn to embody our senses, slow the mental labeling and interpreting of our exteroceptive sensory perceptions, and balance exteroception with turning inward for interoceptive awareness. By slowing and stilling the mental interpretation of the senses, we gain access to more accurate empathetic responsiveness through interoception. By being more consciously connected to the heart and its heartbeat, we develop an ability to relax and to trust our body. We can overcome the potential for spontaneous overreactivity coming from the organism. The brain needs a whole lot more time to sort out input to make the flight simulations much better, with smoother flights and softer landings.

Three Levels of Perception

The three levels of perception in biodynamic practice are classified as ordinary (outer or superficial), subtle (inner or middle), and very subtle (deep). They correspond to similar levels of perception in Tibetan medicine and other Eastern traditions. They refer to:

- *Ordinary:* the physical body of anatomy, physiology, and metabolism
- *Subtle:* the subtle body as depicted in a wide variety of Eastern images of colorful chakras, channels, and wind energies
- *Very subtle:* the very subtle body of pure light

There is linkage between the embryo and Eastern cosmological origin narratives of the human body. The link first appears in an array of rainbow colors associated with the subtle body. These colors generate forms, beams of light consisting of rays of axial orientation and bright points of radial orientation, like stars, similar to embryonic development. The embryo in this way is the subtle body. Light (photons) is refracted through the fluid body of the embryo and organizes around canalization zones of embryonic fluid. Eastern traditions describe a subtle midline channel and two side channels (see fig. 23.1); such images look like the early formation of

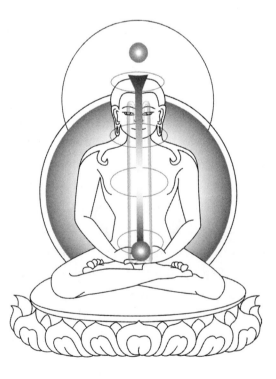

Fig. 23.1. The subtle channels of the body in Eastern traditions

the aorta and neural tube in the human embryo. The midlines and fulcrums of the subtle body then have linkage and manifest in the ordinary body as the heart, the aorta and descending aorta, the neural tube, and the glands associated with a variety of anatomical structures.

Perception of the Five Elements

In Eastern traditions, our anatomy is constructed of five elements, a densification of the colors and light. The elements become the linkage between levels of perception, from the clear light of the very subtle body to the colored form of the subtle body to the five elements of the ordinary body. These are the three levels of perception of the same phenomenon appearing in three different but interrelated ways, like a prism separating clear light into five colors. The elements are said to be infused with wisdom, and so we can see the similarity with the osteopathic notion of the Breath of Life as an innate spiritual intelligence.

In biodynamic practice, the fluid body is composed of the water and earth elements. It is the container for the interaction of the five elements.

PALPATION

From the three levels of perception, we derive the three levels of palpation used in biodynamic cardiovascular therapy. These three levels of palpation are always present when we lay on our hands to bless the client biodynamically. They are called the three springs.

The Three Springs

The three springs are perceptual and palpatory considerations in constructing a unique protocol for clients in every session. Our thinking, feeling hands and heart come into relationship with one or all three springs as our perception expands to include the whole, and our palpation become afferent. In European osteopathy the three springs are categorized according to their correspondence to the three primary embryonic germ layers (ectoderm, mesoderm, endoderm). This is an advanced understanding of the three springs as I learned them from a brilliant French Osteopath Jörg Schurpf. They could also be categorized according to their correspondence with the three levels of energetic perception (ordinary, subtle, very subtle).

First Spring: Tissue/Ordinary

When your fingers are in contact with parts of the vascular tree, the ordinary layer is the fascial connective tissue protecting the artery wall, whose cells are connected to the blood. This is the tissue spring, the outermost edge of the body, including the layers of skin derived from ectoderm embryonically. Palpation of the tissue springs brings us first into relationship with the client's nervous system through the skin-to-skin contact. We wait and observe the client's response and practice attunement to sense our own interoceptive awareness from the contact. We center our initial attention in our third ventricle and synchronize with PR as it moves back and forth, to and from the natural world all around us and out to the horizon. This may or may not lead to a Neutral. It is the time to settle.

Second Spring: Fluid/Subtle

The subtle level is the endothelium, a masterpiece of nature and creation regarding homeostasis in the human body. This is the fluid spring, mostly encompassing the aspects of the body that derive from the embryonic mesoderm. In biodynamic practice this means contact with the fluid body and all the arteries of the vascular tree. The fluid spring includes finding the middle of the blood flow where the dynamic stillness is located biologically. We rhythmically move our attention between our fluid body activity and heartbeat and that of the client. We perceive the buoyant quality of the shared fluid body. The fluid spring breathes in the tempo of PR. We synchronize with the tide moving in and around the fluid spring. This is the Tree of Life, the vast ocean of our embodied existence.

Third Spring: Potency/Very Subtle

The very subtle layer is the potency of the blood flow in the arteries and capillaries. This is the potency spring, encompassing the aspects of the body that derive mainly from the embryonic endoderm. It corresponds to the metabolic potency associated with anabolism and catabolism. It is metabolic potency of heat and fire as mentioned previously. The potency spring deepens into the rhythmic balanced interchange of PR and dynamic stillness. The potency of that tide is the Health.

Practitioner Tip

Doppler radar studies show that the center of blood flow is dynamically still. I doubt if any scan could estimate the exact diameter of that zone of stillness in the middle of the flow. As a practitioner, it is enough to know where the center of blood flow is approximately through buoyant touch and not to overstay your visit.

Integrating Perception and Palpation

Every aspect of our anatomy, physiology, and metabolism has reciprocal movement. The three springs differentiate the intermingled soup of the embryonic germ layers, moving into our hands and away from our hands with different layers of the tide. Thus our hands are rarely static. They are buoyant. Our hands constantly clarify the three springs as the fulcrum of palpation automatically shifts from one spring to another. Our hands ride the reciprocal waves of the three springs while synchronized with PR and resting in our midline of dynamic stillness.

Palpation is a constant attunement synchronized with perception of the whole. The three different springs of elasticity that we feel with palpation gradually synchronize with our inner perception. The blood is moved by the deep wisdom wind of PR residing in the heart, and in this way the artery is a wind instrument, a clarinet, a flute of incredible beauty. We attune to PR, moving back and forth from our heart to the client and then back and forth with cosmos. It seems like a juggling act at first, and then the mechanics of subject-object perception gradually dissolve into one single unified state of *intelligent knowing* extending to the origin of the universe, however briefly. As our teachers constantly remind us: "Be still and know" (Psalm 46:10).

THREE LEVELS OF MIND

Attunement with these levels of the vascular tree involves synchronizing our inner perception with panoramic stillness outwardly. Inwardly, it involves attending to our mind and thoughts until they are quiet enough that we can be aware of gaps in between thought streams, which is mental stillness, however fleeting.

- Thoughts are ordinary mind.
- Gaps between thoughts and resulting stillness are subtle mind.
- Awareness is very subtle mind; it notices both the thoughts and the stillness as a unified whole.

These are the three basic levels of mind for biodynamic practice. It's very easy for a thought stream to build a concept and cause us to lose awareness of the whole. When I'm treating a client, if my mind is very active, I know I cannot visualize colors to have an effective therapeutic effect on the client's metabolism. Visualization practice, whether it is deliberate or spontaneous, is much more effective when the therapist can reduce ideation and discursive thinking. Conscious awareness, which is nonlocal and nonreferential, is enhanced by having fewer thoughts and more periods of stillness. At the same time, such awareness is self-cognizant or self-knowing; it is known by its clarity and lucidity; it is equivalent to the Holy Spirit in some traditions. It is what moves our hands when we are treating a client. Our hands are able to confer a blessing. This is nothing short of Dr. Sutherland's perception of the intelligence of the Breath of Life. It is our innate capacity to knowingly rest in the nonreferential awareness/Holy Spirit/Divine residing in the heart inside the heart. This is spiritual formation enhanced with biodynamic practice.

The three levels of mind—thoughts, stillness, and awareness—can also be described as three levels of the element of space. As described in the osteopathic literature, there is a rhythmic balanced interchange between the elements of space (stillness) and wind (PR). Our sensory perception is built on the element of wind; it is the wind that makes all things alive and move, including our thoughts. This is a deeper level of PR. Being able to switch back and forth between our thoughts and body sensation on a moment's notice is valuable because space and wind are interchangeable elements. As practitioners, we need to develop that level of sensory flexibility and discriminating awareness, making biodynamic practice a contemplative art form.

DEATH AND DYING

The five elements dissolve sequentially in a natural dying process. Earth dissolves first, with accompanying internal images. Then water, then fire, then wind as we take our last breath and dissolve into the element of space. Once the wind element is extinguished, breathing stops and the animating elements of the ordinary body dissipate into the element of space. However, the process of dying continues with the subtle body of colors, sounds, and so forth in one's perception right after death. These brain waves are consistent with cognitive activity.

We've all heard stories of near-death experiences in which survivors remember a sense of separation, a life review, and going to a place that feels like home, in the presence of a spiritual figure, before they recognized the need to come back; these seem to be consistent across cultures. From a biodynamic perspective, the death and dying process is a developmental one. The dying person has the opportunity to dissolve into the very subtle body of clear light, our perceptual home base of originality. But this is true not only after death but in the present moment, with contemplative practice, which is why biodynamic practice must include palliative care.

Multiple levels of consciousness manifest at death, just as in life, and Eastern literature says that after death there can be many train stops on the way to our next destination. Some of those stops go on for other lifetimes. Apparently, it's a long process for some folks to reach clear light, the Breath of Life. We all have our own unique timing for personal spiritual formation based on our conceptual belief systems, religious upbringing, and contemplative practices. Contemporary biodynamic practice enhances and supports spiritual formation—the instinct for self-transcendence—for both the practitioner and the client. If Dr. Sutherland can experience the Breath of Life, so can everyone else. What a gift to practice biodynamically.

AUTOMATIC SHIFTING

Throughout this book, I describe the shifting of the fulcrum of the practitioner's attention. Where does the practitioner's attention land during a session? At the beginning of a session, a practitioner will often deliberately shift their attention from fulcrum to fulcrum—from the third ventricle of the brain to the heart, for example, in order to establish a heart-to-heart connection with the client. Eventually, as the session progresses, shifts in the practitioner's fulcrum of attention become automatic, guided by PR and stillness. For example, the perceptual process of the practitioner will automatically shift between the exteroceptive and interoceptive zones of perception, between the practitioner's own body and the practitioner's hands on the client, and so forth.

Automatic shifting is the essence of constant change mediated by mindfulness and awareness. Our mind and its thoughts are constantly shifting and changing. Life is impermanent. Afferent hands receive impressions in which the client's body is expressing itself in the practitioner's perception. All of this is subject to interpretation, and these explorations in the subsequent chapters are about developing a nonconceptual awareness of the relationship between PR, dynamic stillness, and visionary experiences of the subtle and very subtle body. Awareness is free of interpretation, and that means admitting that we don't know and can't follow a prescribed itinerary for the biodynamic perceptual process.

The Four Embryonic Fulcrums

Biodynamic embryology asserts that there are at least four major embryonic fulcrums from which the various systems of the body unfold. A fulcrum relates to the symmetrical organization of the body and the ordering of its parts. These fulcrums are points of orientation for the movement of growth. Initially they are located in the four fluid cavities seen in the embryo. The first one, associated with the gut, appears a little more than five days after conception. The remaining fulcrums for the heart and blood, nervous system, and bladder arise sequentially starting in the second week. Initially these fulcrums are functional rather than structural. They are simply still points of automatically shifting orientation for growth.

The four fluid cavities and their related fulcrums in the adult are:

1. The yolk sac, the fulcrum of the intestines
2. The chorion, the fulcrum of the heart and blood
3. The amniotic sac, the fulcrum of the third ventricle
4. The allantois, the fulcrum of the bladder

These are fulcrums of attention for the practitioner in biodynamic practice that automatically shift.

The Four Zones of Perception

In biodynamic practice, the practitioner first learns to breath into their abdomen to expand and contract the transversus abdominus muscle. Then the practitioner senses their heartbeat and its potency. Then attention is placed in the fulcrum of the third ventricle to sense PR breathing between the third ventricle and the horizon. Then stillness begins to permeate the environment inside and outside the treatment room.

- Zone A is the body.
- Zone B is the body and the space immediately around the body (the biosphere).
- Zone C is the body, the space around it, and the space in the room (the practitioner's office).
- Zone D is the body, the space around it, the space in the room, and the entire world of nature outside, out to the visible horizon.

These are the zones of perception for the practitioner that I learned from Dr. Jealous.

Perceiving PR

At the beginning of a session, the practitioner works with their own head-righting reflex to orient to the natural world of Zone D. The head-righting reflex refers to the idea that the eyes are designed to orient to the horizon while connected to a stable atlanto-occipital joint space. The attention factor in the brain and nervous system shifts about once a minute from focused to unfocused when we are relaxed, and our attention cycles rhythmically between the third ventricle and the horizon. The practitioner wants to deliberately become aware of and synchronize with this quality of neurological attention, after contemplating the breath and heartbeat. This is, of course, a basic two-dimensional understanding of the tide of PR ebbing and flowing from the front of the body out to the horizon. It is always occurring spontaneously, but the practitioner must begin with a deliberate attempt to synchronize with it.

Gradually the perception of PR becomes more three-dimensional by way of automatic shifting as PR guides the practitioner into all the zones of perception. The practitioner develops a perception of both the inside presence of PR operating within the body or zone A and the outside presence of PR as it is ebbing and flowing through zones A, B, C, and D. PR is the movement of wholeness, and the zones of perception are simple distinctions that are made deliberately in order to orient and synchronize with PR. Gradually these distinctions dissipate during a session into a more wholistic sensibility that is spontaneous and nonconceptual.

In biodynamic cardiovascular therapy, the intention is to explore PR expanding from the pulsating heart, through the entire vascular system, and out to the surface of the skin, and then returning to the heart. PR and the heart breathe together as one thing. This is a subtle and delicate perceptual process of sensing multiple movements at the same time. And here again we have an automatic shifting fulcrum. Since the respiratory diaphragm is attached to the heart, it is a necessary player in this perception of PR. With practice, the movement of the diaphragm becomes included in the synchronizing process of the heart and PR out to the edge of the universe and back. This is an automatic shifting fulcrum of attention that involves visualization practices at the level of the subtle body. We use our breath to enhance the potency of PR as it moves in the vascular system and the whole universe.

Over the course of a session, the practitioner waits for a deepening of the dynamic stillness to occur within the treatment room (Zone C). As the stillness deepens in the room, the practitioner allows the fulcrum of attention to automatically shift between the heart and the stillness. A better way to say this is that the practitioner releases their attention to the stillness with no thought of a return until PR reemerges in its own time. So now PR is moving beyond the skin and Zone B into Zone C (the office room). Gradually this automatically shifting fulcrum generates an even deeper perception of the interchange and relationship between PR, the stillness, and the client.

The practitioner simply sits in the movement of their heart-diaphragm and goes deeper into PR, expanding from that movement to the stillness and returning. Periodically the fulcrum may automatically shift back to the third ventricle as the heart and brain become more balanced within the vascular system. These shifts of the fulcrum are points of ignition as PR is integrating the metabolism of the body with the wholeness of nature into "one taste." This means nonduality in Buddhism. It is the wisdom of impartialness and clarity.

These progressive stages of perception, with the fulcrum of attention automatically shifting under the direction of PR and stillness, are subjective and require contemplative practice to uncover. PR teaches me something different in every session. For any practitioner, it is important to form a personal relationship with PR, the stillness, and the visionary processes. These are the three spiritual aptitudes. Let these automatically shifting spiritual fulcrums be the master teacher. PR only wants to show its wholeness of the universe within the body centered at the heart inside the heart and the stillness of the ocean all around us.

Automatic shifting is the way in which PR opens the heart and empties it rhythmically. The movement of the fulcrum needs to become spontaneous as the practitioner inhabits a greater sense of wholeness in the container of the mind and body in the treatment room. The key point is to learn to release our attention into the open awareness of the dynamic stillness and the bright colors of the world without thought. It is nonlinear and nonconceptual. There is nothing more satisfying than this heart-stillness-visionary connection, especially when our hands are on the client and love becomes transparent and infuses the session.

24

Basic Biodynamic
Cardiovascular Therapy

Please note that a complete view of all the arteries of the body can be seen in the color insert, plates 25–35. These can be reviewed prior to or during the study of the following protocols.

This chapter begins the formal ministry of laying on of hands. Here you'll find demonstrated the basic methods for biodynamic cardiovascular therapy (BCVT), with explicit instructions for the cycle of attunement and palpation, especially of the arteries. You'll also find four basic exploratory protocols to optimize the instinctual metabolism of the contemporary client. This chapter is an essential teaching for all practitioners, no matter what their level of biodynamic practice.

SYNCHRONIZATION THROUGH
THE CYCLE OF ATTUNEMENT

Perception and palpation are blended together in what I call a Cycle of Attunement (COA). The practitioner enters a phase of present-centered attention both while preparing to make contact and while palpating the client. The COA allows the practitioner to remain synchronized or return to being synchronized with PR during the session.

ಕಾ
The Cycle of Attunement
⌁ Part I: Attunement with Oneself ⤳

Let the client know at the beginning of a session that you are going to take a couple of minutes to settle yourself and that you will let them know when you are going to make contact. Take this time to practice these first few steps of mindful attention to establish a calm presence and settle your mind and body in the present moment. The cycle of attunement begins with identifying your own state of mind and body sensation, which prepares the ground for empathy.

1. Begin with correct posture by sitting still and upright, with your knees slightly below the plane of your hips. Sense a midline alignment of the pelvic diaphragm, respiratory diaphragm, pericardium, roof of the mouth, and third ventricle. Your posture should be not too tight and not too loose. It must be authentic and able to accommodate any orthopedic limitations.

2. Begin attending to your breathing. Sense the breath moving into the lower lobes of your lungs so that your abdomen expands upon inhalation. Feel the umbilicus expand during inhalation and relax back during exhalation.

3. Become aware of your thinking and the emotional tones in your mind. Recognize and shift attention away from the stream of wandering mental thoughts of the past, present, and future and toward your breathing.

⁓ Part 2: Synchronizing with the Natural World ⁓

Now you will begin to use your vision and hearing to sense PR in nature.

1. Sense PR moving from the fulcrum of your third ventricle and eyes out to nature and back by looking at the sky outside or at a picture of nature hanging on the wall in the treatment room. This allows nature to participate in the biodynamic therapeutic session. This is a key point of biodynamic practice. I call it horizon meditation. The brain via the third ventricle is subtly and magnetically pulled toward the horizon for about a minute, and then PR changes phase and the brain seems to flow back into the cranium.

2. Use your hearing to listen to the sounds of nature, whether it's birdsong, the wind, or the silence. Use both eyes and ears to sense nature outside the office.

⁓ Part 3: Heart to Heart ⁓

1. Deliberately bring your attention to the trunk of your body and the movement of your heart behind the sternum and above the diaphragm. Now consciously sense your heartbeat, which is a simple mindfulness practice. This ignites empathy.

2. Then become aware of the potency of the heartbeat by sensing the space in the trunk of the body that is occupied by that awareness. This allows empathy to permeate the body and mind.

3. Then sense into the space in front of your sternum, which is the electromagnetic field (EMF) of the heart mixing with the client's heart field (see fig. 24.1). Heart fields tend to synchronize with each other within seconds and exchange information, including PR. Within the heart field is the flow of PR moving back and forth from the client's heart and likewise the return flow from the practitioner's heart to the client. This is the movement of empathy and compassion.

4. Find the back of your heart, meaning the dorsal heart. The dorsal heart

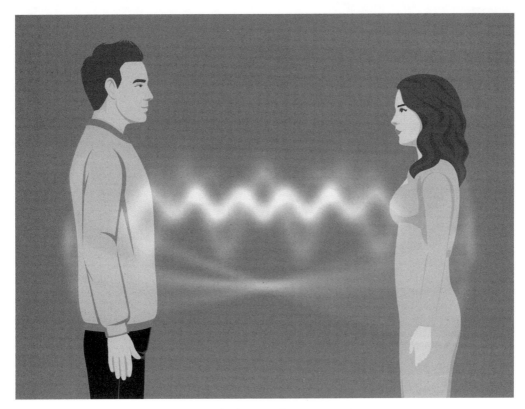

Fig. 24.1. The heart-to-heart connection

and pericardium are relatively fixed anatomically and thus dynamically still. Attunement of embodiment through slowing and stilling resonates with the client through the interpersonal brain and heart systems (see fig. 24.2). As noted throughout, the therapeutic relationship is a two-person biology. Now place your attention in the shared heart field and sense PR moving heart-to-heart. It is a subtle magnetic pull bringing the two hearts in the therapeutic dyad together and then an expansion phase of moving apart. The electromagnetic fields of the hearts are strong, and the sense of PR is like a magnet pushing and pulling the sternum, heart, and pericardium like a pendulum back and forth toward the client in rhythmic phases of PR.

5. Usually a session begins with the third ventricle for perceiving PR and then automatically shifts into the heart fulcrum. It is important to deliberately cycle through both fulcrums to sense the most readily available access point of PR in the moment. Now, let the fulcrum of attunement automatically shift and become spontaneous. The intention is to perceive PR coming from the client through the felt sense of the sternum and anatomical heart area of the practitioner and then returning.

6. In general, the cycle of attunement starts with the perception of PR with the fulcrum of attention inside and then outside in nature from the third ventricle.

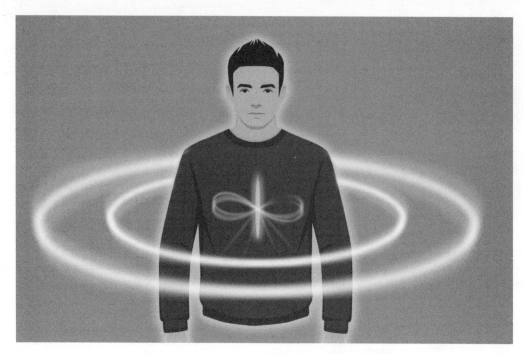

Fig. 24.2. Heart-to-heart with Primary Respiration

Gradually the internal fulcrum automatically shifts into the practitioner's heart for the heart-to-heart connection with the client during the session. Automatic shifting fulcrums happen deliberately and spontaneously. This is balanced in every session.

7. At some point, all fulcrums will synchronize spontaneously into the stillness. All that remains is the heartbeat.

∴ Part 4: Synchronizing with PR ∾

Now you will put attunement of the body and nature together with your hands by asking the client permission to make contact. The cycle of attunement, the movement of attention, is practiced in each hand position. In general, it is important to wait until the client's body signals your hands for more attention. There is a delicate signaling system for bringing contact closer and for removing contact or making more space to avoid unnecessary compression. The core of the cycle of attunement is the capacity of the practitioner to recognize PR in themselves first, followed by its activity in the client.

1. Move your attention toward nature, which may include your hands (the client), and away from nature, which may include your hands (the client), in the tempo of PR. Then move your attention into a heart-to-heart connection in the tempo of PR. Then bring your attention back to your posture, breathing, and heartbeat. This constitutes one basic cycle of attunement (self-nature-other) that is repeated

frequently in a session. (There are variations, which will be discussed later once the practitioner settles their perception into a basic COA.)

2. Gradually your attention becomes evenly suspended between your body and nature so that very little effort is needed to move your attention between those locations. Attention moves automatically with the tide of PR, as it is the glue that holds our perception of the whole together. Allow your attention to rest in the dynamic stillness when you perceive it.

The Tempo of PR

A constant rhythmic balanced interchange is happening between the stillness and PR, as it is between the office space and the natural world. The practitioner is a silent and heartfelt observer of the impermanence of perception. Sometimes students feel like they aren't getting it right because PR seems to fade in midcycle or the stillness is interrupted. And then the practitioner makes efforts to regain awareness of the change of phase of PR. The phase change is just one experience where the healing forces of PR and stillness manifest their potency. Dr. Sutherland told us that PR will lead us to the most important lesion pattern in the client, and I would add the possibility of being led outside the client's body by PR. The world of nature is a primary input in the therapeutic process and must be respected for its potency.

Different tempos in the fluid body, from fast to slow, establish structure and function in the embryo; that's biokinetics. And we are perpetual embryos. The slow tempo of PR is an essential factor that generates order and organization of the whole embryo throughout the life span; this is biodynamics. PR is one of the main factors that provide biodynamic order and organization for growth and development locally and globally.

Practitioner attunement to the slow tempo of PR can potentially dissipate imprinting (a type of stress memory) from the preverbal postnatal time of life. Such dissipation is free of emotional distress. In this way, emotional release is transformed into emotional containment and integration.

Attunement of the Nervous System

The cycle of attunement explores the Health in the practitioner to build self-regulation and self-integration. It is through a commitment to a reliable contemplative practice that the practitioner builds confidence that their treatment does not interfere with the client's therapeutic progression and healing potential. And if there is a side effect from treatment, the practitioner knows how to manage it. Resonance with the practitioner's nervous and cardiovascular systems creates containment for self-regulation in the client's nervous system.

The cycle of attunement has the potential to change the client's nervous system through the perception of being held with safety and trust. Slowness and stillness are the keys to safety. This creates a Neutral for the practitioner and client in which PR is free to choose where support is needed inside or outside the body of the therapeutic dyad. This means that PR is guiding the practitioner's mind and hands as much as it is functioning in and around the client. PR is transparent and moves through the dyad. The autonomic nervous system (ANS) will drop into a settling process in which twitching and vibration might be observed in the client. PR will then help the fluid body into deeper balance and dissipation of stress.

Receptivity and Buoyancy

In biodynamic work, the hands are mostly afferent. Each hand position on the client is called a window. It is a window of observing the activity of the whole body at its surface. This is biodynamic embryology—the sense of the whole embryo still present in the person. There is no intention or effort to look below the surface of the skin in the beginning phases of a biodynamic session. Everything necessary for the practitioner to know is perceived at the surface, under the guidance of PR, with evenly suspended attention that includes the natural world.

When the first part of a cycle of attunement is over, the practitioner asks permission to make contact verbally. This verbal permission is usually done at least once and always at the beginning of a session. It is critical to the establishment of safety and trust in the therapeutic relationship.

Upon contact, the practitioner immediately becomes receptive and repeats a cycle of attunement. This means removing their attention from their hands for a brief period of time in order to sense the therapeutic relationship as a circulatory system and a two-person biology. The majority of perception in any biodynamic session is the practitioner's attunement to their own body-mind-heart rather than that of the client.

The practitioner's hands are buoyant, like a cork floating in water, not so much following the waves as simply accommodating the rise and fall of the client's fluid body synchronized with their respiratory pattern and the constant background or foreground of PR and stillness automatically shifting. The client's fluid body may gradually feel like one large flower opening and closing slowly into the hands with PR.

This has the potential to give the client the space to feel safety and trust in the relationship. This establishes a Neutral. All reliable change associated with integration of the whole mind-body-spirit is synchronized with stillness and PR.

BCVT PALPATION

Following the cycle of attunement, the practitioner begins the work of palpation. That work generally begins with the client's fluid body, and work with the fluid body is integrated throughout the session. This can range from palms up sensing the biosphere around the client's body or palms under the body. A BCVT session can consist of only fluid body exploration. Biodynamic sessions usually begin with the fluid body especially because the blood is 70 percent water. The key principle in BCVT is to always start at the periphery of the cardiovascular system, and the fluid body is the most peripheral at the physical level. Then contact with the artery is made.

BCVT palpation is like playing a flute. The intelligence of the artery and its endothelium needs to be honored through delicate contact that is dynamic in the sense of not being static but responsive to the flow and pressure variations constantly occurring in the cardiovascular system. The finger pads rhythmically modulate pressure to stay at the edge of the artery as it reaches out and recedes in a constant variation of tones, such as pressure, flow, waves, and so forth. The hands are flotation devices on the surface, always accommodating the rise and fall of the arterial waves underneath. The palpation and exploration of an artery is a cross between attempting to play a flute on a living instrument and deciphering the history of ten family generations flowing in the client's blood.

There is a constant story being told via the blood and the vessels that carry it. The blood carries red blood cells for oxygenating the body, but it also carries the immune system and water along with other elements. The endothelium lining all the vessels that carry the blood is a single layer of quiescent cells. (As noted earlier, when these quiescent cells lose their quiescence, it is a marker of heart disease.) In addition, the vessel walls are richly innervated by the sympathetic nervous system. Communication happens not only through the blood and vessel walls but also in molecular signaling between the blood and through the vessel walls via the immune system. There is an enormous amount of activity at the basic physiological and deeper metabolic level in the artery. BCVT palpation tells us the story of all that activity.

Palpation Skills

When it comes to palpation of an artery, there are some simple principles to keep in mind.

Afference: The intention is to maintain afferent, buoyant hands in relationship with the surface tension and pressure in the client's artery and vascular tree. In other words, your hands must already be in receptive mode (afferent) prior to contact. The hands are used to bless as if placing a "feather on the breath of God."*

Initiation and release of contact: Make contact with the tips or pads of the fingers

---

*This is a phrase attributed to Hildegard von Bingen, a twelfth-century abbess known for her mysticism, music, and medicine. There's also a Grammy-award-winning album of her liturgical music under the same name, released in 1982 by Hyperion Records.

of one hand. Once the artery discovers your finger pads or tips, the other hand can explore a different location on the same artery or another artery with your other hand. Likewise, to disconnect, release one hand, pause for a breath, and then release the other hand. Releasing both hands at once can cause a "whiplash" in the vascular tree.

Finger pads, not tips: When palpating an artery, it is recommended that you use the pads of the fingers rather than the tips. Use your fingers not as the talons of a hawk but rather as the footpads of an elephant, which are broad and gentle, without the weight!

Choice of fingers: In traditional Chinese medicine, palpation is done with the index, middle, and fourth fingers resting with even pressure on the length of specifically the radial artery. In biodynamic work, the choice of which fingers is not as important. Occasionally I will use the thumb of one hand on one artery and the pads of the index, middle, and ring fingers of my other hand to sense a different artery. I also find myself frequently using just the pads of the index and middle fingers. Whichever fingers you use on either hand, they need to be lined up along the body of the artery so that the palpation is anatomically correct.

The three springs: The fingers dance gently with the three springs of the pulse. The first layer is the artery wall muscle. The second layer is the endothelium, and the third level is the blood and its core of dynamic stillness.

Micropressure: Any pressure placed into the artery is done only in micro-increments. The formula is: micropressure, pause, microrelease, and attune to each layer and watch the artery. When the artery shows itself, then soften contact to its surface, where the most superficial contact can rest. This contact is not rigid or static; the intention is floatability, buoyancy, and afferent hands. Your hands are buoys floating on the surface of an ocean that is constantly contracting and dilating, ebbing, and flowing.

Support: With all the hand positions on the arteries, it is important to have precise propping of the wrists and arms so that the fingers can be steady. This requires smaller props, especially around the client's head. A sock filled with rice or buckwheat hulls can be an effective prop.

Awareness of trauma: Ipsilateral work is sometimes preferred over bilateral work on the arteries, especially in the neck and shoulders, because of ANS dynamics from the client's trauma history. Regular verbal solicitation of a client's comfort during a session is necessary, especially when working around the neck and shoulders.

Without care and attention to the principles of palpation outlined above, it is possible to alert the protection system of the heart and recruit defensive physiology in both the brain and heart. This most frequently manifests as anxiety, rapid heart rate in the client, nausea, headache, or a sense of deep discomfort. Mindful palpation, on the other hand, is unlikely to recruit the protection system of the heart, which is both a safety system and the heart's innate trauma resolution system for catastrophic injuries. The protection system of the heart is balanced by the pleasure system of the heart. The cycle of attunement engages the pleasure system of the client's heart by raising vagal tone. So, while you are working, regularly practice the cycle of attunement and resynchronize with PR heart-to-heart.

Dynamic stillness rules the artery and its endothelium. The endothelial cells are biologically quiescent. The blood flow has a core of dynamic stillness. Whenever it becomes available, completely and thoroughly rest in the stillness. Hands can become rigid when searching for an artery, and concentration can narrow, possibly inducing a compression in the client's vascular system. Be still and know. Let your hands and body melt into the stillness inherent in the vascular tree by sensing stillness in the room and placing attention out in the natural world. Dynamic stillness spontaneously manifests as the element of space. The element of space is the universe, an extended natural world like a big soup in a soup pot, and the soup pot is simply the element of space. It is Buddha, the Breath of Life, God as light and form. The practitioner completely rests attention there.

The Three Levels of Arterial Palpation

The palpation of the artery at a basic level consists of three objective and subjective palpations done sequentially. Gradually, with practice, a practitioner learns to perform all three within seconds.

1. The first palpation is making contact with the artery superficially or, by gradual increments, deeply, pressing gently and slowly, pausing occasionally, using micrograms of pressure into the artery in order to feel its potency, which is a subjective palpation. Superficial palpation uses the contact of the finger pads on the surface of the skin, with no pressure applied. We let the artery come to us rather than immediately searching for it. Deep palpation uses pressure by the finger pads not only to occlude the artery very briefly but to sense any bones that are adjacent to the artery. Then we lighten the pressure of our fingers to a superficial unobtrusive level. Gradually more of the artery will tell its story, and we keep adjusting our contact to stay at the superficial edge of the artery. From this place we can hear the story the blood and artery are telling. On the one hand, this palpation is mechanical and objective, but on the other hand, it is also a subjective palpation

regarding its response to the contact. This is the initial handshake. We may need several attempts at positioning our fingers to find the sweet spot of the artery. This is normal in the process of finding the right finger placement.

2. The second palpation again explores the superficial aspect of the artery. Does the artery seem fast or slow? This is both an objective and a subjective palpation. It is quite possible that a client has a normal heart rate (sixty to seventy beats per minutes), and yet when you contact that client's artery, it appears to be beating much faster or, in some cases, much slower. This is just part of the evolving storyline that is constantly flowing through the client's body.

3. The third palpation is also done from the superficial sweet spot of the artery. Does the artery seem strong or weak? Once again, this is a subjective palpation, and it must be remembered that this is not a diagnosis. Frequently men have stronger pulses and women have softer pulses. This is quite normal.

Typically these three levels of palpation are done with each arterial contact. Thus, as the session unfolds, whether it is exclusively cardiovascular work or bridging between the fluid body, heart, and body, a coherent narrative can unfold over the whole session. The story at the end of the session may be different from what it was at the beginning. In this way the practitioner can begin to get a sense of an unwritten story in the cardiovascular system of the client. Palpation of the artery is a listening skill first and foremost.

Bridging

Bridging happens when the practitioner switches attention from one physiological system of the body, such as the ANS, to another physiological system, such as the fascia, or from physiology to metabolism. It may occur in every session. The sequence of bridging begins with a cycle of attunement. On principle, the ANS becomes active especially upon palpation and is always a part of the therapeutic equation. Bridging might happen more specifically when, for example, one hand of the practitioner is oriented to an artery and the other hand to a cranial structure. The practitioner then waits for PR to synchronize the two hands, thus completing the bridge.

The Story in the Artery

The arteries have a story that they tell constantly. To hear the story, we need ultra-sensitive ears in the pads and tips of their fingers. When we palpate an artery, we explore not only its endothelium and the tension gradients in the fascia holding the artery, but also the flow dynamics in the lumen of the artery. Pressure waves, microcurrents, and so forth are only a part of the many elements associated with the story that unfolds in an artery. The artery and its endothelium are connected to every endothelium in the body. The blood moving through the artery is connected everywhere in the body, all the way through the capillary beds and out to the biofilm on the surface of the teeth and skin. Frequently, when we are working with an artery bilaterally, the artery expresses itself and then disappears. That is normal. Do not chase after an artery if it disappears from sensation in your fingers. Just wait for the next part of the story to unfold with PR and stillness.

Dynamic stillness is very important in the palpation of the cardiovascular system, as mentioned. This is not only because the heart develops embryonically around a core of slow metabolism, but also because the endothelium of arteries contains the quiescent cells that must be dynamically still for the arteries' normal function. The perception of stillness in the treatment room is of vital importance because when it appears, we must recognize it and connect it to the movement of our heart and our client's artery. This means allowing a cycle of attunement to rest and abide in the stillness. It is a high priority to connect the cardiovascular system of the client with the dynamic stillness. This is a big story.

The following four basic protocols are essential practice in learning BCVT. As a beginner it is important to have a sequential learning that is safe for the client to experience. It is also important at the beginning of learning BCVT to practice each of these protocols individually until the practitioner's hands and heart inform him or her that some steps may not be necessary or can be combined in different ways. This is an individual aptitude to be discovered with the skills being taught here. The focus is on safe practice since almost every client has a vascular problem, and this is an optimal roadmap for helping the vascular system to heal.

Pietà

I usually begin with all my clients by making contact with the fluid body. I call this the pietà. The fluid body is made up of the elements of water and earth. It is made up of every living atom and molecule in the human body. Everything that makes us human is dissolved and dissipated throughout the fluid body. Thus, we are contacting the totality of the human body and its metabolic level. Pietà is effected through attunement, as described earlier in this chapter. It is a preparatory contact made at the beginning of a session since it will take several minutes for both nervous systems of the therapist and client to synchronize and for safety to be established in the attunement process.

ʘ

The First Protocol:
Primary Respiration (PR) and the Fluid Body

For this first protocol, the client is supine.

⌁ 1. Pietà ⌁

Place your receptive hands under the client's leg and shoulder (see figs. 24.3–5). Practice a cycle of attunement (with your attention moving to self-other-space and then the reverse). Come into relationship with the client heart-to-heart, then attend to your hands, then back to yourself, synchronizing with PR. Wait to be called to pay attention to your hands by the sense of the client's body melting gently into them.

Wait for the melting and then the breathing of PR in your hands.

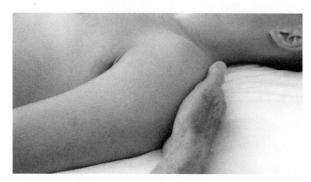

Fig. 24.3. Pietà 1

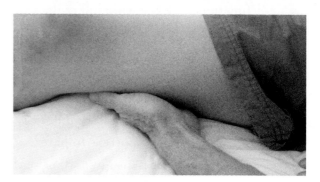

Fig. 24.4. Pietà 2

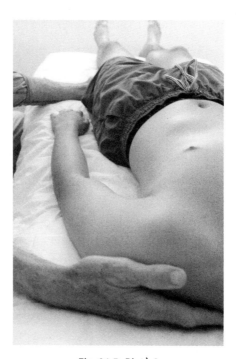

Fig. 24.5. Pietà 3

◌ 2. Fluid Body and Zone B ◌

While practicing the pietà, synchronize with your fluid body. Sense and visualize your body as a three-dimensional, transparent, living continuum of fluid. Imagine your body as one drop of crystal-clear water extending beyond the skin and, via evaporation, forming a warm wet cloud—Zone B or the biosphere—above the surface of your skin. This shape extends and fills the space around your body.

Practitioner Tip

To sense Zone B, begin by sensing the total surface area of the skin. This establishes an orientation to your fluid body as a single shape apart from musculo-skeletal anatomy.

The Fluid Body

The fluid body can be sensed as a moving, living ocean within and all over and above the surface of the skin. It fills the space around the body, extending out from the body by up to fifteen inches or more. Dr. Jealous called this Zone B; Dr. Becker called it the biosphere. Zone B is literally a warm, wet, electric cloud surrounding the body, just as it was in the embryo (which was surrounded by an amniotic sac and a chorionic sac). The embryo is a transparent living fluid body. Ninety-nine percent of the molecules in the body are water molecules, then and now. This is the original intelligent body and it is still present within us. Humans are perpetual embryos connected to the universe.

There are three sensory aspects of the fluid body:

- **Transparency.** PR passes through the fluid body without stopping at a fulcrum.
- **Dissipation.** When we put our hands on the client and become receptive, any stress in the client's fluid body will dissipate into the practitioner's fluid body. The practitioner simply allows the client's trauma or stress to move through their own body as a nonthreatening vibration.
- **Buoyancy.** The melting described earlier leads to a sense of the whole fluid body breathing with PR.

Note: These three aspects are discussed in greater detail in my book *The Biodynamics of the Immune System.*

⌁ 3. Cranial Cycle of Attunement ⌁

1. Sit at the head of the table, with your body at least two feet from the client's head, and be still.
2. Connect with the back of your body and feel PR gently pulling your spine and nervous system backward.
3. Breathe up and down your midline between the heart and spine.
4. Make a heart-to-heart connection with PR.

⌁ 4. Shoulders ⌁

1. Sit at the head of the table and practice a cranial cycle of attunement, as just described.
2. Contact the top of the client's shoulders bilaterally, with your palms up or down (see figs. 24.6–7). Feel the client's breathing and perhaps their fluid body beginning to breathe with PR.

Practitioner Tip

If your face is close to the face of the client, turn your head slightly to one side to avoid breathing directly on them. The practitioner's head must not be in the same plane as the client's head. If a client senses the practitioner's breath on their face, they likely will not rebook another session. One time when I was teaching for the Upledger Institute in 1986, I sent my mom to get a session from Dr. John, as he was fondly called. When she got home, I asked her how it went. She was visibly upset and just said one word: "halitosis." He was breathing into her face the whole session with bad breath.

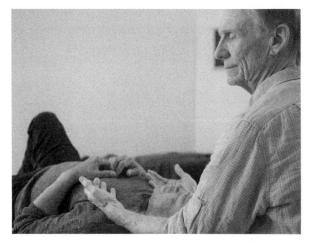

Fig. 24.6. Palms up on the shoulders

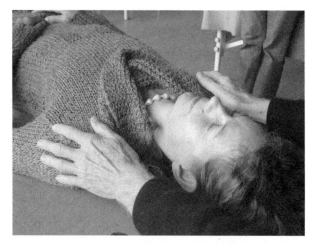

Fig. 24.7. Palms down on the shoulders

∿ 5. Heart Fulcrum (C3–C4) ∿

1. Sit at the head of the table and again practice a cranial cycle of attunement, as described on page 320.

2. Place your hands under the client's neck, around the level of C3–C4, with the longest of the fingertips on each hand touching (see figs. 24.8–10). This was the initial location of the embryonic heart. Your fingers may be invited toward a subtle motion of floating up (toward the ceiling) and down (back to the table) at the rate of PR.

3. Reestablish a heart-to-heart connection with PR or allow the client's fluid body to decompress into the stillness.

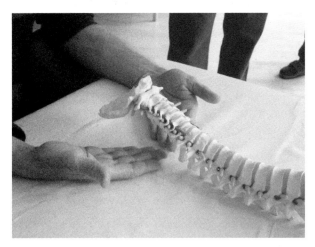

Fig. 24.8. Heart fulcrum 1

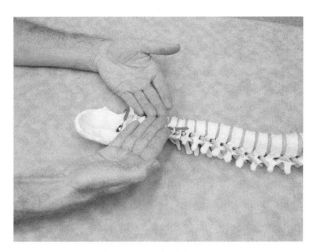

Fig. 24.9. Heart fulcrum 2

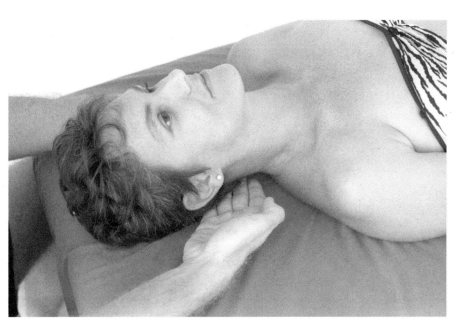

Fig. 24.10. Heart fulcrum 3

❧ 6. Coccyx, Diaphragm, and Umbilicus ❧

1. Approach from the side, by the gluteal fold. Place one hand under the respiratory diaphragm. With the third finger (or longest finger or most comfortable finger) of the other hand, contact the space between the coccyx and the sacrum (sacral sulcus; see figs. 24.11–12). This is gentle contact that does not involve any lifting of the sacrum. Practice a cycle of attunement. Wait for the respiratory diaphragm and pelvic diaphragm to synchronize with the client's breathing.

2. Move the hand under the diaphragm to a position over the umbilicus, with the palm up or down (see figs. 24.13–15). If the client's breathing does not lift the hands by the expansion of their abdomen, then ask the client to breathe into the point of contact several times. The practitioner may sense the space all around and in the sacrum breathe and come alive with PR, like a flower opening and closing. Practice several cycles of attunement.

3. Wait for both hands to synchronize with PR simultaneously.

This sequence helps normalize the autonomic nervous system (ANS) of the client. This means that the ANS needs to have a relative amount of equilibrium for PR to express its healing priorities. This is the Neutral when PR is free to move toward enhancing the capacity for self-healing of the client. It also allows the client to become conscious of PR's activity and subtlety in the abdomen or space between the two hands. Every system and function of the body holds stress in its own way and dissipates it in its own way. The most important instruction for the practitioner is to wait, watch, and wonder, as Dr. Jealous said.

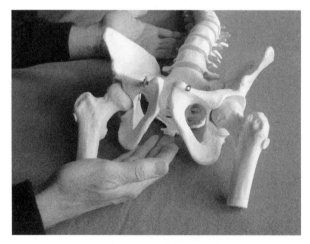

Fig. 24.11. Coccyx and diaphragm 1

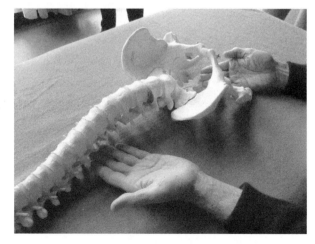

Fig. 24.12. Coccyx and diaphragm 2

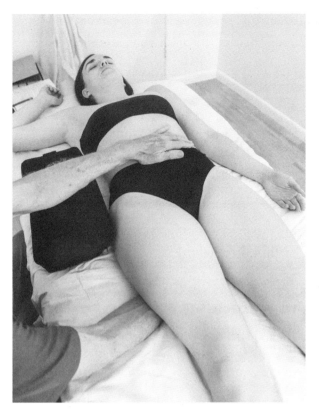

Fig. 24.13. Coccyx and umbilicus

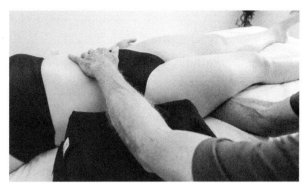

Fig. 24.14. Coccyx and umbilicus, palm down

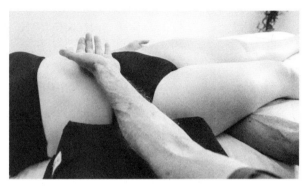

Fig. 24.15. Coccyx and umbilicus, palm up

◡ 7. Bilateral Anterior Tibial Artery ◡

1. Sit at the foot of the table. Practice a cycle of attunement.
2. Hold the client's heels in the palms of your hands. Notice any dissipation of the client's fluid body into yours.
3. Using the pads of the index and middle finger of each hand, contact the anterior tibial artery on each of the client's feet (see figs. 24.16–17). Depending on the size of your hands and the client's feet, you might use one, two, or three fingers

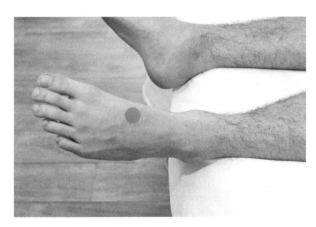

Fig. 24.16. Anterior tibial artery 1

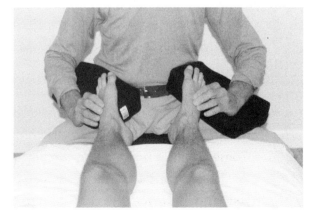

Fig. 24.17. Anterior tibial artery 2

on each foot. Practice a cycle of attunement by sensing your own heartbeat synchronizing with the client's arterial pulse. Then synchronize your attention with PR in the heart field.

Practitioner Tip

Use cushions to support your wrists and arms to stabilize the arterial contact. In a session the hands are rarely suspended without such support.

IGNITION AND MIDLINE

ଚଙ

Accessing the Third Ventricle

This is an enhancement practice for perceiving PR and stabilizing the head on the neck for the practitioner.

1. Sit in a comfortable meditative posture. Make sure your posture is not too tight and not too loose. Do a body scan from the feet to the head and begin to sense the entire surface volume of the skin three-dimensionally.

2. Gradually bring your attention to the way your head is resting on your neck. Sense heaviness in your elbows and allow your shoulders to soften.

3. Bring your attention to the occiput in the back of your head. Imagine your head is like a bobble-head doll and let yourself experience more weight in the occiput in such a way that your head extends slightly (chin lifting slightly) with micromovement. Spend several minutes sensing the slowness of the occipital bobble head.

4. Bring your attention around to your face. Feel the weight of your face and let your nose fall slightly forward with gravity. Spend several moments sensing the slowness of the facial bobble head.

5. Bring your attention into the space between the occiput and your face. This is generally in and around the third ventricle. Sense the central stillness from this place.

When this meditation is coupled with sitting and looking at the horizon, it becomes a deeper form of an atlanto-occipital joint recalibration in the practitioner. Consequently, it is ideal to do this practice while outside in nature.

To assist in the sensory acquisition of the third ventricle, it is helpful to close your eyes, allow your eyes to roll up to the middle of your forehead, hold for several seconds, and then relax the eyes. This puts a very slight tug on the anterior third ventricle via the optic chiasm. Practice this movement occasionally until it feels like it is easier to rest your attention in the third ventricle. You may experience an ignition and permeation of potency releasing from the third ventricle when your eyes are rolled up to the middle of the forehead, so it is important to hold your eyes in this position only for several seconds at a time.

When biodynamic work is correct, your attention will naturally rest in the third ventricle and the heart together, whether you are a practitioner or a client. Thus, the ability to access and rest in the third ventricle is a barometer of the restorative function of biodynamic work with PR. As a client, when a biodynamic practitioner has stopped trying to help me, I can access and rest in my third ventricle and in this way help myself and allow the practitioner's relationship with PR and stillness to function unobstructedly and for the potency of PR to increase. I can also tell when a practitioner is too close to me because if I try to access my third ventricle, I sometimes literally get bounced out of it. Then I have to let the practitioner know I need more space.

∞

Synchronizing Primary Respiration and Secondary Respiration

The basic principle at work here is that Primary Respiration generates secondary respiration, meaning physiological breathing. Breathing is largely an unconscious phenomenon, especially when we are sleeping. We might say that the body breathes itself. There are many ways in which our breath can be unconsciously imprinted, especially with stress, which interferes with our physiological function. People all too often think that they can master their breathing based on the host of breathing exercises available on the internet. This is only half the case; the more important half is restoring the natural synchronization between our breath and PR.

I offer the following explorations as a method for regaining the normal and natural relationship of PR with breathing for the practitioner, but also for the practitioner to gently practice while in contact with a client to give a spark of potent breathing in the hope of igniting a therapeutic process under the direction of PR.

1. Sit still and sense the surface of your skin from your feet to your head and out to your fingertips. This is a simple body scan but with a focus on the total awareness of the surface of the skin. Remember that biodynamic practice begins with the acquisition of embodied wholeness. Simply sensing the whole surface of the skin initiates this process and invites a gradual awareness of PR, which itself is the movement of wholeness. If you find that you cannot sense the total surface of your skin from head to foot, stay with the trunk of your body, where the skin moves the most while you breathe.

Practitioner Tip

To sense the total surface of your skin, visualize it as if you are seeing the surface of the water from underneath. Or, alternatively, visualize the surface of the body from the outside, as if you are looking at a globe that is transparent. Or, another option, if the globe is solid, then in your mind's eye, turn your body around slowly so that you see, in turn, the front, one side, the back, then the other side. I learned to do this by looking at an actual globe of the Earth and memorizing each continent until I could spin the globe around in my mind and see every continent and ocean. I then brought that same concept to my body.

2. Bring your attention to the rise and fall of your breath, breathing normally. Narrow your focus to the movement of the respiratory diaphragm and its effect on the skin, especially around the trunk and shoulders. Such attention may generate an awareness of a wavelike movement in the spine with each up-and-down excursion of the diaphragm. Perhaps sense the spine as seaweed in the ocean.

3. Such attention on the diaphragm consciously accesses the pulsation of the heart. The heart is attached to the respiratory diaphragm, and so the heartbeat is part of the diaphragmatic movement; they form one unified motion. Allow yourself to feel that motion. Sensing their motion together as one generates a greater sense of embodied wholeness, first as a potency (called the sea of chi in Taoism) and then as a type of potency radiating from this cardiac-respiratory center of the body. This location is the fulcrum of PR in these protocols.

4. Take several minutes to soften through the abdomen and rib cage and allow your breathing to start to slow down as the unified motion of the diaphragm and heart becomes more three-dimensional. The accessory muscles of respiration need to become active, and that means with each inhalation the transversus abdominus muscle expands. It should feel like your belly button is expanding out with each inhalation and relaxing back with each exhalation. Then the scalene muscles in the neck, with the pleura suspended from them, can also respond, allowing the lungs much more freedom to fill and empty as if the entire contents of the trunk, abdomen, and pelvis are a single water balloon.

5. As the trunk softens with the abdomen, gently toggle some of your attention back and forth from the diaphragmatic movement to the surface of the skin. Gradually observe the motion of breathing from the point of view of the skin. It is a delicate perceptual shift of the fulcrum of attention that is evenly suspended between the diaphragm and the skin. It is from the vantage point of the skin

that the relationship of breathing to PR can be observed. From here onward, if you have any confusion while practicing this method, simply return to this stage of the practice and maintain mindfulness of the whole body, heart, and breath.

6. Notice the end point of your exhalation, and as inhalation begins, gently move some attention to the surface of the skin and observe if PR is starting or continuing to expand. Is this phase in coordination with the inhalation of the diaphragm? Now, of course the inhalation of secondary respiration is much faster than PR, so the caveat here is to avoid holding your breath while observing PR. Just continue to breathe normally, with attention on the skin, the breath, and direction of PR. But with each inhalation, notice if the direction of PR is coordinated or synchronized with your breath.

7. If you do not sense PR expanding out through the skin during successive cycles of diaphragmatic inhalation, resettle some extra attention back to your diaphragmatic movement. Pay attention gently to the end point of your inhalation, start to exhale, and then gently move some attention to the surface of the skin. Notice if PR continues to come in through the skin toward the fulcrum of the diaphragm-heart. (This is the same as in the previous instruction except in the opposite direction.)

8. Now for the point of the practice: Synchronization occurs when, having observed the coordination of the breath and PR through the skin, the urge to take a deep breath occurs. This urge will occur at the beginning of the expansion phase of PR. This occurs regularly while breathing unless there is a loss of potency, and this practice reignites the potency, which is very important for Health to manifest. The sense is a mild to moderate shift in your breathing at the end point of either inhalation or exhalation. A spontaneous deep breath occurs. This is synchronization and ignition of the therapeutic potency of PR. I usually wait for two or three experiences of synchronization before leaving this exploration.

PR may then direct your awareness more locally or globally in your body or that of the client. This is to be expected, as PR continues to enhance embodied wholeness. So, at this point the practitioner leaves the instructions and becomes spontaneously guided by what Dr. Becker called "the will of PR." This would be a natural transition point or ending for this phase of synchronization.

Practitioner Tip

Practice this first stage of synchronizing PR with secondary respiration on your own, rather than with a client, until you are very familiar with it. In this practice, the quality of your attention is lightly suspended between the middle, surface, and external environment of the body. This is a delicate and subtle relationship that is important to build in your body awareness before working with a client because of the need to reignite the potency of PR in its therapeutic mode in the client. When you are using this practice with a client, the client may take a deep breath or, on the other hand, contract if it is too deep for them. You must be able to sense this, and while the breathing of the client is easy to observe, the contraction of their whole fluid body might be elusive until you have gained more practice

---

∾ Building the Potency of Primary Respiration ∾

There is a next step in this meditation that can be done after some initial practice with the steps outlined above. After noticing the synchronization of PR and secondary respiration several times and opening to the priorities of PR, the practitioner can enhance the potency of PR. This is done by consciously coordinating a slightly deeper but shorter sip of air while inhaling during the expansion phase of PR. Since the natural inhalation is three to five seconds, this short sips is maybe a microsecond in length before exhalation begins. It is a microboost in the volume of air being inhaled but done in conscious coordination with PR to enhance its potency.

The same process can be explored during the exhalation of diaphragmatic breathing, with a microboost of exhaling air for a microsecond and noticing the effect on PR as it moves through the skin toward the diaphragm-heart. The potency of PR is not limited to either of its phases but rather operates in both. This is an air volume exercise; it is a gentle practice of adding a little extra air that is focused and concentrated within the action of the respiratory diaphragm while perceiving PR. The practitioner can then observe whether the potency of their own PR has increased and its effect on their body or that of the client.

Now at this point the practitioner has a lot of balls in the air, so to speak, regarding perception of this powerful yet subtle relationship. So, it is best to try it once or twice and then wait and sense the effect holistically in the body or in the sense of PR. It is not a technique like yogic pranayama that would be continually and repetitively practiced for a long period of time. It is a balancing act of the physiology of breathing and its reference point of PR. This relationship is constantly changing. I find that five minutes of periodic microboosts in either the inhalation or the exhalation is enough.

Once this exploration becomes second nature to the practitioner, then less time is needed to recognize synchronization and induce a little potency into the practice. It becomes easy and second nature. It must be remembered that the potency of PR is the so-called Health spoken of in biodynamic osteopathy. Thus, this skill enhances the therapeutic outcomes in clinical practice.

◡ Awakening to the Instinct of the Natural World ◞

There is yet a third level to this practice that is of equal importance: exploring the synchronizing processes outside in nature. Begin by practicing horizon meditation, noticing PR moving from the heart and brain out to the horizon and back. While sitting comfortably (and at a time when the wind is not blowing excessively), now repeat the above steps but include awareness of the movement of the air and wind against your skin. Sense how the movement of the air wraps around the contours of your body. Sense the different variations in speed and potency as the air speeds up or slows down. Notice the direction the wind is coming from. The PR inherent within the movement of air in the atmosphere of the planet will change phases regularly in its base tempo of about once per minute. During this phase change, the air will stop periodically, signaling a clear stillpoint in the natural world. Follow the principles outlined above to coordinate diaphragmatic breathing, PR, and the wind of the natural world into one living continuum of wholeness. The value in this practice is that it wakes up the instinctual healing intelligence of the body in relationship to the natural world.

⌘

The Second Protocol: Ignition and the Midline

For this second protocol, the client is supine.

◡ 1. Pietà Palms Up ◞

Place your hands with the palms up on the client's shoulder and leg (see fig. 24.18). Practice a cycle of attunement, as described at the beginning of this chapter.

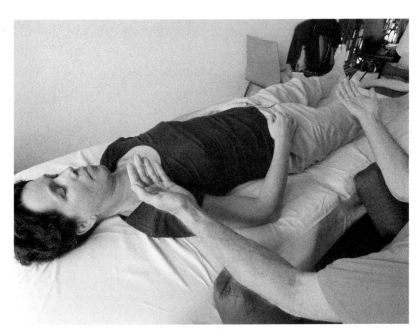

Fig. 24.18. Pietà, palms up

✌ 2. Dimensions of the Diaphragm ✌

1. Sit at the side of the client's pelvis. Explores a cycle of attunement and synchronize PR and your breathing, as described on page 235.

2. Place one hand under the coccyx, with finger pad contact, and wait (see figs. 24.11–12, page 322). Place your other hand under the respiratory diaphragm. Allow the two diaphragms to synchronize their motion with PR.

3. Place both hands under the respiratory diaphragm (see figs. 24.19–21). Sense the three-dimensionality of the diaphragm, noticing the lateral and anterior-posterior movements. Is the abdomen visibly expanding during inhalation and receding upon exhalation? This settles the heart.

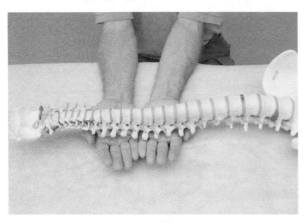

Fig. 24.19. Diaphragm 1

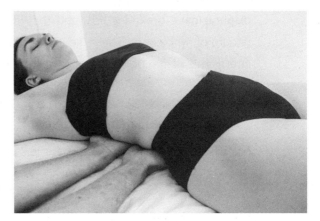

Fig. 24.20. Diaphragm 2

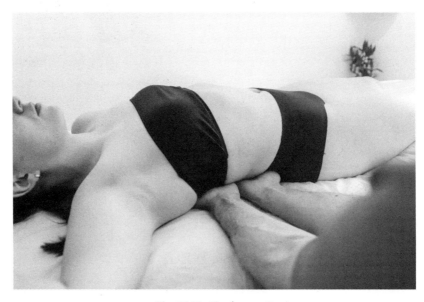

Fig. 24.21. Diaphragm 3

◠ 3. Rostral Midline via the Nasal Cartilage ◡

1. Sit at the client's head. Place your hands palms up several inches lateral of the client's head (see fig. 24.22). Explore a cycle of attunement.

2. Make contact with the shoulders bilaterally, palms up (see fig. 24.23).

3. Verbally negotiate contact, and then place your hands bilaterally over the client's frontal bone, with your thumbs contacting the area of the ethmoid bone under the glabella of the frontal bone (see figs. 24.24–25).

4. Shift so that the medial sides of the pads of your index fingers fit in the depression of the nasal cartilage (see figs. 24.26–30). Be sure to support your arm and elbows to allow the pads of the index fingers to be stable. The hands should not rest upon or compress any part of the client's frontal bone or other cranial structures. There can be skin contact, but it is floating rather than resting. Bring attention to your own coccyx and notochordal (spinal) midline and then orient with the central stillness in your body.

5. The practitioner waits to sense the client's midline lengthening from the nose, through the ethmoid bone and sphenobasilar space down to the coccyx with PR.

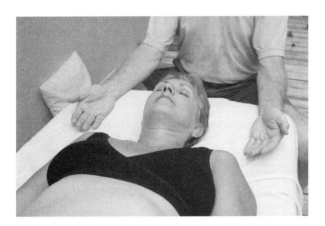

Fig. 24.22. Palms up lateral of head

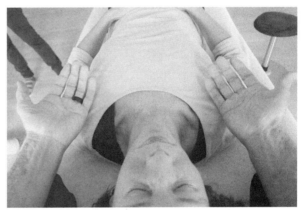

Fig. 24.23. Palms up on shoulders

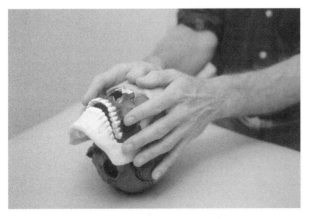

Fig. 24.24. Glabella-ethmoid 1

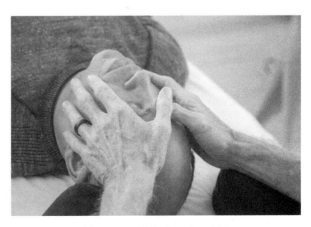

Fig. 24.25. Glabella-ethmoid 2

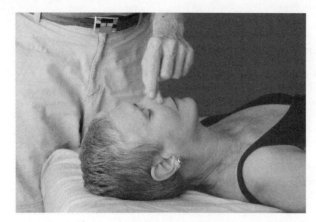

Fig. 24.26. Nasal cartilage 1

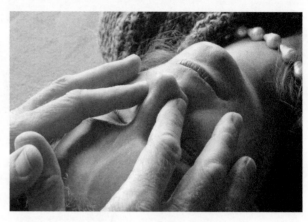

Fig. 24.27. Nasal cartilage 2

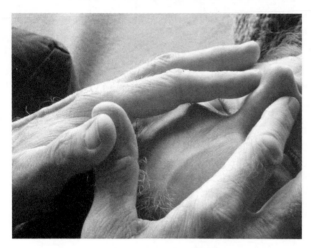

Fig. 24.28. Nasal cartilage 3

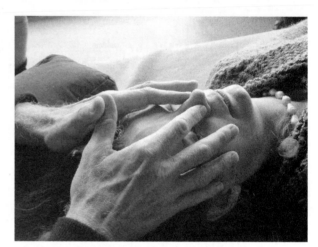

Fig. 24.29. Nasal cartilage 4

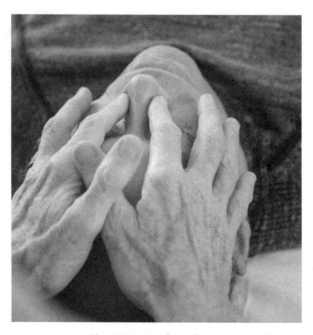

Fig. 24.30. Nasal cartilage 5

When bringing attention to your fingers and the client's nasal cartilage, sometimes you might offer one or two micrograms of traction on the nasal cartilage inferiorly or caudally toward the client's feet and ceiling of the treatment room. There is a sweet spot in which the midline lengthens. The traction is the gentlest of offerings. Bring attention to the whole fluid body expanding with PR at the end.

∼ 4. The Anterior-Posterior Fluid Fields of the Face ∼

1. Sit at the client's side, perpendicular to the head. Place one hand under the client's head, allowing the client's occiput to rest on your palm and/or fingers. The client's external occipital protuberance should be situated between your ring finger and middle finger (see fig. 24.31). In this position, your hand is holding the transverse sinus of the client, with the fulcrum of the external occipital protuberance being the intersection of the straight sinus and transverse sinus. In this way, your middle finger approximates the posterior attachments of the superior leaf of the tentorium. Your ring finger approximates the inferior leaf of the client's tentorium. (It is fine to use other fingers depending on the size of your hand.) Wait until you can sense a spreading or gapping of the superior and inferior leaves of the tentorium.

2. Upon sensing the spreading of the tentorium, contact the upper fluid field of the client's frontal bone with your free hand (see fig. 24.32). Position your hand so that the pad of the thumb and pad of the middle finger are in light contact with the lateral portion of the client's frontal bone. Wait to feel PR breathing between your two hands.

3. Then shift your hand from the frontal bone to the maxilla in order to sense the same dynamic (see figs. 24.33–34).

4. Then switch your hand from the maxilla to the mandible, with similar bilateral contact as the frontal and maxilla (see fig. 24.35).

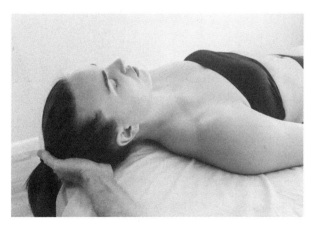

Fig. 24.31. Transverse sinus

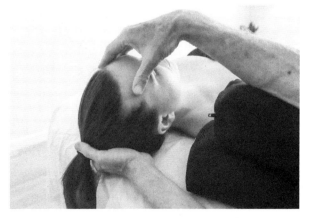

Fig. 24.32. Frontal bone

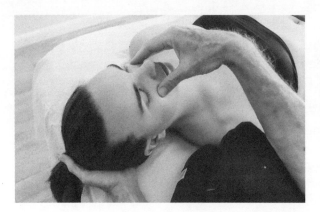

Fig. 24.33. Maxilla 1

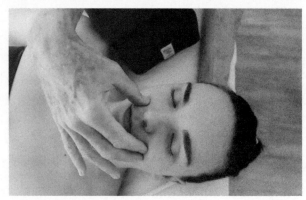

Fig. 24.34. Maxilla 2

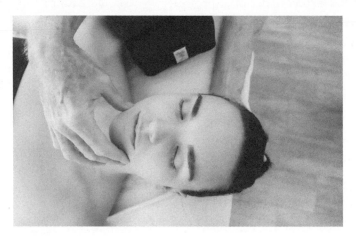

Fig. 24.35. Mandible

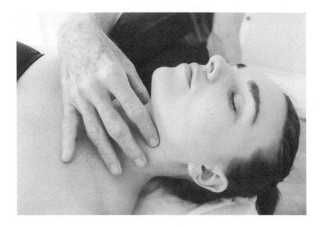

Fig. 24.36. Hyoid 1

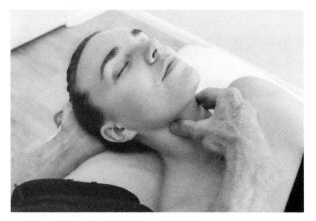

Fig. 24.37. Hyoid 2

5. Finally, shift your hand from the mandible to the hyoid bone bilaterally (see figs. 24.36–37). These windows are related to ignition and the importance of the face in inducing growth and development of the brain and heart embryonically.

ᴗ᛬ 5. Longitudinal Fluctuation at the Coccyx ᛬ᴗ

1. Sit at the client's side, facing the client's head and neck. Negotiate permission to make contact, and then place the middle finger of the hand closest to the client on the space around the coccyx and sacral sulcus, between the coccyx and sacrum (see figs. 24.11–15, pages 322–23). The finger lightly touches the bone in that area without any lifting. Rest your other hand in your lap, without contact. Synchronize your attention with the health and wholeness (PR) of the client through a heart-to-heart connection. Visualize the anatomical space in your own body from the coccyx up through the dural tube all the way to the third ventricle. Imagine a tube several inches in diameter with a color of your choice. This is the space of the vagus nerve in the center of the body. Wait to sense the movement of PR as a longitudinal fluctuation in the client's spinal dural space. This is a electromagnetic fluid stream of information that Dr. Sutherland called the direct current. PR is its most stable rate, though it is sometimes perceived at a faster rate.

2. Upon sensing the longitudinal fluctuation, with PR as a guide, move your attention to the central stillness within the longitudinal fluctuation. Wait for the potency and permeation of the longitudinal fluctuation of PR to clarify and/ or amplify its therapeutic intention. Gradually, move your attention out to the horizon and synchronize with the interchange between stillness and PR.

Practitioner Tip

The longitudinal fluctuation is diagnostic in the sense that it is frequently missing in the contemporary client due to traumatic stress, lifestyle, the use of prescription medications, and chronic inflammatory conditions. It needs to be checked early in some sessions and then again at the end of some sessions. When it is unavailable, the focus becomes allowing the whole three-dimensional fluid body to breath with PR in both Zones A (the body) and B (the space around the body).

ᴗ᛬ 6. Bilateral Posterior Tibial Artery ᛬ᴗ

Finish by holding the posterior tibial arteries of the feet bilaterally. The posterior tibial artery wraps around the inferior border of the medial malleolus. It is deep to the flexor hallucis longus and the flexor digitorum longus. Rest the pads of your fingers on the tendons until the artery presents itself into your awareness (see figs. 24.38–42; the dot indicates the anatomical location for palpation of the posterior tibial artery).

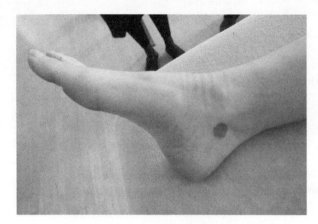

Fig. 24.38. Posterior tibial artery 1

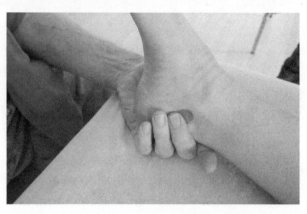

Fig. 24.39. Posterior tibial artery 2

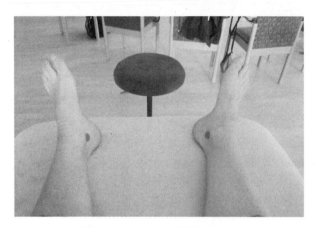

Fig. 24.40. Posterior tibial artery 3

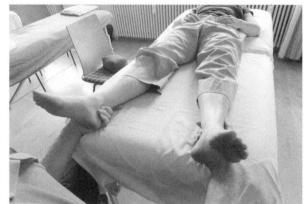

Fig. 24.41. Posterior tibial artery 4

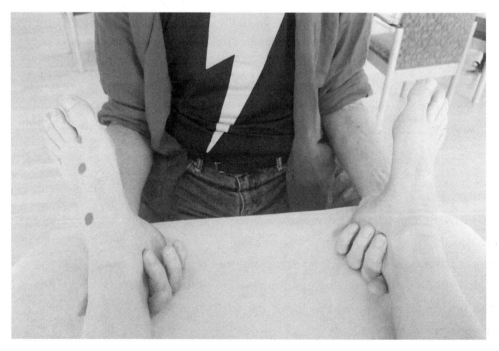

Fig. 24.42. Posterior tibial artery 5

ᘒᘒ
The Third Protocol: Basic Neck and Face

For this third protocol, the client is supine.

ᘐ I. Pietà ᘓ

Place one hand under the client's shoulder and the other hand under the leg (see figs. 24.43–44). Make sure the hand under the leg is not reaching too far, so you remain sitting up straight. Practice a cycle of attunement, as described at the beginning of this chapter. Sense the fluid body breathing into your hands with PR.

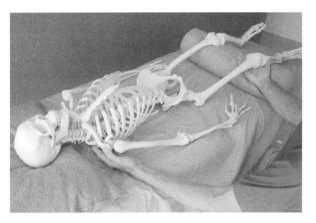
Fig. 24.43. Pietà 1

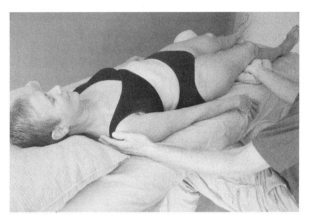
Fig. 24.44. Pietà 2

ᘐ 2. Umbilicus ᘓ

Place your hands, palm up, above and below umbilicus for sensing Zone B (see figs. 24.45–46). Sense PR flowing back and forth through your hands and arms, as if through an umbilical cord.

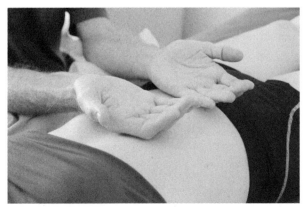
Fig. 24.45. Umbilicus, palms up 1

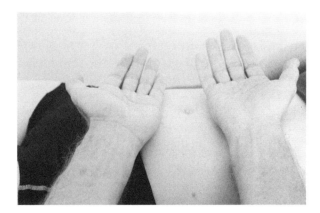
Fig. 24.46. Umbilicus, palms up 2

❧ 3. Synchronizing the Pelvic-Respiratory Diaphragms
with the Radial Artery ❧

1. Sit on one side of the client, facing the client's face at an angle. Observe the client's breathing.

2. Comfortably position the finger pad of one or two fingers under the coccyx. Wait a minute, and then position the other hand comfortably, palm up, under the floating ribs (see figs. 24.11–12, page 322). Wait for pelvic and respiratory diaphragms to synchronize their motion. Sense the motion of the breath coming into your hands and observe it visually. Then, wait for the fluid body to breathe as one drop with Primary Respiration (PR). Sometimes this feels like your hands are opening and closing slowly, like a flower.

3. Leave one hand on the coccyx, and with your other hand contact the radial artery on the side where you are sitting (see figs. 24.47–48). Allow PR to connect your two hands through the vascular tree or fluid body.

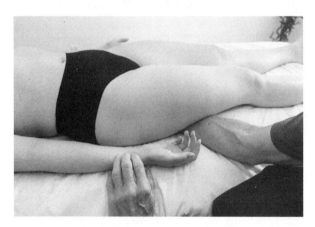
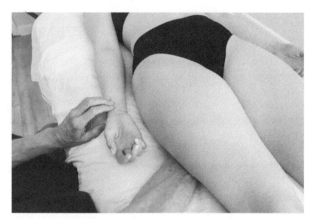

Fig. 24.47. Coccyx–radial artery 1   Fig. 24.48. Coccyx–radial artery 2

❧ 4. Bilateral Anterior Tibial Artery ❧

1. Contact one foot slightly lateral of the tendon of the big toe. The artery is several centimeters long and can be contacted anywhere on the length of the dorsum of the foot. Closer to the big toe, the artery changes names and becomes the dorsalis pedis artery. No need for a helicopter landing; it may take five or ten micro-adjustments with your finger pads to sense the artery.

2. Place your other hand on the anterior tibial artery of the other foot (see figs. 24.16–17, page 323). Now sense your own heart pulsing with the client's artery. Then feel a heart-to-heart connection with PR. The heart-to-heart connection with PR ignites the vascular tree and helps dissipate stress in the tree, especially from surgery. Remember to use cushions under your hands and forearms.

∿ 5. Heart Fulcrum ∾

1. Sit at the head of the table and settle with your hands palm up lateral of the client's head (see fig. 24.49). Practice a cranial cycle of attunement, as described on page 320.

2. Bring attention to your spine. Allow PR to move your spine back and forth. This separates your nervous system from the client's nervous system.

3. Place your hands under the client's neck, around the level of C3–C4, with the longest of the fingertips on each hand touching (see figs. 24.50–52). This was the initial location of the embryonic heart. Intermittently focus on the client's and then your own whole body, feeling the heart and the capillaries under the skin as a three-dimensional network. This is the interface with the fluid body. Is the client's fluid body able to breathe with PR? Your fingers may be invited toward a subtle motion of floating up (toward the ceiling) and down (back to the table) at the rate of PR.

   The Heart Fulcrum balances the client's cranial-facial-cardiac area as one field of embryonic activity and influences the client's dorsal and ventral vagal system to produce an anti-inflammatory response. Alternatively, you can allow the client's fluid body to dissipate its stress through your own fluid body.

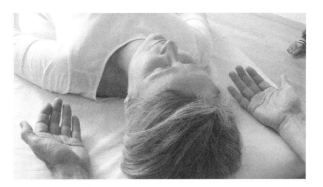

Fig. 24.49. Hands palm up lateral of head

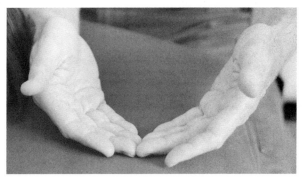

Fig. 24.50. Heart fulcrum 1

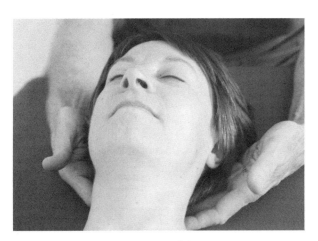

Fig. 24.51. Heart fulcrum 2

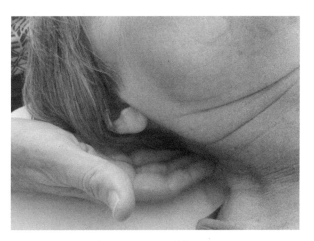

Fig. 24.52. Heart fulcrum 3

⤳ 6. Bilateral Subclavian Artery ⤳

1. Place your hands with the palms up or down on the client's shoulders. Practice a cranial cycle of attunement, as described on page 320. Bring your attention to your spine and allow PR to move your spine back and forth.

2. With your right thumb or another finger, find the midpoint of the clavicle and place the pad of the finger around the top and posteriorly under the clavicle. Wait for the subclavian artery to come into your finger. Ask your client if they are comfortable. If they are not comfortable, remove your finger. If they are comfortable, now place your left thumb or other finger on the left subclavian artery (see figs. 24.53–55).

3. Now sense your own heart pulsing with the client's artery. Then feel a heart-to-heart connection with PR.

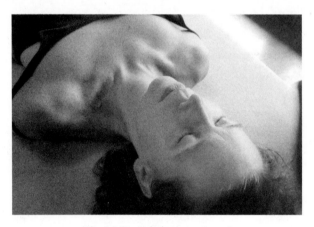

Fig. 24.53. Subclavian artery 1

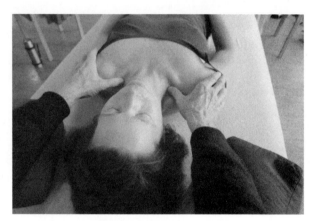

Fig. 24.54. Subclavian artery 2

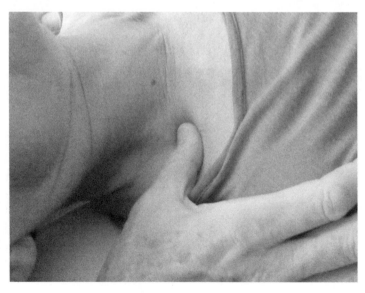

Fig. 24.55. Subclavian artery 3

❧ 7. Carotid Sinus and Lower Fluid Fields
of the Face and Neck ❧

1. Contact the belly of the sternocleidomastoid (SCM) muscle on either the right or left side of the client's neck at the very midpoint of the muscle between the mastoid process and the head of the clavicle (see figs. 24.56–57). I prefer to use the pad of my middle finger, and then my other fingers contour to the shape of the client's SCM without any compression.

2. Ask the client if they are comfortable; if they are not, remove your hand. If they are comfortable, place the finger(s) of your left hand on the belly of the SCM muscle on the left side of the client's neck (see fig. 24.58). Again, ask the client if they are comfortable.

3. Now sense your own heart pulsing with the client's artery. Then feel a heart-to-heart connection with PR.

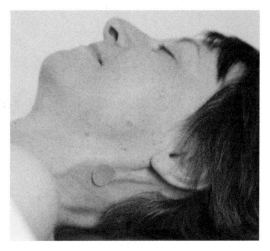

Fig. 24.56. Carotid sinus 1

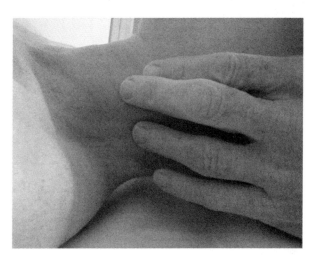

Fig. 24.57. Carotid sinus 2

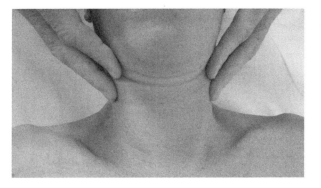

Fig. 24.58. Carotid sinus 3

Practitioner Tip

The carotid sinus is where the carotid artery bifurcates into the internal and external carotid arteries. At that junction there is also a cluster of cells associated with cranial nerves 10 and 11 that register the pH of the blood. They are known as baroreceptors and are important in regulating blood pressure.

∽ 8. Facial Artery and the Upper Fluid Fields of the Face ∽

1. Find the facial artery as it crosses the lower edge of the mandibular arch. It is directly on the diagonal line of the nasal labial fold (see fig. 24.63). Use the edge of your index and middle fingers to sense the edge of the bone where the artery is located (see figs. 24.59 and 24.61).

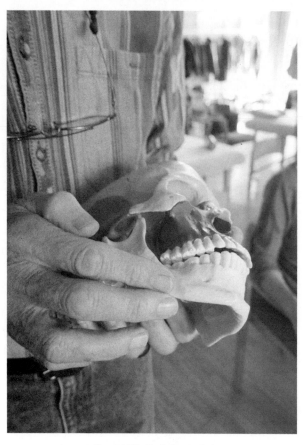

Fig. 24.59. Facial artery 1

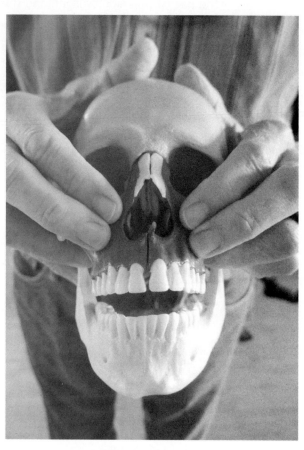

Fig. 24.60. Facial artery 2

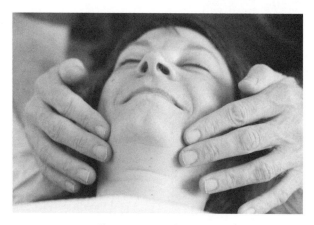

Fig. 24.61. Facial artery 3

2. Now find the facial artery as it crosses the nasal labial fold. Here you will use the tips of one or two fingers lateral of the nose, between the zygomatic bone and the maxilla (see figs. 24.60 and 24.62). Remember that deep arteries from the circle of Willis emerge around the nose and eyes and meet the facial artery. This is also a pulse location in classical Chinese medicine for balancing the chi in the head.

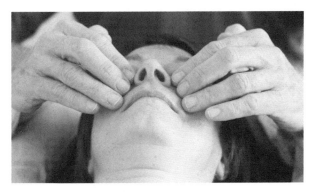

Fig. 24.62. Facial artery 4

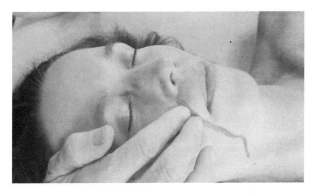

Fig. 24.63. The path of the facial artery between the mandibular arch and the nasal labial fold

◡ 9. Bilateral Posterior Tibial Artery ◡

1. Find the easiest way to position a finger pad to sense the artery under the tendons surrounding the medial malleoli. The precise location is the acupuncture point called kidney #3. Then find the posterior tibial artery on the other foot (see figs. 24.38–42, page 336). Although arteries do follow bones, you can palpate this artery more superiorly on the tibia if there is too much fascia around the ankle.

2. Now sense your own heart pulsing with the client's artery. Then feel a heart-to-heart connection with PR.

ба

The Fourth Protocol:
Basic Visceral Vasculature

Please study the map of abdominal arteries shown in figure 24.64. For this fourth protocol, the client is supine.

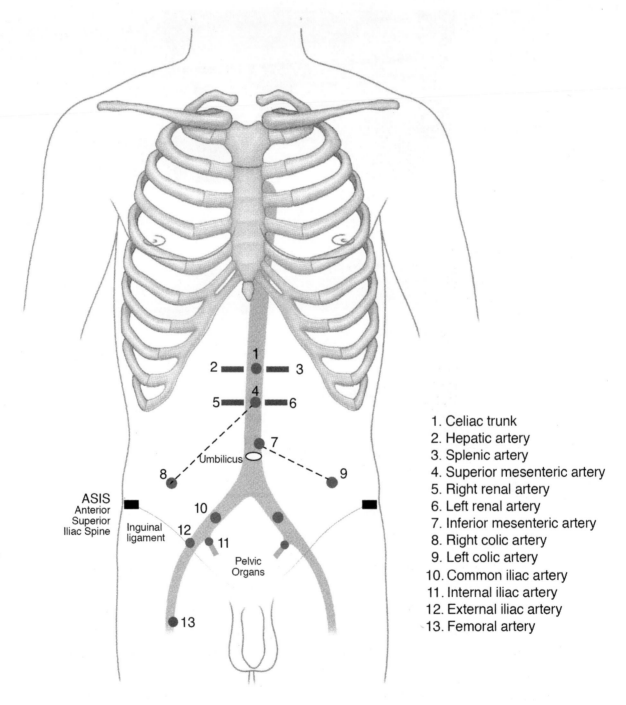

1. Celiac trunk
2. Hepatic artery
3. Splenic artery
4. Superior mesenteric artery
5. Right renal artery
6. Left renal artery
7. Inferior mesenteric artery
8. Right colic artery
9. Left colic artery
10. Common iliac artery
11. Internal iliac artery
12. External iliac artery
13. Femoral artery

Fig. 24.64. Abdominal pulses

⌁ 1. Pietà Palms Up ⌁

1. Sit at the side of the client. Practice a cycle of attunement, as described earlier in this chapter. Orient and synchronize with the natural world. Bring attention to your heart-diaphragm movement. Bring attention to your vascular tree via your heartbeat and its potency spreading throughout your body (see fig. 24.65).

2. Shift your attention to your hands, palm up on top of the client's shoulder and leg. Feel Zone B like a warm, wet, electrically charged cloud breathing with PR. This is the fluid body in its continuity with Zones A and B.

3. Finish with the pietà contact to see if the client's vascular tree is moving with PR.

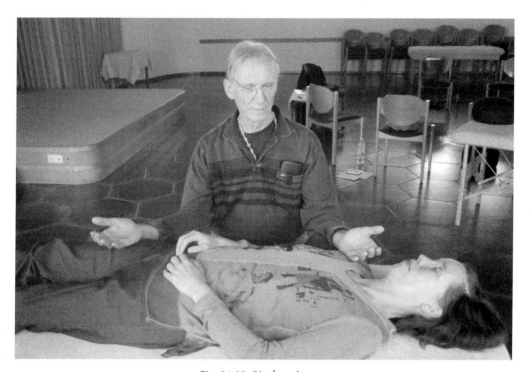

Fig. 24.65. Pietà, palms up

⌁ 2. Vascular Tree ⌁

1. Contact the radial artery on the right side of the client with one hand (see figs. 24.66–69). Then contact the anterior tibial artery with your other hand (see figs. 24.70–71). Practice a cycle of attunement heart-to-heart. This ignites the vascular tree.

2. Feel the whole tree move with PR. It is as if a breeze is blowing the tree. The vascular tree has the same basic motions as the sphenobasilar synchondrosis: flexion-extension, side-bending rotation, torsion, and shearing. Listen to the silence when it arrives. The center of the blood flow spiral is dynamically still.

3. The next step would be to repeat this sequence on the left side, but I recommend waiting several sessions with a new client before exploring the vascular tree on the left side of the client's body.

Practitioner Tip

The basic rule of thumb for BCVT is to stay in the peripheral end of the vascular tree since the vascular system in the embryo develops from the periphery to the center. *In general, always start on the right side.* This is the side of the vascular tree farthest away from the heart. PR will guide you to the left side of the client's vascular tree.

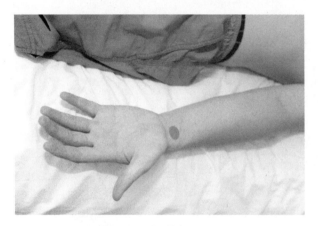

Fig. 24.66. Radial artery 1

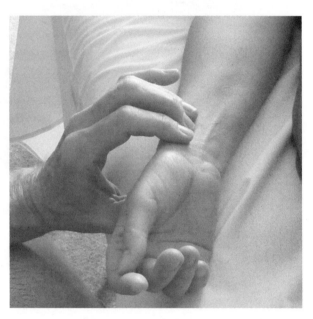

Fig. 24.67. Radial artery 2

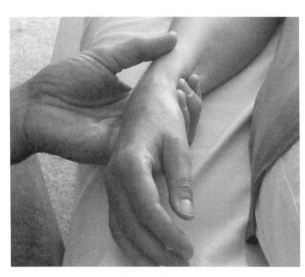

Fig. 24.68. Radial artery 3

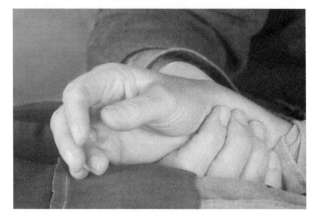

Fig. 24.69. Radial artery 4

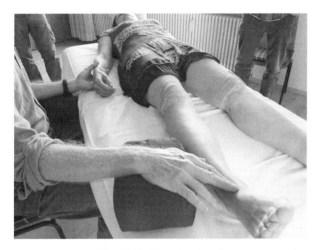

Fig. 24.70. Vascular tree 1

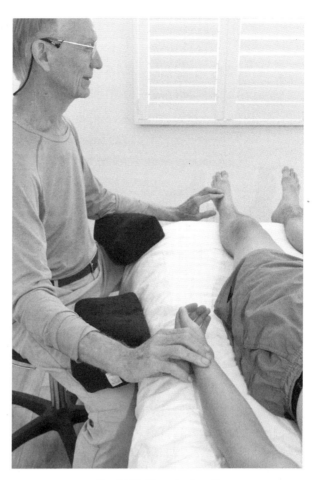

Fig. 24.71. Vascular tree 2

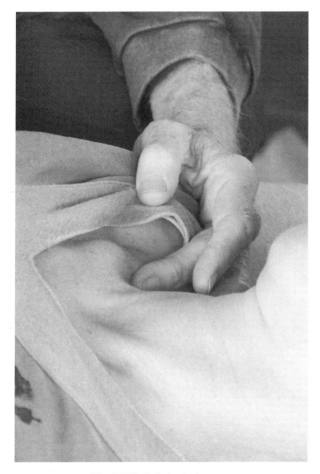

Fig. 24.72. Subclavian artery

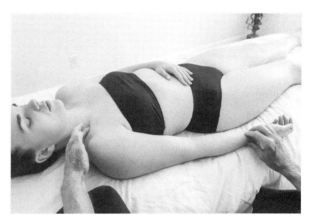

Fig. 24.73. Radial and subclavian arteries

4. Now explore a branch of the vascular tree between the radial artery and sub-
    clavian artery. Find the subclavian artery first, and then the radial artery (see
    figs. 24.72–73). This is invaluable for women who have had a mastectomy or had
    lymph nodes removed from their axilla.

Practitioner Tip

The vascular tree holds stress and trauma just like all the other systems of the body. Igniting the vascular tree discharges such stress. This is valuable for clients who have had heart surgery of any kind. Wait six months after such surgery to treat client's vascular tree. If you are not sure whether to proceed, get a release from the client's doctor.

---

3. Subclavian Artery

1. Sit at the head of the table. Place your hands bilaterally over the shoulders and upper arms of the client, either palm up or palm down (see figs. 24.74–75). Synchronize with PR. Practice a cycle of attunement. Sense your spine breathing out the back of your body with PR.

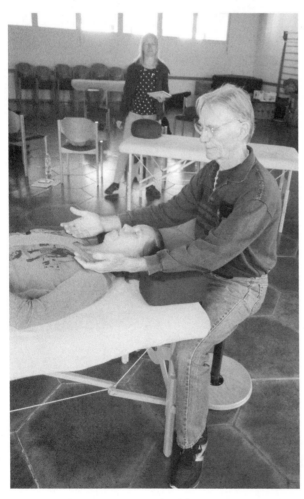

Fig. 24.74. Shoulders 1

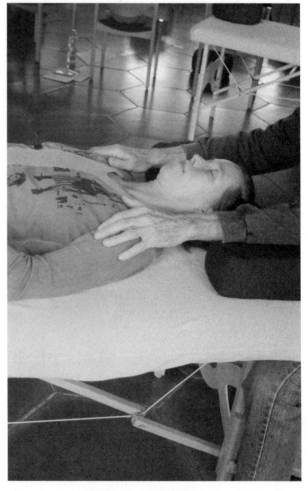

Fig. 24.75. Shoulders 2

2. This area of the neck is rich in ANS innervation, and some clients are very sensitive here, so it is important to solicit the comfort of the client while making this contact. Begin contact ipsilaterally, starting on the right side. Use one hand to contact the radial artery. Then use your other hand to contact the subclavian artery, close to the midclavicle and under the clavicle from its superior border (see figs. 24.53–55, page 340). The connective tissue of the neck at that area of the clavicle is like a sling or a hammock. Using the pad of your index or middle finger, roll gently over and under the clavicle until there is no more slack in the connective tissue. Then slightly release your finger, raising it a millimeter or two up from the clavicle, while maintaining a slight pressure, and the subclavian artery will come into your finger. (Sometimes no pressure or rolling of the finger is necessary to palpate the subclavian artery.)

3. Repeat on the left side of the client. If a client is very comfortable with the contact, make contact somewhere else for comfort on the client's vascular tree.

Practitioner Tip

Initially you may not sense the artery but must wait until the artery comes to your fingers. It is wrapped in the inferior cervical sympathetic ganglion, plus it is connected to the vagus nerve. Arteries are often sensed as a flow rather than a pulsation, and they will vary in terms of sensation from side to side. Wait for PR to synchronize the heart, the hands, and the vascular tree. Rest awareness in the stillness while sensing the movement of the heart(s).

⌁ 4. Inferior Common Carotid Artery ⌁

1. Still sitting at the head of the table, place your hands bilaterally over the shoulders and upper arms of the client, either palm up or palm down (see figs. 24.74–75, page 348). Synchronize with PR. Practice a cycle of attunement. Sense your spine breathing out the back of your body with PR.

2. Starting on the client's right side, place the pad of your index finger on the medial or lateral border of the sternocleidomastoid muscle (SCM) several millimeters above its attachment on the clavicle (see figs. 24.76–77 on page 350). Sometimes the common carotid artery can be found on top of the SCM. Gently palpate that area until the pad of your index finger senses the artery. Maintain this contact and then use your other hand to repeat on the client's left side.

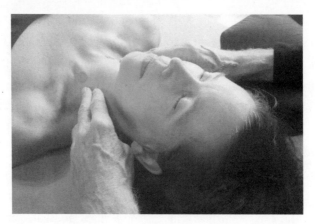

Fig. 24.76. Common carotid artery 1

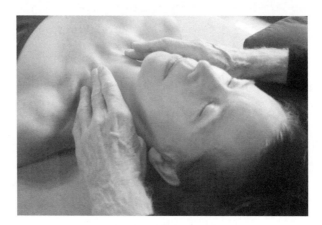

Fig. 24.77. Common carotid artery 2

Practitioner Tip

Sensing the pulse of the common carotid artery is valuable in lowering the tone of the ANS. This is because the contact is located close to the vagus nerve under the manubrium. This creates the potential for safety.

The common carotid artery is different from right to left. Specifically, the right common carotid artery arises from the subclavian artery, whereas the left common carotid artery comes directly from the aortic arch. Occasionally you may sense the flow of PR through the entire vascular system of the client, and the client may sense this as well. Some clients report feeling the flow of grace or love in their body. The cycle of attunement maintains the constant potential for igniting the vascular tree. Sometimes I ask clients to put a slight smile on their face when they sense this level of wholeness.

∿ 5. Abdominal Aorta ∿

1. Approaching the client from the side, place one or both hands, palms up or down, above and below the client's umbilicus (see figs. 24.78–80). Sense the client breathing. During inhalation, the client's transversus abdominus muscle expands and the umbilicus lifts up toward the ceiling. Upon exhalation, the abdomen relaxes back. If the client is not able to expand and lift your hands during inhalation, verbally direct the client to breath into your hands for several cycles. This reminder can be given as often as necessary for the client to learn proper anatomically correct breathing. This is an important way to move abdominal lymph and tone the vagus nerve.

2. Beginning close to the umbilicus, place both hands so they span the width of the rectus abdominis muscle, with the tips of the thumbs on one edge of the rectus abdominis and the remaining fingers on the opposite edge of the muscle (see fig. 24.81). Gently and slowly allow your hands to move toward the client's spine while reciprocally having your hands make a lifting motion, periodically

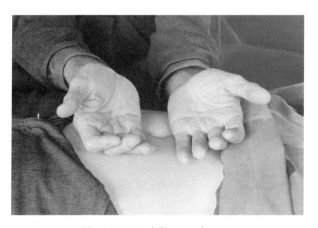

Fig. 24.78. Umbilicus, palms up

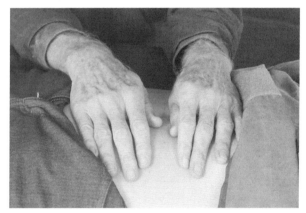

Fig. 24.79. Umbilicus, palms down

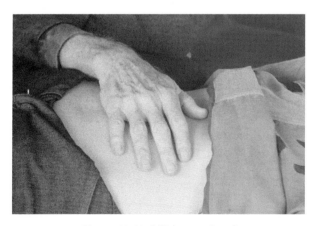

Fig. 24.80. Umbilicus, one hand

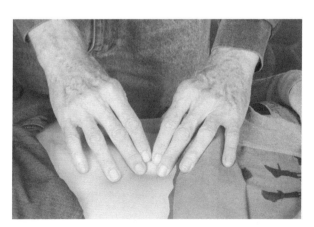

Fig. 24.81. Abdominal aorta

stopping and listening for the big pulse of the aorta. Once you feel contact with the aorta, then simply listen, and resynchronize with PR.

3. Ask the client to bend their knees, which puts slack in the core muscles and makes it easier to lift the mesentery. Then, with your hands, begin to lift the whole mesentery (see figs. 24.82–83). The mobility of the mesentery is important as it is an original embryonic structure and must be assessed in all abdominal exploration.

4. Now move your hands to several inches below the umbilicus and repeat the palpation (see fig. 24.84). This is the inferior end of the abdominal aorta, where it bifurcates into the common iliac arteries.

Through this sequence we are, at the same time, holding the web of the abdominal ANS plexuses and their mesentery. Always attune to the client breathing into your hands.

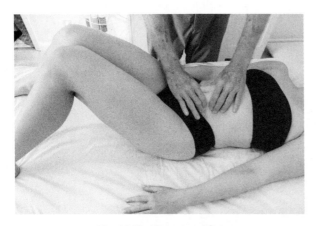

Fig. 24.82. Mesentery lift 1

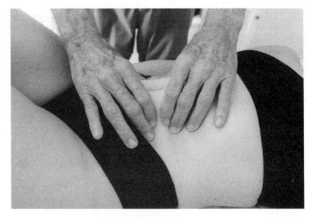

Fig. 24.83. Mesentery lift 2

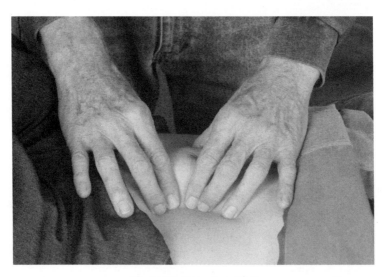

Fig. 24.84. Mesentery lift 3

∻ 6. External Iliac and Femoral Arteries ∻

1. Sit on the right side of the client. Place a hand over the client's anterior superior iliac spine (ASIS) and ask them to slightly bend their knee. The crease of the inguinal ligament (see figs. 24.85–86) will deepen and can easily be palpated.

2. Approach the location of the external iliac artery using the middle of the inguinal ligament as a landmark (see fig. 24.87). It is above the superior border of that point at an angle toward a point several inches below the umbilicus. The pads of the fingers of your left hand line up above the inguinal ligament, palpating the external iliac artery. These finger pads are actually lined up together as if you were playing a flute (and no contact with the thumb is used). The pads of the fingers of your right hand are inferior to the inguinal ligament, palpating the femoral artery (see fig. 24.88). The femoral artery is the continuation of the iliac artery as it goes below the inguinal ligament. As it comes under the inguinal ligament it angles slightly toward the medial side of the knee in the neurovascular bundle of the femur. This palpation unlocks imploded fight-or-flight responses in the neurovascular bundle in the extremities and is very grounding.

3. Repeat on the left side of the body using opposite hands.

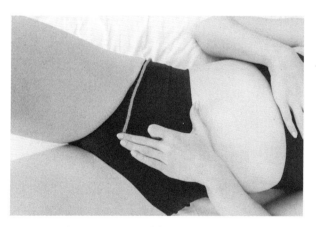

Fig. 24.85. Inguinal ligament location 1

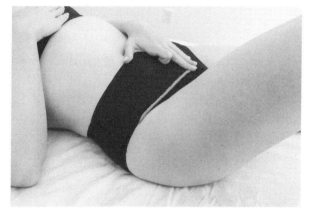

Fig. 24.86. Inguinal ligament location 2

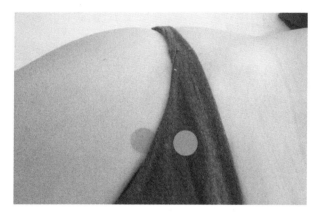

Fig. 24.87. External iliac and femoral arteries 1

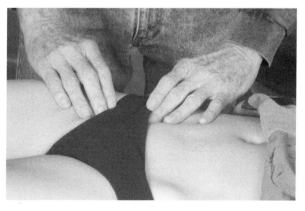

Fig. 24.88. External iliac and femoral arteries 2

Practitioner Tip

The pads of the fingers of both hands are lined up above and below the inguinal ligament that they form a V shape. This is because the iliac artery is at an angle coming from the lower abdominal aorta and the femoral artery angles back toward the medial side of the knee. This area is rich in lymphatic vessels, and the palpation is beneficial for moving the lymph.

⌇ 7. External Iliac-Femoral and Anterior Tibial Arteries ⌇

1. Contact the external iliac artery on the left side with your left hand on the anterior tibial artery and your right hand on the external iliac artery, slightly superior to the inguinal ligament (see fig. 24.89).
2. Switch to the other side. Contact the femoral artery on the right side with your left hand on external iliac artery and the anterior tibial artery with your right hand (see fig. 24.90).
3. Repeat steps 1 and 2 on the opposite sides.

Gradually the silence arrives. When it does, drop the cycle of attunement and rest awareness in the silence while sensing the movement of PR between and through the heart(s).

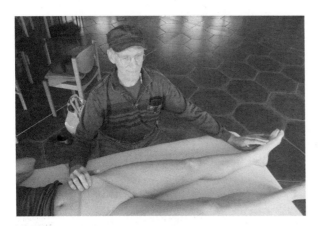

Fig. 24.89. External iliac and anterior tibial arteries

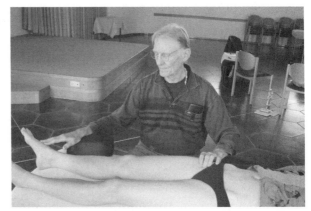

Fig. 24.90. Femoral and anterior tibial arteries

⌁ 8. Coccyx and Diaphragm and/or Tibial Arteries ⌁

Finish with coccyx-diaphragm and/or the tibial arteries.

This completes the introduction to the basic practices of biodynamic cardiovascular therapy. Remember that these are teaching and learning protocols that must be gradually adapted for the reader's clinical practice.

25

Intermediate Biodynamic
Cardiovascular Therapy Skills

Please note that a complete view of all the arteries of the body can be seen in the color insert, plates 25–35. These can be reviewed prior to or during the study of the following protocols.

Now that we have covered the basic skills for biodynamic cardiovascular therapy (BCVT) in the preceding chapter, we will explore intermediate skills that allow us to observe different layers of the client's metabolism. The starting point is always the cycle of attunement and synchronization with Primary Respiration (PR). In these intermediate skills with BCVT, there is greater focus on resting in the heart-to-heart connection with PR.

ଚଙ

Intermediate Facial Protocol

◡ 1. The Vascular Tree ◡

1. Sit at the side of the table. Practice several cycles of attunement without contact and then the pietà window (see figs. 24.3–5, page 318).

2. Negotiate permission to contact the vascular tree of the client. Contact the radial artery with one hand, cupping under or over the wrist of the client, and use your other hand to contact the anterior tibial artery (see figs. 24.70–71, page 347). Now both hands are in contact with the peripheral ends of the cardiovascular system. Focus attention on your own belly breathing, counting your own heartbeats to seventy and listening to silence. Vary the depth of contact in both hands with intermittent micropressure and release.

3. Lightly bring your attention to the heart field between you and the client. Wait for PR to breathe heart-to-heart. Feel the heart swing toward the client and away as if the pericardium is a big pendulum. You, the client, or both of you may experience an accelerated heart rate. In some cases, this is simple awareness, even though the heart is not moving faster. In other cases, the heart may actually be moving faster, if this is happening in your client, direct the client to take

a slow breath into the abdomen to lower the heart rate. This is the autonomic nervous system going through a process that leads to stabilization.

～ 2. Facial Artery ～

1. Sit at the head of the table and make gentle bilateral contact with the client's shoulders, with your palms either up or down (see figs. 24.6–7, page 320). Practice a cranial cycle of attunement, as described on page 320. Synchronize with PR.

2. Make contact with the facial artery of the client bilaterally, using three or four fingers of each hand. Follow the line of the nasal labial fold over the edge of the mandible; this is where to place the contact (see fig. 24.61, page 342). Sense the activity of the facial artery as it extends from the external carotid artery and wait for PR to breathe the fluid fields of the face.

3. Now move to the nasal labial fold bilaterally (see figs. 24.62–63, page 343). Make contact bilaterally, with two or three fingers of each hand in the nasal labial fold.

～ 3. Supraorbital and Supratrochlear Arteries ～

1. Place the finger pads of both hands over the frontal bone (see fig. 25.1). This is where the internal and external carotid artery reconsolidates (anastomosis). Sense the capillaries under the skin breathing in the tempo of PR. These are the leaves of the vascular tree.

2. Ask permission from the client to place your fingers bilaterally around the supraorbital ridge of the frontal bone above the eyes. The location of the supraorbital and supratrochlear arteries is shown by small dots in figure 25.2. Make contact on one side first, allow the client time to settle, and then make contact with the opposite supraorbital ridge. (You may want to say something like "Now I am going to make contact around your other eye.") The supratrochlear artery is located where the lacrimal bones meet the frontal bone and is more

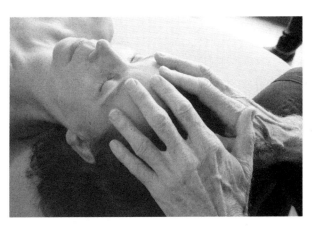

Fig. 25.1. Frontal anastomoses

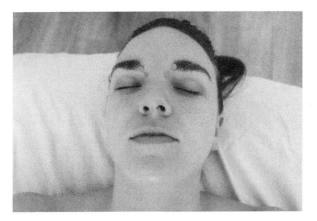

Fig. 25.2. Location for supraorbital and supratrochlear eye arteries

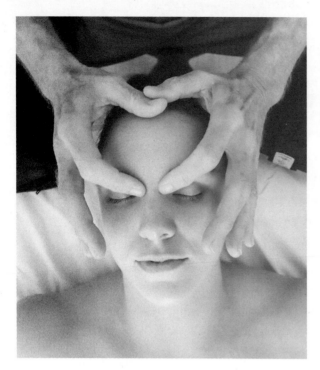

Fig. 25.3. Palpation of supraorbital and
supratrochlear eye arteries 1

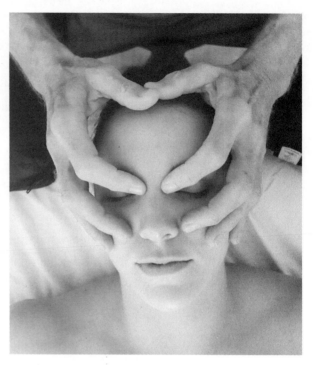

Fig. 25.4. Palpation of supraorbital and
supratrochlear eye arteries 2

medial than the supraorbital. Contact is made more laterally on the supraorbital ridge for the supraorbital artery (see figs. 25.3–4). Frequently the practitioner's finger pads contact both arteries simultaneously.

Depending on the size of your hands and comfort level with correct props for the hands, you can palpate these two arteries around the eyes on each side at the same time or one at a time starting with the lateral supraorbital artery.

Practitioner Tip

Palpation of the supraorbital and supratrochlear arteries is a very good way to work with the social nervous system. It is especially helpful for the contemporary client who sits in front of a computer or smart phone all day in order to relieve eyestrain and resulting headaches. These arteries derive from the ophthalmic artery, which derives from the circle of Willis, which derives from the vertebral and internal carotid arteries.

∽ 4. Transverse Facial and Maxillary Arteries ∾

1. Figure 25.5 shows the relative location of the two arteries superior and inferior to the zygomatic ridge of the temporal bone. Make bilateral contact with the zygomatic process of the client's temporal bones, using the tips or pads of two, three, or four fingers, depending on the size of your hand (see fig. 25.6). Find the transverse facial branch of the external carotid artery directly on, above, or below the zygomatic process. This is a way to explore the temporal bone and TMJ. It is possible to sense the zygomatic process rotating as the entire temporal bone rotates.

2. Place your fingers bilaterally up to a centimeter inferior of the zygomatic process (see fig. 25.7). Make contact with the tendon of the masseter muscle. Gently press into the muscle and release. Wait until the maxillary artery comes into your fingers. Then practice a cycle of attunement, including sensing your own heartbeat. Make sure to solicit the comfort of the client.

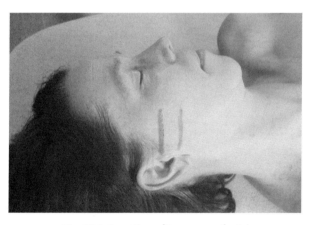

Fig. 25.5. Location of transverse facial and maxillary arteries

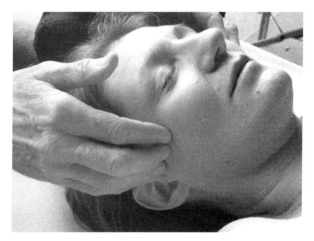

Fig. 25.6. Palpation of transverse facial artery

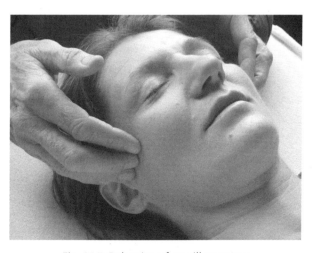

Fig. 25.7. Palpation of maxillary artery

ᵕ 5. Internal Carotid Artery and the Carotid Canal
of the Temporal Bones ᵕ

1. Gently make bilateral contact with the ears (see fig. 25.8). The intention is to tune in to the temporal bone and stimulate the vagus nerve.

2. For the internal carotid artery, make bilateral contact with the mastoid processes of the temporal bone with the most convenient finger under the ear (see figs. 25.9–10). The temporal bones may be sensed moving in their typical pattern of what cranial osteopaths refer to as a "wobbly wheel." The motion of the temporal bone is eccentric because the carotid canal has several sharp bends in it. Wait to sense the pulse of the internal carotid artery through the bone. The bone forms around the artery. Let the fluid fields of the cranium breath with PR.

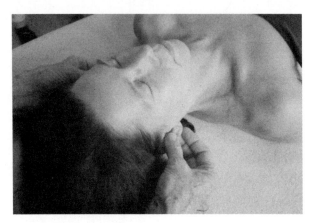

Fig. 25.8. Mastoid process and carotid canal 1

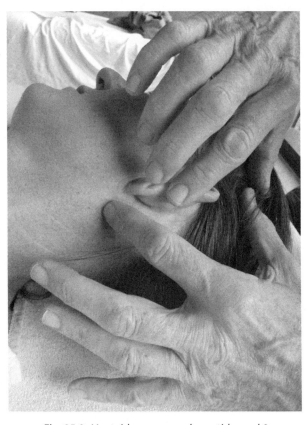

Fig. 25.9. Mastoid process and carotid canal 2

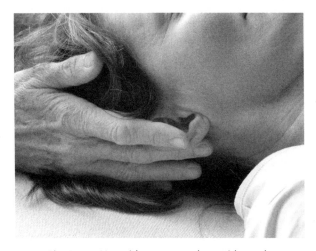

Fig. 25.10. Mastoid process and carotid canal 3

❧ 6. Bilateral Anterior Tibial Artery ☙

1. Sit at the foot of the table. Using the pads of the index and middle finger on one hand, contact the tibial artery on the corresponding foot of the client. Use your other hand to contact the tibial artery on the other foot (see figs. 24.16–17, page 323). Depending on the size of one's hands and the client's feet, one, two or three fingers may be used on each foot.

2. Synchronize attention with PR.

❧ 7. Bilateral Posterior Tibial Arteries ☙

1. Contact the posterior border of the tibia with one hand in order to contact the posterior tibial artery close to the medial malleoli. Use your other hand to contact the same on the other foot (see figs. 24.38–42, page 336). Usually two or three fingers of each hand are used to palpate these arteries.

2. Synchronize attention with PR.

ෝ
Heart Ignition Protocol

Please refer to the anatomical images in the color insert for more detail on cardiovascular anatomy.

This is the first formal protocol on connecting more directly with the heart itself. As mentioned earlier, the cardiovascular system develops from periphery to center. We have so far learned the techniques for palpation in the periphery of the vascular tree, and now we will formally approach the heart, the center of our being. This requires that our hands are both afferent and connected to our own heart via Primary Respiration (PR). We now contemplate that our biodynamic hands are capable of offering a blessing to ignite the instinct for self-transcendence. That instinct has an intimate connection to the heart inside the heart, as we have discussed. We must bear in mind that the heart is also an organ of emotional safety and an important nexus for the vagus nerve, the autonomic nervous system, and breathing via pulmonary circulation. We maintain an attitude of sacredness to make as much space as possible for everything that the human heart is capable of holding in life and death. We simply cannot know what our client holds in their heart. Our hands are used in the position of a sacred gesture called the gesture of invocation.

❧ 1. Cycle of Attunement with a Focus on Invocation ☙

1. Begin by settling without contact. Then inform the client that you are about to make contact.

2. The client is supine. Practice the pietà, palms up, over the client's shoulder and

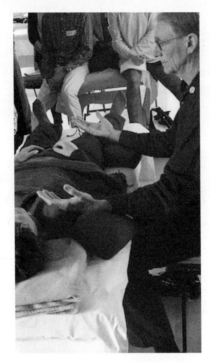

Fig. 25.11. Pietà, palms up

leg (see fig. 25.11). This is the gesture of invocation used when contacting the heart. It is also an exploration of Zone B, sensing the warm, wet, electrically charged biosphere around the client's body breathing with PR.

Attunement

It is important to establish stillness and a heart-to-heart connection with PR to ignite the heart and vascular tree. This cycle of attunement begins with sensing your fluid body, the feeling of breathing into the abdomen, the movement and potency of the heart, and the space at the back of the heart. Gradually you expand your awareness of the movement of the heart throughout the entire trunk of your body and beyond.

Stillness is the way in which the heart develops. It is the center of blood flow, and the cycle of heart attunement includes the perception and deepening of dynamic stillness. When you sense this depth of stillness, fully rest your attention in the stillness at the back of the heart and connect it to the stillness in the room and outside in nature. This is deeply restorative to the cardiovascular system.

PR may also begin to breath in the vascular system between your hands like an accordion opening and closing or torsioning rhythmically. Numerous developmental perceptional processes can occur under the guidance of PR and stillness.

❧ 2. Radial and Axillary Arteries ❧

1. Sit at the right side of the table and practice a cycle of heart attunement.

2. Contact the radial artery with one hand and place your opposite hand palm up on the same shoulder to contact the fluid body (see figs. 25.12–13).

3. Turn the hand on the shoulder over, so it is palm down, to make direct contact with the axillary artery (see fig. 25.14). This is a good way to stabilize the heart-brain-connection, breathing, and even the fascial system locally via the subclavian artery. It also is valuable for releasing fascial restrictions from mastectomies, especially those that involved removal of lymph nodes from the axilla.

4. Repeat this sequence on the other side of your client's body. Patients with serious heart conditions should receive medical clearance to have biodynamic cardiovascular therapy sessions.

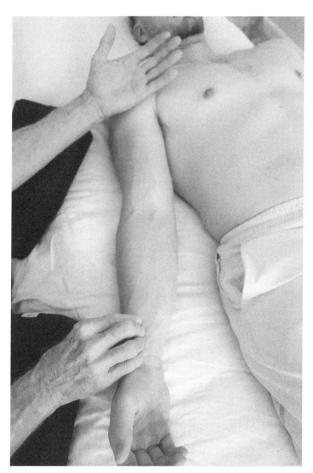

Fig. 25.12. Radial artery and shoulder 1

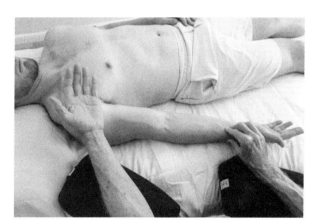

Fig. 25.13. Radial artery and shoulder 2

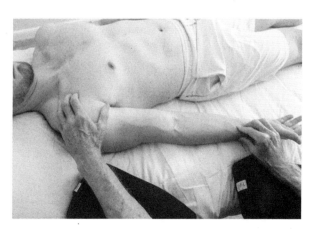

Fig. 25.14. Radial artery and shoulder 3

∿ 3. Heart and Cardiac Developmental Movement ∿

Review the anatomical location of the adult heart and pericardium. Note that the heart is attached to the diaphragm via the pericardium, slightly to the left of the midline of the sternum. The heart lies on an axis roughly between the right shoulder and spleen.

1. Sit at the left side of the client's trunk. Place both hands palm up over the sternum between the xiphoid process and the manubrium (see figs. 25.15–16). This is the sacred gesture of invocation. In biblical terminology it is the invocation of the Holy Spirit, the sacred. Wait for PR to begin breathing in the fluid body around the client.

2. Place one hand under the client's rib cage, approximating the position of the posterior portion of the heart (see fig. 25.17). Take time to sense the heartbeat and its four developmental movements: transparency like an open fish net, stretching into a tube, looping and torsioning into an S shape, and bending and folding upside down within the context of PR, with stillness at the center of the folding (see plates 10–13 in the color insert for reference).

3. Now place your other hand palm up or down on top of and in the middle of the sternum (see figs. 25.18–19). Be sure to configure your hands comfortably to

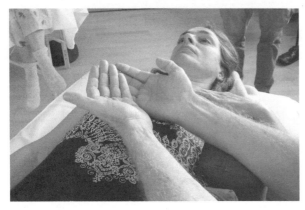
Fig. 25.15. Heart invocation 1

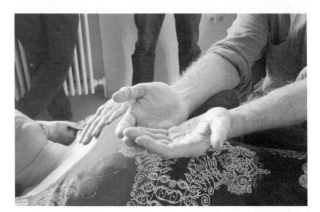
Fig. 25.16. Heart invocation 2

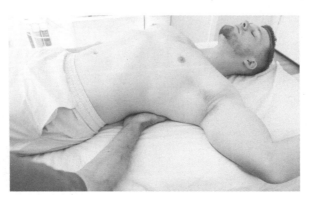
Fig. 25.17. Hand under the heart

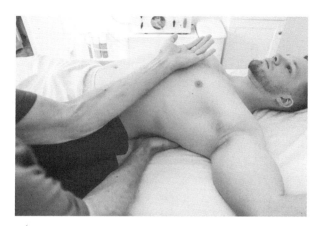

Fig. 25.18. Heart hold 1

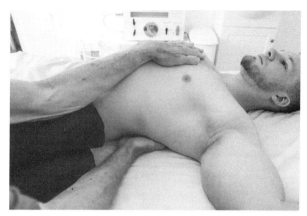

Fig. 25.19. Heart hold 2

prop up your wrists and arms as needed. It is up to the practitioner to decide which hand goes where because the practitioner must be comfortable.

4. Remember that the axis of the heart is on a line to the tip of the right shoulder. When the left ventricle ejects its contents into the aorta, the blood moves in a counterclockwise direction due to the spiral arrangement of the myocardial muscle cells. Upon diastole, the heart moves in a clockwise direction. Explore the spiral movement of the heart.

Embryologically, the heart develops what are called primary and secondary heart fields from two different types of mesodermal cells. The primary heart field cells originate from *lateral plate mesoderm*. The secondary heart field can be subdivided into an anterior and posterior field because of the influence of extracardiac neural crest cells moving from the posterior portion of the neural tube along the aortic arch vessels and into the inflow and outflow tracks of the heart. These cells become the autonomic innervation of the heart. The inflow and outflow vessels are formed from *splanchnic mesoderm*. This means that the cells making up the posterior heart are more fixed and the primary fields are more operating in a dilation field (ballooning) of expansion. In addition, there is a structure in the embryo, called the spinae vestibuli, that attaches the posterior heart to the posterior body wall or coelom of the embryo. Thus, the hand in back of the heart will sense more resistance, while the front hand over the sternum will sense more freedom. The hands palm up on either side of the heart can sense the heart opening and closing like a lotus flower in the tempo of PR.

The intention of this stage is to come into relationship with the heart at three levels:

- The primary and secondary heart fields
- The four developmental movements of the heart (see fig. 19.1 on page 239 and color insert)
- The spiral movement of the heart

Practitioner Tip

The intrathoracic pressure between the diaphragm, the lungs, the pericardium, and the left ventricle of the heart come into balance via the spiral motions of the heart as it pumps blood. This balance can be affected by an impact trauma to the trunk of the body. Such an impact causes a type of a whiplash of the pericardium. This has the potential over time to constrict the ventricles of the heart and cause heart disease, specifically myocarditis and pericarditis, which are also symptoms of long COVID.

∿ 4. The Aortic Arch ∿

1. Practice a vascular tree contact on the right side (see figs. 24.70–71, page 347).

2. Sit at the left side of the table facing the neck and shoulders of the client. (Or, alternatively, if it is easier for you, sit on the right side.) Place the finger pads of one hand, palm up, under the client's neck at C3–C4 (see figs. 25.20–21). Place the other hand palm up or down over the shoulder, with the fingertips approaching the aortic arch close to the sternoclavicular notch but not on the tissue over the thyroid gland (see figs. 25.20–23).

3. Make gentle contact with the spinous processes of the vertebra, using only a finger pad or two. This is known the heart fulcrum window. Find the back of the heart and the stillness. Wait for the tide of PR.

4. Practice a cranial cycle of attunement, as described on page 320, and wait to be invited into the client's aorta by PR.

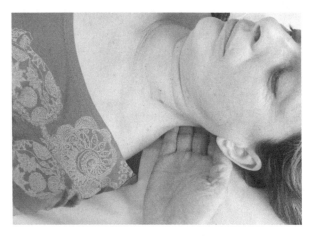

Fig. 25.20. Aortic arch 1

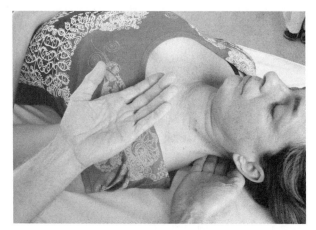

Fig. 25.21. Aortic arch 2

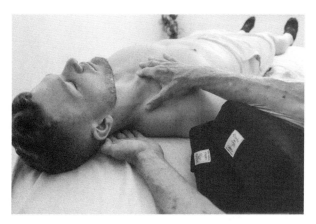

Fig. 25.22. Aortic arch 3

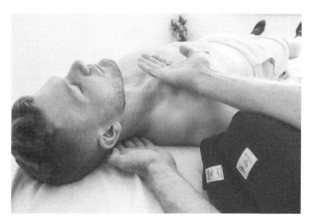

Fig. 25.23. Aortic arch 4

This stage is very beneficial for balancing the autonomic nervous system (ANS) since the aorta is innervated by both branches of the ANS. The hand position can be awkward, however. It is critically important to have props for the wrists and arms in order to support afferent palpation with the hands. Choose which hand positions work best for your comfort and ease. The potency of PR will lift your hands off the client.

∿ 5. Cerebrovascular Balancing of the Carotid Artery and Superior Sagittal Sinus ∿

1. While the client is still supine, place the pads of the fingers of one hand under the heart fulcrum of C3–C4. Place the other hand palm up over the shoulder (see fig. 25.23). Synchronize with PR.

2. Now ask the client to lie on their right-hand side. Decide the direction from which you will approach the client. A practitioner usually approaches the client from the back of their head and neck. This requires propping of the arms to stabilize the hands. It is possible but not preferable to approach the client from the front of their neck and face; sometimes approaching the client face to face can activate the client's ANS. I recommend that the therapist decide based on what they know about the comfort level of the client. Or the therapist can simply ask the client which position they prefer for this level of contact.

3. It is important to use a preparatory hand position. Place one hand over the shoulder of the client and the other around the top of the client's head, but without contact (see figs. 25.24–26).

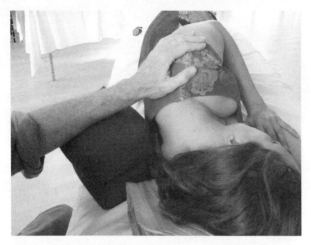

Fig. 25.24. Cerebrovascular balancing 1

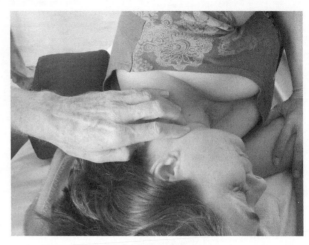

Fig. 25.25. Cerebrovascular balancing 2

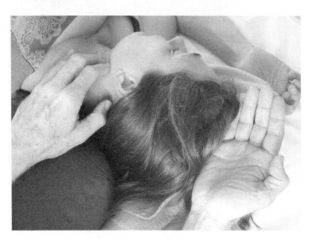

Fig. 25.26. Cerebrovascular balancing 3

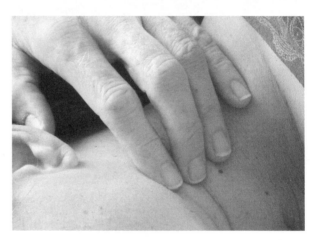

Fig. 25.27. Cerebrovascular balancing 4

4. Use the fingers of the hand that is over the client's shoulder, especially the index, middle, and ring fingers, to contact the midbelly of the sternocleidomastoid muscle (SCM). The carotid sinus is under the SCM. Contact is made at the junction of the common carotid and internal carotid artery (see figs. 25.25–28). This is the location of the carotid sinus. Since the carotid artery crosses under the SCM, the practitioner will find the area of the carotid sinus halfway down the SCM. The pads of the fingers simply contact the belly of the SCM gently.

5. Place your other hand lightly over the superior sagittal sinus of the client's cranium (see figs. 25.29–31). My hands are shaped to show underlying location. Now you have both branches of the vascular system (venous and arterial). Begin to sense the entire vascular system of the cranium breathing with PR. These arterial skills help the flow of oxygen into the brain.

6. Finish by leaving one hand on the superior sagittal sinus and moving your other hand to the sacrum.

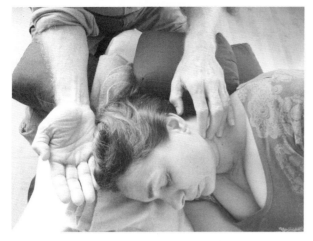

Fig. 25.28. Cerebrovascular balancing 5

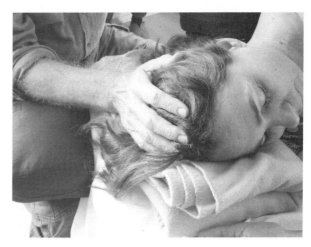

Fig. 25.29. Cerebrovascular balancing 6

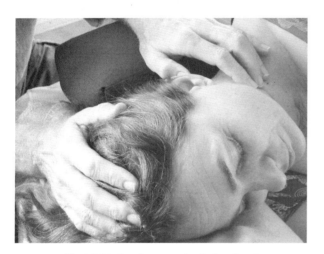

Fig. 25.30. Cerebrovascular balancing 7

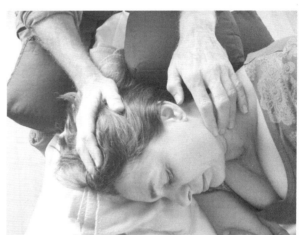

Fig. 25.31. Cerebrovascular balancing 8

❧ 6. Bilateral Anterior or Posterior Tibial Artery ❧

1. The client is supine. Sit at the foot of the table. Use the pads of the index and middle fingers on one hand to contact the anterior tibial artery on the corresponding foot of the client. Do the same with the other hand on the other foot (see figs. 24.16–17, page 323). Depending on the size of your hands and the client's feet, you might use one, two, or three fingers on each foot.

2. Practice a cycle of attunement by sensing your own heartbeat synchronizing with the client's arterial pulse. Then synchronize attention with PR in the heart field.

    Alternatively, you can practice the cycle of attunement with the posterior tibial artery by holding the client's heels in the palms of your hands in such a way that your index and middle fingers are just inferior to the medial malleolus see figs. 24.38–42, page 336).

The traditional foot contact is an option any time. It is to simply hold the heels of the client's feet without contacting the vascular system.

ᎧᎧ

Intermediate Visceral Metabolic Protocol Part I

Before beginning to read through this protocol, take a few moments to review the geography of the abdomen in figure 25.32 and the vascular anatomy shown in plates 32–33 in the color insert.

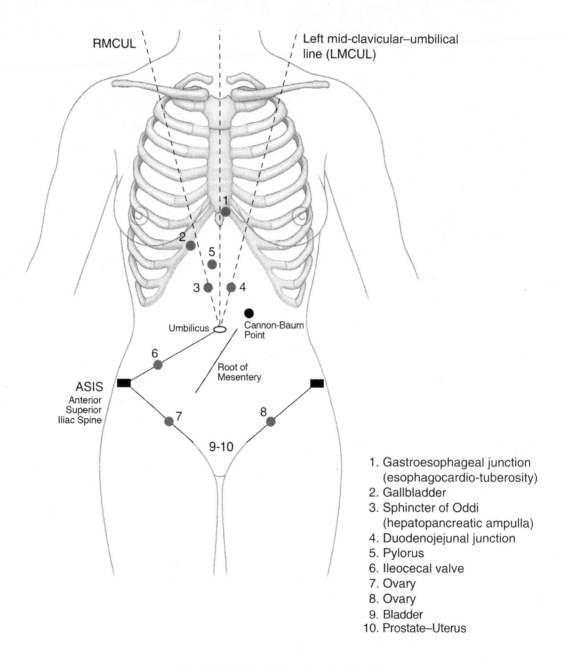

RMCUL

Left mid-clavicular–umbilical line (LMCUL)

Umbilicus

Cannon-Baum Point

Root of Mesentery

ASIS
Anterior Superior Iliac Spine

9-10

1. Gastroesophageal junction (esophagocardio-tuberosity)
2. Gallbladder
3. Sphincter of Oddi (hepatopancreatic ampulla)
4. Duodenojejunal junction
5. Pylorus
6. Ileocecal valve
7. Ovary
8. Ovary
9. Bladder
10. Prostate–Uterus

Fig. 25.32. Abdominal anatomy landmarks

The practice of using the hands palm up either singly or doubly is a repeating theme with all artery work. It involves knowing the relationship of Zones A and B. The vascular system derives from the fluid body, and the fluid body must be treated first and then intermittently throughout a session of artery work. In this way, biodynamic practice can bridge between the fluid body, cardiovascular system, and nervous system in each session. This is the sequence of how a body unfolds as an embryo. The intention is to find the Health in the viscera with PR.

For this protocol, the client is supine.

⤳ 1. Fluid Body, Umbilicus, Creation ⤳

1. Sit on one side of the table facing the client. Synchronize with PR and then make a heart-to-heart connection.

2. Negotiate permission to make contact. Then place both hands palm up over the umbilicus (see fig. 25.33). The location is specifically over the umbilicus where the creation energy of PR comes and goes in a spiral. Depending on the degree of inflammation in the client's abdomen, one hand is above the umbilicus and the other below. If the inflammation is severe enough, only one hand is necessary; the other hand rests without contact. Both hands synchronize with PR through the umbilicus. Practice a cycle of attunement out to nature and then into a heart-to-heart and then a heart-hands-heart connection with PR. Wait, watch, and wonder.

3. If the client is comfortable, place the tip of an index or middle finger directly and perpendicularly into the entrance of the umbilicus (see fig. 25.34). Direct the client to breathe directly into your fingertip at least three times or until your finger is allowed to deepen slightly into the umbilicus. Stop when you sense the abdominal aorta and resynchronize with PR. Wait for the client's potency or breath to push your finger out.

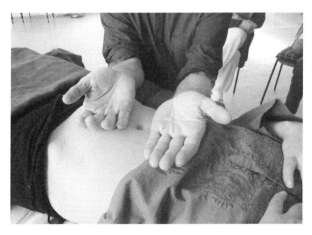

Fig. 25.33. Umbilicus 1

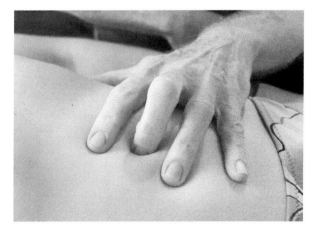

Fig. 25.34. Umbilicus 2

⌇ 2. Synchronizing Abdominal Heat with PR ⌇

1. Stand or sit on one side of the client's abdomen. Using your dominant hand, begin to make multiple hand placements, palm down, around the client's umbilicus in a clockwise direction (see figs. 25.35–38). The hand pauses for several seconds before moving. The territory covered is approximately the outline of the large intestine.

2. Using the base of the thumb—the most sensitive area in the palm for sensing heat—begin to sense variations in heat coming from the intestines and viscera. Make a mental note of which areas are warm, hot, or neutral. Stop in locations that magnetize the contact, and synchronize the heat and your hand with PR. Go around the umbilicus several times until the heat seems evenly distributed.

PR is the movement of abdominal fire and all the elements. After you contact the heat with PR, PR contacts the arteries. The arteries and blood are of the water element.

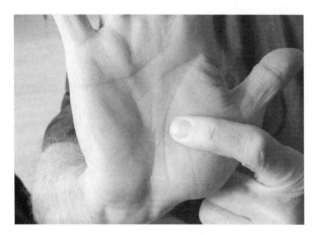

Fig. 25.35. The sensitive base of the thumb

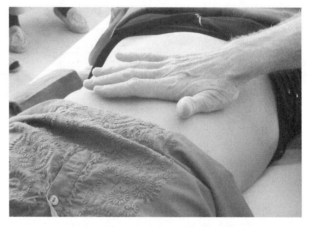

Fig. 25.36. Synchronizing abdominal 1

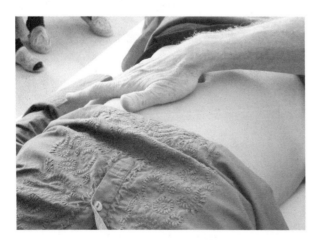

Fig. 25.37. Synchronizing abdominal 2

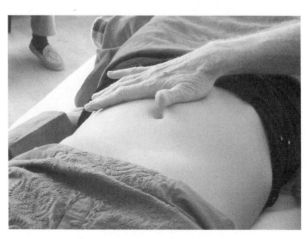

Fig. 25.38. Synchronizing abdominal 3

⌇ 3. Developmental Liver Movement and Truncus Coeliacus Artery ⌇

1. Sit on the right side of the client in such a way that you can place one hand under ribs 9, 10, and 11 (see fig. 25.39) and use the other hand to contact the truncus coeliacus artery several inches below the xiphoid process (see fig. 25.40). Take a few moments to synchronize with the truncus coeliacus. The hepatic artery originates here and carries the superior branch of the dorsal vagus to the liver. The dorsal vagus monitors glucose metabolism and the metabolic function of the liver. Synchronize with PR between your hands. Differentiate the artery from the abdominal aorta.

2. Keeping the hand below the ribs in place, move the top hand from the artery to the area over the costal arch approximating the location of the entire liver (see figs. 25.41–42). The liver moves on a mechanical axis from a point just below the nipple of the left breast. As best you can, use the middle fingers of each hand above and below to approximate that axis. The liver can rotate

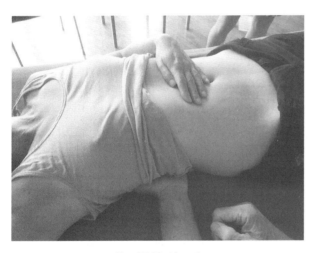

Fig. 25.39. Liver 1

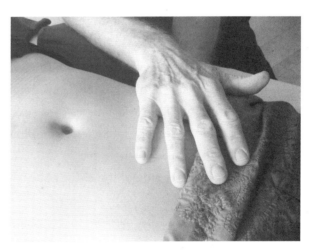

Fig. 25.40. Liver 2

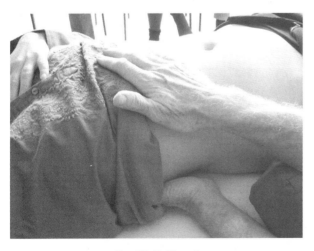

Fig. 25.41. Liver 3

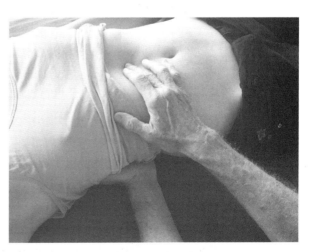

Fig. 25.42. Liver 4

around that axis with breathing and its own natural motility. It can also swing like a pendulum toward the umbilicus and back. Its developmental motion is a breathing-type motion toward the heart with PR. The motion feels almost like bellows used to fan a fire.

Synchronize with the liver's developmental motion and begin to sense this movement in the tempo of PR.

↭ 4. Radial and Subclavian Arteries ↝

1. Sit at the side of the table and practice a cycle of attunement.
2. Contact the radial artery with one hand and place your other hand palm up on the same shoulder (see figs. 25.12–13, page 363).
3. Switch the hand on the shoulder from palm up to contact with the subclavian artery (see fig. 25.14, page 363). This is a good way to stabilize the heart-brain connection via the subclavian artery.

↭ 5. Superior Mesenteric, Radial, Subclavian, and Tibial Arteries ↝

The superior mesenteric artery branches from the abdominal aorta about three client fingers' width above the umbilicus, emerging from the abdominal aorta in between the right and left renal arteries (see fig. 25.43). Note the relative location of both the superior mesenteric and inferior mesenteric arteries in figure 25.44.

1. Sit at one side of the client's abdomen. Practice belly breathing and synchronize with PR.
2. Negotiate permission to contact, then use one hand to make contact with the radial artery. With your other hand, make light contact with the area of the superior mesenteric artery, three fingers' width above the umbilicus (see fig. 25.45). Observe the rise and fall of your client's transversus abdominus muscle. Differentiate the abdominal aorta from the superior mesenteric artery. Gradually allow the pads of your fingers to sink very slowly until they contact the pulse or flow of the superior mesenteric artery. Once you've made contact, resynchronize with your own sense of PR—natural world, heart-to-heart and heart-to-hands. Wait until PR is expressed between the two arteries. This may involve sensing the total contents of the mesenteries to move in a clockwise and counterclockwise motion. This is the original embryonic developmental motion that occurred around the mesenteric artery.
3. Have one hand stay in contact with the superior mesenteric artery, and use your other hand to contact the subclavian artery (see fig. 25.46). Sense PR in this branch of the vascular tree moving like an accordion between your hands.

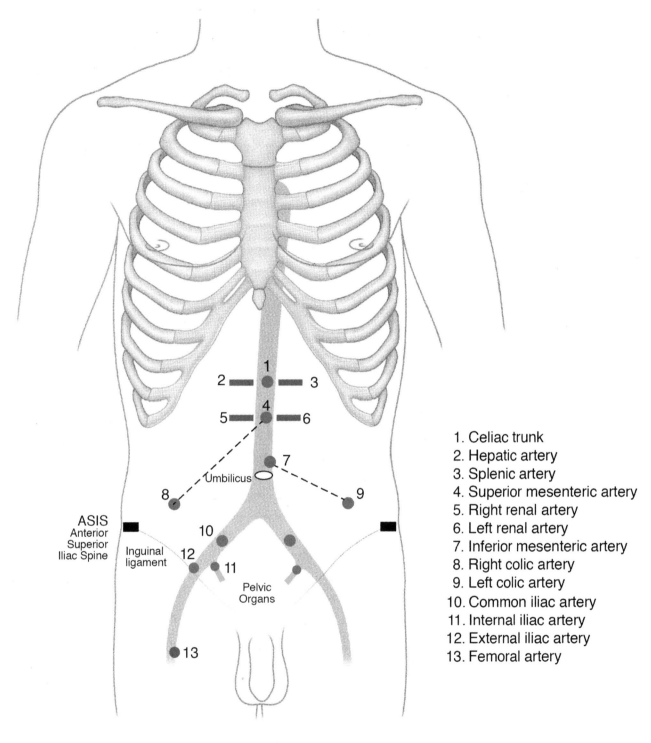

Fig. 25.43. The abdominal pulses

1. Celiac trunk
2. Hepatic artery
3. Splenic artery
4. Superior mesenteric artery
5. Right renal artery
6. Left renal artery
7. Inferior mesenteric artery
8. Right colic artery
9. Left colic artery
10. Common iliac artery
11. Internal iliac artery
12. External iliac artery
13. Femoral artery

4. Shift the hand in contact with the subclavian artery to the anterior tibial artery (see figs. 25.46–48). You will need to change hands on the superior mesenteric artery to do this. Attempt to sense PR breathing in this part of the vascular tree. PR breathes between your hands like an accordion opening and closing.

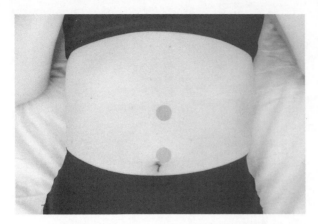

Fig. 25.44. Location of superior (upper dot) and
inferior (lower dot) mesenteric arteries

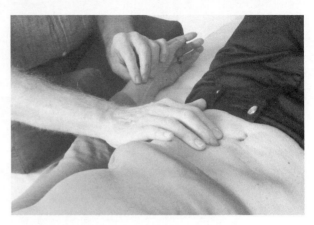

Fig. 25.45. Superior mesenteric and radial arteries

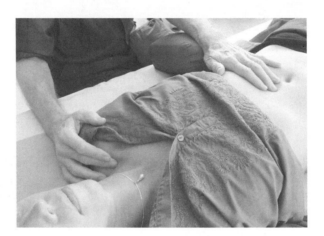

Fig. 25.46. Superior mesenteric and subclavian arteries

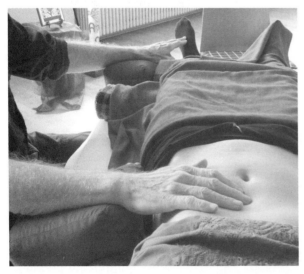

Fig. 25.47. Superior mesenteric and
anterior tibial arteries 1

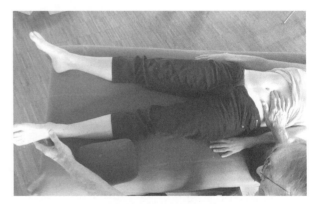

Fig. 25.48. Superior mesenteric and
anterior tibial arteries 2

◌ 6. Right Colic and Superior Mesenteric Arteries ◌

The dots on figure 25.49 show the relative locations of the superior mesenteric and right colic arteries.

1. Sit at the right-hand side of the client's abdomen. Use your right hand to gently palpate the shape of the ascending colon, which is directly underneath the anterior abdominal wall or musculature.

2. Use as many fingers as possible from your right hand to find the medial edge of the ascending colon, where the right colic artery and other branches of the superior mesenteric artery are located. This artery is located approximately at the midpoint of the ascending colon on its medial side. Use your left hand to contact the superior mesenteric artery, the originating source of the right colic artery (see fig. 25.50).

3. Synchronize attention with PR between your hands as the artery and its blood flow breathes with PR. The large intestine may also begin to expand, contract, and rotate on its clockwise and counterclockwise developmental axis in the tempo of PR.

Many clients have functional constipation, and this palpation may be helpful when combined with a more optimal lifestyle.

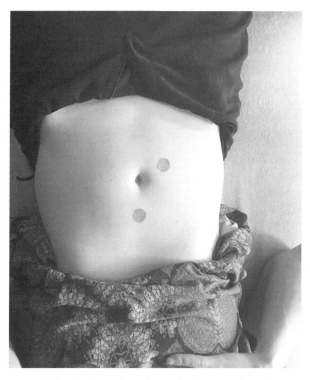

Fig. 25.49. Location of superior mesenteric and right colic arteries

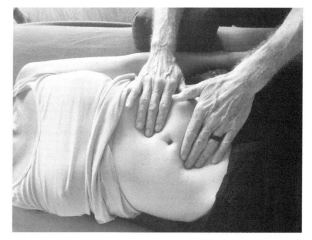

Fig. 25.50. Palpating the superior mesenteric and right colic arteries

◂ 7. Left Colic and Inferior Mesenteric Arteries ◂

The dots on figure 25.51 show the location of the inferior mesenteric and left colic arteries.

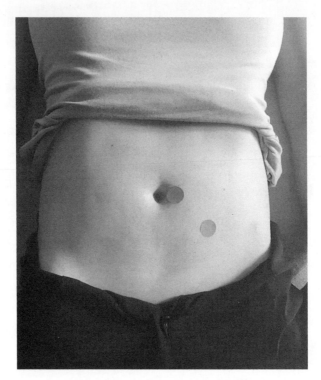

*Fig. 25.51. Location of inferior mesenteric and
left colic arteries*

1. Sit at the left-hand side of the client's abdomen. Use your left hand to gently palpate the shape of the descending colon, which is underneath the small intestine. Since the left colic artery is deeper than the right colic artery, palpation must be done slowly, with the fingers delicately moving down toward the artery in a pendulum type of motion.

2. Use as many fingers as possible from your left hand to find the medial edge of the descending colon, where the left colic artery and other branches of the inferior mesenteric artery are located. This artery is located approximately at the midpoint of the descending colon on its medial side. Use your right hand to contact the inferior mesenteric artery, the originating source of the left colic artery (see fig. 25.52). It is located within an inch above or to the left side of the umbilicus.

3. Synchronize attention with PR between your hands as the artery itself breathes with PR (see figs. 25.53–54). The large intestine may also begin to expand, contract, and rotate on its developmental axis in the tempo of PR.

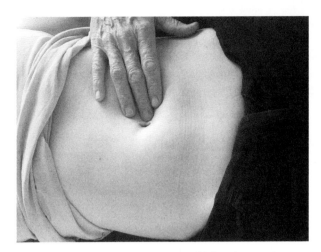

Fig. 25.52. Inferior mesenteric and left colic arteries 1

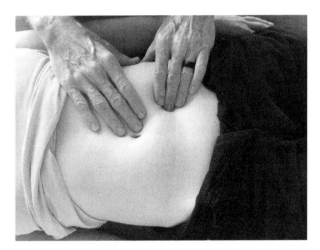

Fig. 25.53. Inferior mesenteric and left colic arteries 2

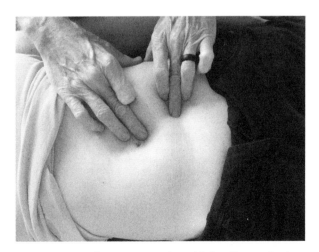

Fig. 25.54. Inferior mesenteric and left colic arteries 3

∾ 8. Coccyx: Three Variations ∾

1. The relative location of the sacrum is shown in figure 25.55. Approaching from the side, place your dominant hand under the client's leg by the gluteal fold. Use your middle finger (or longest finger or most comfortable finger) to gently contact the coccyx and then relax adjacent to the coccyx. Do not lift the sacrum. Reorient, resynchronize, and practice a cycle of attunement.

2. Place your free hand in one of three locations:

• **Variation 1:** Place the middle finger of your free hand in the umbilicus (see fig. 25.56).

• **Variation 2:** Contact the radial artery of the client with your free hand (see fig. 25.57).

• **Variation 3:** Place your free hand palm up or down over the umbilicus

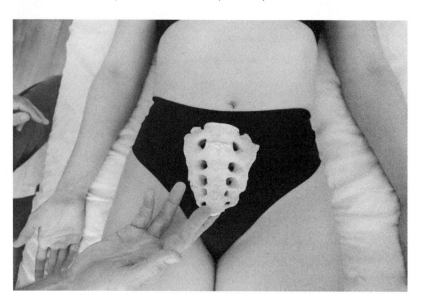

Fig. 25.55. Coccyx

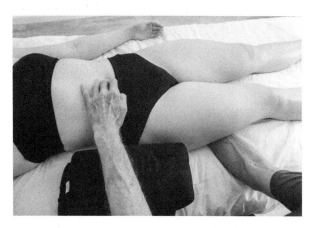

Fig. 25.56. Variation 1: coccyx and umbilicus

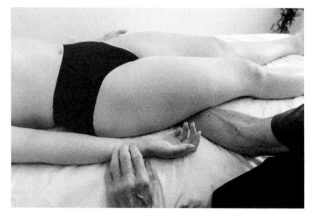

Fig. 25.57. Variation 2: coccyx and radial artery

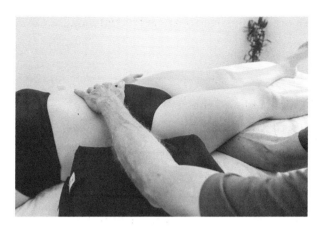

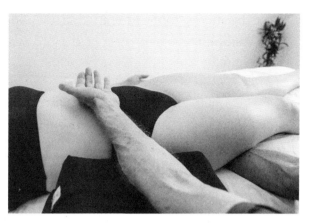

Fig. 25.58. Variation 3: coccyx with palm down over umbilicus

Fig. 25.59. Variation 3: coccyx with palm up over umbilicus

(see figs. 25.58–59). You may sense the space all around and in the sacrum breathe and come alive with PR like a flower opening and closing. Practice several cycles of attunement. Wait for both hands to synchronize with PR simultaneously by igniting heart-to-heart with PR. Remember that palm up is a method for holding Zone B of the client. At the same time, it is a gesture of invocation. In Taoist cosmology, the universe enters and exits the umbilicus. The energy of the entire ancestral lineage constantly moves through the umbilicus.

Practitioner Tip

Double-sheeting makes it much easier to contact the coccyx in a session; you simply slide your hand between the sheets to comfortably contact the coccyx. For the sake of showing a more precise location of the contact in the photos for this sequence, I did not double-sheet. And sometimes I forget to double-sheet, in which case I ask the client to flex their knee and press down on their foot to lift their pelvis to make it easier to find the coccyx.

These windows help normalize the ANS of the client. They function to harmonize the sacral outflow of the parasympathetic nervous system (PNS) and its connections to the vagus nerve via the hypogastric plexus in the abdomen and the vascular tree at the radial artery. This means that the ANS needs to have a relative amount of equilibrium for PR to express its healing priorities (or for PR to automatically shift from its maintenance mode to repair mode). Every system and function of the body holds stress in its own way and dissipates it in its own way, especially the fluid body. The most important instruction for the practitioner is to continually synchronize with PR by attuning to the natural world, the abdominal breath, the heartbeat, and its potency, and resting in awareness of stillness when it appears.

How to Determine Which Side of the Abdominal Arteries to Contact

It is not always necessary to work both sides of the arteries, especially the iliac arteries or vascular tree. Even the arteries in the neck can be worked ipsilaterally, especially if the ANS of the client is not resilient. In clinical practice, the side to work on can be determined with bilateral contact on either of the tibial arteries. Direct palpation of the abdomen can also indicate which side is preferred. Or a side can be chosen based only on the intuition of the therapist. If time permits and the client is resilient, working both sides of an artery is okay.

Ꮛᴏᏻ

Intermediate Visceral Metabolic Protocol Part 2

⌁ 1. Styloid Process and Vagus Nerve ⌁

The location of the styloid process can be seen in figures 25.60–61.

Sit at the head of the table, sensing your heart moving back as your arms stretch forward. Make delicate contact with the tips or pads of the index fingers near but

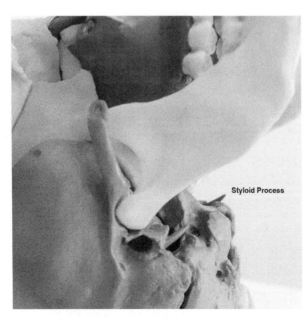

Fig. 25.60. Location of the styloid process

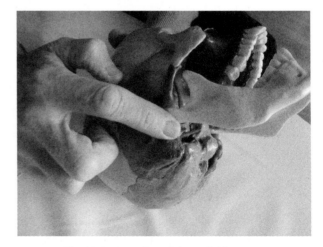

Fig. 25.61. Location of the styloid process

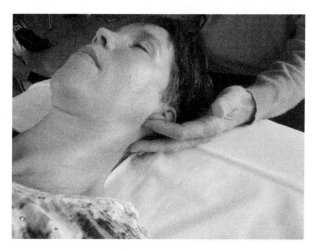

Fig. 25.62. Styloid process and vagus nerve

not directly on the styloid process bilaterally (see fig. 26.62). Sense the stillness in the jugular vein. Practice several cycles of attunement until the stillness permeates the client's vascular tree. The intention is to stimulate the vagus nerve to stimulate an anti-inflammatory response in the abdomen.

⌁ 2. Coccyx and Respiratory Diaphragm ⌁

Place the fingertips of one hand under the client's body close to the coccyx. Place your other hand under the floating ribs below the diaphragm (see figs. 24.11–12, page 322). Wait for the pelvic and respiratory diaphragms to synchronize. Then if PR starts to move in the fluid body, melt your hands into the table to synchronize with the stillness.

This type of synchronizing is important at all phases of biodynamic cardiovascular therapy. The stillness is a deep part of the cardiovascular system, especially the center of blood flow. All molecules in the visible universe must achieve a stillpoint for transformation. We synchronize with the stillness to restore optimal metabolic function.

⌁ 3. Portal Vein and Mesentery ⌁

The anatomy of the portal vein area can be seen in figure 25.67 on page 385.

1. Approaching the client from the side, use both hands to span the width of the rectus abdominis muscle on either side of the umbilicus. Place the tips of your thumbs on one edge of the rectus abdominis and the remaining fingers on the opposite edge of the rectus abdominis. Sense the developmental motion of the intestines in their clockwise and counterclockwise motions around the umbilicus in the tempo of PR.

2. Gently and slowly allow your hands to lift the whole mesentery. Conduct a motion test by moving your hands mechanically in a clockwise and counterclockwise motion (see figs. 25.63–66).

3. The root of the mesentery is on a diagonal line from the approximate location of the inferior mesenteric artery to the ileocecal valve at the beginning of the large intestine (see fig. 25.68). The inferior mesenteric artery is close to the duodenojejunal junction (DJJ), where the duodenum merges with the small intestine.

Approach from the left side of the client. On this diagonal line, starting by the left anterior superior iliac spine (ASIS), gradually scoop, lift, or push the mesentery toward the liver to flush the portal vein system (see figs. 25.69–74). Do not go beyond any tissue barrier palpated in either position. Use at least four hand positions, as the intention is not to do a fascial glide all the way to the liver but rather to move a segment at a time to maximize the therapeutic benefit for both the mesentery and portal vein system. Let the client's breath contact with the heel of your hand and sense if the breath invites a deeper palpation with the exhalation phase, without going beyond a tissue barrier.

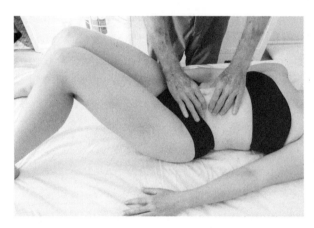

Fig. 25.63. Mesentery lift 1

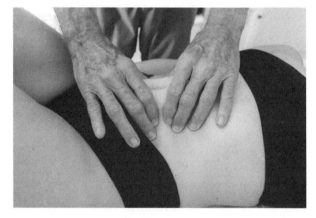

Fig. 25.64. Mesentery lift 2

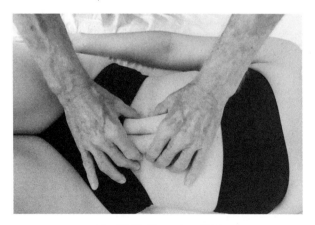

Fig. 25.65. Mesentery lift 3

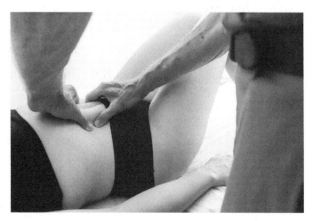

Fig. 25.66. Mesentery lift 4

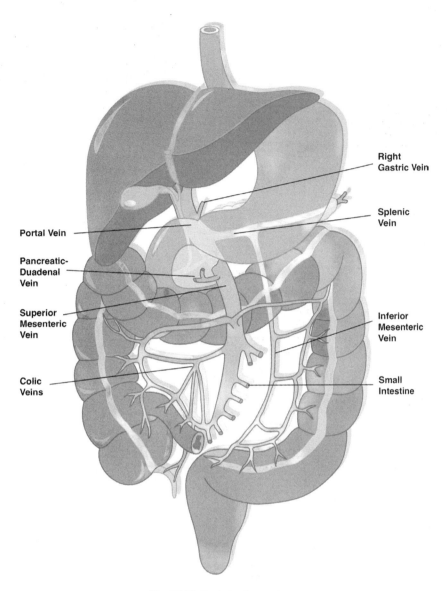

Fig. 25.67. Portal vein anatomy

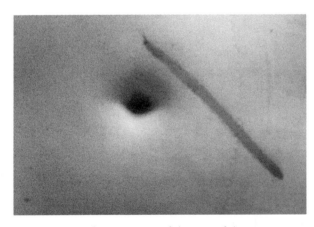

Fig. 25.68. Surface anatomy of the root of the mesentery

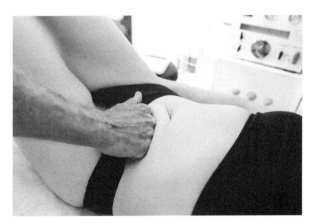

Fig. 25.69. Mesentery and portal vein 1

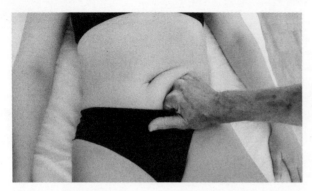

Fig. 25.70. Mesentery and portal vein 2

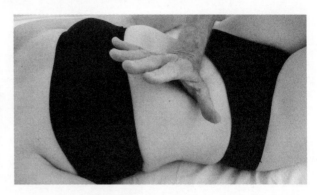

Fig. 25.71. Mesentery and portal vein 3

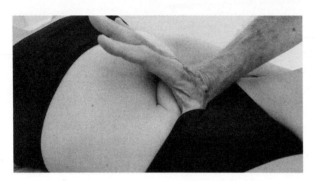

Fig. 25.72. Mesentery and portal vein 4

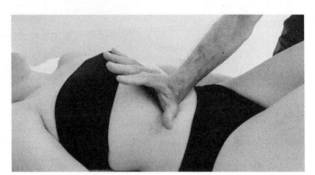

Fig. 25.73. Mesentery and portal vein 5

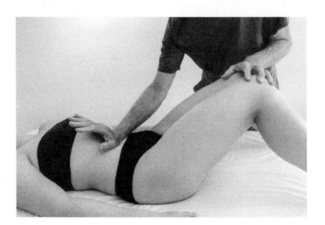

Fig. 25.74. Mesentery and portal vein 6

This practice also treats all the ANS abdominal plexuses, including the vagus nerve embedded in those plexuses. It also treats the abdominopelvic lymphatic system.

⌁ 4. Superior and Inferior Mesenteric Arteries ⌁

The dots in figure 25.75 indicate the relative locations of the superior and inferior mesenteric arteries. I am using my index finger to point out the relative locations of these two arteries in figures 25.76 (superior) and 25.77 (inferior).

Approach from the left side of the client's abdomen. The client's knees can be

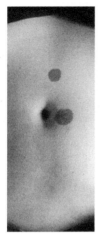

Fig. 25.75. Location of superior and
inferior mesenteric arteries

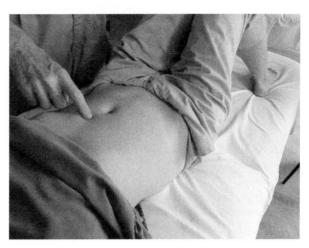

Fig. 25.76. Location of superior mesenteric artery

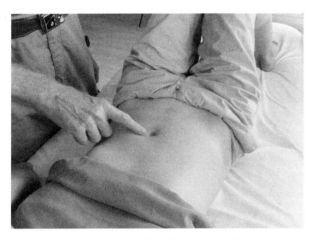

Fig. 25.77. Location of inferior mesenteric artery

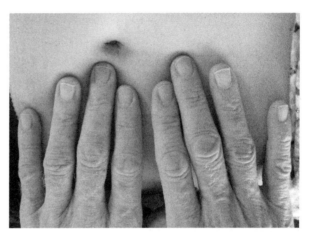

Fig. 25.78. Superior and inferior mesenteric arteries

flexed, relaxed, and together, with the feet spread laterally if necessary. Abdominal arteries are palpated using a broad surface of the pads of the fingers while making a slow circular motion down toward the artery. Pause every few seconds and listen for the pulse. Contact the superior mesenteric artery first and differentiate it from the abdominal aorta. Use your free hand to then contact the inferior mesenteric artery (see fig. 25.78). At the same time, wait for the client's breath to come into the point of contact with your fingers. Wait for the exhalation to pull your fingers deeper into contact with the artery.

∻ 5. Inferior Mesenteric, Radial, Subclavian, and Tibial Arteries ∾

1. Approach from the left side of the client's abdomen. The client's knees can be flexed, relaxed, and together, with the feet spread laterally if necessary. To contact the inferior mesenteric artery, use the pads of the index and middle fingers of one hand to contact the abdominal aorta and slowly withdraw until

the artery is sensed. Alternatively, start at the surface around the umbilicus and slowly search with incremental micropressure spirals. The inferior mesenteric artery is deeper than the superior mesenteric artery. It is located on a plane within an inch above or to the left side of the umbilicus.

2. Once you have contacted the inferior mesenteric artery, use your free hand to contact the radial artery on the left wrist (see fig. 25.79). Practice a cycle of attunement.

3. Switch from the radial to the subclavian artery on the left. Practice a cycle of attunement (see fig. 25.80).

4. Finally, contact the inferior mesenteric and anterior tibial arteries with the finger pads of each hand. Practice a cycle of attunement (see fig. 25.81).

∽ 6. Differentiating Common, Internal, and External Iliac Arteries ∽

1. The client's knees can be flexed and resting together. Bilaterally or ipsilaterally, gently trace the pathway of the lower abdominal aorta to the bifurcation of the common iliac artery. Then palpate the common iliac artery to the

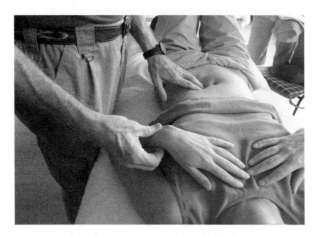

Fig. 25.79. Inferior mesenteric and radial arteries

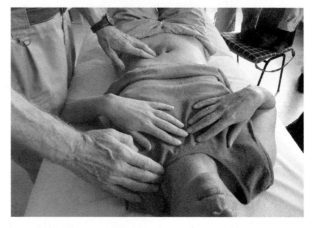

Fig. 25.80. Inferior mesenteric and subclavian arteries

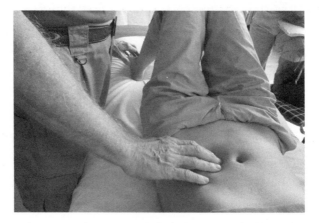

Fig. 25.81. Inferior mesenteric and anterior tibial arteries

bifurcation of the internal iliac artery (see figs. 25.82–85). This is usually at the level of the sacroiliac-joint space; the basic landmark is the line that bisects the anterior superior iliac spines (ASIS), although the abdominal aorta could end above that line in some clients. Figure 25.86 shows the palpation of the common iliac arteries.

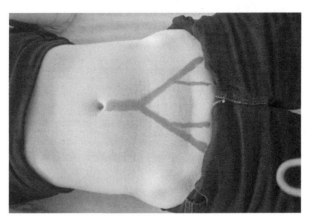

Fig. 25.82. Iliac arteries

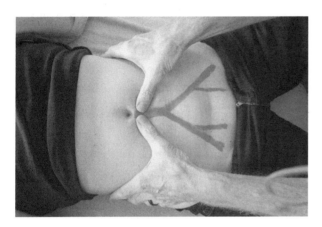

Fig. 25.83. Abdominal aorta to common iliac arteries 1

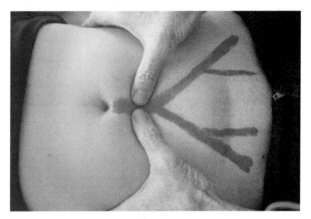

Fig. 25.84. Abdominal aorta to common iliac arteries 2

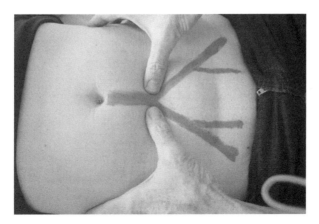

Fig. 25.85. Abdominal aorta to common iliac arteries 3

Practitioner Tip

Figure 25.82 shows the basic surface anatomy for the iliac arteries. If you are new to this palpation, begin exploration ipsilaterally, starting on the right side of the client's abdomen. Using the finger pads of one or both hands, find the bifurcation of the common iliac artery at the distal end of the abdominal aorta. This is usually at the level of the ASIS and the fourth lumbar vertebra. I use what I call the three-breath rule of thumb. I have the client breathe directly into the point of contact. I wait three breaths for the client's breath to contact my fingers and invite me deeper. This usually happens within three cycles of the client's breath.

2. Locate the internal iliac artery, which branches into the pelvic floor midway between the terminating point of the abdominal aorta and the inguinal ligament (see figs. 25.87–88). The majority of the blood supply to the pelvic floor is coming from the internal iliac artery. This is also the location of the hypogastric

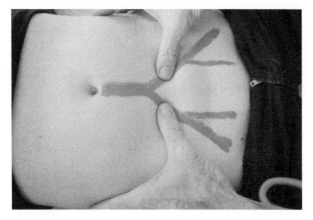

Fig. 25.86. Common to internal iliac arteries 1

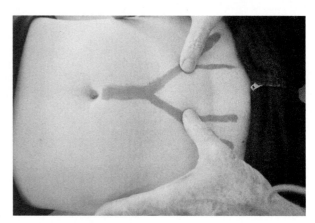

Fig. 25.87. Common to internal iliac arteries 2

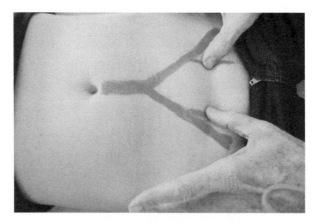

Fig. 25.88. Internal iliac arteries 3

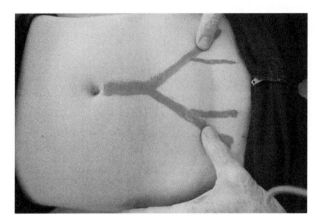

Fig. 25.89. External iliac arteries 1

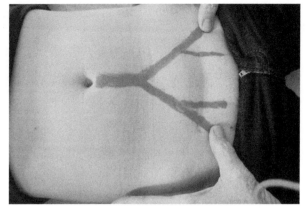

Fig. 25.90. External iliac arteries 2

plexus and its transition zone with the sacral outflow of the PNS between the abdomen and pelvis. Use the three-breath rule of thumb and have the client breathe directly into the point of contact.

3. Now palpate the external iliac artery, which is close to the inguinal ligament (see figs. 25.89–90).

The iliac arteries represent a transition zone between the abdominal and pelvic vascular systems. In addition, there is a transition in the fascial planes and an area of lymph nodes by the inguinal ligament.

⌁ 7. Inferior Iliac, Femoral, and Tibial Arteries ⌁

1. Contact the inferior iliac artery with one hand. Use your other hand to contact the femoral artery at midthigh rather than near the inguinal ligament (see figs. 25.91–92). Here the femoral artery is in the septum between the quadriceps muscle and the adductor muscle. As above, wait for the client's breath to contact your fingers and invite them deeper. Practice a cycle of attunement.

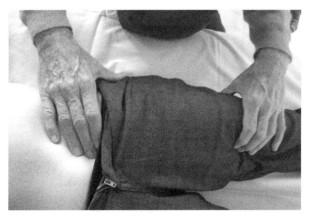

Fig. 25.91. Internal Iliac and femoral arteries 1

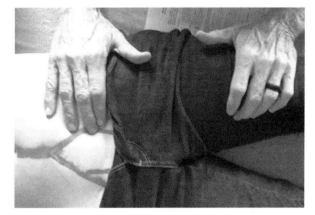

Fig. 25.92. Internal iliac and femoral arteries 2

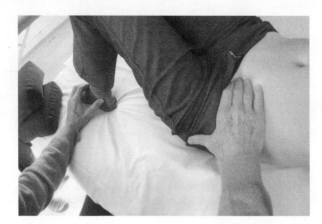

Fig. 25.93. Internal iliac and anterior tibial arteries

2. Shift from the femoral artery at midthigh to the anterior tibial artery on the same side (see fig. 25.93).

Practice on both sides if you are inspired to do so. Usually one leg has more lymphatic congestion than the other; choose the side that has the most congestion to start.

If the internal iliac artery is too difficult to palpate, such as with a client who is obese, then palpate the external iliac arteries as they surface by the inguinal ligaments. This can be done bilaterally or ipsilaterally. If ipsilaterally, then use your free hand to palpate a convenient artery, especially the femoral artery, as described here.

⁓ 8. Bladder ⁓

Place one hand palm down or palm up on the superior border of the pubic symphysis, with your fingers pointing toward the client's head (see figs. 25.94–95). Sense

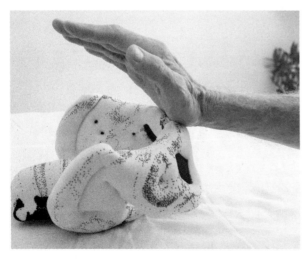

Fig. 25.94. Bladder 1

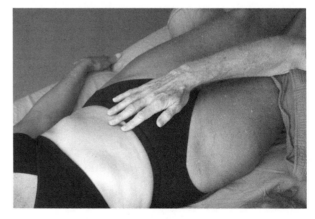

Fig. 25.95. Bladder 2

the rocking movement of the bladder and the uterus or prostate. Wait for PR. Your other hand may palpate the radial artery or simply rest without contact.

◅ 9. Coccyx and Cannon's Point ◃

Figure 25.96 shows the relative location of the superior and inferior mesenteric arteries in relation to Cannon's point. Contact the coccyx with one hand. Use the finger pads of your other hand to contact Cannon's point, close to where the stomach attaches to the transverse colon (see figs. 25.97–98). This is the point where the vagus nerve terminates and the sacral PNS begins. This is where the superior mesenteric artery ends and the inferior mesenteric artery begins. Practice a cycle of attunement and wait for the client's breath to invite you deeper.

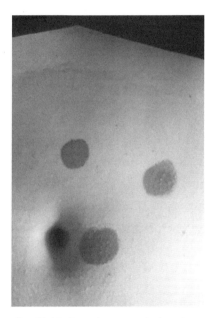

Fig. 25.96. Superior mesenteric artery,
inferior mesenteric artery, and Cannon's point

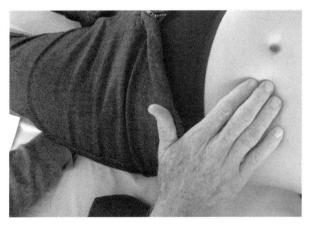

Fig. 25.97. Coccyx and Cannon's point 1

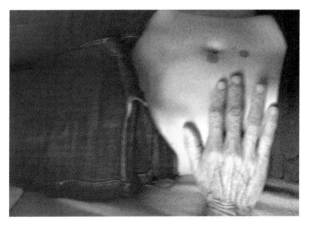

Fig. 25.98. Coccyx and Cannon's point 2

The Obese Abdomen

With an obese client, it is unlikely that the abdominal aorta and its arteries can be palpated. In these clients, skin-to-skin contact can be made over the abdomen to sense and synchronize with the blood flow under the skin in PR. This can be done directly over the umbilicus. Holding the liver from the right side, with one hand on top and the other below the liver, is also valuable; sense PR breathing the liver and its vascular tree.

Another option is to have one hand under the liver and the other hand contacting the femoral artery below the inguinal ligament. Yet another option is to have one hand under the liver and the other hand contacting the subclavian artery at the level of the midclavicle. Finally, I recommend contact around the inguinal ligaments and costal arch because of an increase in fascial tension and lymphatic restriction there. It is appropriate to explore fascial release in those areas.

Now that I have demonstrated the basic and intermediate biodynamic cardiovascular protocols, we can turn our attention to an advanced understanding of BCVT. This next chapter by K. Michelle Doyle, a gifted midwife, demonstrates BCVT with a pregnant mom. What follows now is advanced work. Practitioners must be familiar with these last two chapters before proceeding in clinical practice, especially with pregnant moms.

26

Biodynamic Cardiovascular Therapy during Pregnancy

K. Michelle Doyle

K. Michelle Doyle is both a certified nurse midwife and a certified biodynamic craniosacral therapist. Weaving these two professions together provides Michelle with unending joy.

Please note that a complete view of all the arteries of the body can be seen in the color insert, plates 25–35. These can be reviewed prior to or during the study of the following protocol. Of special interest is the embryology of the heart, as shown in plates 1–24, which should be studied before any biodynamic practice with a pregnant mom. In addition, chapters 6, 7, and 8 must be read before practicing the following work.

This chapter explores biodynamic cardiovascular therapy (BCVT) with a pregnant mom. My model in the photographs is Amie. She is thirty-seven weeks pregnant. You can see the smile on her face at the end of the session (fig. 26.1).

There are several considerations for exploring this protocol. First, be willing to create a narrative and explain to mom where you are and what you are doing in simple, brief statements as the session unfolds. Always be sure there are pauses and stillpoints in the narrative to allow the health of Primary Respiration (PR) to manifest its unerring potency. This requires the practice of a regular cycle of attunement. The practice begins with the perception of your own internal states of mind and body. Your own posture, breath, and heartbeat are the basis of interoceptive awareness to ignite empathy and to allow PR to manifest its therapeutic movement between your heart, the client's heart, and, in the case of a pregnant mom, the baby's heart as well. You will make a heart-to-heart connection with PR as a regular phase of the cycle of attunement. Mom's blood volume has increased by some 50 percent during her pregnancy, and this protocol can really help balance mom's metabolism by supporting her cardiovascular system.

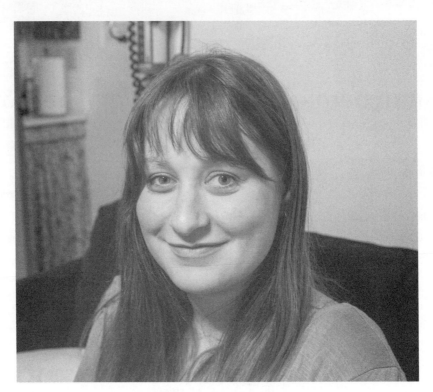

Fig. 26.1. Happy mom

Second, sometimes the baby will become active during a session, and of course the intention with the protocol is that mom and baby become more deeply synchronized to support optimal vascular and metabolic well-being. It is really okay if baby becomes active and excited by the unerring potency of PR. Some babies like to dance with PR. In addition, baby's heart rate variability (HRV), a measure of vagal tone in the developing heart and vascular system, is synchronized with mom's HRV. A BCVT session will optimize baby's and mom's HRV. How wonderful to have a resilient heart. You can speak directly to the baby and acknowledge the activity as playful. Mom can also acknowledge baby's activity. She knows her baby's movements, and this protocol includes teaching mom how to palpate her baby's vascular system for deeper, more optimal heart synchronization to manifest. Therapeutic relationships throughout life are largely based on the prenatal development of the baby's heart and its reference point of mom's heart and blood.

Third, the session is about establishing a flow that includes multiple cycles of attunement as all three members of the session are synchronized at the heart level of safety and spirit manifesting in the deep heart.

Last, remember that the goal is to create a safe therapeutic space where mother and baby can deepen into their synchronistic relationship supported by PR. The following protocol is not a road map to be strictly followed but merely the suggestions of an experienced tour guide. Enjoy!

ᘒᘒ
Metabolic Protocol for Pregnant Moms

⌁ 1. Kidney Breathing, Fascial Tension, and Interstitium ⌁

1. Practice a cycle of attunement (see page 320).

2. Invite mom to be mindful with her breathing. Take several minutes with this.

3. Gently contact the kidney 1 meridian point bilaterally on the client's feet (see figs. 26.2–5).

4. Invite the client to imagine that she is inhaling and exhaling through the bottom of her feet.

5. Gradually invite the client to imagine the breath is coming up her legs, through her pelvis, and wrapping around her kidneys. Point out to the client that the kidneys are in back of the intestines and so forth. The fascial system gets engaged and can be felt in this location on the plantar fascia of the feet.

6. Invite the client to imagine that as she is exhaling, the breath is leaving her kidneys, going down her legs, and exiting from the bottom of her feet. Fascial tension may manifest as a variety of movements perceived by your thumbs.

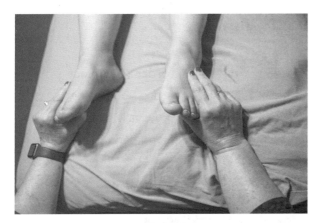

Fig. 26.2. Kidney breathing and fascial tension 1

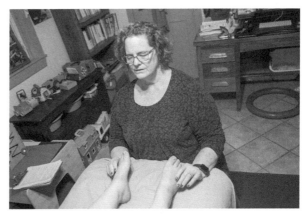

Fig. 26.3. Kidney breathing and fascial tension 2

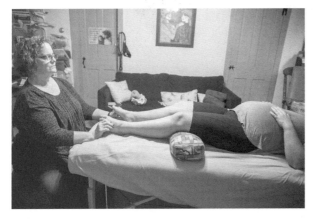

Fig. 26.4. Kidney breathing and fascial tension 3

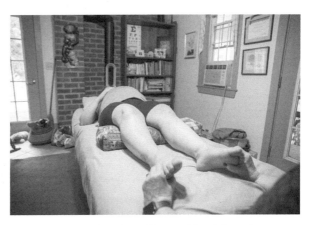

Fig. 26.5. Kidney breathing and fascial tension 4

7. Invite the client to do this practice slowly, with a six-second or longer inhalation and a six-second or longer exhalation. When the breath slows down even a little, the autonomic nervous system (ANS) of the client can rebalance gently.

8. Now move your thumbs inferiorly on the plantar fascia to a point on the edge of where the central and lateral pads of the plantar fascia insert on the calcaneus. The heel bone is covered with a dense pad of fat, and your fingers are bilaterally on the edge of that pad of fat in the central portion of the pad. From here, put your attention on the interstitium of mom's body. The interstitium is the total of all biological water outside all the cells in the body and bounded by the fascial system of the body. The interstitium is a major player in the optimal function of the fascia and the immune, lymphatic, and cardiovascular systems. When synchronized with PR, the interstitium floats and makes gentle waves. It is an organ of detoxification as well, and mom has a lot of waste products she is dealing with in her body from her and her baby. This is a gentle way to promote the drainage of waste products metabolically.

9. Finish the practice by removing your hands and asking the client to be mindful of her breathing, this time not focusing on her feet.

⌁ 2. Bilateral Posterior Tibial Artery ⌁

1. Sit at the end of the table.

2. Use one hand to contact the posterior border of the tibia in order to contact the posterior tibial artery close to the medial malleoli. Then use your other hand to contact the same on the other foot (see figs. 26.6–7). Usually two or three fingers are used with each hand to palpate the arteries. You can choose which parts of the artery to connect with.

3. Synchronize attention with PR.

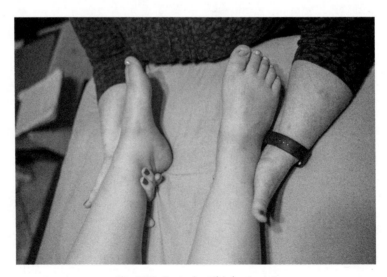

Fig. 26.6. Posterior tibial artery 1

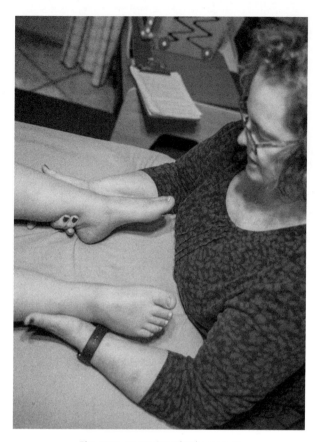

Fig. 26.7. Posterior tibial artery 2

When working with women who are pregnant, the posterior tibial artery can be very supportive to the kidneys and the whole vascular tree.

Practitioner Tip

Mom can easily get tired standing on her feet, and consequently these initial phases of a session support her low back and lower extremities. You can choose which specific parts of the posterior and anterior tibial arteries to connect with while you are working heart-to-heart with PR.

⌁ 3. Bilateral Anterior Tibial Artery ⌁

1. Sit at the foot of the table.
2. Use the pads of the index and middle fingers on one hand to contact the anterior tibial artery on the corresponding foot of the client. Use your other hand to do the same on the other foot (see figs. 26.8–9).

3. Differentiate between the anterior tibial artery and its distal end toward the big toe, called dorsalis pedis. Choose which is the easiest part of the artery to contact. Depending on the size of your hands and the client's feet, you might use one, two, or three fingers on each foot.

4. Synchronize attention with PR and notice mom settling, as seen in figure 26.10.

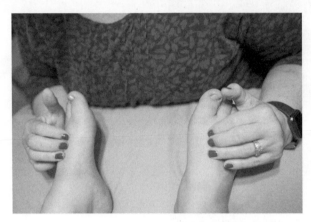

Fig. 26.8. Anterior tibial artery 1

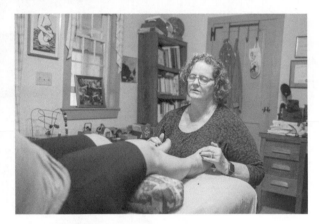

Fig. 26.9. Anterior tibial artery 2

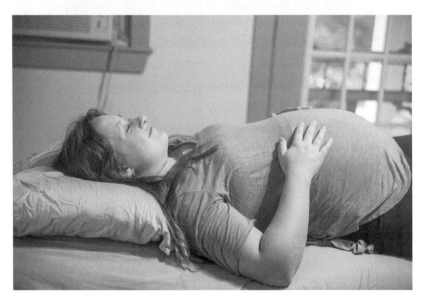

Fig. 26.10. Mom receiving treatment

⌁ 4. Heart and Birth Canal ⌁

1. The pregnant mom will need to be in a semireclining (supine) position. Lots of pillows will be needed to prop her up, especially in the later stages of her pregnancy.

2. While sitting at the client's feet, make bilateral contact with whichever tibial artery is easier to contact.

3. Practice a cycle of heart attunement in which you sense PR moving through your heart and toward the birth canal of the pregnant mom. PR has a strong movement through the birth canal (midline), and the infant will be attracted to orient to that midline for birth. While you are sensing PR through your own heart, contact both the mother's PR coming through her birth canal and the synchronized heart-to-heart connection between the mother and her baby.

4. When you feel that you have reached the end of this practice, invite the pregnant mom to be mindful of her breathing to finish.

⌇ 5. The Vascular Tree ⌇

1. Practice several cycles of heart attunement with the hands palm up over the leg and shoulder in a modified pietà position to contact the fluid body above the client. Then switch to palms under the shoulder and leg (see figs. 26.11–12).

2. Sit at the side of the table, and after settling with a cycle of attunement, negotiate permission to contact the vascular tree of the client.

3. Make contact with the radial artery with the finger pads of one hand cupping under or over the wrist of the client. Place the fingers of your other hand over the lower leg, just above the ankle, to contact the anterior tibial artery. Now both hands are in contact with the peripheral ends of the entire arterial system (see figs. 26.13–15).

4. Focus attention on your own heart and your own fluid body while holding the pulse of the client's vascular system under your hands.

5. Focus on receiving and listening to the movement of the artery. This listening is done through the micromovements of your fluid body, respiratory diaphragm, and heart pulsation. As much as possible, continue to expand your awareness of the area or space in which you perceive the movement of your heart. If at any time the heart movement activates the defensive system of the heart, slow your breathing and reconnect with PR, especially out to the horizon in back.

6. Lightly bring attention to your own heart, sensing PR from the heart and pericardium.

7. Once you have perceived PR, place your attention on the buoyancy of the tree, as if it were merely floating on the wind of PR. This is connected to the stillness function of the endothelium and the blood cells themselves.

   The vascular tree is held in its matrix of PR. This means that the practitioner senses the breathing motion of PR as if the tree extended beyond the vascular system and into the fascia that holds it and lymphatics that it is connected to.

8. At this point, PR is perceived not as having a specific tempo or rate but rather a more global living presence that could be expressed in spiritual terms or experiences.

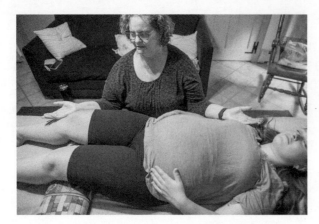

Fig. 26.11. Pietà with palms up

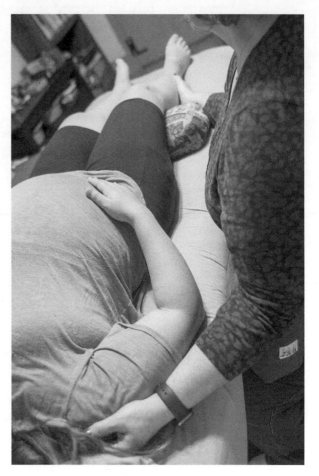

Fig. 26.12. Pietà with hands under the body

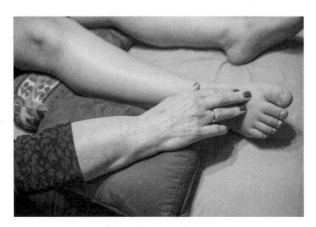

Fig. 26.13. Radial artery

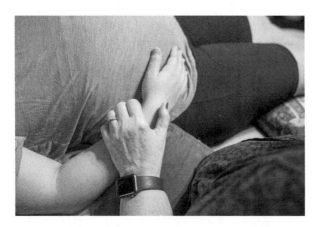

Fig. 26.14. Tibial artery

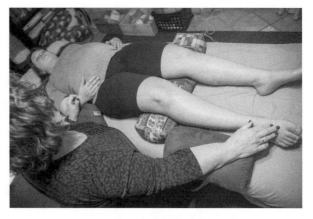

Fig. 26.15. Vascular tree

⌁ 6. Maternal Inguinal Ligament ⌁

1. If mom is comfortable, she can remain supine (see fig. 26.16). More likely, she will want to lie on her side—support whichever one is more comfortable for her.

2. While standing or seated, make contact with the inguinal ligament. Position the mother's legs so that it is comfortable for you to contact the midway point of her inguinal ligament with one hand. Use your other hand to make contact with mom's low back for support and relaxation (see figs. 27.17–20).

3. Repeat on the other side if it feels necessary.

In general, this practice softens and relaxes the trunk and pelvis to create more space for the baby.

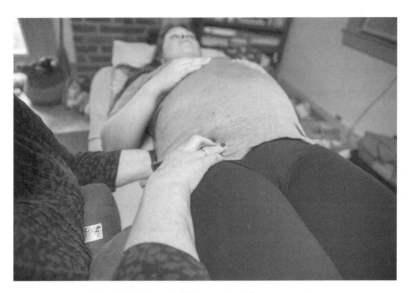

Fig. 26.16. Inguinal ligament with mom supine

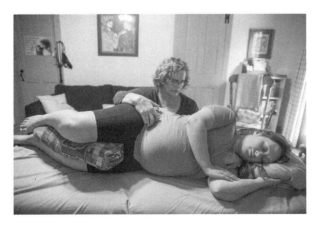

Fig. 26.17. Inguinal ligament with mom on her side 1

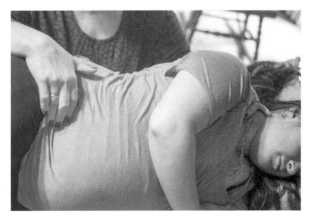

Fig. 26.18. Inguinal ligament with mom on her side 2

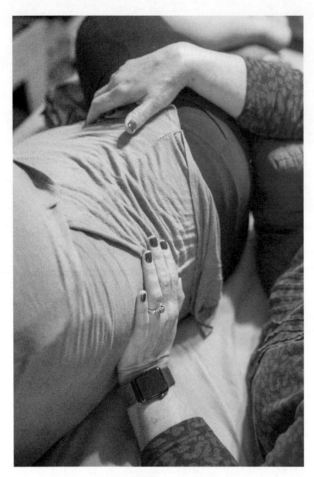

Fig. 26.19. Inguinal ligament and low back 1

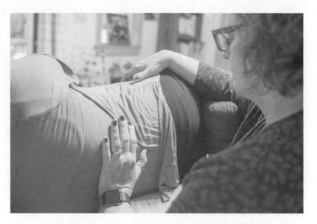

Fig. 26.20. Inguinal ligament and low back 2

❧ 7. Holding the Feet ❧

Finish the session at mom's feet (see fig. 26.21).

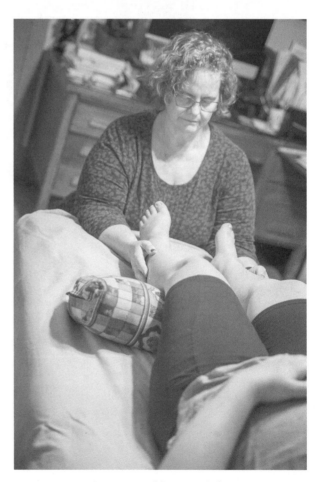

Fig. 26.21. Holding mom's feet

A Practice for Mom
Contacting the Fetal Pulse

For this practice, the mother can be seated or lying down on her back. Her hands are resting over her umbilical area, with her fingertips close together but not touching (see figs. 26.22–25). She gently moves her finger pads below her umbilicus to the lower curvature of her pregnant abdomen and then rests her finger pads there and senses the shape of her baby. She gently explores with micropressure the structure of her baby to find a pulse. Then she moves several inches up toward her umbilicus, repeating the same process several inches at a time until she gets to the xiphoid process. Then, replacing her hands and fingers over her umbilicus, she repeats the exploration, first going to the right and then to the left. Finally, she explores the diagonal line from one ASIS to the liver and the other ASIS to the spleen. She gently explores any location containing a

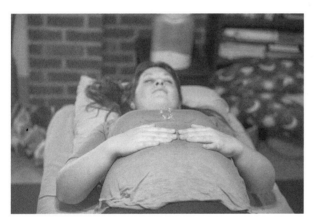

Fig. 26.22. Directed baby palpation 1

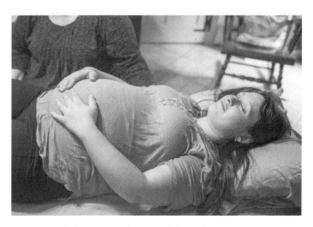

Fig. 26.23. Directed baby palpation 2

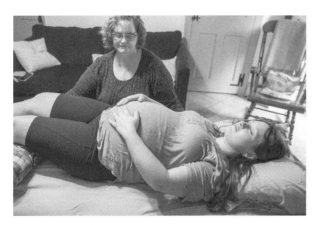

Fig. 26.24. Pietà while directing palpation. One variation is for the therapist to hold space with a simple hold like Pietà while the pregnant client contacts with fetal pulse.

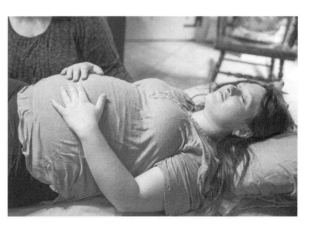

Fig. 26.25. Directed baby palpation 3

discernible pulse of her baby. At any location, when she perceives the pulse, she stays there and synchronizes her attention with her own heartbeat while sensing the pulse of her baby. She then enters a period of prayer and contemplation of loving kindness. This can include a nurturing conversation with her baby, introducing the baby to the whole family the baby is about to enter. She repeats this process as often as possible. And maybe the actual heart of the baby and its beat can be discerned.

Prayer of Loving Kindness for Pregnant Moms

Mom repeats each line slowly, with or without the therapist. It can be said out loud or silently. Repeat as many times as is comfortable during the day.

For Mom

May I be safe and protected,
May I be healthy in body and mind,
May I be happy,
May I live with ease and in peace.

For Baby

May you be safe and protected,
May you be healthy in body and mind,
May you be happy,
May you live with ease and in peace.

Together: A Circle of Love

May you and I be safe and protected,
May you and I be healthy in body and mind,
May you and I be happy,
May you and I live with ease and in peace.

27

The Breath of Life and Fire in Biodynamic Practice

Please note that a complete view of all the arteries of the body can be seen in the color insert, plates 25–35. These can be reviewed prior to or during the study of the following protocols.

Dr. Sutherland's reference to the Breath of Life in his writings was his perception of a bright light in the client's body (Paulus 1999). The integration of color visualization, rooted in both biblical and Eastern traditions, in biodynamic practice derives from Dr. Sutherland's visionary mystical experiences. The Breath of Life as clear light radiates from the heart inside the heart. Figure 27.1 shows the center of the embryonic heart, where spirit resides. It is an empty space surrounded by form. Plate 13 in the color insert shows a full-color drawing of the embryonic center. I amplify Sutherland's experience to include Tibetan medicine and both Buddhist and

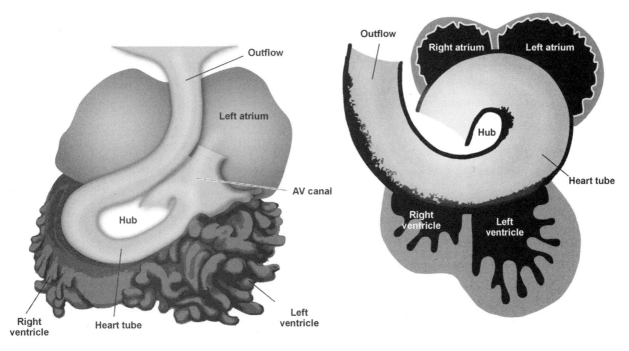

Fig. 27.1. The heart inside the heart

ayurvedic tantric practices. As mentioned in previous chapters, there are three biodynamic spiritual aptitudes. As practitioners, we are familiar with the perception of Primary Respiration (PR) and dynamic stillness. This chapter focuses on the third aptitude of visualizing Health.

The body's metabolism is as complex as the entire universe and thus is a mirror of the external universe. Visualization associated with the origin of the universe, such as the Breath of Life, is an adjunct to biodynamic practices associated with embryology and its originality. Two sources of originality are now integrated into biodynamic practice: the embryo and the cosmos. This is needed because of the unhealthy metabolism of the contemporary client. A mind full of thoughts and emotions cannot practice such visualization; our mind needs to be supple and relaxed. Recognize the activity of your mind. If your mind is active, focus on moving attention to the breath and heartbeat to stabilize the mind, or turn to the practice of wisdom eyes (see page 443). Thoughts are not the enemy, nor can they be extinguished. They must be recognized in their innate capacity to naturally dissipate sooner or later. As is said by many meditation masters, thoughts naturally self-liberate when the practitioner can rest in open awareness of space, the essence of dynamic stillness.

The perceptual spiritual spectrum of biodynamic cardiovascular therapy (BCVT) is mediated by stillness (space), PR (wind), and form (color). A therapeutic container of wholeness is built with the perception of PR, stillness, and color visualization, the originality of the universe and the voidness at the end of the previous universe. Such origin is perceived by synchronizing with PR. Such voidness is perceived with dynamic stillness. It is a spontaneous origin that is synchronized within BCVT. This is because PR provides the spark that ignites the self-healing instinct every fifty seconds. This rate is merely a doorway to the deeper essences of PR. It is superficial and an important portal to liminal space, which is sacred space.

The following visualization skills associated with the third biodynamic aptitude are nonlinear perceptual processes; I call them a biodynamic buffet. They are biodynamic enhancements to access the subtle body and very subtle body of the client with the intention of synchronizing with the Health. These bodies are but one body with three aspects. BCVT is a laying-on-of-hands ministry in the same mystical tradition as Judeo-Christianity and all other spiritual traditions. Our hands bless the client.

PRINCIPLES OF
BIODYNAMIC VISUALIZATION PRACTICE

1. Color visualization is medicine. In biodynamic practice, it is medicine for the metabolism of the client. All cells in the body emit biophotons and are sensitive to light.

2. Visualizing color has the potential effect of reconnecting the client to the cosmological origin of the universe.

3. The practice begins as a deliberate visualization and gradually becomes spontaneous. Many clients report seeing colors in a session.

4. The power of the mind is used to manifest color. The hands synchronize with the mind to perceive PR homogenized with the color or the stillness changing the texture and tone of the color.

5. Rely on the tide, the stillness, and the light, to direct your session. And remember these foundational principles.

6. There are three types of eye gazing in BCVT: (1) the *gaze of humility*, in which the eyes rest open, looking at a point on the floor several meters in front; (2) the *gaze of compassion*, in which the eyes look at the horizon and sense PR moving back and forth from the third ventricle of the brain to the horizon; (3) the *gaze of wisdom*, or sky gazing, in which the eyes observe a point suspended in space ten degrees or so above the horizon; this ignites the creative mode of PR between heart and cosmos.

7. Sense micromovement spiraling. First it seems as if a pearl is rotating around the diameter of the abdomen on a plane below the umbilicus. Then the pearl is rotating around the pleura at the plane of the atria of the heart. Then imagine the eyes are rotating around the third ventricle. All these rotational movements access the inherent spiral of PR. The rotation moves clockwise, and then PR changes phase and the movement automatically shifts to counterclockwise.

8. Sense the spiral of the heart in the palms of the hand at the point Pericardium 8. The hands are able to synchronize with the client's inherent spiraling in any fulcrum.

9. Periodically visualize the Breath of Life as a light in your heart after synchronizing with PR heart-to-heart and allow it to radiate out into the blood and body. Then allow its radiance to move out to the edges of the universe and back. The light can be visualized as a spiritual figure from any tradition. While you are working, that spiritual essence may become a second pair of hands moving inside your hands.

THE FIRST VISUALIZATION PROTOCOL

The following three protocols gradually introduce visualization as a foundation skill to integrate, when appropriate, during a biodynamic treatment. Practice will allow the visualizations to become spontaneous and free flowing.

As with any BCVT session, the cycle of attunement, discussed in chapter 24, begins each protocol. Sit and settle. Let the client know you are settling and that you will let them know when you are going to make contact. Recognize your own state of mind and body. Then begin the pietà with the fluid body, the original embryonic body that is now a metaphor for the great ocean of the universe. Then sense into and synchronize with PR in the vascular tree, which completes the cycle of attunement.

This first protocol incorporates visualization into the cycle of attunement and a basic exploration of the client's metabolic condition.

ಐಃ

Visualization in the Cycle of Attunement

The client remains supine for this protocol.

~ 1. Attunement to Oneself ~

1. Sit and settle. Identify your state of mind and body. Adjust as necessary.
2. Drop your breath into your lower abdomen at a point between your umbilicus and pubic bone. Sense the sides of your diaphragm expand laterally like a jellyfish.
3. Sense your heartbeat.
4. Sense the potency of the heartbeat expanding throughout the trunk and extremities.
5. Synchronize with the tide of PR heart-to-heart. PR is initiated in the back of the heart and moves the blood. It also spreads throughout the electromagnetic heart field. Now both your own and the client's cardiovascular systems are synchronizing.

~ 2. Oceanic Pietà of the Medicine Buddha ~

1. Sit at the client's right side. Place one hand under the client's shoulder and your other hand under the client's leg (see figs. 27.2–4). You are holding the interstitium, the aquarium, the interface between the fluid body and the cardiovascular system. You are holding the whole ocean, both with your palpation locally and with your perception globally. Hold the whole fluid body with the Tide moving between your third ventricle and the horizon and then between your heart and the client's heart.
2. Practice several cycles of attunement while your hands are in the position of the pietà. Establish which fulcrum of PR is accessible in that moment, the third ventricle or the heart. Remember that the fulcrum may shift automatically.
3. With your eyes closed or open, visualize the entire contents of the client's body as a deep blue ocean of lapis lazuli. It is not static. Perceive the tide of PR, the waves, and the currents with the color of the deep blue ocean. It moves in the color. Practice a cycle of attunement. Imagine seeing a colorful lava lamp.

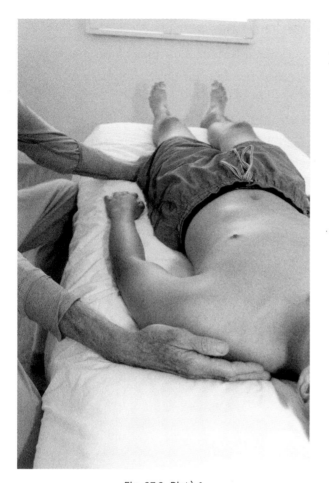

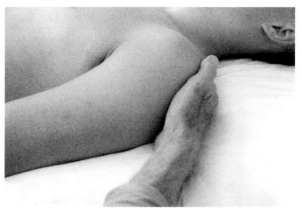

Fig. 27.3. Pietà 2

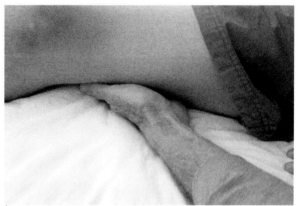

Fig. 27.2. Pietà 1 *Fig. 27.4. Pietà 3*

4. Imagine a time when you saw the color of a large body of water, such as the ocean, glistening aquamarine in the sunshine. Now visualize the entire contents of the client's body being a beautiful clear aquamarine light moving with the tide, the waves, and currents. It has a shimmering, radiating quality to it. It is the color that projects from the forehead of the Medicine Buddha to heal all sentient beings. Over time you will sense an immediate response in the client.

5. The most deeply healing color is that of pure water, without any earth element. The crystal-clear level of the fluid body is associated with the element of space from which the universe appeared originally as clear light. Start by visualizing the entire contents of the client's body as the color white, as above. Then allow the white to disappear and become a transparent crystal-clear living whole.

At any time, the dynamic stillness will exchange places with PR. That is the signal to drop all effort and all visualization and rest in the vast expanse of the stillness as it extends to the edge of the universe. Sometimes only one color is needed.

ᘏ 3. The Vascular Tree: The Tree of Life ᘏ

1. I usually start on the client's right side and then in subsequent sessions on the left as shown by making contact with the radial and anterior tibial arteries (see figs. 27.5–7). Visualize the Tree of Life or the life channel, as it's called in some traditions (see fig. 27.8). As you synchronize with PR and the stillness, imagine

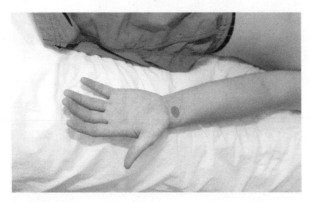

Fig. 27.5. Radial and anterior tibial arteries 1

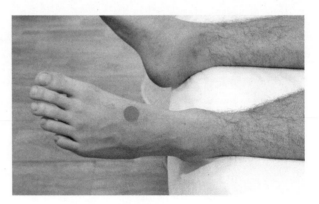

Fig. 27.6. Radial and anterior tibial arteries 2

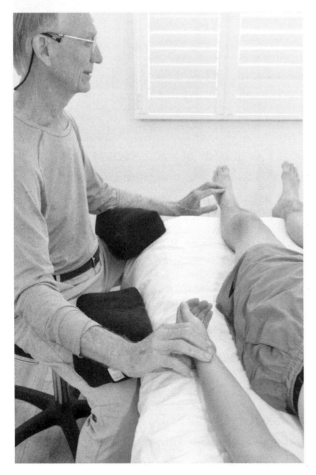

Fig. 27.7. Radial and anterior tibial arteries 3

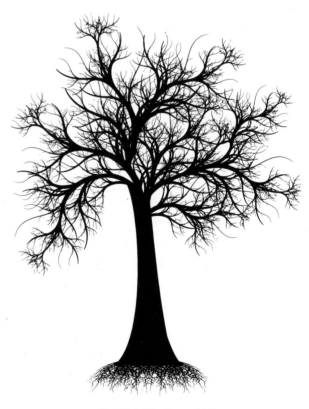

Fig. 27.8. The Tree of Life

your whole vascular tree and the client's gently moving with the breeze of PR. Notice if any color is available. Deliberately visualizing a color for several seconds may ignite the spreading of the color in yourself and the client. Many practitioners see color without knowing its potential for healing.

2. Wait for the Tree of Life to move. It usually moves in a torsion pattern. If the vascular system is holding a trauma, such as heart surgery or an impact injury to the chest, the tree may shake strongly for a moment as it discharges its constricted tone.

On the top of the Tree of Life (a metaphor for midline) a bird is perched seen in many creation stories. It represents the Breath of Life. Bird song is the Breath of Life in many indigenous cultures. As mentioned, Drs. Sutherland and Still were already working with the originality of the universe in the beginnings of Osteopathy and the Cranial Concept. I now call it the Cranial Cosmos Concept. It is already built into our biodynamic explorations every time we orient to PR and the stillness. Spirit, the sacred, manifests as a movement of the Breath of Life in the blood and lives in the heart that is unencumbered by constantly polarizing emotions. The sacred manifests with every breath. It is the preexisting condition of all beings. Whenever we take a spontaneous deep inhalation, that is the PR synchronizing with our metabolic instincts of self-healing and self-transcendence.

Our ordinary breath becomes interconnected with the sacred when synchronized with the perception of stillness and PR in any one of its five (wind) fulcrums.

THE FIVE FULCRUMS OF THE WIND ELEMENT
Pineal–Third Ventricle
Hypoglossal plexus
Posterior heart fields
Superior mesenteric plexus
Hypogastric plexus

These five fulcrums of PR maintain and support healing for all structure and function of the physical body.

We are always in direct connection with the sacred via our senses, without the need for an intermediary or ministerial representation. It is innate and intrinsic as a human being to have such direct experience, and it confers continual spiritual authority.

Direct connection to Originality is the essence of biodynamic practice, and it begins with the perception of PR and the stillness relating to the cardiovascular system.

⌣ 4. Umbilical Origin ⌣

Place your fingers on the anterior midline of the client's body, with one finger always in the umbilicus (see figs. 27.9–10). Sense the location of the abdominal aorta, the superior and inferior mesenteric arteries, the umbilical arteries, and the hypogastric plexus between the umbilicus and pubic bone. Imagine playing a piano.

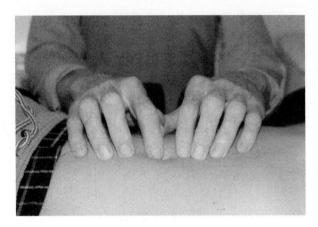

Fig. 27.9. Umbilical origin 1

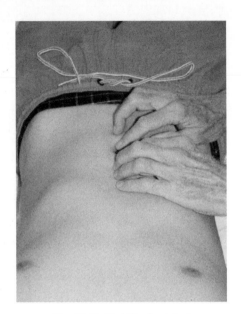

Fig. 27.10. Umbilical origin 2

⌣ 5. Lung Ignition ⌣

Make bilateral contact with the subclavian arteries, which sit below the midclavicular area and branch into the internal thoracic artery feeding the muscles of respiration (see figs. 27.11–13). I typically use my thumb pads, but any finger pads are okay. I also tend to move slightly medial toward the carotid arteries if the client is able to get to Neutral from this palpation.

A strong spontaneous deep breath may occur in both the therapist and the client. This is synchronized with PR. This is lung Ignition. It may also be a recapitulation or repair of the first breath after birth. If you intuit that this might be the case, explore the inferior and superior thyroid arteries, as neonatal breathing is coregulated by the thyroid.

Notice the pleural dome and the effect of PR expanding and contracting the lungs in the tempo of the Tide. Are the ribs breathing internally? Does the dynamic stillness of the subclavian vein move into your perception? Do your hands feel as if they are entering the blood flow in the tempo of PR?

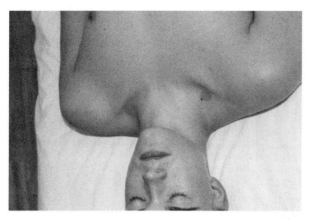

Fig. 27.11. Lung Ignition 1

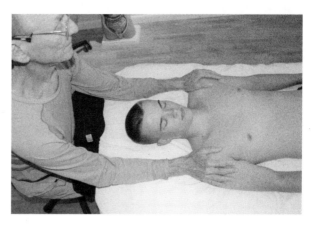

Fig. 27.12. Lung Ignition 2

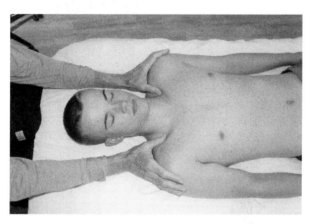

Fig. 27.13. Lung Ignition 3

↭ 6. Hypogastric Plexus ↭

1. Hold the coccyx-sacrum with the finger pads of one hand for the sacral outflow of parasympathetic nervous system (PNS). Place the fingertips of your other hand on the midline between the umbilicus and pubic bone of the client to affect the posterior vagus via the hypogastric plexus (see fig. 27.14). Place the

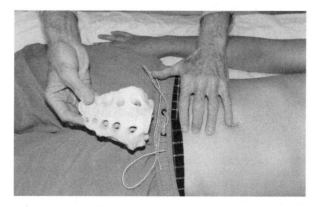

Fig. 27.14. Hypogastric plexus

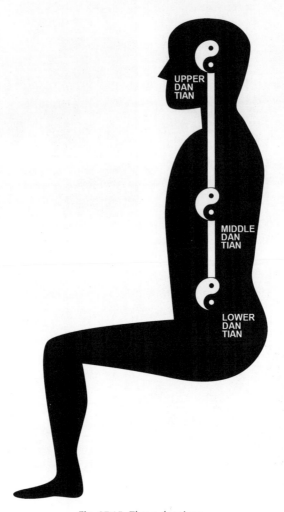

Fig. 27.15. Three dantians

pad of your middle finger on the specific acupuncture point Ren 6, for the lower dantian, a part of the hypogastric plexus. The lower dantian relates to our subtle body in classical Chinese medicine. It is the engine of our metabolism.

The palpation depth, if permitted by the quality of relaxation when the client exhales, is midway between abdominal surface and L2. It is in the vicinity of the bifurcation of the abdominal aorta into the common iliac arteries. This is where the hypogastric plexus and lower dantian are suspended. Visualize the lower dantian as a ball about the size of a golf ball with either of the five primary colors (see fig. 27.15). Some prefer to visualize it as gold or a pearl.

2. Invite the client to breath into your hands. It is quite enough to stay at the surface, allowing your fingers to gently vibrate the Ren 6 point on the anterior midline between the umbilicus and pubic bone.

3. If you like, shift the hand under the coccyx-sacrum to the depression below the spinous process of L2. This is Du 4 (Mingmen, the Gate of Life). Sense the

spiral of PR moving clockwise anteriorly through the umbilicus or Ren 6. At the second lumbar vertebra the spiral moves counterclockwise. Help the spiral synchronize with PR. Is there a color in the spiral?

⌁ 7. Earth Pulses and the Second Pair of Hands ⌁

1. Make contact with the tibial arteries, whether anterior, posterior, or both, bilaterally or ipsilaterally if the client needs it (see figs. 27.16–18). These are the earth element pulses, and they are the first to disappear in the dying process.

2. If appropriate, visualize a healing image to finish the protocol. Invite a benevolent second pair of hands if appropriate. Allow the second pair of hands to be an image, a real person alive or dead who represents a spiritual healing presence and is safe, without generating any fear. The second pair of hands may take over and move through your own hands from the center of the heart.

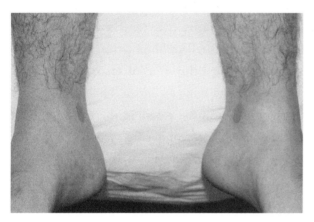

Fig. 27.16. Earth pulses 1

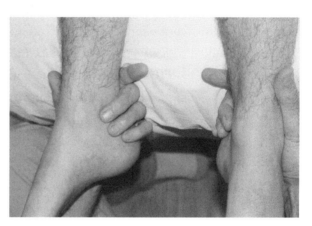

Fig. 27.17. Earth pulses 2

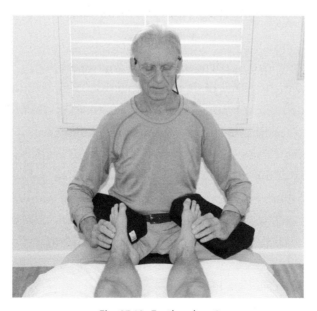

Fig. 27.18. Earth pulses 3

THE SECOND VISUALIZATION PROTOCOL

In the first protocol above, we learned to bridge our contact between the fluid body, the vascular tree, visualization practice with the Indo-Tibetan elements, and discrete acupuncture points. This is a newly emerging exploration necessary for the metabolic conditions of the contemporary client. The intention in this second exploration is to affect the client's metabolism positively by stimulating the vagus to send anti-inflammatory signals to the body and increase interoceptive awareness in the core of the body. PR and the stillness can then increase their potency for repair. Reliable embodiment depends on clear signals from the body's interoceptive systems that begin in the gut and end in the brain. We will now continue the integration of color visualization with biodynamic practice to affect the body's metabolism at the core of its interoceptive systems.

We will use the five colors of the rainbow that the five elements came from in Buddhist cosmology. Each color has a specific spiritual significance; together, they are called *wisdom colors*. Once again, PR is the key to this visualization practice. Each element has PR attached to it. Consequently, they are called the wind of space, the wind of wind, the wind of fire, the wind of water, and the wind of earth. The wisdom colors exist in the subtle body, especially the heart, and the colors of the wind elements relate to the physical body, making the body an interconnected system of the five elements. Biodynamic practice builds a bridge between these two aspects of our whole body.

ళ౬

Visualization Practice:
Exploring the Wisdom Colors

⸱ 1. Beginnings ⸱

1. Settle into abdominal breathing and feeling your heartbeat.

2. Synchronize with PR at any of its wind fulcrums and then settle into your heart. Make a heart-to-horizon connection with PR, shifting the focus of your heart fulcrum to the cosmos, the natural world, via the horizon.

3. With your eyes closed or open, begin to visualize your own heart with the wisdom colors of the rainbow sequentially: white, blue, yellow, red, and green. Take a few minutes to visualize each color as a light that radiates from inside your heart or to visualize the heart itself as that color. It takes a few moments to find the visualization that is correct for your sensibility.

4. Practice several cycles of attunement. Then synchronize a heart-to-heart connection with the client via PR.

5. Now you will begin to make the bridge between the wisdom colors and the wind

elements. Imagine the entire body of the client and yourself as pearlescent white for several seconds. The color always radiates from your heart. Wait.

6. Visualize the dyad as a deep ocean blue for several seconds. Wait.

7. Visualize the dyad as bright yellow, a golden sun, for several seconds. Wait.

8. Visualize the dyad as blood red for several seconds. Wait. This is the potency of PR—the Health.

9. Visualize the dyad as emerald green for several seconds. Wait.

10. Synchronize with the Tide, the waves, and currents.

Sometimes visualizing only one color is enough, and blue is a spacious color to initiate visualization. Always resynchronize with the potency of the Tide, which is the color red.

Palpation

Regarding palpation with visualization, attention needs to be made with your whole body to take a backward step with your hands, arms, spine, and intention. This means to extend, lengthen, and stretch the space between the physical contact of your hands on the client's body and your spine and nervous system. This energizes the heart meridian through the arms and opens the window of all possibilities in the heart meridian. Too frequently our mind, hands, and arms are like a tight spring and need softening and lengthening to avoid compressing the client, both mechanically with our touch and subtly with the visualization of color.

⌣ 2. Oceanic Pietà ⌣

1. Begin with the pietà, with one hand under the upper leg and the other supporting the shoulder and scapula on the left side of the client. This is the opportunity to practice several cycles of attunement and find the midline between the third ventricle, the heart, and the lower dantian.

2. The lower dantian is a fulcrum between the umbilicus and the second lumbar vertebra. Imagine that midline between those three areas is connected to the descending and abdominal aorta and extending up through the neck and out the top of the head. It is a tube the color of soft radiant blue. This is a visualization of the vagus nerve.

    The other option is to practice all or part of the Medicine Buddha visualization (dark blue ocean, aquamarine ocean, and clear crystal water). The fluid body is an ocean that is vast.

⌣ 3. Cosmic Vascular Tree ∿

1. Contact the vascular tree on the left side of the client by contacting the radial and tibial arteries. In the cycle of attunement, we generally move the automatic shifting fulcrum of attention for PR from the third ventricle out to the horizon and back and/or from heart to heart. Here, allow your attention to move beyond the horizon into the universe, and imagine connecting with the North Star or any planet or galaxy in the cosmos.

2. Sense the middle core of the vascular tree trunk, allowing your fingers to gently sink into the very middle of the blood flow in each artery. The center of blood flow in every artery is a cone of dynamic stillness, the element of space. Be sure that your fingers remain buoyant. They gently explore vasodilation and vasoconstriction of the artery and the blood while synchronized with PR. Imagine your fingers are playing a flute of the most beautiful music. PR invites your fingers to move out to the surface of the artery and then rhythmically invites them back into the stillness in the middle of the blood flow. Take some time to practice this palpation until the midline of dynamic stillness fills your six senses, including your mind, with nonconceptual awareness.

⌣ 4. Mesentery: The Root of Embodiment ∿

1. Position yourself on the left-hand side of the client's body by their anterior superior iliac spine (ASIS). Place the thumbs of both hands (or just one hand) underneath the sigmoid mesentery. Take up slack with a gentle scooping motion until you feel the tension at the root of the mesentery, which is surrounded by the hypogastric plexus, where the posterior vagus nerve terminates (see figs. 27.19–20). This is on a diagonal line between the two ASIS points.

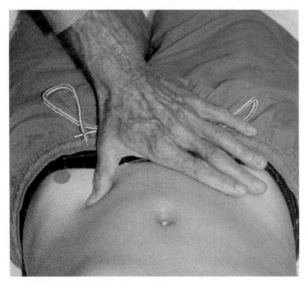

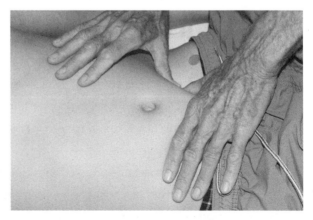

Fig. 27.19. Mesentery 1   *Fig. 27.20. Mesentery 2*

2. Leaving one hand in place, shift your other hand to contact the superior mesenteric artery, three client fingers' width above the umbilicus. When you perceive PR starting to move, your hands will sense a large steering wheel turning clockwise and counterclockwise. It is the deep spiral of creation.

The superior mesenteric artery and mesenter are the first two structures that differentiate from the endoderm and mesoderm in the peritoneal cavity of the embryo. The mesentery is an organ system, and it mediates the inflammatory process in the abdomen metabolically. This practice infuses it with the rhythmic balanced interchange of PR and the dynamic stillness to stimulate the vagus for its anti-inflammatory properties. At the same time, your hands are influencing the portal vein system (see fig. 27.21).

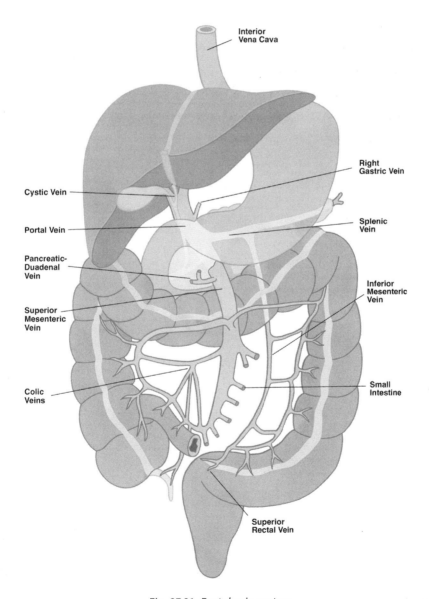

Fig. 27.21. Portal vein system

✌ 5. Lung Ignition ∿

The intention here is to contact the ribs over the lung fissures. The left lung has only one fissure, under the fifth rib at an angle that bisects the ventral costal arch. The right lung has two fissures. Contact is initially made with the superior fissure under the fourth rib, which is nearly horizontal. The right inferior fissure is under the fifth rib and at an angle bisecting the ventral costal arch (see fig. 27.22).

1. Have the client lie on one side.
2. Settle into the contact approximating the location of the lung fissures on either side of the rib cage (see figs. 27.23–24). Synchronize with the rhythmic balanced interchange of PR and dynamic stillness from the treatment room to the horizon and beyond to the North Star. This is the center of the universe and thus its origin from a Taoist view.
3. The root of the lung, at the junction of the heart and lungs, is where the major blood vessels for pulmonary circulation are located. The cardiac and pulmonary plexuses of the autonomic nervous system are located here, including both branches of the vagus nerve (dorsal and ventral). The blood vessels entering

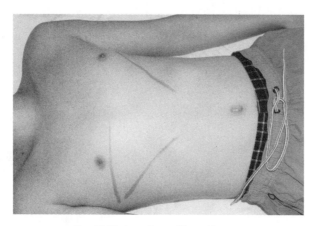

Fig. 27.22. Location of lung fissures

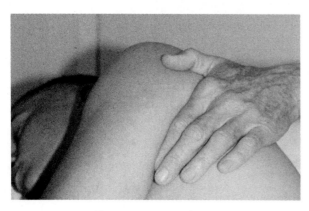

Fig. 27.23. Lung Ignition 1

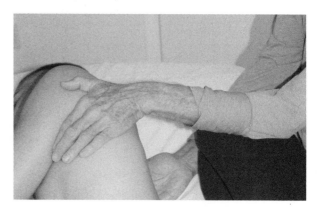

Fig. 27.24. Lung Ignition 2

and exiting the root of the lungs are in the shape of a cross, horizontal and vertical. At some point PR will allow you to feel the cross and its vibrancy. Wait until there is a sense of expansion not only with respiration and pulmonary circulation but also with the tide.

4. While holding the heart in this way, begin to imagine the heart being each of the five colors of the rainbow, one at a time. Alternately, you can settle into one color that appears to you through the potency of PR.

The wind of wind element in the Indo-Tibetan system is green. That is the basic elemental color of PR. It is a beautiful emerald. We know from our biodynamic practice that PR and the dynamic stillness have multiple levels of depth and consequently their color will change. Color visualizations are a living process, not a static one. Changes in the colors of PR frequently indicate a deepening potency in the Health.

∻ 6. Blue Vagus ∻

1. Contact the sacrum-coccyx with the finger pads of one hand and place your other hand underneath the fifth thoracic vertebra (see figs. 27.26–27). This connects the sacral outflow of the parasympathetic nervous system with the main network of the entire vagus nerve in the heart.

2. Visualize the vagus nerve as a tube of light blue between your hands. It is important to visualize it as a blue tube to maintain subtlety with PR moving in that blue tube. The blue tube is the central channel in the subtle anatomy of the body in Eastern traditions (see fig. 27.25). (Over the sequence of this protocol, we contact the entire length of the vagus nerve and both of its branches at the physical and subtle levels.)

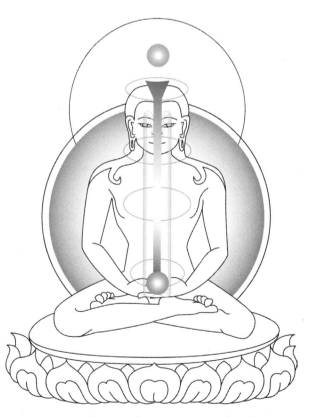

Fig. 27.25. The central channel of the subtle body

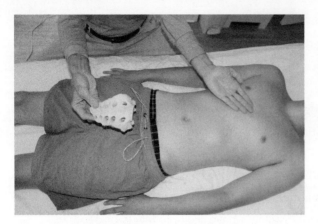

Fig. 27.26. Blue vagus 1

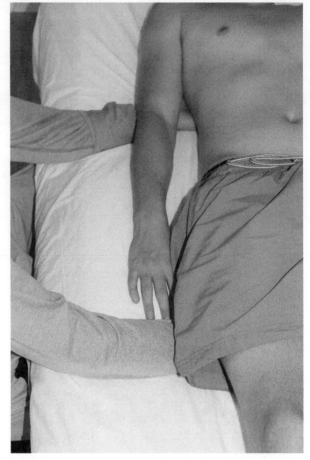

Fig. 27.27. Blue vagus 2

↫ 7. Earth Pulses ↬

1. Make contact with the tibial arteries, whether anterior, posterior, or both, bilaterally or ipsilaterally if the client needs it (see figs. 27.16–18, page 417). These are the earth element pulses, and they are the first to disappear in the dying process.

2. If appropriate, visualize a healing image to finish the protocol. Invite a benevolent second pair of hands if appropriate. Allow the second pair of hands to be an image, a real person alive or dead who represents a spiritual healing presence and is safe, without generating any fear. The second pair of hands may take over and move through your own hands from the center of the heart.

THE THIRD VISUALIZATION PROTOCOL

Fire is the essence of the Ignition process in biodynamic practice. Dr. Jealous taught that it begins with a spark that jumps between two objects, such as the skin of the client and the hands of the therapist. Such a spark needs a gap of space between the client's skin and the therapist's hands. This protocol is specifically about the element of fire and its relationship with PR (the wind of fire) to Ignite the water element, unify Zones A and B of the fluid body, and Ignite the possibility of the client's metabolism returning to a natural state of harmony with the universe. Our hands maintain buoyancy while continually synchronizing with Zone B and Zone A.

One of the last teachings that Dr. Jealous gave before he died was on the biodynamics of the fire element. He said that fire is the very nature of potency, and potency has different levels of intensity. For example, the fire in the digestive system is a smoldering fire. The fire in the heart is a torch that melts metal. The fire of inflammation is a wildfire. The fire of sexuality is a great hot magnetism. The Sanskrit literature talks about sexual magnetism, or energy, as kundalini, which is associated with the creation—meaning not just human conception but the creation of the entire universe. Kundalini as a form of sexual energy is enlightening, and misuse of its energy can lead to spiritual crises and can even psychosis. And the abuse of sexual energy can burn badly. Does the client-therapist relationship naturally express magnetism?

The fire in the eyes sees the whole universe. Metabolic fire allows us to sense how the body's natural processes are breaking down molecules and creating energy and, at the same time, when we synchronize with PR, how PR is a fuel for the fire that thermally regulates the body. The felt sense of fire is heat. Heat is released in all metabolic processes. It is the deepest potency of embodiment. The wind of fire drives the metabolism of the body. It delivers all nutritional molecules (glucose or ketones) to the mitochondria in every cell and helps removes all cellular waste products when the body's metabolism is in balance. Consequently, together with PR, fire expresses a life force known as the potency in osteopathy. It is this potency that generates growth and development in the universe of the embryo through the life span. Dr. Jealous called the potency of PR the Health.

When we make physical contact, our hands begin to conduct heat through the clothing or skin of the client. We are always literally in touch with the heat. Sometimes we can feel beads of sweat trickling down our spine, under our armpits, or down the brow of our face. Sweat linked to thermal regulation comes from the blood. We will explore making minimal contact with the client's skin or clothing to allow the spark to initiate Ignition, the essence of fire. The skin has differential rates of heat escaping from it as well as thermal spikes, like flames, that can repel the therapist's hands. Our hands can function like a spring, always ready to be pushed off the client's body. Dr. Jealous said that this sensation of heat is the most fundamental release or discharge in a biodynamic session.

Biodynamic practice is metabolic practice. As a Nike ad once said, "Go for the burn." Most contemporary clients have a very combustible inflammatory process going on in their body in which the fire of creation in the abdomen and pelvis has been misplaced to the heart and brain. There is a significant difference between combustion and Ignition! This misplacement and dysregulation of the fire element creates metabolic syndrome, an internal wildfire, and the inflammation transported through the blood vascular system further dysregulates the endothelium and its glycocalyx. This turns off vasodilation and upregulates the immune system so the artery can protect itself. The waste products of inflammation then back up in the interstitium, fascia, and lymphatic system. The body becomes a barrel of toxicity full to overflowing. Could it be that long COVID and mRNA vaccine side effects are the preexisting full barrel of toxicity now overflowing? The priority in these metabolic protocols is to support the reorganization of the fire element with the help of the other four elements, including their colors, and opening the metabolic pathways of detoxification. The cycle of attunement allows the therapist to gently resynchronize with PR and the stillness, which dissipates the excessive tone in the client's autonomic nervous system (ANS) through the therapist's body and mind.

We use caution when we explore this fire protocol with visualization. These five colors from the Indo-Tibetan palette are not in balance in many contemporary clients. This means the contemporary client is not in harmony with the universe externally and internally. Recall that the external universe is represented by the body's internal metabolism with its trillions upon trillions of molecules and cells. When we visualize a color in our work with a client, the client's body is likely to have an immediate response. If that response is contraction, then it may be the wrong color or the wrong time. If the response is an expansion, then observe the living quality of the shape being perceived. The expansion becomes a living, moving reality under the direction of PR. In other words, the visualization will grow on its own as if the therapist is watching a movie. It is the very movement of spontaneous originality and the unfolding of the universe.

⏾⏾

The Fire Element Protocol

From the Tibetan medical point of view, the fire element has five fulcrums in the body. This protocol explores these fulcrums.

THE FIVE FULCRUMS OF THE FIRE ELEMENT

Skin

Superior mesenteric and renal arteries

Liver

Heart

Eyes

⌁ 1. Umbilical Origin ⌁

Place your hands palm up over the umbilicus (see fig. 27.28). Contact with the umbilicus is light. Settle into PR heart-to-heart.

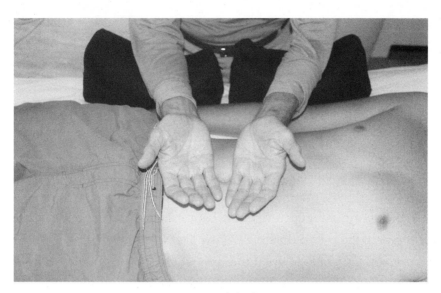

Fig. 27.28. Umbilical origin

⌁ 2. Pietà ⌁

1. Begin with the pietà, with one hand under the client's shoulder and your other hand under the client's leg (see figs. 27.2–4, page 411). You are holding the fluid body, which runs continuously from Zone A (the body) to Zone B (the space around the body, or biosphere). Zone B includes electricity and infrared heat. It holds the heat that escapes the body along with the water that evaporates from the blood.

2. Settle yourself and practice several cycles of attunement, allowing your hands to simply notice heat and noticing any changes in the heat of your own body. Know that this heat is moved by the cardiovascular system from the core of the body to the skin, especially with the venous system. Does a color spontaneously come into your mind in or around the client's body?

Practitioner Tip

It may help to feel your heartbeat and breath below the level of the abdomen, between the umbilicus and pubic bone. This will help recenter the fire of creation in the abdomen or Hara, as it is called in the East when referring to cosmology. In Taoism, the center of the universe is the umbilicus.

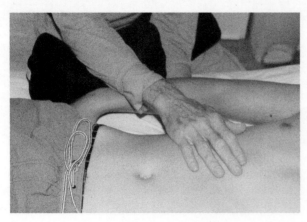

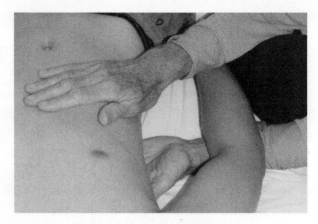

Fig. 27.29. Liver suction field 1   *Fig. 27.30. Liver suction field 2*

⌁ 3. The Liver Suction Fields ⌁

1. Using the area of acupuncture point Pericardium 8 on the palm of one hand, slowly search the surface anatomy of the liver for heat. Rest your palm (specifically the Pericardium 8 point) at the spot where it registers the most heat from the client's liver. Place the other palm under the liver (see figs. 27.29–30).

2. Now place the hand from under the liver with the palm down over the xiphoid process (not shown in above images). Embryonically, the liver develops in what is called a suction field since it is attached to the developing respiratory diaphragm. Slightly cup each hand in such a way that the palms can flatten during the client's inhalation and cup during the client's exhalation. Synchronize this suction motion with PR. Then a suction field gently takes over the hands. Gradually the flat palm/cupped palm reciprocal motion will settle. Pay attention to any heat from the liver. Wait for dissipation or a fountain of potency from the liver to push the hands off. Feel PR breathing through both Pericardium 8 points while monitoring the client's breathing. You can ask the client to breath into the lower lobes of their lungs if you feel this will help the general movement around the liver and diaphragm.

3. Then visualize the entire liver as emerald green. This green is an evaporation of heat, a green mist that expands outside the body like a cloud. The cloud can dissipate naturally, or if you are inclined and comfortable with the visualization, you can allow this green cloud of mist to dissipate out through Zone D into a beautiful forest of trees.

⌁ 4. Metabolic Fire: Superior Mesenteric and Renal Arteries ⌁

Water-fire balance is located between the kidneys. This is the primary fulcrum of heat in the body because of its digestive capacity and potency (wind of fire) to move metabolites throughout the body. The acupuncture point Ren 11 lies over the superior mesenteric artery, which is marked by the middle dot in figures 27.31–32. The superior mesenteric artery lies three fingers' width above the umbilicus. The other two dots on either side of the superior mesenteric artery are the locations of the right and left renal arteries. Altogether this is an area of high potency due to the fire element.

1. Place both hands, stacked on top of one another, palm down, and a little space between the hands for the spark of the fire element to be able to jump and ignite over Ren 11. Align Pericardium 8 on each palm with Ren 11 on the client. Use the arrangement of cupped hands to sense the suction fields present, as you just did with the liver. Pericardium 8 breathes with PR coming from the back of the heart, the source of the spiritual PR. Wait until you sense PR breathing between and through those two points. It prefers to move in a spiral pattern.

2. Line up your fingers on the client's abdomen, with the tips of your index fingers together on Ren 11 (see fig. 27.33). The tips of your index fingers should be in contact with the tips of the middle fingers, which are aligned over the renal

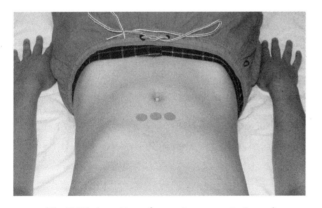

Fig. 27.31. Location of superior mesenteric and renal arteries

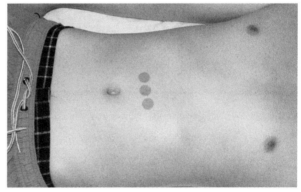

Fig. 27.32. Location of superior mesenteric and renal arteries

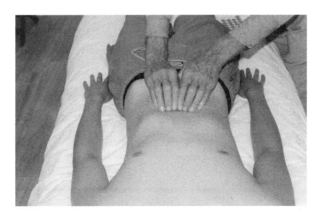

Fig. 27.33. Superior mesenteric and renal arteries

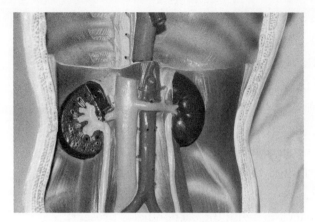

Fig. 27.34. Anatomy of superior mesenteric and
renal arteries

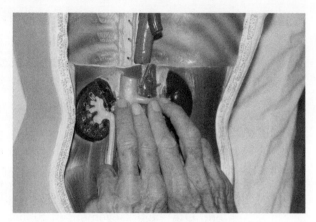

Fig. 27.35. Anatomy of superior mesenteric and
renal arteries

arteries. Feel the client's breathing. Upon the client's exhalation, wait for the fingers to be invited toward the space between the kidneys to sense the superior mesenteric and renal arteries. Remember that the left kidney is more superior than the right and both kidneys are on the psoas muscle, which may invite the fingers to be on a slight diagonal line (see figs. 27.34–35). Tune in to PR. Rest in the warmth and heat of your own body, and notice temperature variations in yourself. Wait for the client to breathe into your fingertips or direct them to do so at least three times. The repelling potency of the fire element will push your fingers out.

If the client is overweight and this anterior abdominal contact cannot reach the kidneys, place your hands under the floating ribs of the client and sense into the space between the kidneys from the eleventh and twelfth ribs.

Note: In your intake assessment with any client, confirm whether they have a preexisting kidney problem. If they do, stay with the superior mesenteric artery only, unless you have clinical experience treating clients with kidney conditions.

Practitioner Tip

You can give your client homework to place their hands palm down over their lower abdomen while lying down and practice breathing into their hands so that during inhalation their abdomen lifts and during exhalation it simply settles back. This greatly facilitates the relationship of the wind element with the fire element. And it moves a lot of lymph.

⌇ 5. The Heart Fire ⌇

1. Stack the hands, palm down but slightly separated, with the Pericardium 8 points aligned with each other and over the acupuncture point Ren 17 on the client's sternum, between the fourth and fifth costal cartilage joint space (see fig. 27.36). Keep a little distance between your bottom hand and the client's skin. Allow the hands to become buoyant, sensing the heat discharging from the client's heart. Some clients may need to feel your hands making contact, which is fine; the hands maintain their transparency in either case. Or play with making contact and making space between your hands and the client's skin.

2. Place one hand underneath the trunk of the client's body to make very gentle contact with the spine above the respiratory diaphragm. This is the area of the esophageal plexus, where the dorsal vagus joins the sympathetic plexuses after it descends from the heart. Place your other hand on the client's chest, spanning the bottom of the sternum, including the xiphoid process, to sense the rise and fall of the diaphragm and the expansion/contraction of the pericardium (see fig. 27.37). The pad of the longest finger should contact Ren 17 as above. Follow the rise and fall of the client's breath. Practice a cycle of attunement and come into direct heart-to-heart relationship with PR moving between your heart and the client's heart.

3. If you like, begin to visualize the client's heart in the color white and then blue. This visualization can be balancing for the client's cardiovascular system.

4. If you like, use the mudra shown in figures 27.38–40 to balance the fire element associated with the heart. The mudra does not make contact with the skin of the client. It remains in Zone B, one to several inches above Ren 17. Fire needs a spark to jump the distance between the mudra and the skin to balance that element, especially in the heart, the holder of the principal side effect of the majority of metabolic problems. This sequence has the potential to reduce inflammation but not eliminate it unless there is deep repair of the intestines,

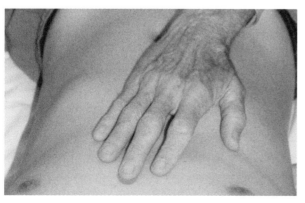

Fig. 27.36. Ren 17

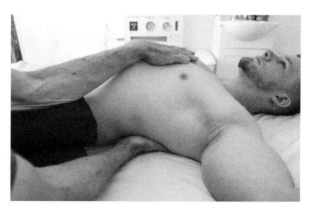

Fig. 27.37. Heart fire

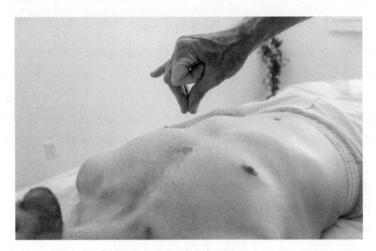

Fig. 27.38. Fire mudra 1

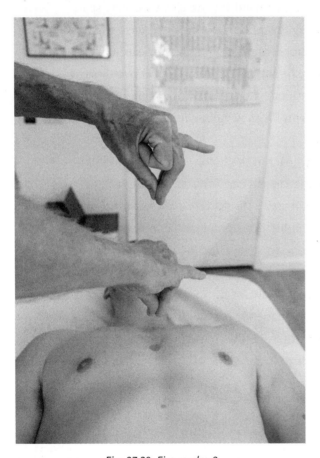

Fig. 27.39. Fire mudra 2

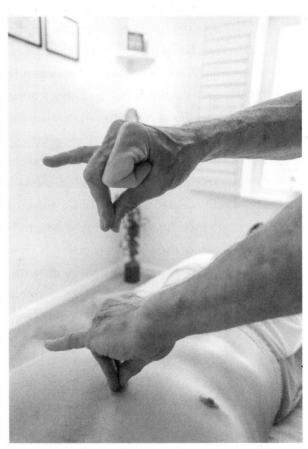

Fig. 27.40. Fire mudra 3

where the blood is built. Hold the mudra for several minutes, playing with the right distance between the two hands and the distance between the hands and the skin of the client. There is a sweet spot where chi aligns and flows from Ren 17.

↜ 6. Heart-Cosmos Connection ↝

If possible, complete three cycles of the following practice during the last segment (4) of the heart fire sequence above.

1. Start with the felt sense of PR moving your heart, pericardium, and trunk toward the client in a heart-to-heart connection. Visualize the Breath of Life in your heart. Is it a light? Is it a holy person or some other symbol radiating a luminosity and brightness throughout your body and then expanding to fill the room you are in? Be with that visualization and felt sense of your heart.

2. Allow your perception to expand beyond the room (Zone C) in small increments to include Zone D to the horizon and way beyond. This image of PR becomes spiritual PR from the heart. It is the wisdom wind. This wisdom wind of PR changes phase outside of time and completely returns to the center of your heart. The beginning of the universe is now spontaneously located in your heart, ignited by the wisdom wind. The heart in this moment expresses a total originality.

3. Explore visualizing the colors of different planets, moons, and the sun of our solar system. Then expand to include the whole Milky Way and beyond. Stay in the tempo of PR being expressed from all its fulcrums with a felt sense of peacefulness, love, and beauty. The practice of wisdom eyes (page 443) is the short version of this heart-cosmos practice.

Attend to your perception of PR from your heart, with or without a color, to expand out to the horizon and beyond. Attempt to see PR and its color breathing out through the universe and back to your heart. The heart-to-heart connection with PR expands to become a heart-cosmos connection. It may simply feel as if the circumference of the trunk of your body expands during the phase changes of PR. The spiritual PR from the back of the heart radiates a shimmering blue color from a white or crystal-clear core in your literal heart. The heart-cosmos connection is simply a mirror of wisdom. The universe is reflecting its spiritual essence to the center of the heart. The center of the heart reflects this originality back to the universe. It is interconnected as one unified whole. (See figure 27.41 as an aesthetic to consider for the heart-cosmos connection; I call it *Look into the Void*.)

At a deeper level, consider that the reflection from your heart as it radiates out is actually generating the client, the natural world, and all visible and invisible structure in the universe. Imagine the client has disappeared and the radiance from your heart creates the client, the natural world, and all that is

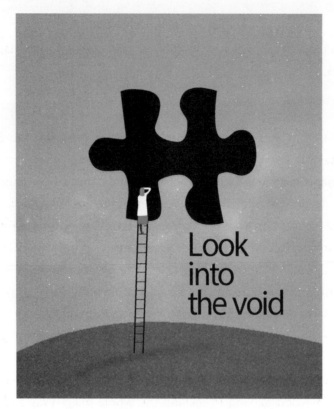

Fig. 27.41. Look into the Void

visible to the eyes and heard with the ears. The universe is a blank canvas, and your heart paints the universe with the radiance of the Breath of Life always residing in your heart. When PR changes phase, the entire universe including the client dissolves and dissipates back into your heart. Wait and rest in the Breath of Life until it decides to spontaneously radiate the universe into existence. From this perspective the heart is *mirrorlike wisdom*. This is a deep compassion practice to continually create the client in their original wholeness.

⌣ 7. Heaven's Gate ⌣

1. Sit at the head of the table for a few moments and settle without contact.
2. Contact the client's shoulders for a few moments.
3. Make bilateral contact with the bifurcation of the carotid arteries into the internal and external carotid arteries (see figs. 27.42–43). This is an important acupuncture point called Heaven's Gate (Large Intestine 18). This has a beneficial influence on the vagus nerve as it is next to the carotid artery. Synchronize with PR inside the arteries and note the difference between the two carotid arteries. Then synchronize with PR heart-to-heart.

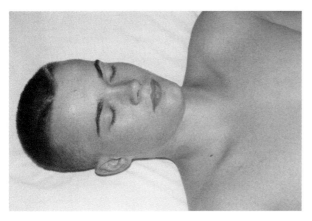

Fig. 27.42. Location of Heaven's Gate
(Large Intestine 18)

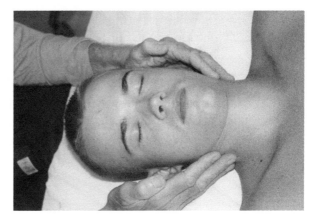

Fig. 27.43. Heaven's Gate palpation

⌇ 8. The Gaze of Compassion ⌇

1. Sitting at the head of the table, allow your spine to move backward as if being magnetically pulled by PR toward the horizon. Also feel the sides of your body move laterally. Allow your hands to gently contact the client's shoulders for several moments.

2. Negotiate permission to contact the inside corner of the client's eyes, above the nose. This is the top of the vascular tree. The internal carotid artery passes through the temporal bone, goes to the circle of Willis, and spreads from there, including the ophthalmic artery around the eye. The upper inside corner of the eye, marked in figure 27.44, is where the supratrochlear and supraorbital branches of the ophthalmic artery wrap around the frontal ridge of the frontal bone. Both are small arteries.

3. Using the pads of your index fingers, which fit perfectly in the corner of the eye, very gently feel the space between the skin and the frontal bone and the pulse of the supratrochlear and supraorbital arteries (see fig. 27.45). Once your hands

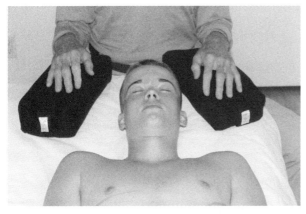

Fig. 27.44. Location of palpation for the supraorbital and
supratrochlear arteries

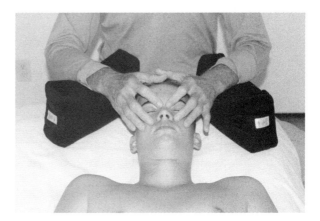

Fig. 27.45. Gaze of compassion palpation

are settled, lift your gaze to the horizon and sense PR moving from your third ventricle to the horizon and back in its slow tempo. This is the gaze of compassion. You can lower the fulcrum to your heart and sense PR moving from your heart to the horizon and back. Notice if your perception automatically shifts back and forth between the heart and third ventricle.

When you gaze at the horizon without being captured by your thoughts, you are looking at the whole planet and all sentient beings living on it. PR becomes the movement of compassion, which extinguishes all fires.

Practitioner Tip

There are several acupuncture points and deep arteries related to the immune system and the eyes on or around the greater wing of the sphenoid. Bilateral contact in that area may be more effective for some clients.

↷ 9. Earth Pulses ↶

1. Make contact with the tibial arteries, whether anterior, posterior, or both, bilaterally or ipsilaterally if the client needs it (see figs. 27.16–18, page 417). These are the earth element pulses, and they are the first to disappear in the dying process.
2. If appropriate, visualize a healing image to finish the protocol. Invite a benevolent second pair of hands if appropriate. Allow the second pair of hands to be an image, a real person alive or dead who represents a spiritual healing presence and is safe, without generating any fear. The second pair of hands may take over and move through your own hands from the center of the heart.

This chapter introduced basic biodynamic visualizations and imagining color as metabolic medicine. First, color is offered deliberately but only for several seconds to see if the spark of that color ignites a more spontaneous spreading and luminosity. Often one color is enough until familiarity is gained with this aptitude. The color offered can change quickly to many shades and hues or transmute into a completely different color. White and blue are the most basic healing colors to begin with. These practices last several seconds to maybe a minute or two before fading into the stillness or PR. When initially offering a color, attention is also placed on the hands because color travels at the speed of light and there can be an instantaneous vibration in the cellular metabolism of the body perceived by the hands. As mentioned, all cells in the human body emit biophotons and the heart emits the most. We are always affecting the cosmos with our luminosity. This luminosity contains the intelligence of the Breath of Life. Practice the protocols from this chapter before moving to the next.

28

The Five Fulcrums of the Water-Earth Elements

Please note that a complete view of all the arteries of the body can be seen in the color insert, plates 25–35. These can be reviewed prior to or during the study of the following protocols.

The fluid body contains all five fulcrums of the water and earth elements. Water and earth are combined in Tibetan medicine because water always contains earth minerals unless it is distilled. Blood is considered the water element in both the Indo-Tibetan and Sino-Tibetan systems of elements. The Sino-Tibetan system views the water element to be primary, while the Indo-Tibetan system sees the element of space as primary.

THE FIVE FULCRUMS OF THE WATER-EARTH ELEMENTS

All twelve major joints of the body

Trunk

Tongue-thyroid

Cranium

Stomach-spleen

Therapeutically, these fulcrums coregulate the metabolic flow of nutrients, waste removal, and the building of blood from real food.

The following biodynamic practices and protocols are deep repair for the fluid body. They begin with a Cycle of Attunement (COA). In this COA, the element of space is the dynamic stillness. We sit still and become present for the relationship. We place our hands in the pietà for sensing the whole. We then palpate the vascular tree to contact the Tree of Life cosmologically. We tune in to our posture, breath, and heartbeat as the ground of practice. We then make a heart-to-heart connection with PR to ignite the Tree of Life and the blood, the element of water. The following protocols are designed to be practiced sequentially in clinical practice. Each protocol encompasses one or more of the five fulcrums located in the body with the water and earth elements. It is important to work with only one or two of these fulcrums in any session of BCVT. The fulcrums link to the metabolism of the body, and each fulcrum activates a degree of potency that must be given time to express its healing priorities.

BIODYNAMIC VISUALIZATION PRACTICES TO ENHANCE THERAPEUTIC POTENCY

1. Synchronizing perception and palpation with *heart-in-hand* spiral meditation with the pericardium meridian (PC-8) as the principal fulcrum in the palm of our hands for PR.

    Heart-in-hand practice involves sensing a deep spiral from the belly through the heart and eyes that translates into PC-8.

2. The *heart-cosmos* practice with PR from the previous chapter is expanded with sky gazing practice and seeing the fulcrum of the element of space to calm the mind. This sky gazing practice develops wisdom eyes capable of seeing clearly inside and outside the body.

3. An internal second pair of hands can be visualized emerging from your heart based on the heart-cosmos visualization taught in chapter 27 and continued here. The internal second pair of hands can be Jesus, Buddha, Mary, Green Tara or any compatible spiritual figure who acts as a spiritual guide for you. Such a visualization is spontaneous rather than deliberate. Simply ask your heart who and what is necessary in the moment as it arises in the therapeutic process. And most times a void with light is all that appears and all that is necessary in the moment.

4. Visualization of the five primary colors are medicinal to repair the metabolism of the body as noted in the previous chapter.

5. Most of the palpation is done with finger pads rather than fingertips. The fingers are not static but subtly sensing three levels of the artery muscular wall, the endothelium, and the blood. Together these three levels are called the three springs and can be applied in any palpation.

6. These enhanced biodynamic processes function better when the mind is calm, and we are able to move our attention from our thoughts to open awareness of space thus allowing thoughts to self-liberate naturally. Always begin a session with a cycle of attunement. Stop mentally labeling sights and sounds.

ஓௗ
The First Water-Earth Elemental Protocol— The 12 Joints of the Body and Trunk Fulcrums

⌣ 1. Sit without Contact and Attune ⌣

1. Find your upright posture.

2. Notice the activity of your mind. Move attention into the space of stillness, where thoughts naturally dissipate on their own or are simply in the background.

3. Notice your breath and heartbeat. Ignite empathy.

4. Feel a heart-to-heart connection with PR. Ignite your vascular tree.

5. Find a heart-cosmos connection with wisdom eyes from the previous chapter. (see page 433), looking five to ten degrees above the plane of the horizon, being sure to lift your eyes without extending your head.

⤳ 2. Pietà ⤳

The client is supine. With one hand under the shoulder and one hand under the upper leg, sense the fluid body (see fig. 28.1). Visualize the fluid body as a deep blue.

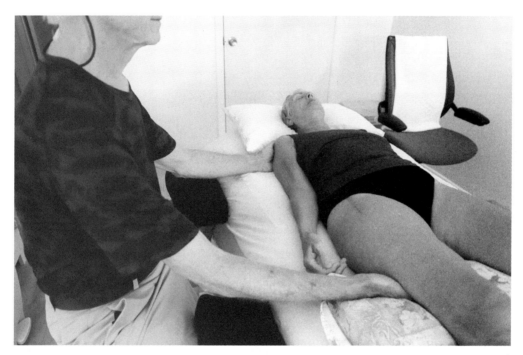

Fig. 28.1. Pietà

⤳ 3. Vascular Tree:
Igniting a Heart-to-Heart Connection with PR ⤳

Make contact with the client's radial and anterior tibial arteries (see fig. 28.2). Sense the vascular tree through the tone of autonomic nervous system (ANS) in the arteries. Metabolic problems cause the vascular tree to stiffen; it loses vasodilation with metabolic problems, which most clients have. The capillaries are the leaves, the arteries are the branches, the cerebral arteries are the top of the tree, and the heart and aortas are the trunk of the tree. Remember that the vascular tree forms from the periphery to center, while the heart develops from the center out.

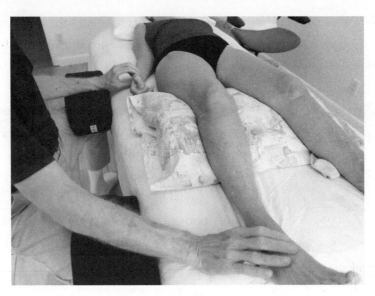

Fig. 28.2. Sensing the vascular tree

～ 4. The Fulcrum of the Twelve Joints ～

The first fulcrum of the water-earth element consists of the twelve major joints of the body, which are associated with the upper and lower extremities. These joints are like a constellation of stars. It is as if the cosmos is the fluid body, made of the water and earth elements. Each contact in the constellation of joints in the fluid body is ipsilateral except for the heart fulcrum. You are simply tracing a path through a unique cluster of stars as if the extremities were part of the Milky Way or any other of the billions of galaxies in the universe.

The blood is the deepest level of the fluid body and the water element in the physical body. Sensing the pulse is sensing the blood. Sensing the vascular tree is sensing the totality of the blood. These contact points will all be close to an acupuncture point. The intention is to contact these points as if they were a constellation in the Milky Way. Each of us has a unique constellation in the same way that each of us has a different natal chart in astrology. Our constellation reveals our relationship with the cosmos. Maintain attunement heart-to-heart to ignite the constellation therapeutically and then integrate the enhanced perceptual processes when appropriate.

It is up to you to choose which side of the body to begin with. Then make each of the subsequent contacts, crisscrossing back and forth from one side of the body to the other as follows:

1. Ipsilateral anterior tibial and popliteal arteries (fig. 28.3)
2. Ipsilateral popliteal and external iliac arteries (fig. 28.4)
3. Ipsilateral subclavian and brachial arteries (fig. 28.5)
4. Ipsilateral axillary and ulnar arteries (fig. 28.6)

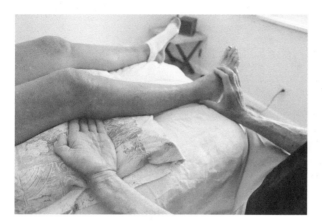

Fig. 28.3. Tibial and popliteal arteries

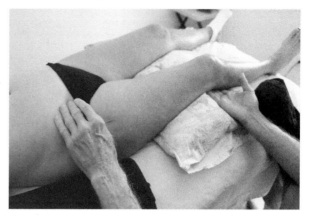

Fig. 28.4. Popliteal and external iliac arteries

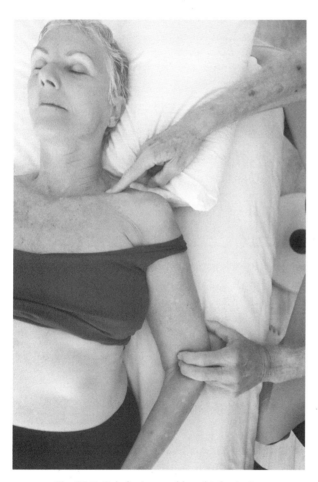

Fig. 28.5. Subclavian and brachial arteries

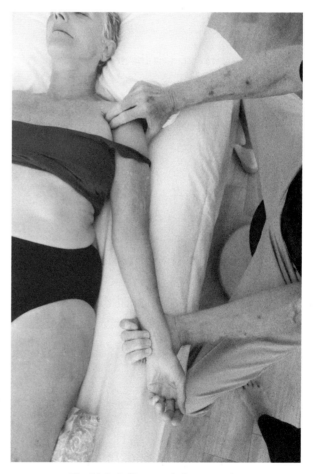

Fig. 28.6. Axillary and ulnar arteries

⌁ 5. The Trunk Fulcrum ⌁

Use one hand to contact the celiac trunk artery just below the xiphoid process and the other to contact the sternomanubrial notch (see fig. 28.7). Sense the aorta. Wait for PR to breath the trunk.

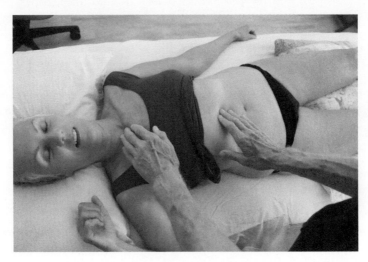

Fig. 28.7. Trunk contact

The trunk is the second fulcrum of the water-earth elements. We will also revisit it later.

My contact is with the celiac trunk artery with the finger pads of my right hand and the aorta with the fingers of my left hand. Settle and visualize a blue tube of liquid light flowing under your hands, as if the tube is resting in the client's spine. Let the liquid light be moving in the tempo of PR in both directions. It is like a lava lamp with its quality of movement.

⌒ 6. Coccyx and Heart ⌒

My contact is with the coccyx using the finger pad usually of my middle finger. The finger pads of my right hand are under the fourth, fifth and sixth thoracic vertebrae (figs. 28.8–9). Let your hands be soft and afferent. Settle into a cycle of attunement and continue to visualize a blue tube of light in front of the spine between both of your hands. Let Primary Respiration flow heart to heart.

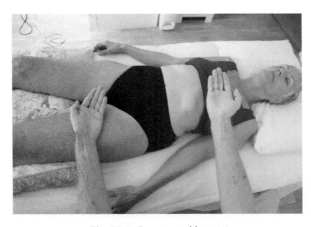

Fig. 28.8. Coccyx and heart 1

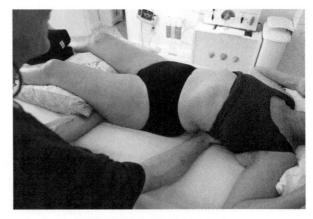

Fig. 28.9. Coccyx and heart 2

Practitioner Tip

"Settle" is a brief but important instruction. Always synchronize with PR heart-to-heart to activate the potential for visualization that stabilizes and integrates the entire ANS via the vagus nerve.

ॐ

The Second Water-Earth Fulcrums Protocol— The Tongue, Cranium, and Heart Fulcrums

◡ 1. Wisdom Eyes ◡

When we practice with our eyes open, frequently we gaze down at our client, and this is called the *gaze of humility*. To synchronize with PR, we gaze at the horizon, and this is the *gaze of compassion*. The practice called the *gaze of wisdom* involves the following.

1. Sit in a still posture with your eyes open.
2. Orient your breath to a spot between the umbilicus, pubic bone, and second lumbar vertebra.
3. Consciously feel your heartbeat and its potency. This ignites empathy.
4. Look ten to fifteen degrees above the plane of the horizon. Keep your head on the plane of the horizon, so only your eyes are lifted, which places a gentle tug on the third ventricle of the brain. Simultaneously maintain wide peripheral vision.
5. Between your physical eyes and the farthest-away object you can see in front of you, visualize a ball of space about the size of an orange or grapefruit. Initially this ball of space seems transparent, but it can become darker. It could even become a black dot or disk. Even rainbow colors could appear in that fulcrum. It is the fulcrum for seeing the origin of the universe in Eastern meditation practices.

You'll use this gaze of wisdom, or wisdom eyes, practice periodically when treating a client. If that means simply looking at an object on the wall of your office close to the ceiling, that's perfect. Simply visualize the ball or disk suspended in space between your eyes and the farthest object in front of you in your office. It's also important that you include the right and left corners of your peripheral vision in this practice. It's as if you are trying to see the entire visual field available to your eyes and at the same time differentiate this small ball-disk slightly above the plane of the horizon. You are creating a fulcrum to see the origin of the universe. This practice allows you to see more deeply into the vascular tree on the inside of your body and the client's body.

It takes time to synchronize with PR in a session. The good news is you can drop directly into the dynamic stillness at any time with wisdom eyes. Move your attention away from your thoughts, concepts, and emotions into open space visually. It stabilizes the mind and body. The exploration of wisdom eyes is an immediate experience of a stillpoint. You suddenly shift all your attention to that ball in space. It's simple, though it takes practice to master. Thoughts will come and go, and they mainly just go if we do not chase after them. You are looking at the vastness of the universe through a fulcrum attached to your third ventricle. Imagine having the capacity to shift your entire physiology and metabolism on a moment's notice.

◡ 2. Heart-Cosmos Connection ◡

Follow the steps outlined on page 433 to establish a heart-cosmos connection.

◡ 3. Heart Fulcrum ◡

The client is supine. Make contact with the heart fulcrum at the level of the spinous processes of C3–C4 (see figs. 28.10–11). Wait for PR to breathe into the embryonic fulcrum of the heart from this original location of the heart.

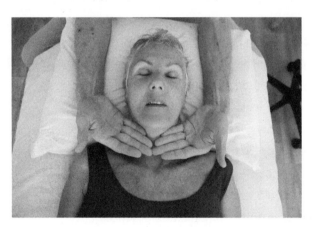

Fig. 28.10. Heart fulcrum 1

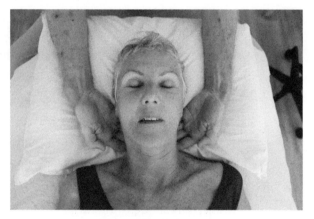

Fig. 28.11. Heart fulcrum 2

Practitioner Tip

Whenever we sit at the head of the table, before making contact, we allow PR to move our spine, occiput, and brainstem posteriorly. This is finding the back of the body. Our nervous system must expand backward because of how close we are to the client's brain. Then we find the space between our heart and our spine with our breath. This is a temporary midline established by the breath and space. Abdominal breathing expands very gently to surround the heart and relax the heart and dorsal pericardium in the core of the body. Then we bring our attention to the sternum and anterior heart fields, breathing with PR heart-to-heart with our client. This is a cranial cycle of attunement, as described in chapter 24. Typically, the first contact would be a gentle palm down contact on the shoulders and then reattunement in order to not activate or trigger the autonomic nervous system of the client.

❧ 4. The Fulcrum of the Tongue-Thyroid ❧

1. The tongue-thyroid is the third fulcrum of the water-earth elements. Sit at the head of the table and use the tips or pads of your index fingers to make gentle contact bilaterally with the tendon of the sternocleidomastoid muscle (SCM). Sense the carotid arteries and the lateral borders of the thyroid gland where the inferior thyroid arteries enter the thyroid (see fig. 28.12).

2. Make gentle contact between the greater horns of the hyoid bone and the septum of the SCM anteriorly. This also effects the laryngeal branch of the vagus and the connection to the pharyngeal plexus (see fig. 28.13–15). Sense the superior thyroid and laryngeal arteries coming from the carotid artery. Wait for the hyoid to soften and expand laterally.

3. Shift your finger pads to contact the external base of the tongue. The genioglossus, mylohyoid, digastric, and geniohyoid muscles attach to the sublingual and digastric fossa of the body of the mandible. The contact is on the anterior midline close to the body of the mandible (see fig. 28.16–17). Gentle three-spring pressure can be used if the base of the tongue is tight. Explore the fulcrums of tension. Wait for the tongue to soften.

4. Check the facial artery where it crosses over the mandible (see fig. 28.18).

5. Check the tension of the styloid process bilaterally if necessary (see figs. 28.19–21).

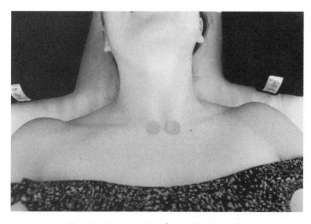

Fig. 28.12. Location for palpating the inferior thyroid arteries

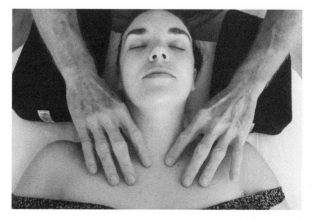

Fig. 28.13. Inferior thyroid arteries

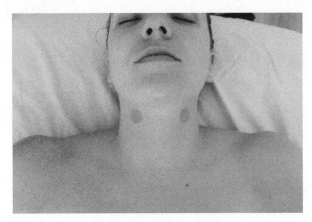

Fig. 28.14. Location for palpating the superior thyroid and laryngeal arteries

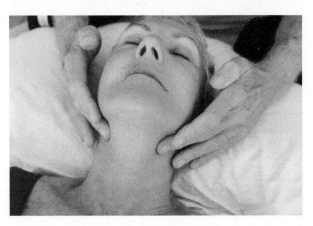

Fig. 28.15. Contact on the hyoid bone and superior thyroid and laryngeal arteries

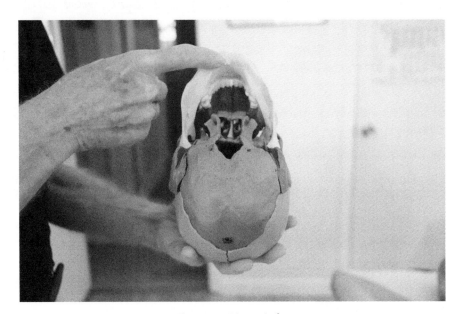

Fig. 28.16. Digastric fossa

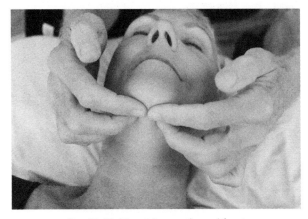

Fig. 28.17. Digastric muscle and fascia

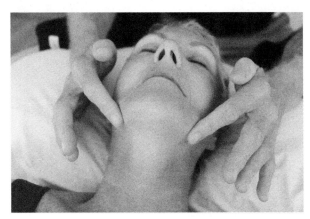

Fig. 28.18. Facial artery

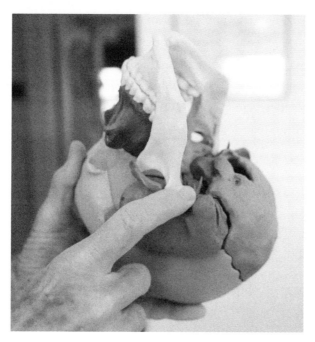

Fig. 28.19. Styloid process 1

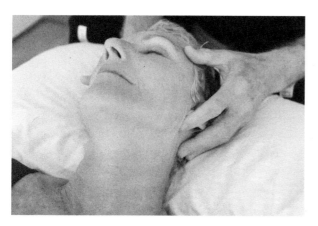

Fig. 28.20. Styloid process 2

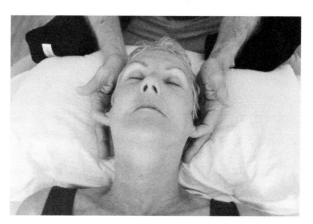

Fig. 28.21. Styloid process 3

☙ 5. The Fulcrum of the Cranium on Three Axes ☙

1. The cranium as a whole is the fourth fulcrum of the water-earth elements. Begin with wisdom eye practice (see page 443). Then contact the client's cranium with overlapping thumbs on Du 20 (see figs. 28.22–23). Be sure to stabilize your wrists with cushions. This is the vertical axis of the central channel of the subtle body. Visualize a light blue tube extending from Du 20 vertically down through the aorta and terminating at the lower dantian. The blue tube also extends several centimeters above the head, merging into a pinkish red shimmering light. Alternatively, visualize the brain itself as the color white.

2. Contact the horizontal axis through the parietal ridge (see figs. 28.24–26). This

axis includes the anterior and posterior commissures adjacent to the third ventricle. The parietal bones are the most metabolically active bones in the cranium. Move your fingers along the ridge until you sense the sweet spot of the anterior commissure. If necessary, ask the client to roll their eyes up to the middle of their forehead for just a moment and then relax them. This stretches the anterior commissure, and you'll feel a wave through the parietal ridge in the

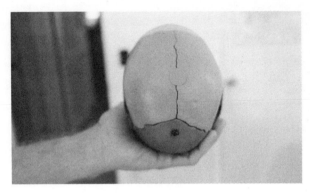

Fig. 28.22. Location of Du 20

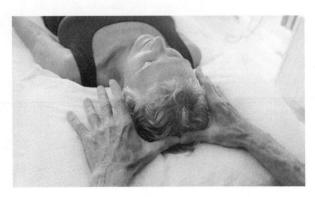

Fig. 28.23. Du 20 contact

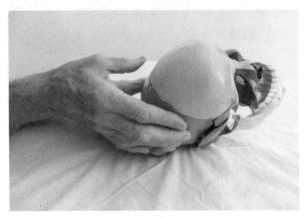

Fig. 28.24. Parietal ridge 1

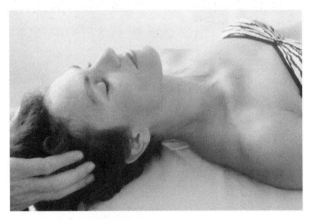

Fig. 28.25. Parietal ridge 2

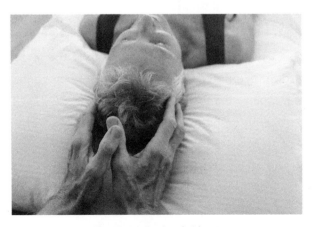

Fig. 28.26. Parietal ridge 3

pads of your fingers, indicating the correct location. Visualize this axis as white or any color that comes to mind or is shown to you.

3. Have the client lie on their side. Contact the longitudinal axis. It is a front-to-back axis. This begins an exploration of Sutherland's fulcrum located on this axis at the Great Vein of Galen. Place the finger pads of one hand on the external occipital protuberance, the inion. Imagine the longitudinal axis as a line through the straight sinus and extending to a point where it exits around the bregma. Place the finger pads of your other hand here (see figs. 28.27–28). Sense the fulcrum automatically shift and the line between your two contacts breathing in the tempo of PR. Notice if the third ventricle or the pituitary radiates a light. Engage a second pair of hands (see page 451) if available.

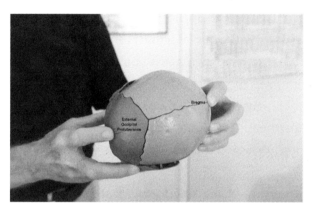

Fig. 28.27. Sutherland's fulcrum 1

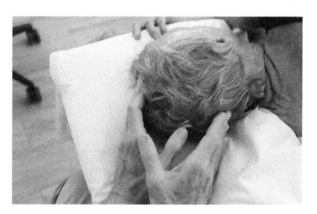

Fig. 28.28. Sutherland's fulcrum 2

⌁ 6. Core Link: Sacrum and Occiput ∿

Finish by finding PR between the sacrum and occiput while client is lying on their side (see fig. 28.29).

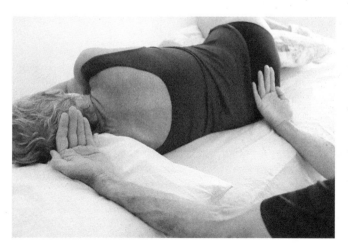

Fig. 28.29. Core link

ᏬᏬ
The Third Water-Earth Fulcrums Protocol—
The Stomach-Spleen Fulcrum

ᴗ 1. Sit without Contact and Attune ᴗ

Find your midline of stillness, rest your mind, and notice your breath and heartbeat. Feel a heart-to-heart connection with PR. This is the cycle of attunement. Then find a heart-cosmos connection with wisdom eyes, looking above the plane of the horizon without extending your head.

ᴗ 2. Heart in Hands ᴗ

Rest your hands, palms up, on your legs and bring your attention to Pericardium 8 by the medial border of the thenar eminence (see fig. 28.30) for the location of Pericardium 8 and Heart 8 indicated by the dots. Feel your heartbeat, and know that with every contraction of the left ventricle, the heart twists in a counterclockwise direction, and when the heart relaxes, it moves in a clockwise direction. Sense this movement with PR moving in and out of your hands. Allow PR to breathe through Pericardium 8 while sensing your heartbeat. It is a spiral motion and may even radiate a color. Are your hands glowing? Which color is radiating? Is it the Breath of Life?

This is how to train to sense the spiral movement of the blood with PR through Pericardium 8 in the palms of your hands. Your hands now become an instrument of blessing. It is a benediction of the Holy Spirit living in the heart inside the heart.

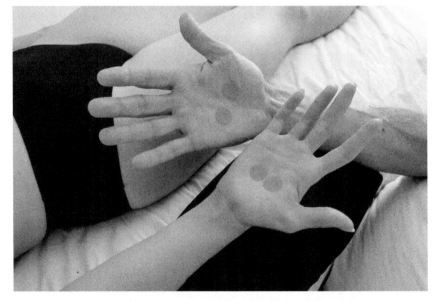

Fig. 28.30. Heart in hand

The Internal Second Pair of Hands

The second pair of hands involves two possibilities. One is that at any time during a session, and especially at the end, we can invite a benevolent, healing figure to enter the room and place their hands on the client. This practice derives from the osteopathic lineage. It is an invitation for a sacred presence to assist the treatment by placing their hands on the client. The therapist simply observes and remains in communion with the benevolent other without interrupting.

For twenty years I could sense the benevolent other in my treatment room, and frequently clients would say they felt a second pair of hands on them. About ten years ago, this benevolent presence became a visionary apparition. Usually it was Jesus, manifesting with either water or blood coming from the stigmata in his hands and pouring over or into the client. It's a baptism of blood and water. When Jesus appeared in sessions while I was treating two of my nieces, I told them about it and they verified that their experience was exactly what I was seeing.

The other possibility with a second pair of hands is to place attention on a divine light combined with a sacred image, such as Jesus, Medicine Buddha, or others that we may be spiritually compatible with. The radiant energy of that light as a beam coming from the spiritual image moves from our heart and down through our pericardium meridian into the palms of our hands. At this point, whether it remains a light or transforms to a spiritual figure, the radiant divine light appears as divine hands that move through the chest, shoulders, and arms into the therapist's hands. There is a pause, and then the sacred hands move into the client's body as if it is transparent. As Dr. Sutherland discovered, PR will choose the most important site it wants to engage and heal. As biodynamic therapists, we simply watch where this second pair of hands as divine light and spiritual wisdom goes into the client. We call this wisdom that is rooted in the Breath of God Primary Respiration. We can observe its activity, resolution of the chosen fulcrum, and disengagement within moments.

As many of my clients are Christian, Jesus spontaneously appears in my heart during my laying-on-of-hands ministry. I see him as a bright light with different hues of the rainbow. I feel his hands emerge from my heart, go through my arms, and gently merge into my hands, at which point they continue inside the client's body to a location only Jesus can know. I am the willing observer. His hands then generate a clear bright light and whatever anatomical object he is holding turns to pure light. Sometimes I am allowed to see what structure he is holding and remain in his presence without interfering. When he is finished, his being and essence return to my heart as a powerful light capable of illuminating the universe. With some female clients, Mary, the mother of Jesus, appears from my heart. With others, multifaith sacred images of the feminine come alive in my heart and spontaneously move through my arms and hands.

It starts with seeing a bright light in your heart, and most often that is the only necessary appearance of the sacred. Allow it to radiate everywhere.

⌇ 3. Pietà ⌇

With one hand under the client's shoulder and one hand under the upper leg, sense the fluid body. Visualize the fluid body as a deep blue.

⌇ 4. Vascular Tree ⌇

Sense the vascular tree as the Tree of Life. The capillaries are the leaves, the arteries are the branches, and the heart and aortas are the trunk of the tree. Visualize the Tree of Life floating in a vast ocean of dark blue and ignite heart-to-heart with PR.

⌇ 5. The Trunk Fulcrum ⌇

1. The trunk is the fourth fulcrum of the water-earth elements. Place the pads of one or two fingers in the client's sternal notch to access the vagal bodies. Place the pads of one or two fingers of your other hand in contact with the client's celiac trunk a couple of centimeters inferior of the xiphoid process (see fig. 28.31).

2. Listen to the client's breathing. Notice if the client has paradoxical breathing, which is too much breath in the upper lobes of the lungs while the abdomen is not expanding on inhalation. Verbally direct the client to breathe into the point of contact on the abdomen. Watch for PR in its spiral.

3. Shift the contact from the vagal bodies to the celiac artery, and shift the hand that contacted the celiac trunk to the umbilicus (see fig. 28.32). Practice a spiral to synchronize with PR.

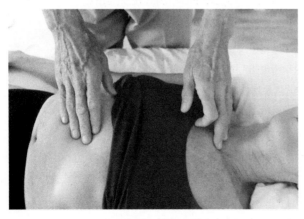

Fig. 28.31. Trunk

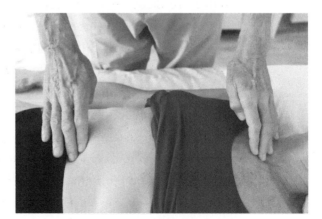

Fig. 28.32. Trunk

⌁ 6. The Stomach-Spleen Fulcrum ⌁

The spleen, with its paired meridian of the stomach, represents the earth element in the Sino-Tibetan system. Within the Indo-Tibetan system, the stomach and spleen are both water and earth combined and comprise the fifth fulcrum of the water-earth elements. Water and earth generously provide the nourishment we need to live and thrive. The stomach and spleen within us receive the drink and food we consume, make it into a proper digestive mixture, and transport its essence to fuel every organ, function, and system of the body. Figure 28.33 shows the location of the splenic artery.

1. Sitting at the left-hand side of the client, place Pericardium 8 of your right hand over the spleen. Place Pericardium 8 on the palm of your left hand over the stomach at the point where the most heat is radiating (see fig. 28.34).

2. With the pads of the index and middle fingers of your left hand, find the celiac trunk. With the pads of the index and middle fingers on your right hand, feel the splenic artery approximately midway between the celiac trunk and the spleen (see fig. 28.35). The splenic artery bisects the stomach, usually in the

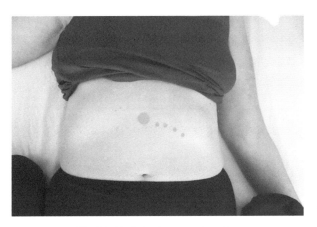

Fig. 28.33. Splenic artery location

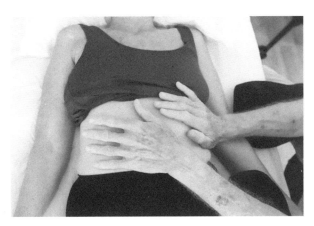

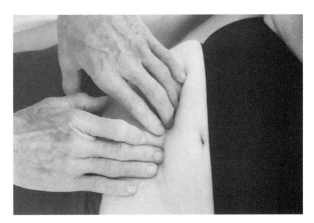

Fig. 28.34. Splenic artery 1   *Fig. 28.35. Splenic artery 2*

upper half, depending on stomach ptosis and the contents in the stomach.

3. Synchronize with PR and visualize a mist of color floating from the stomach up through the trunk of the body, out the trunk of the body, and into the earth. It is like a gentle mist, or rain, simply falling to the earth. Then repeat step 1 if necessary. Sense PR moving between the stomach and spleen.

⌁ 7. Sacral Outflow of PNS—Terminal Dorsal Vagus ⌁

Contact the coccyx to begin this process. The other hand has options for contact posteriorly or anteriorly on the client's body. In general I prefer my free hand to contact the terminal ends of the dorsal vagus at either the hypogastric plexuses or Cannon-Baum point. There are options depending on the practitioner's sense of what is needed in the moment. Please review the hand positions for the coccyx and abdomen in chapters 24 and 25. Review figure 25.33 (page 371) and figure 25.44 (page 376) for the relative location of the abdominal pulses and landmarks. See figures 28.36–38 for the individual hand positions. These are designed to stabilize the entire neurovascular system of the abdomen and pelvis.

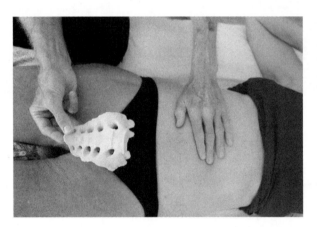

Fig. 28.36. Coccyx and Cannon's point

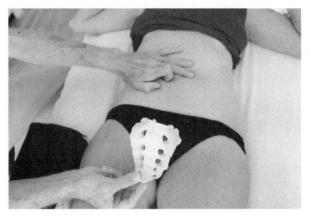

Fig. 28.37. Coccyx and umbilicus

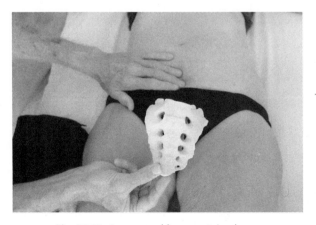

Fig. 28.38. Coccyx and hypogastric plexus

29

Biodynamic and Trauma-Informed Care for Concussions

Please note that a complete view of all the arteries of the body can be seen in the color insert, plates 25–35. These can be reviewed prior to or during the study of the following protocols.

I would like to thank a couple of people in particular for their assistance with this chapter: Sue Wozniak, for integrating biological gender differences, and Margery Chessare, for her willingness to edit and make suggestions for greater clarity. I am grateful to both of you for your help.

Concussions are a community challenge because of their increasing prevalence in contemporary culture. It is likely that everyone reading this essay and most of the clients we treat have a history of concussions. I will explore this territory with you from a biodynamic point of view. *Traumatic brain injury* (TBIs) describes the traumatic event and immediate neurological consequences to the head. The term *concussion* refers to a mild form of TBI. There are numerous symptoms of reduced or impaired function somatically, neurologically, and psychophysiologically that occur after a TBI (Romeu-Mejia et al. 2019, Signoretti et al. 2011). Throughout this chapter, I will use the terms *TBI* and *concussion* interchangeably.

A TBI interferes with molecular signaling between neurons and the endothelium of the cerebrovascular system, thus making it difficult for the brain to get the vascular nutrition it needs to function physiologically and metabolically, locally and globally throughout the soma. It also makes it difficult to remove the waste products of neuroinflammation and cell metabolism. This results in a subsequent loss of function physiologically and metabolically. Severity depends on the vector of the injury to the cranium and previous history of head trauma. The brain can rebound violently against the cranial bones and dura mater, ripping and tearing hundreds of thousands of neurons. Even one TBI can have long-lasting consequences (Zhou et al. 2013).

Brain tissue takes the longest of any body tissue to heal, so knowing how many concussions a client has sustained in their life is important; there may be an experience of headache pain associated with the trauma or memories of past trauma, for example. I know this one personally, having sustained at least six TBIs in my life, starting at age ten. As complete a history as possible of the client's TBIs must be known before beginning to explore this territory in biodynamic practice.

Interest in TBI is peaking due to publicity around the devastating effects of concussions on professional athletes. While going through the magazine rack at an airport departure lounge I saw "Play football = die!" on a headline in a newspaper. There is a deeply embedded "no pain, no gain" ethic in the family culture of contact sports, especially American-style football and international hockey. The incidence of TBIs among these professional athletes leads to chronic traumatic encephalopathy (CTE). It is known that almost 100 percent of athletes in these two professions who sustain multiple TBIs will likely end up with debilitating and chronic neurologically based physical and mental health issues as they age (Mez et al. 2017). Former players also experience a high rate of suicide.

The incidence of TBIs has increased among all ages and populations because of the sheer speed at which people lead their lives and drive their bodies with inputs like high-energy drinks and Starbucks (and these are by no means the only two ways in the way people speed up and disconnect from their body). Pediatric TBIs have seen a substantial and alarming increase in the past decade, a particular concern due to children's delicate developing brains (Ledoux et al. 2022). There was a 60 percent increase in concussion incidence from 2007 to 2014 in adolescents (Zhang et al. 2016). TBIs sustained prior to adolescence are potentially worse for long-term health outcomes. Our work is so valuable for children who suffer a TBI, including infants. I have treated numerous infants with TBI. Infants and children should receive cranial treatments from a pediatrically trained biodynamic craniosacral therapist or craniosacral therapist.

Research has shown that there are gender differences in the neurological expression of genes and in the healing response times of TBIs. In other words, males and females express different proteins in their brains following an TBI (Valera et al. 2021). As of a few years ago, researchers did not know why this is so. Much more research needs to be done, especially since girls and women may have longer healing response times from an TBI than boys and men (Mollayeva et al. 2018, 2019).

Domestic violence is the third most frequent cause of concussion, after motor vehicle accidents and sports injury (Doctor and Shiromoto 2009). Poorer outcomes for women from concussions have been correlated with particular phases of the menstrual cycle at the time of concussion. The follicular phase represents the first half of the cycle up to ovulation and features higher estrogen levels, while the luteal phase that follows tends to feature higher progesterone levels. Some studies found women had worse postconcussion symptoms when the injury was sustained during the luteal phase compared with concussions occurring during the follicular phase (Giordano et al. 2020). Also, the preexistence of depression or anxiety may be associated with the outcomes and prevalence of postconcussion syndrome (Martin et al. 2020). The type of persistent postconcussion symptoms tends to vary by biological sex. Males report sleep disturbance, aggression, and substance abuse, while females report headache, anxiety, and depression (Giordano et al. 2020). The pathophysiology of concussions thus varies and includes numerous symptoms (Romeu-Mejia et al. 2019, Signoretti et al. 2011). The Rivermead Post-Concussion Symptoms Questionnaire is readily available online, and I find it the easiest to work with. The CDC also publishes a Signs and Symptoms of Concussion Checklist that is very comprehensive.

COMORBIDITY

Metabolic syndrome is a significant risk factor in delaying the healing response time from TBIs. Eighty-eight percent of the U.S. population has metabolic syndrome (Araújo et al. 2019) and its associated condition known as "leaky gut," a chronic degradation of the epithelium of the gut lining in the small intestine. A TBI can generate leaky gut overnight by disrupting the barrier function of the epithelium (Bansal et al 2009). This upregulates the immune system, causing chronic, systemic inflammation via the portal vein, the liver, and the endothelium in much of the cardiovascular system. The result is a greater potential for inflammation to reach the brain via the vascular endothelium of the blood-brain barrier (Patterson and Holahan 2012) and a decrease in cerebral blood flow (Wang et al. 2016, Meier et al. 2015). This makes concussions a metabolic syndrome. A concussion can also exacerbate leaky gut for someone whose immune system is already compromised by further weakening the immune system and increasing gut pain. The good news is that this challenge to the viscera activates the anti-inflammatory response of the vagus nerve (Pavlov and Tracey 2012). The vagus nerve is a key player in treating concussions and metabolic syndrome.

In addition, 90 percent of the bacteria in the gut produce neurotransmitters that coregulate neurological functioning and directly correlate to a wide variety of psychological and functional problems from behavior to cognition. The most significant metabolic pathway from the gut microbiome to the brain are the blood vessels and the dorsal portion of the vagus nerve (Kolacz and Porges 2018). This further illustrates that concussions are a significant metabolic problem involving the quad of gut-liver-heart-brain.

Since the brain needs high-quality fatty acids to function properly, from the mitochondria all the way down to the myelin sheath, the ketogenic diet and the metabolic pathways of ketogenesis, in which fats are converted to ketone energy for the brain, can be a helpful healing component (D'Andrea et al. 2019, Gross et al. 2019). The brain prefers ketones over glucose for its mitochondria. When the mitochondria are more efficient, they secrete fewer waste products that can be difficult to remove if neuroinflammation is present. This means clients can dietarily reduce the metabolic pathway of glycolysis in which carbohydrates, especially from processed foods and added sugars, are used to provide such energy to the brain. Ketogenic diets have been used since the 1920s to help children with brain dysfunction. All the children I worked with in my fifty-year career who had mild, moderate, or severe developmental delays, which included significant brain damage, improved on a ketogenic diet specifically formulated for each child. Even a child on a feeding tube can have a tablespoon of organic linseed oil placed in the shunt once or twice a day and see some improvement.

Healing needs to happen not only at the mitochondrial/ATP cycle level of the axons in the brain but also in the body, including the liver and myofascial system. The fascia makes up so much of the body's integrity and its proprioception, so its capacity to dissipate impact trauma must be addressed in any long-term concussion rehab program as well as in other forms of the manual therapeutic arts, especially biodynamic craniosacral therapy and colon hydrotherapy, fields in which both my wife and I are licensed to perform in the state of Florida. My wife Cathy teaches medical personnel internationally in the correct use of colon hydrotherapy. The cellular recycling and waste removal systems of the body need to be functioning well to heal an TBI. The first requirement is a reduction in dietary carbohydrates, especially added sugar (the main fuel of the inflammatory process and significant feeder of cancer cells) to heal more efficiently from TBI (Agrawal et al. 2016). This makes metabolic syndrome a major comorbid factor in concussions. Plus, as mentioned, metabolic syndrome is already present in most Americans. No wonder COVID was so lethal for so many, especially those who are obese (Popkin et al. 2020).

Post-traumatic stress disorder (PTSD) is also a comorbid factor in TBIs (Combs et al. 2015). TBIs, many of which have a traumatic origin, can cause PTSD. Likewise, for those who already have PTSD, healing from a TBI may be greatly delayed and thus exacerbate preexisting symptoms such as dysautonomia driven by the autonomic nervous system (ANS) both physiologically and metabolically (Doctor and Shiromoto 2009). Biodynamic treatment for concussions must be trauma-informed. As biodynamic therapists, we must remain synchronized with Primary Respiration (PR) and its healing intentions. We must stay centered in the midline of dynamic stillness. Knowing our own trauma and concussion history is vital. I still receive cranial treatments for my history of concussions to this day.

TRAUMA-INFORMED CARE (TIC)

Trauma-informed care honors the wide variety of intersecting identities and stories that each of us humans have. First and foremost therapeutic work is about honoring our client's humanity and avoiding retraumatization. We all must be sensitive to side effects, even from the most gentle touch. A critical factor mentioned throughout this book and in my previous books is the necessity to have a safe and trustworthy container in the therapeutic relationship. As practitioners of any therapeutic modality, we must generate trust, collaboration and empowerment because ultimately, the client is the master of their own experience (Yamasaki 2024). This is what I have learned in my journey starting with chapter 1 of this book.

Three Tenets

I work with what are called the three tenets of compassion for TIC. It begins *first* with the gate of not-knowing and letting go of theory. Typically we try to find out what's wrong with the client. The reality is that we need to ask, "How did this happen?" As biodynamic therapists, we listen to our client's narrative and begin to get a sense of somatic empathy. Frequently we can taste and touch the fear that our client is experiencing not only at the level of their brain but also the level of their gut and heart. As biodynamic therapists we may frequently encounter our own sense of anxiety and fear once we begin the treatment. We may fear that somehow the theory we learned in class or a book will melt away into the stillness. We can only be present for that moment and wait for its door to open.

The door opens to the *second* process of trauma-informed care. We stabilize in our ability to bear witness and rest in our own midline of stillness mentally and emotionally. This develops emotional empathy and is greatly facilitated by the interoception of consciously sensing our own heartbeat (Chen et al. 2021, Heydrich et al. 2021, Fukushima et al. 2011). Biodynamically, we rest in our breath and heartbeat. How simple is that.

Then it is possible to experience the *third* tenet of compassionate response. It is important to differentiate between reaction and response. Frequently, there is the urge to move things along in the therapeutic treatment. It is important to resist that urge and not be reactive but rather to wait for the appropriate compassionate response. In biodynamic terminology this means resting in the rhythmic balanced interchange of PR and dynamic stillness.

Polyvagal Neutral

Knowledge of polyvagal theory, social safety, and the neuroception of safety is also important for TIC. The key point in the context of treating concussions is to avoid the side effect of eliciting defensive physiology in the ANS. As Dr. Rollin Becker used to say, "The therapeutic process does not begin until the will of the patient yields to the will of Primary Respiration." The will of the patient is the activated ANS arising from head trauma. Our hands and our presence communicate safety until a Neutral is perceived. This is a settling in the ANS of the client. This facilitates PR shifting from its maintenance mode to its therapeutic mode and thus the "will of Primary Respiration" begins the treatment. We must also recall that Dr. Sutherland said that respect and reverence for the self-healing mechanism of PR must become an aspect of every treatment.

Cycle of Attunement

The perceptual process of facilitating a Neutral in biodynamics is the cycle of attunement. As biodynamic therapists, we regularly reverse attention during a session for a phase of resynchronizing with our own fluid fields, the tide of PR, and the dynamic stillness in our own internal awareness and external perception of the natural world. The cycle of attunement is always the basic unit of perceptual work in a biodynamic session. It is biodynamic mindfulness/awareness practice! It supports the three tenets of compassion in building somatic and emotional empathy.

Fluid Body, Fluid Fields, Fluid Brain

In biodynamic practice we perceive PR and its rhythmic balanced interchange with dynamic stillness. We initially palpate the fluid fields of the whole known as the fluid body, and then we approach the unique fluid fields of the cranium that mark the boundaries between the face, vault, and base. Working with the fluid nature of the body is always the starting point in a biodynamic session. And it may be particularly crucial to recovery from TBI. New research indicates the brain itself communicates through fluid waves (Gepshtein et al. 2022). The traditional view of brain function describes brain activity as an interaction of neurons. However, brain activity is better described as the interaction of waves. Both views are needed to understand how the brain functions. As the Salk Institute describes it, "The researchers hypothesize that the same kinds of waves are being generated—and interacting with each other—in every part of the brain's cortex, not just the part responsible for the analysis of visual information. That means waves generated by the brain itself, by subtle cues in the environment or internal moods, can change the waves generated by sensory inputs" (Salk Institute 2022). This speaks to the efficacy of biodynamic cardiovascular therapy in the treatment of TBI.

The Health

In all the courses I teach, the relationship of PR to the dynamic stillness is fundamental and is directly related to the Health. "Find the Health, anyone can find disease," as A.T. Still, founder of osteopathy, famously said. Biodynamic trauma-informed care is fundamentally based on Dr. Still's prescription to "Find the Health." We orient to the perception of dynamic stillness as a treatment enhancement for TBI. The Health becomes the endpoint of a biodynamic session, according to some biodynamic osteopaths. They say the Health is perceived by an increase in the potency of PR and the depth of the dynamic stillness nonconceptually and nonreferentially. This is the deep beauty of our midline internally and externally.

Dynamic stillness internally is intrinsic to the venous system, especially in the cranium. It seeks to balance itself with PR, as expressed in spiral or helical blood flow and endothelial function. This translates into a connection with the Dynamic Stillness inherent in the venous sinus system of the cranium, balancing it with the midline of the carotid and vertebral arteries. The dynamic stillness, called cellular quiescence in biology (in reference, for example, to the cells of the vascular endothelium), is critical to the entire metabolism of the body. The center of the spiral blood flow is dynamically still, the endothelium cells are quiescent, and all molecules in the body and in nature must undergo a stillpoint for a higher or deeper level of transformation to occur. This is grace woven into all layers of cranial structure and function. Our therapeutic perceptions of the fluid body and its fluid fields together with PR are fulcrums of orientation for the Health to manifest in clients with concussions. Thus, "wholeness is the smallest subdivision of life," as Dr. James Jealous said.

KEY POINTS IN TREATING CONCUSSIONS

1. Regarding the bones, it is important to have a sense of the beveling of the major cranial sutures, especially the occipitomastoid suture (OMS). According to Dr. Becker, the occiput has its greatest range of motion between the OMS bilaterally (occipital squama), and the OMS is hard-wired into the fourth ventricle for proper distribution of the cerebrospinal fluid (CSF) into the subarachnoid space of the brain and spinal cord. The atlanto-occipital joint (AOJ) must also be explored because it houses links to both the orienting and the head-righting reflexes that are compromised in an TBI.

2. It's important to know different skills for interacting with the bones of the vault derived from membrane, the bones of the face derived from the foregut endoderm of the embryo, and the bones of the cranial base derived from cartilage. These three embryonic derivatives can provide doorways into concussion symptoms. The fluid fields of these three aspects of the cranium can be sensed in order to integrate them into the cranium's preexisting wholeness.

3. The movement of the reciprocal tension membrane (RTM) system of the cranium must be observed. My favorite listening station is the inferior lateral angle of the parietal bones, where both layers of the tentorium can be sensed.

I call this the "side door" to the midline and sella turcica, the seat of the pituitary.

4. The ram's horn movement of the neural tissue itself, as noted by Sutherland and by embryologists, must be observed with sensitive fingers and hands.

5. The fluctuation of CSF especially in the third and fourth ventricles as well as in the core link connection of the dura mater from the sacrum to the occiput must be observed.

6. The cerebrovascular drainage system may be compromised due to the likely displacement of Sutherland's fulcrum, also known as the great cerebral vein or the vein of Galen, at the anterior end of the straight sinus and more importantly connected to the pineal recess in the posterior third ventricle. This also includes the space of the superior sagittal sinus because of the uptake mechanism of the CSF in the arachnoid villi in that area of the cranium.

7. The relationship of blood flow to the endothelium of both the arteries and veins must be palpated with the sensitivity and perception of the Tide. Research shows that TBIs cause a reduction in blood flow to the brain. This is an important entrance point in assisting the restoration of function to the brain.

8. Midline skills for the embryonic notochord are essential. This structural midline appears as a snakelike movement in its development and terminates rostrally with the cartilage of the nose. This midline is deeply associated with dynamic stillness.

9. Facilitating a therapeutic response with the tide of PR can minimize the effects of certain symptoms of the heart itself. Some types of TBIs concuss the heart via the pericardium. Resulting conditions could be pericarditis of the parietal pericardium or myocarditis of the visceral pericardium. The vagus nerve must be approached regularly.

10. Belly breathing must be an essential part of the healing process for both the practitioner and the client. The transversus abdominus muscle interdigitates with the diaphragm. Concussions may cause a startle reflex in the diaphragm. It spasms and tightens, forcing more breath to fill the upper lobes of the lungs. But the breath needs to return to the belly and lower lobes of the lungs to better oxygenate the brain and keep the lower lobes of the lungs functioning at a higher level because the highest concentration of oxygen receptors is in the lower lobes. Breathing primarily in the upper lobes, known as paradoxical breathing, puts too much pressure on the heart. In the Eastern traditions, the breath must be able to rest in the lower dantian, a source of profound energy located anterior to the bifurcation of the common iliac arteries and abdominal aorta. Belly breathing primes the energy of the lower dantian.

Cranial Structure Palpation

Biodynamic craniosacral therapy in general is known anecdotally to be helpful for the effects of concussions by reducing symptoms more quickly, probably due to increasing circulation in the brain (Meier et al. 2015). When dealing with post-concussion clients, the traditional Sutherland/Still osteopathic anatomical layers of the bones, dural membrane, neural tissue, cerebrospinal fluid, and blood must all be considered for palpation. This is important, as the impact of TBI on the cranium dissipates its force vector through all the different layers of structure and function. Dr. Upledger's release of the "energy cyst" is another good example of a skill that may help relieve concussion symptoms. I was in Dr. Upledger's first teacher certification training in 1986, and I learned so much from him about concussions.

PALPATORY SKILLS FOR TRAUMATIC BRAIN INJURIES

As biodynamic therapists, we always work within the perception of the rhythmic balanced interchange of Primary Respiration (Ignition) and dynamic stillness (midline). The physical pressure used makes no difference when synchronized with this interchange. Pressure is a negotiation between our hands and the client's tissue. And safety must be established for all styles of biodynamic practice to access the Health (the potency of Primary Respiration). The art of biodynamic practice is always returning to this interchange when our attention is captured mentally or emotionally. We practice the cycle of attunement regularly, placing our attention out to the horizon and back in the tempo of PR or sensing PR heart-to-heart with the client. The natural world always participates in the biodynamic process.

The following three explorations are each built around an easy-to-follow protocol. The three protocols are designed to be sequential and afford the practitioner the opportunity to help the client resolve deeper issues embedded from concussions. The guide is PR and the activity of the client's autonomic nervous system (ANS). Activation of the ANS for a client with TBI is difficult to avoid, and we must treat the side effects if the client has a reaction.

Let PR determine the pace and length of each session in union with skillful observation of the client's ANS for skin color changes in the face, eyes glazing over, rapid or shallow breathing, and fasciculation activity (shaking or trembling centrally or peripherally in the extremities). The pace is slow, and verbal contact with the client periodically during treatment is necessary.

☙

First Palpatory Protocol for
Traumatic Brain Injury

↜ 1. Cycle of Attunement ↝

Practice a cycle of attunement (COA) while sitting and settling without client contact. Tell the client you will verbally let them know when you are going to make contact. (Please refer to chapter 24 for a detailed explanation of the basic COA and chapters 27 and 28 for description of the advanced COA.)

↜ 2. Pietà ↝

The client is supine. Settle into contact under the shoulder and hamstring muscle for several minutes to mutually settle each other's fluid body and synchronize with PR and the dynamic stillness (see figs. 24.3–5, page 318).

↜ 3. Coccyx and Diaphragm ↝

1. Move to hold under both the coccyx and the respiratory diaphragm of the client (see figs. 24.11–12, page 322). This is not new to many biodynamic practitioners and is an essential beginning to monitor the client's breathing pattern and, if possible, allow it to balance between the respiratory and pelvic diaphragms. One symptom of concussion is a tight diaphragm caused by the startle reflex mechanism. This skill helps balance the fluid body of the client and the fulcrum for the fluid body, the abdominopelvic cavity (kidney-bladder).

2. Place the fingertip of one hand close to the sacral sulcus (between S5 and the coccyx). Contact with the coccyx is enough if the sulcus cannot be differentiated. The sacral outflow of the parasympathetic nervous system (PNS) emerges here. It meets the two subdiaphragmatic dorsal vagus nerve branches at Cannon's point on the distal transverse colon and the inferior hypogastric plexus.

3. Place your other hand under the crura of the diaphragm. Wait for the pelvic and respiratory diaphragms to synchronize, if possible, after several breaths. The intention is to balance the ANS throughout the body via the vagus/PNS and sympathetic cardiovascular connections. Wait for the respiratory diaphragm and the breath to synchronize in yourself and the client; you'll note a spontaneous deep breath, our experience of the Breath of Life.

   This type of synchronizing is important in all phases of treating concussions. Local changes in the body need to be synchronized with the breath gradually, especially at the end of a session. This maintains balance and integration in the client's autonomic nervous system.

◡ 4. Umbilical Breathing ◠

1. Approaching from the side, place the palm of your dominant hand over the top of the umbilicus. Wait for several moments, then place your bottom hand or several fingers under the second lumbar vertebra (see fig. 29.1). Allow the top hand to feel the rise and fall of the client's breath. You can ask the client to gently breath into their abdomen. The transversus abdominus muscle interdigitates with the respiratory diaphragm and should rise and fall with each breath as the umbilicus lifts on the inhalation and falls back on the exhalation.

   The client's knees can be flexed or not for comfort. Ideally, there should be some slack in the abdominal tissue.

2. As the bottom hand remains with L2 in the palm or finger pads, shift the top hand so the tip of the middle finger is gently in the client's umbilicus (see figs. 29.2–3). Feel the breath of the client as if the breath is making a pointed direct contact with the hand. Wait for an instinctual breathing response in the client as if they're trying to push against your finger and/or take a spontaneous deep breath.

   This sequence involves contacting three deep layers of abdominal fascia

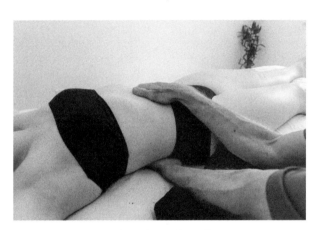

Fig. 29.1. Umbilical breathing 1

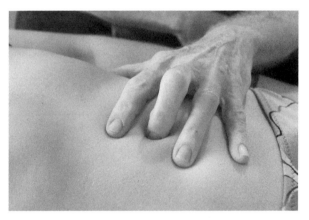

Fig. 29.2. Umbilical breathing 2

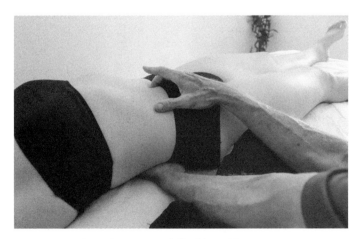

Fig. 29.3. Umbilical breathing 3

(peritoneum, mesentery, and transversalis), allowing the instinctual intelligence of the breath to guide your hand. The hands may be invited by the exhalation to sense the central peritoneal space anterior to the abdominal aorta and possibly the abdominal aorta itself, from which the renal arteries and all the visceral arteries arise. Remember that the research indicates a direct relationship of concussions with the intestines.

Ideally, the endpoint occurs at the end of a third deepening of the hand with an exhalation. This may need to be repeated over several sessions. Slowly remove your hand from over the umbilicus. Then remove your lower hand. The key here is the relationship of the breath to your hands and the three levels of the abdominal breathing system.

⌁ 5. Jugular Vein and Superior Sagittal Sinus ⌁

1. Have the client lie on their right side. Sit behind the client and gently place your hand on the client's shoulder (see fig. 29.4) before contacting the jugular vein. Then contact the jugular vein at midneck (see fig. 29.5). The jugular vein is directly adjacent to the sternocleidomastoid muscle (SCM) in the carotid sheath. Contact the SCM at its posterior border, with fingers palpating at an angle underneath the

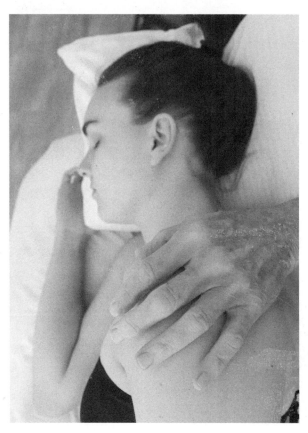

Fig. 29.4. Shoulder contact

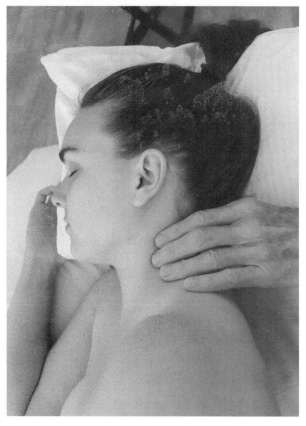

Fig. 29.5. Jugular vein contact

SCM, to contact the carotid sheath and gently sense the jugular vein between the carotid artery and the SCM. The vagus nerve is also present in the sheath bilaterally. This contact generates more blood retention in the brain and consequently more blood perfusion, which protects and nourishes the brain from concussions. Research has shown this is very helpful (Weihong et al. 2021).

2. Place your other hand over the superior sagittal sinus of the client to contact the dynamic stillness inherent in that venous sinus (see figs. 29.6–7). The length of the middle finger (that's the one I use for this palpation) is attracted to the dynamic stillness as the element of space.

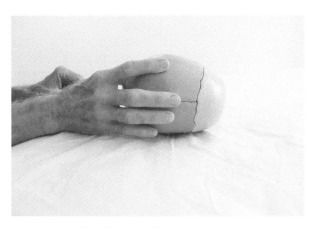

Fig. 29.6. Superior sagittal sinus

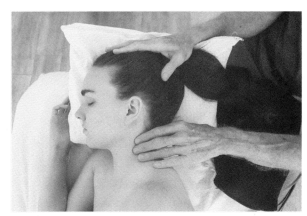

Fig. 29.7. Jugular and superior sagittal sinus contact

⌁ 6. Parietal Ridge and the Third Ventricle ⌁

1. The parietal bones (see figs. 29.8–9) are the most metabolically active bones in the cranium, having the most red marrow of all the cranial bones. While the client remains on their right side following the preceding sequence, approach from the top of the head and place the fingers of both hands under the right parietal ridge of the client's cranium. In this way, the client's parietal bone is

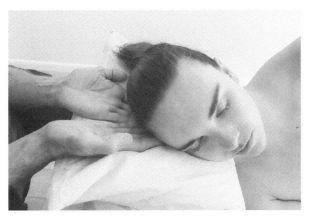

Fig. 29.8. Parietal ridge 1

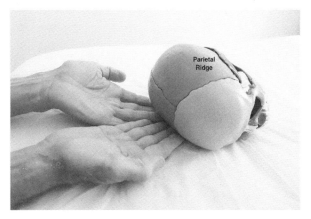

Fig. 29.9. Parietal ridge 2

resting on your finger pads (see figs. 29.10–11). This begins to interface with the third ventricle of the client. Gently shift your fingers posteriorly along the ridge until you sense more of a stillness in or around the third ventricle. This initiates a rebalancing of Sutherland's fulcrum, which gets displaced with concussions.

2. Now shift one of your hands to make gentle contact with the left parietal bone of the client, so that now one hand is under the right side and the other is on top.

3. Repeat the above steps with the client lying on their left side. This contact begins to affect the anterior and posterior commissures that interconnect the hemispheres of the brain.

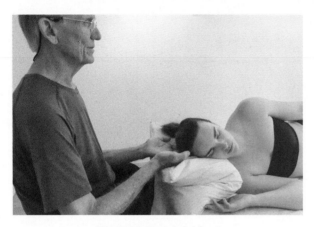

Fig. 29.10. Parietal ridge 3

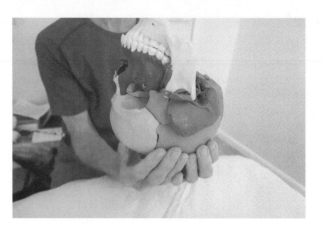

Fig. 29.11. Parietal ridge 4

⌇ 7. Occipital Mastoid Suture (OMS) ⌇

1. The client remains lying on one side. Figure 29.12 shows the location of the OMS between the edges of my two fingers. Placing the pad of your index or middle finger directly on the OMS bilaterally, position your hand in a V spread

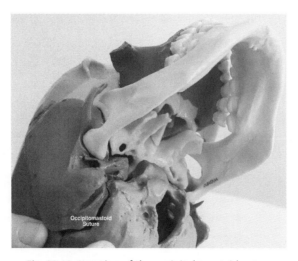

Fig. 29.12. Location of the occipital mastoid suture

(see figs. 29.13–14). As I learned it from Dr. Upledger, the V spread involves sensing the flow of chi or energy between the fingers of two hands. This leads to a sense of expansion and natural movement of the structures between the fingers and hands.

The greatest range of motion of the occiput is medial-lateral motion of the occipital squama. This is the transition zone from cranial base to cranial vault embryonically. Dr. Becker felt that the OMS is the most important suture in the cranium. especially given its association with a vaginal birth and ignition of the brain and cerebrospinal fluid.

2. Now shift and sit behind the client and contact both OMS as shown in figures 29.15–16.

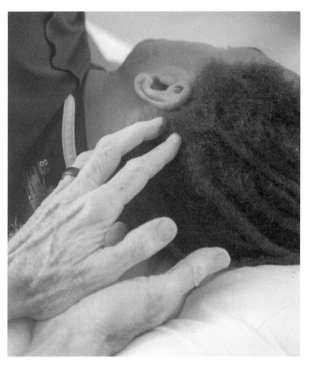

Fig. 29.13. Occipital mastoid suture 1

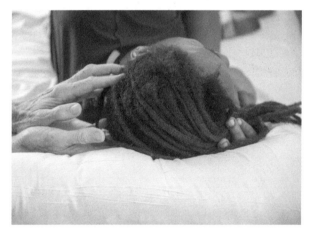

Fig. 29.14. Occipital mastoid suture 2

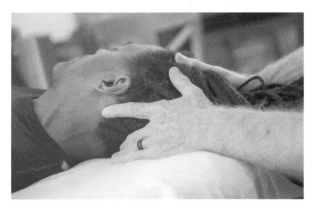

Fig. 29.15. Occipital mastoid suture 3

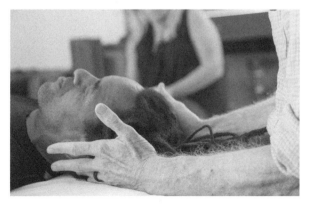

Fig. 29.16. Occipital mastoid suture 4

∿ 8. Subclavian Arteries and Lung Ignition ∿

The client is supine. Sitting at the head of the table, make bilateral contact with the client's subclavian arteries under the midpoint of the clavicle (see figs. 29.17–20). Use this as the starting point, then move the hands and fingers about a centimeter medial, closer to the origin point of the vertebral artery as it exits from the subclavian artery. The subclavian artery relates to lung and pulmonary ignition, which is critically important since biological breathing must be restored in a client with trauma.

The scalenes, too, may need input. The scalenes are accessory muscles of respiration, and depending on the nature of the TBI, they can be very tight, causing the client to breathe in only the upper lobes of the lungs.

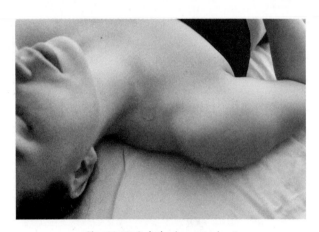

Fig. 29.17. Subclavian arteries 1

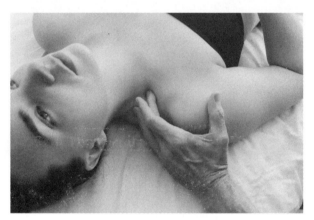

Fig. 29.18. Subclavian arteries 2

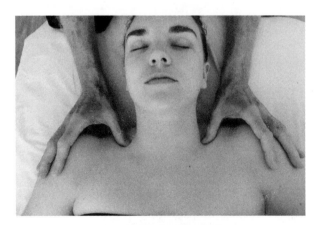

Fig. 29.19. Subclavian arteries 3

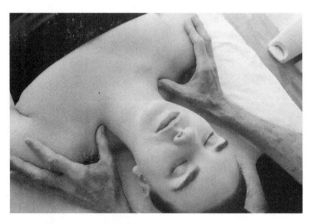

Fig. 29.20. Subclavian arteries 4

ༀ 9. Atlanto-Occipital Joint (AOJ) ༀ

1. With the fingertips or finger pads, depending on the client's sensitivity, contact the suboccipital triangle, creating a fulcrum between the occiput and C2 (see figs. 29.21–23). Gradually the suboccipital triangle will soften, the cranium may gently unwind, the vertebral artery will pulse into the fingertips, and the flexion/extension developmental movement of the occiput will ignite. Being able to sense the vertebral artery is key, as it supplies 20 percent of the brain's blood. Dr. Becker was fond of saying that the AOJ is the "gateway" to the cranium.

2. In addition, from this fulcrum, evaluate the lymphatic system. If there is edema in the AOJ, it must be drained as part of this concussion protocol. The embryonic lymphatic system originates in the carotid sheath. A lymphatic pump for the thoracic duct may need to be applied; Dr. Sutherland did this for most of his patients.

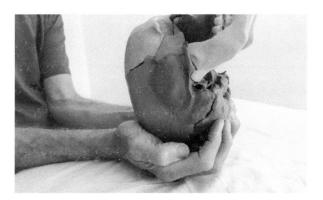

Fig. 29.21. Location of the atlanto-occipital joint

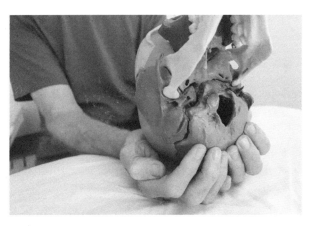

Fig. 29.22. Atlanto-occipital joint 1

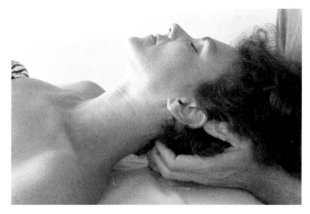

Fig. 29.23. Atlanto-occipital joint 2

ༀ 10. Sutherland's Fulcrum and the Transverse Sinus ༀ

1. Place the pads of most of your fingers in alignment with the transverse sinuses, located bilaterally, slightly inferior to the external occipital protuberance (inion), along the superior nuchal line (see figs. 29.24–28). Note the lateral-medial

movement of the occipital squama on either side—this is the greatest range of motion in the occiput—and sense the dynamic stillness in the transverse sinus.

2. Using one or two finger pads from each hand, gently contact the external occipital protuberance (inion). From here, bring awareness to the anterior end of the straight sinus, known as Sutherland's fulcrum. Sutherland's fulcrum is located in the area between the anterior end of the straight sinus and the pineal recess

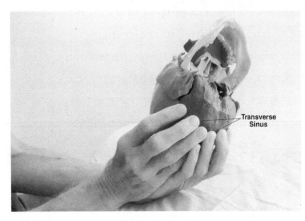

Fig. 29.24. Transverse sinus 1

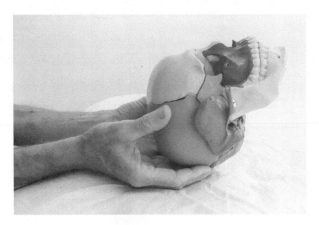

Fig. 29.25. Transverse sinus 2

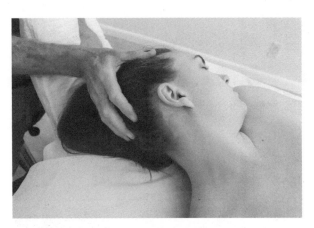

Fig. 29.26. Transverse sinus 3

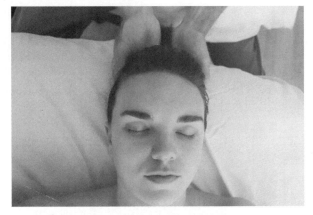

Fig. 29.27. Transverse sinus 4

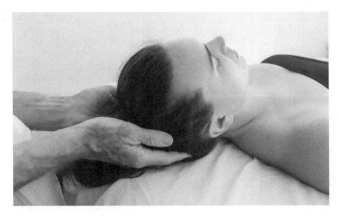

Fig. 29.28. Transverse sinus 5

of the third ventricle. Sutherland's fulcrum is the great cerebral vein (or vein of Galen) that drains into the straight sinus from the posterior third ventricle. In general, there will be a felt sense of gyroscopic motion as Sutherland's fulcrum automatically shifts to its natural fulcrum. You might also sense other motions.

⌁ 11. The Cycle of Completion ⌁

The end of the session begins obviously when you are running out of time on the clock. However, the end of a session can also be marked by the manifestation of Health. Health in a biodynamic perspective is an increase in the potency of PR.

The end may also be sensed by finishing at the coccyx and diaphragm and/or the feet. Repeat the coccyx and diaphragm palpation from page 454 and then hold the feet.

ⵣⵣ
Second Palpatory Protocol for Traumatic Brain Injury

⌁ 1. Cycle of Attunement ⌁

Practice a cycle of attunement. (Please refer to chapter 24 for a detailed explanation of the basic COA and chapters 27 and 28 for a description of the advanced COA.)

⌁ 2. Abdominal ANS Plexuses ⌁

The client is supine. Sit or stand at the side of the client. Place the fingertips or pads of both hands in a line equally above and below the umbilicus (see figs. 27.9–10, page 414). Wait for client's breath to contact your fingers. Remember that many concussions cause the epithelium of the intestines to loose proper barrier function. This is a short treatment to support the epithelium.

⌁ 3. Pericardium Motility ⌁

1. Sit at the left side of the client. Place your left or right hand located between R3 and R5 on the lower sternum, with your fingers pointing toward the client's neck (see fig. 29.29).

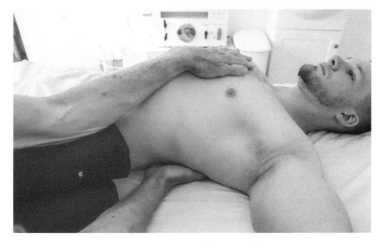

Fig. 29.29. Pericardium motility

2. Place your other hand under the client's diaphragm. Attune to the client's breathing and synchronize with PR heart-to-heart.

4. Atlanto-occipital Joint and Glabella

1. Sitting at the head of the table, practice a cranial cycle of attunement, as described on page 320. This explores sensing the spine being pulled backward by PR as you subtly extend your arms and contact the client's shoulders with your hands, either palm up or down (see figs. 29.30–31). Uncoil the springs of your arms so they lengthen. Then make a heart-to-heart connection via PR.
2. Place the fingertips of both hands in the center of the heart fulcrum of C2–C3 (see figs. 24.8–10, page 321).
3. Then make bilateral contact with the mid-SCM for the carotid sinus (see fig. 29.32).

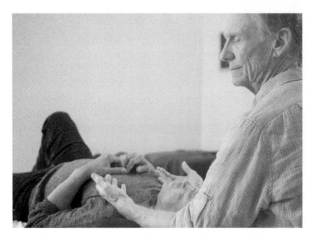

Fig. 29.30. Contact with the shoulders, palm up 1

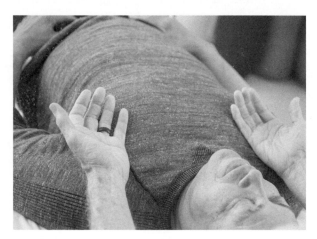

Fig. 29.31. Contact with the shoulders, palm up 2

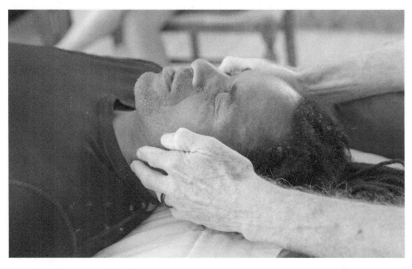

Fig. 29.32. Mid-SCM jugular vein

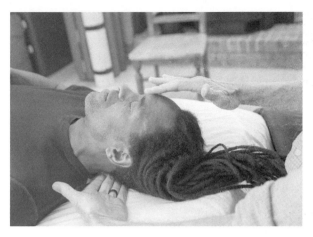

Fig. 29.33. AOJ and glabella 1

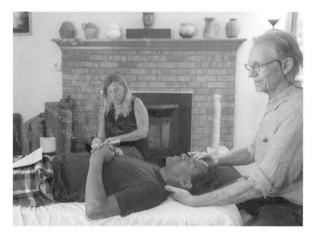

Fig. 29.34. AOJ and glabella 2
(Hospice nurse Kelli Foley observing)

4. Sitting at the head of the table, place the finger pad(s) of one hand in the center of the AOJ. With the finger pad(s) of the other hand, contact the glabella, the axis of rotation of the cranial base (see figs. 29.33–34). This line breathes with PR. The basic embryonic motions of the cranial base may manifest.

⌁ 5. Styloid and Mastoid Processes and Carotid Canal ⌁

1. Gently make bilateral contact with the styloid processes (see figs. 29.35–37; note that the styloids are the pointed toothpick-appearing small projections inferior to the ear canal in fig. 29.35). Direct contact is not required. Simply be close to each one. This is the embryonic point of origin for the lymphatic vessels, and the vagus nerve is also located here.

2. Styloid-aorta for vagus stabilization (see fig. 29.38). Repeat on other side.

3. Gently make contact bilaterally with the mastoid processes of the temporal bone (see figs. 29.39–41). Synchronize attention with the axis of rotation of the temporal bones. Then synchronize with the pulse of the carotid arteries in the carotid canal. Sense the relationship with the petrous temporals and the cranial base flexion/extension in PR. Then sense the circle of Willis floating on the cranial base.

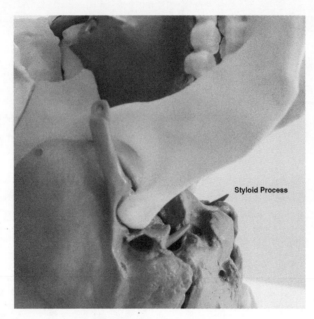

Fig. 29.35. Styloid process 1

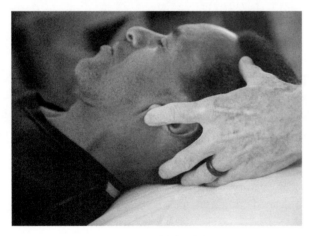

Fig. 29.36. Styloid process 2

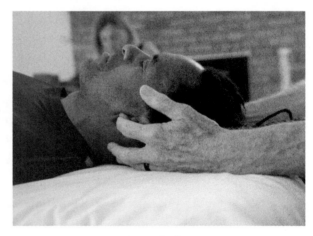

Fig. 29.37. Styloid process 3

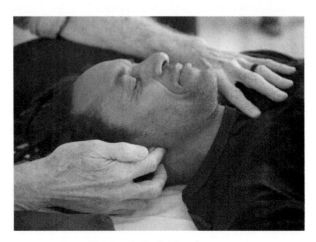

Fig. 29.38. Styloid and aorta

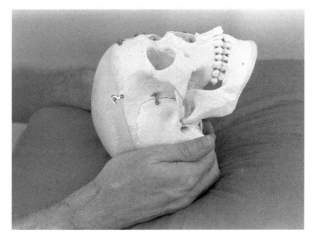

Fig. 29.39. Mastoid process 1

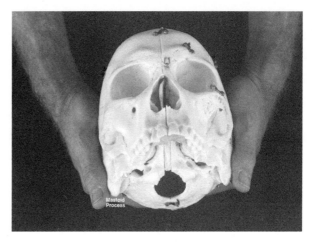

Fig. 29.40. Mastoid process 2

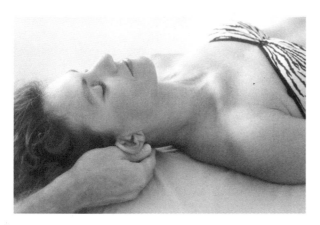

Fig. 29.41. Mastoid process 3

⌇ 6. Temporomandibular Joint (TMJ) ⌇

1. Have the client lie on one side. Figure 29.42 shows the position on the top side of the client's cranium for the location of your hands when placed underneath the client's cranium. Place one hand on the masseter-temporalis muscles supporting the client's cranium and your other hand on the OMS (see fig. 29.43). Imagine you are holding a bowl of water. Verbally solicit your client's comfort.

2. Repeat on the other side.

   Now determine which side is most comfortable for the client. Remain on that side for the balance of the session.

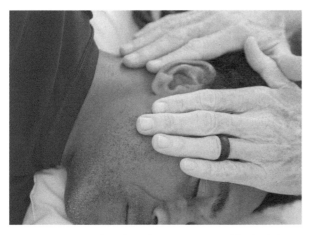

Fig. 29.42. Hand position for temporomandibular joint

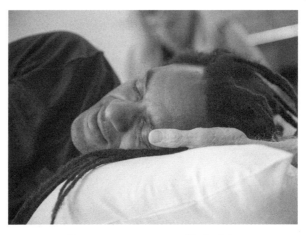

Fig. 29.43. Temporomandibular joint

∿ 7. Sutherland's Fulcrum ∿

1. With your client still lying on one side, place one or two finger pads of one hand on the external occipital protuberance. Place the finger pads (or palm) of your other hand on the bregma (approximately). The line running between the two points of contact is the axis of rotation for Sutherland's fulcrum (see figs. 29.44–46). The fulcrum may be displaced outside the body. Consider this for impact and other strong traumatic concussions.

2. Allow either or both hands to be raised just off the body, and wait for the hands to be drawn closer by PR.

3. Wait for the fulcrum to automatically shift. Make space for the third ventricle to radiate PR and remain spacious and gentle.

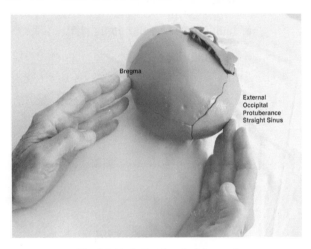

Fig. 29.44. Sutherland's fulcrum 1

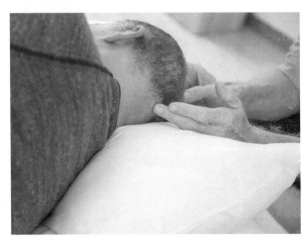

Fig. 29.45. Sutherland's fulcrum 2

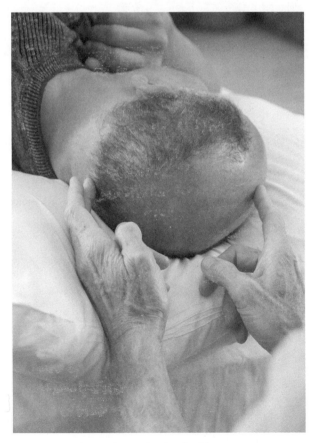

Fig. 29.46. Sutherland's fulcrum 3

⌣ 8. Core Link: Sacrum and Occiput ∿

With your client still lying on one side, contact the sacrum with one hand and the occiput with the other. Use either the palm or the back of each hand (see figs. 29.47–48). Synchronize with PR in the dural tube.

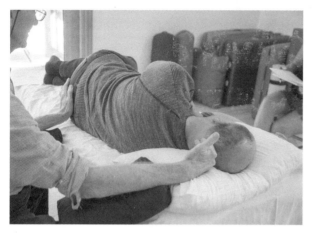

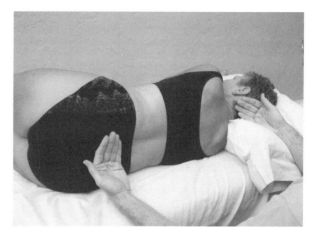

Fig. 29.47. Core link 1   *Fig. 29.48. Core link 2*

⌣ 9. Embryonic Link: Sacrum and Ethmoid ∿

With your client still lying on one side, contact the sacrum with the palm or the back of one hand. Then contact the glabella/ethmoid with just a finger pad (see figs. 29.49–50). Let PR breath between those contacts.

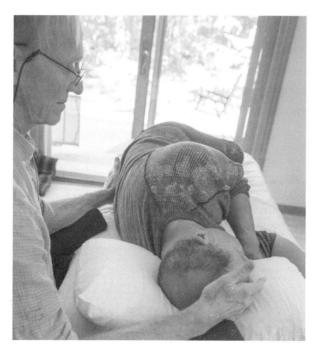

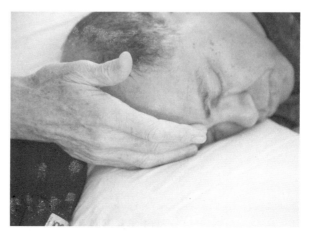

Fig. 29.49. Embryonic link 1   *Fig. 29.50. Embryonic link 2*

⌇ 10. Coccyx and Diaphragm ∿

Finish with the client in supine position. Contact the coccyx and respiratory diaphragm (see fig. 29.51).

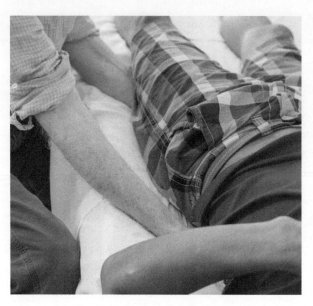

Fig. 29.51. Coccyx and diaphragm

Facial Bones: Interosseous Motion Dynamics

Think of the hard palate as a group of interrelated motion dynamics. These relationships are called the sphenomaxillary complex. They are:

- flexion/external rotation and extension/internal rotation torsion
- side-bending
- shearing

As the sphenoid bone expresses flexion, a series of motion dynamics occur. The palatines are taken into external rotation via their articulation with the sphenoid at the pterygoid processes. The palatine bone glides between the pterygoid processes and is taken inferiorly and laterally by them to express external rotation. Dr. Sutherland called the palatine bones speed reducers. The palatines act as intermediate gliding structures that reduce the strength of the potency of PR in its expression through the hard palate. This also works the other way around as the strength of chewing and talking is not directly fed into the cranial base. The horizontal plates of the palatines are an integral part of the hard palate and express a lowering and widening in their external rotation phase.

The maxillae are moved by the sphenoid via the vomer and the palatine bones. The arch of the hard palate flattens and widens in external rotation, and this is further encouraged as the palatines transfer their motion to the maxillae from the pterygoid processes of the sphenoid.

The vomer is moved by the body of the sphenoid. Its articulation with the sphenoid is gliding. The flared superior aspect of the vomer, called its rostrum, articulates with the inferior aspect of the body of the sphenoid. As the sphenoid expresses flexion, the vomer rotates in the opposite direction and there is a gliding action between them. The vomer also acts as a speed reducer. As the vomer expresses flexion, it descends inferiorly at the rear of the hard palate. This helps lower and widen the arch of the hard palate.

The action of the sphenoid is transferred to the hard palate via the motions of the palatines and vomer. When the sphenoid goes into flexion, the vomer descends on the hard palate and the maxillae and palatines rotate externally.

၆၈

Third Palpatory Protocol for Traumatic Brain Injury

Interoral work may be indicated for TBI, and some of the skills in this series describe that work. Any trauma directly to the face will require that all facial bones be evaluated, depending on the severity of the trauma. In addition, many clients have had traumatic dental work, especially as children, that can benefit from interoral work. Interoral work is special and delicate, requiring constant permission from the client and a signaling system for when the client needs a break and to have the practitioner's fingers removed from their mouth.

SOME CONSIDERATIONS FOR INTRAORAL AND FACIAL WORK

- Our first contact with the world, our environment, and society is with our face.
- Awareness of the visceral system and the superior end of the gastrointestinal tract.
- Facial and dental trauma-speed reducers.
- Face as persona in depth psychology.
- Emotional communication via the vagus nerve and facial PNS.
- Fascial connections to neck and arms via the TMJ.
- Facial ganglion role in the ANS.
- Cranial nerves and sensory function.

⁓ 1. Cycle of Attunement ⁓

Begin with a cycle of attunement, pietà, and vascular tree. (Please refer to chapter 24 for a detailed explanation of the basic practices and chapters 27 and 28 for more advanced practices.)

⁓ 2. Becker Vault Hold ⁓

The sphenoid bone can be seen in the rear of the orbit of the eye in figure 29.52. The greater wings of the sphenoid are under my thumbs bilaterally in figures 29.53–54.

The client is supine. Use your thumbs to contact the greater wings of the sphenoid bilaterally and the little and ring fingers to contact the occiput (see fig. 29.55). Allow the fluid fields of the face to move with PR and note how the sphenobasilar joint (SBJ) is expressing itself.

The SBJ has the following embryonic motions in the tempo of PR: flexion/extension, torsion, side bending with rotation, lateral strain, and vertical strain and/or compression.

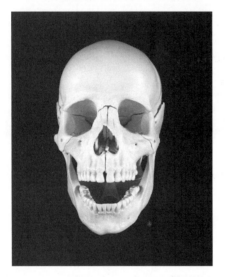

Fig. 29.52. Facial bones

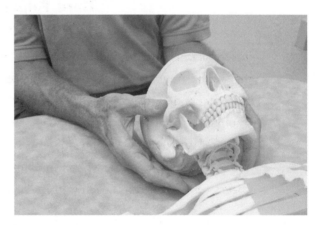

Fig. 29.53. Becker hold 1

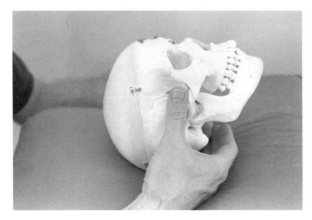

Fig. 29.54. Becker hold 2

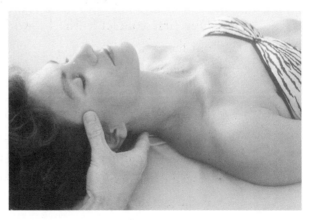

Fig. 29.55. Becker hold 3

ᴗ 3. Facial Bones ᴗ

1. Spread your fingers on the frontal bone (see fig. 29.56). Test the spring of the capillary beds subcutaneously. Wait.

2. Place a thumb over the glabella just above the nasal bones, and place the other thumb over the first . At the same time, place the other fingers along the lateral aspects of the frontal bone (see fig. 29.57). Sense a spreading and expansion across the ethmoidal notch and movement in the relationship between the frontal bone and ethmoid bone.

3. While standing or seated at the side of the client, contact the nasal bones near their articulation with the frontal bone with the thumb and index finger of one hand. With your other hand, gently stabilize the frontal bone at its lateral aspects. The bones move as if the face is cylindrical. The motion testing involves inducing a gentle shearing motion; it is not a linear back and forth laterally but rather a twisting motion around the cylinder (see figs. 29.58–60).

4. Now shift one hand to contact the maxillae bilaterally; keep your other hand on the frontal bone to stabilize it (see figs. 29.61–62). Begin to sense motion in relationship between the frontal bone and the maxillae. Notice a shearing motion. Wait for a stillpoint. Tune in to any irregular patterns.

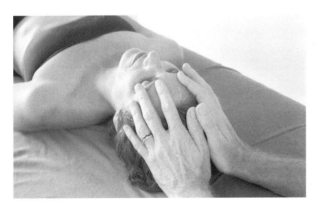

Fig. 29.56. Frontal spread

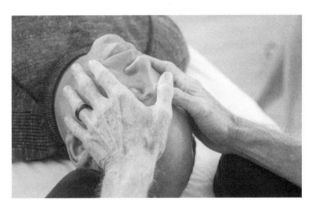

Fig. 29.57. Thumbs on the glabella

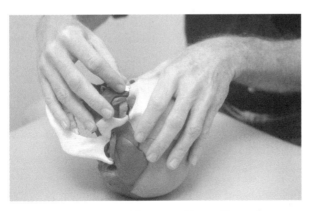

Fig. 29.58. Nasal bones and frontal bone 1

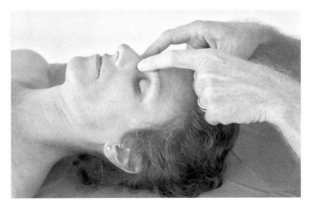

Fig. 29.59. Nasal bones and frontal bone 2

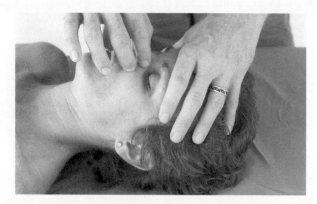

Fig. 29.60. Nasal bones and frontal bone 3

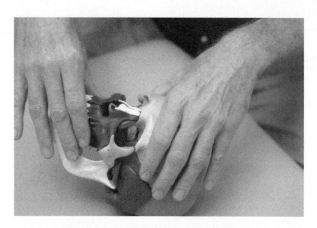

Fig. 29.61. Maxillae and frontal bone 1

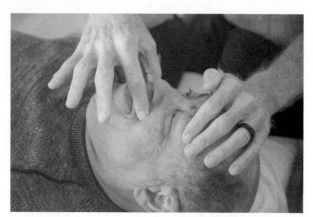

Fig. 29.62. Maxillae and frontal bone 2

⌇ 4. Bird in the Ventricle ⌇

1. Repeat the glabella contact from the preceding sequence, with your thumbs on the glabella and hands over the client's face lateral of the nose (see fig. 29.57). The orbits of the eyes have seven articulating bones: frontal, sphenoid, maxillae, zygomae, palatines, ethmoid, and lacrimals. Allow the seven sets of bones and their interosseous connections to float and manifest movement. Solicit the client's comfort and check for ANS activation and abdominal breathing. Let the ethmoid frontal bones breath with PR.

2. I call this contact "The Bird," a nod to the reference made by Dr. Jealous of the "bird" in the third ventricle. Its wings are the lateral ventricles, and its tail extends down through the fourth ventricle into the terminal ventricle. He also said that the contact at the bregma is lighter than a nanogram.

    Sit at the head of the table and practice a cycle of attunement. Negotiate permission to make contact, then place the pads of your index and middle fingers bilaterally on the greater wings of the sphenoid (see fig. 29.63). The length of the index fingers are positioned along the coronal suture and the thumbs are positioned around or on top of bregma. This is the location of the anterior dural girdle, a reduplication of the dura present after birth for a short time.

3. Now, if they are not already, bring the pads of the thumbs together so they are crossed on top of one another or have their tips touching, depending on the size of your hands (see figs. 29.64–66). No pressure is placed on the bregma. I frequently hover in the hair line a millimeter above bregma.

4. Synchronize your attention with PR in the client's fluid body and then the fluid fields of the cranium. The greater wings of the sphenoid will tend to move laterally for fifty seconds, while the bregma depresses inferiorly for fifty seconds. Then the cycle reverses itself. The perception of this motion must be precise. These are the wings of the bird in the lateral ventricles expressing themselves.

The bregma may begin to feel as if it is breathing on a line down through the

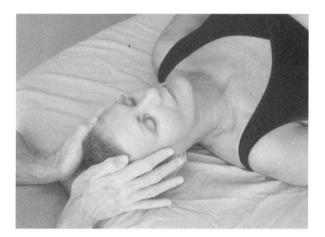

Fig. 29.63. Anterior dural girdle

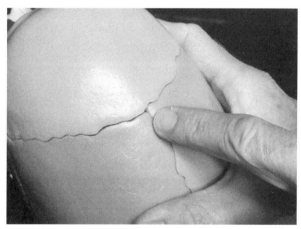

Fig. 29.64. Bregma bird location 1

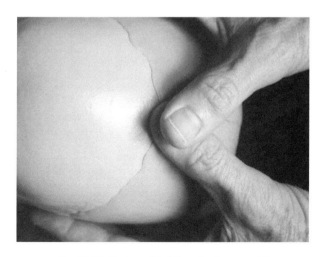

Fig. 29.65. Bregma bird thumb placement 2

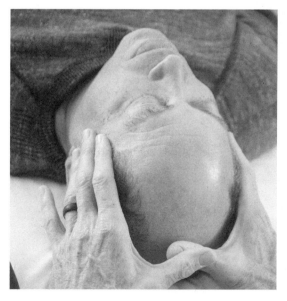

Fig. 29.66. Bregma bird 3

third and fourth ventricles. Gradually PR will express itself more fully and there may be a sense or an image of a bird in flight. When I teach this in class, I ask each student to imagine the image of a real bird and to name the bird during our feedback session.

5. Following this contact for the third ventricle, the sacrum and feet must be contacted in the ways elaborated in previous chapters and the whole Health of the client must be allowed to expand with the potency of PR. This may include checking the longitudinal fluctuation.

⌣ 5. Ethmoid Relationships ⌣

The ethmoid's primary relationship is with the sphenoid bone. Figure 29.67 shows their relationship. The patterns of movement between them are compression, torsion, side bending, and shearing. Think of the sphenoid as the keystone of the cranial base. The patterns between the sphenoid and ethmoid and the sphenoid and occiput compensate and mirror each other, especially in TBI. Contact with the ethmoid happened with the thumbs over glabella in figure 29.57 (page 483). Now we will investigate deeper. This is preparation for the intraoral work that follows.

1. Sit at the side of the client. Place the thumb and middle finger of one hand on either side of the nasal bones near their articulation with the frontal bone. Place the index finger of the same hand over the frontal bone at the glabella near the bridge of the client's nose. Place your other hand over the lateral aspects of the frontal bone and the greater wings of the sphenoid (see fig. 29.68). If your hands

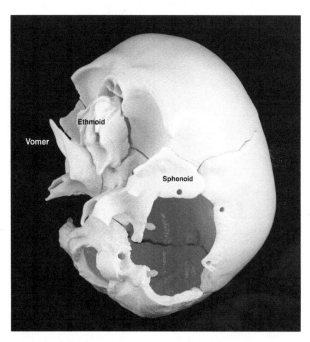

Fig. 29.67. Vomer, ethmoid, and sphenoid

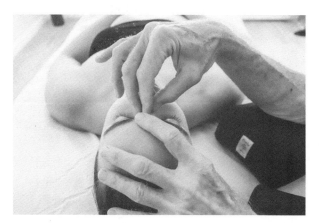

Fig. 29.68. Ethmoid and frontal bones

are not big enough, you can stabilize the greater wings via the lateral aspects of the frontal bone.

2. Sense motion in the relationship of the sphenoid and ethmoid. The ethmoid in its flexion phase rotates in the opposite direction to the sphenoid bone. Note any patterns and help the system access a Neutral.

3. You can suggest an anterior traction toward the ceiling at the nasal bones while stabilizing the sphenoid. At the same time, via your index finger, also gently suggest a posterior pressure at the glabella. This will help disengage the ethmoid from any compression at the ethmoidal notch of the frontal bone.

◦∴ 6. Ringing the Ethmoid Bell ∴◦

1. Take a moment to look at the ethmoid-vomer relationships in the skull shown in figure 29.67. Place one finger toward the rear of the hard palate under the vomer. Place the thumb of your other hand over the glabella near the bridge of the client's nose (see figs. 29.69–70). Follow the motion. As the frontal bone expresses external rotation and the ethmoid rotates posteriorly in flexion, the glabella deepens posteriorly. As this occurs, the vomer will rotate inferiorly at the rear of the hard palate and the hard palate will flatten and widen. In extension, the opposite will occur.

2. In the flexion phase, follow the glabella with a gentle suggestion of posterior motion. Sense the vomer descending inferiorly toward your finger in the client's mouth. Continue following the motion. You are rocking the ethmoid via its articulations with the frontal and vomer bones. Continue to ring the ethmoid bell until a Neutral is achieved.

3. Finish with a coccyx and diaphragm contact.

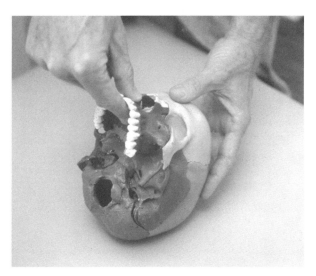

Fig. 29.69. Ethmoid bell 1

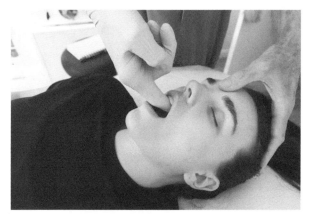

Fig. 29.70. Ethmoid bell 2

∿ 7. Vomer Decompression ∿

1. Using a vault hold (see figs. 29.71–72) or Becker hold (see figs. 29.53–55, page 482), sense your way into the hard palate. There are three particular motions you might feel: a sense of pulling, a sense of compression in the inter-palatine suture, or a blocklike lack of motion. The vomer forms a thirty-degree angle between the sphenoid and maxillae (see fig. 29.67). In the following work, we will be approximating this thirty-degree angle with the horizontal plane of the hard palate.

2. Stand or sit at the side of the table. Place one hand at the greater wings of the sphenoid via the lateral aspects of the frontal bone, with your thumb relating to one greater wing and your index finger relating to the other. Place the thumb of your other hand externally on the midline of the upper lip at the alveolar ridge and your index finger of that same hand on the alveolar ridge internally behind the upper teeth (see figs. 29.73–74). The finger in the mouth is on the midline of the hard palate. Approximate a thirty-degree angle with your two fingers and sense motion relationships between the sphenoid and vomer.

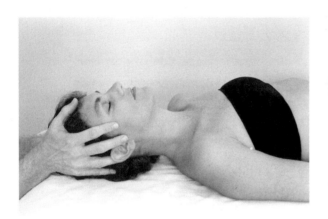

Fig. 29.71. Vault hold 1

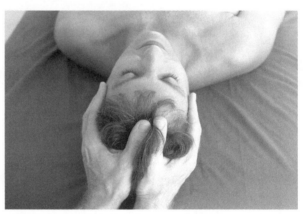

Fig. 29.72. Vault hold 2

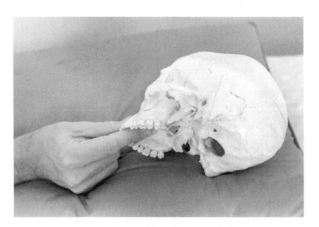

Fig. 29.73. Vomer 1

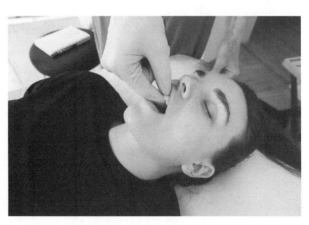

Fig. 29.74. Vomer 2

3. You can stabilize the sphenoid and then decompress the vomer along a thirty-degree angle. Although figure 29.74 does not show my other hand spanning the frontal bone to stabilize the sphenoid, that is easy to accomplish even if your fingers do not span the frontal bone enough to contact the greater wings of the sphenoid. See figure 29.78 (page 490) for the position of the hand on the frontal bone. Be very precise in searching for the right glide path. Follow any compression as necessary and wait for a Neutral. Because of trauma, the angle of decompression may be greater or lesser than thirty degrees. Suggest decompression within the range of the thirty-degree axis in an anterior/inferior direction. Allow your finger inside the mouth to move farther back on the hard palate. Stay on the midline, sense any motion dynamics, and wait for a Neutral.

4. Maintaining the same hand position as above, now test for torsion. Here your finger is at the midline of the hard palate under the rear of the vomer, and you're simply rotating your fingertip around a vertical axis at the inferior pole of the vomer. Sense the direction of ease and wait for a Neutral to appear.

5. Test for side bending of the vomer. Stabilize the sphenoid bone and subtly glide your finger on the hard palate back and forth on the anterior/posterior axis. Follow the direction of ease and wait for a Neutral.

6. Test for vomer lateral shear. With your finger on the midline of the palate, suggest a lateral movement one direction or the other. Find the direction of ease and wait for a Neutral.

ᴥ 8. Maxilla and Zygomatic Bones ᴥ

1. Use a traditional vault hold (see figs. 29.71–72) and sense the quality of potency in the maxilla through the fluid fields of the face.

2. Make bilateral contact with the zygomatic bones (see fig. 29.75). Check their capacity for flexion and extension. These bones are very important to explore in clients with facial trauma.

3. Stand or sit at the side of the table. Place one hand on the greater wings of the sphenoid via the lateral aspects of the frontal bone. Place the palmar surfaces of the index and middle fingers of your other hand along the biting surfaces of the upper teeth (see figs. 29.76–78). Make sure you are over the rear molars. Monitor flexion/external rotation and extension/internal rotation. Remember that as the sphenoid flexes and dives anterior and inferior, the maxillae descend and widen. Follow the motion and wait for a Neutral.

4. Test for torsion. The greater wing on one side will be relatively superior, while the maxilla on the opposite side will be superior. Torsioning occurs around an A–P axis (anterior–posterior). This pattern is always due to trauma of some kind and commonly from the birth process. As one maxilla rises superior relative to

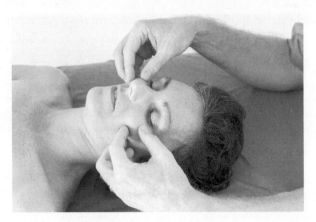

Fig. 29.75. Zygomatic bones

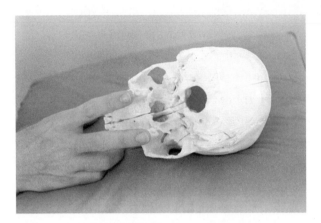

Fig. 29.76. Maxillae interoral 1

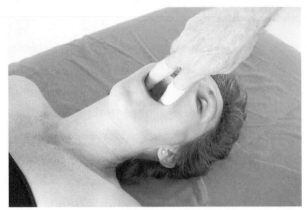

Fig. 29.77. Maxillae interoral 2

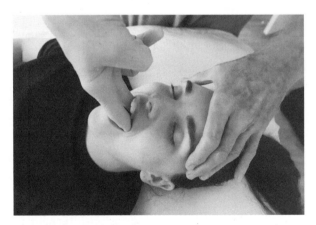

Fig. 29.78. Maxillae interoral 3

the other, this causes a side bending in the vomer. The vomer becomes bent between the sphenoid and maxilla. Test for torsion in the maxillae and wait for a Neutral to appear. Always follow the motion in the direction of ease. This is an up/down motion.

5. Test for side bending by rotating the maxillae first in one direction and then the next around a vertical axis. Follow the system into ease and wait for a Neutral and expansion of the fluid fields.

6. Test for shearing and sense if the maxillae have sheared or shifted laterally in their relationship to the sphenoid. This will cause a shearing across the structure of the vomer. The vomer will take on an S shape as its superior aspect is pulled one way by the sphenoid and its inferior aspect is pulled the other way by the maxillae.

Let PR guide the system into its direction of ease and wait for a stillpoint.

⤳ 9. Palatine Relationships ⤳

1. Use a vault hold and sense your way into the palatines.

2. Ask the client to lie on their side. From the side of the table, place your hands under the client's face (see figs. 29.79–80). You are now on the horizontal plate of the palatine bone. Sense the direct relationship to the sphenoid bone in the center of the facial bones. Wait for a Neutral.

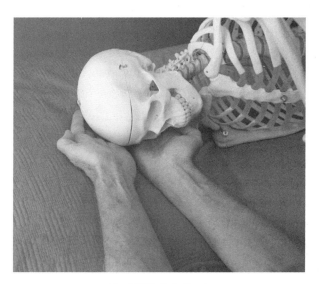

Fig. 29.79. Palatine 1

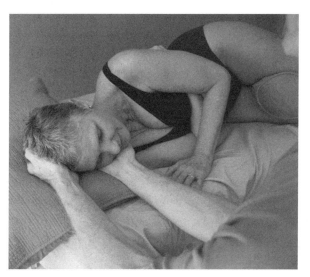

Fig. 29.80. Palatine 2

Traditionally the palatine bones are palpated intraorally. However, in my clinical practice over the years, especially with TBI and associated dental trauma, I have found that holding the cranium on the side, as shown here, is safer and more effective for rebalancing all the bones of the face, vault, and neurocranium.

⤳ 10. Coccyx and Diaphragm ⤳

1. Move to hold under both the coccyx and respiratory diaphragm of the client (see figs. 24.11–12, page 322).

2. Place the fingertip of one hand close to the coccyx. The other hand goes on the floating ribs under the diaphragm. Wait for the pelvic and respiratory diaphragms to synchronize. Then, if PR starts to move in the fluid body, melt your hands into the table to synchronize with the stillness.

⌁ 11. Bilateral Anterior Tibial Arteries ⌁

Be cautious and slow when treating clients with concussions. As mentioned earlier, only two or three of any of the skills detailed in the three protocols may be enough. Keep your eyes on the activity of the client's ANS to support safety and avoid retraumatization.

It is essential when treating concussions, including dental work trauma, that it be based on trauma-informed care (TIC). There must be an agreed-upon signal system with the therapist and client regarding modifying any therapeutic touch. The therapist must regularly check in with the client, verbally soliciting their well-being by saying something like "How are you with this?" Never ask "What are you feeling?" The Neutral as discussed throughout this book is perhaps the most difficult state to achieve for the client with impact trauma. The autonomic nervous system (ANS) must be honored and respected. The therapist must maintain an eagle eye and hand for any visible and palpatory signs of ANS distress. Shaking and trembling, exaggerated breathing, histamine responses in the skin, crying, and fluttering eyes are only some of the visible and palpatory signals from a client's potentially distressed ANS. Furthermore, it is contraindicated to actively seek out an emotional response from the client. As mentioned earlier in this book, the best advice regarding emotional release, is "seek not, forbid not." TIC in manual therapy means regular removal of the hands from the client, observing several cycles of breathing, periodically soliciting comfort, and then taking the next step with the therapeutic engagement manually for proper integration of change process within the ANS. The client absolutely needs to be empowered and given the opportunity to self-regulate internally by the pacing, tempo, and timing of the therapeutic session. Slowly is Holy!

30

Reclaiming the Mystical
Origins of Biodynamics

Divinity Serves Divinity

BILL HARVEY

BILL HARVEY has been a Rolfer for forty years and a practitioner of Biodynamic Craniosacral Therapy for over thirty years. Most recently he has been given the distinction of Master Teacher by the University of Sufism.

The story of how Dr. Sutherland discovered biodynamic craniosacral therapy after fifty years of research into the cranial concept downplays one crucial detail: Dr. Sutherland and his circle of practitioners were Christian mystics. The word *mystic* means to experience the unseen, such as angels, or heaven, or God, for oneself, rather than to have an intellectual understanding of these concepts. The importance of this detail did not become clear to me until I had been studying the mysticism of Sufi healing intensively for about four years. Though it is possible to adhere to any religion and still be a Sufi, the particular type of Sufism that I've been studying follows the guidelines and cosmology of Islam. In Islam there are many different realities, and entering each of those worlds has a distinct phenomenology or body-feel to it. In a similar way to it being easy for each of us to recognize that we have entered a room where an argument has recently taken place, each of these realities has a different sense of spaciousness, lightness, and qualities of light. One of the worlds in the Islamic cosmology is called the Jabarut. In this world it is possible to contact specific Divine Qualities, such as Divine Mercy or Divine Compassion. Once I had the experience of entering this world, I immediately realized that I visit this world every working day. This is the world where biodynamic craniosacral therapy takes place, and this is where my consciousness goes to do cranial work. By the way, the translation for the Arabic word *jabarut* is potency. In the Islamic cosmology, the Jabarut is the world of Divine Qualities. In other words, the human concepts of compassion and mercy are but a shadow of what Divine Compassion and Divine Mercy would be. In the Jabarut we can experience those qualities, and in the process our own capabilities in those areas can be enhanced. In turn, we can offer a greater sense of those qualities to our clients.

Once I realized that the Jabarut is the world where the healing properties of biodynamics occur, I quickly realized that adding the Divine Qualities that are available in the Jabarut to the work that we are doing with PR makes our work vastly more effective and powerful. Accordingly, I realized that this is the work that Dr. Sutherland was doing all along in his context of Christian mysticism. Primary Respiration is the beacon that lets us know we're in the right place/space to gain access to the kind of healing that can only come from a source greater than ourselves. But to make it acceptable in the world of biomechanics, Dr. Sutherland's work was taught in a way that omitted nearly all of the spirituality that made such powerful healings possible except by a very few osteopaths. Thus, I began the task of reverse engineering the mystical origins of biodynamic craniosacral therapy.

In this meditative exploration we will take the attunement aspect of our preparation for a session to a much deeper level by explicitly going to the Jabarut and accessing both Divine Qualities and our own divinity. This attunement will in turn enhance our ability to perceive the inherent divinity of our client. In this way we can move beyond "fixing" or "helping" our client to directly serving our client's divinity with our own divinity. Let's begin by exploring.

ༀ

Three Paths to Primary Respiration

1. Settle for a moment and experience your own breathing. As your breath deepens, let your eyes soften and become aware of the deepest part of your eye socket. Allow your gaze to settle just below the horizon. Allow your ears to widen as though you could hear the sounds in the adjoining rooms. Become aware of your heartbeat and the slightest tugging or pushing pressure on your heart and your eyes. This miniscule tugging or pushing pressure is Primary Respiration (PR), which is the movement of the self-healing process.

2. Let's start with the vyaghra mudra. To do this mudra, with both hands, place your thumbs at the base of the little fingers, then fold your fingers over your thumbs.

3. Place your hands on your lap with the fingers pointing toward each other and close your eyes. Within three or four breaths you may feel an awareness of your central channel moving from your base to your crown. Within a minute or two you may have an awareness of your calvarian seam, approximately a half inch above the top of your ears and encircling your cranium. This awareness in turn gives you access to your left and right cerebral hemispheres. Gently lift

these hemispheres. When your body gives you the signal of an involuntary deep breath, notice that you are able to effortlessly perceive PR.

4. Place your right hand over your physical heart and feel your own heartbeat. The simple act of feeling your own heartbeat automatically increases both compassion and empathy for yourself and others. Now, imagine some living thing that you are grateful for. For this exercise to work you must actively be grateful, it's not effective if you're pretending. Put your right hand over the middle of your sternum, the location of our thymus gland. This is the location of your spiritual heart. Notice that the sensation of gratitude immediately transfers to this spot. In addition to feeling gratitude, conjure a feeling of adoration and unconditional love for someone alive or dead. Again, the key is to actually feel this unconditional love. Take a few moments to allow this feeling to permeate your being.

5. Now imagine that you are lifting both your cerebral hemispheres and the upper chambers of your physical heart into the space of PR. You will feel your spiritual heart ascend. The goal of the ascension is to reach the Jabarut, the world of the soul. In the Taoist cosmology this would be the world of the heart within the heart. You will feel a different sense of gravity and a different sense of light. The Divine Name for unconditional love is *Wadude*. As you breathe in, your physical heart uncoils in a counterclockwise direction as the descent of the diaphragm takes the bottom of the pericardium with it. As you inhale, imagine the quality of Wadude entering through your crown and traveling into your spiritual heart. As you exhale, as your heart moves in a clockwise direction, imagine Divine Unconditional Love traveling with the blood throughout every part of your body. Feel the Divine Love as it encounters hard, stuck places within you. With each succeeding breath feel the internal permeation of love.

6. Now imagine breathing Wadude into the pores of your skin. With each inhalation, Divine Love enters your skin, and with each exhalation, that love joins your capillary bed. Within a short amount of time your entire body tingles with this love. As you touch your client, your capillary bed contacts the capillary bed of your client and becomes one field of Divine Love. And the clockwise and counterclockwise motions become an embodied spiral filling your body without left-right symmetry. All organs and fluids, especially the blood, become a living spiral of the spiritual ascension of the heart.

As "healers," our spiritual evolution is never finished. There are many higher realms of reality above the Jabarut. To reach and inhabit those realms requires spiritual development and spiritual maturation. Once those realms are attained, accessing complete healing for the deepest personal wounds and the healing of generations of lineage trauma becomes possible for ourselves and for the world.

31

Igniting the Spiritual Heart

The spiritual journey lives as a potential in the human heart. It is ignited through contemplative practices, which clear a space inside the physical heart for divinity to live and express its virtue as a radiance throughout the blood, body, and cosmos. The spirit can radiate the universe from the heart inside every heart. This originality lives in a formless subtle dimension preexisting in the physical heart, yet that dimension must be clear of emotional debris and the conceptual excrement pervasive in our contemporary culture. It is with this intention to engage the various levels and stages of potential spiritual maturation that the following biodynamic cardiovascular therapy explorations are offered as a ministry of laying on of hands. The primary heart meridian channel from a Taoist perspective is a description of the spiritual maturation process during the lifetime of a human being. The Taoists believed you had to finish our spiritual maturation in this one life. Therefore, these skills are a deep spiritual heart Ignition protocol for biodynamic practitioners and their clients. They ignite the instincts for self-transcendence and self-healing.

THE FOUR CHANNELS OF THE HEART

In their classic work *The Manual of Acupuncture* (2016), Peter Deadman and Mazin Al-Khafaji offer great detail on the meridians and channels of the body from the perspective of traditional Chinese medicine. Of particular use to the field of biodynamic cardiovascular therapy are the insights they offer regarding the four channels of the heart.

Primary channel: The nine points of the heart meridian in the arm for one channel called the primary channel. It originates in the heart from the coronary arteries and descends through the diaphragm to connect with the small intestine. A branch goes superiorly adjacent to the esophagus across the face and connects with the tissues around the eyes. Another branch goes directly from the heart to the lungs to emerge in the axilla as the Heart 1 point. It follows the axillary, brachial, and ulnar arteries, has a point in the palm of the hand, and terminates at the little finger. Each of the nine points is named for a step in the spiritual maturation of the individual in Taoist philosophy.

The Nine Points of the Heart Meridian

HT-1   This is the beginning of the spiritual path filled with infinite possibilities.

HT-2   This part of the spiritual path is to cleanse and purify limitations and to see the pathway of one's life and personal destiny.

HT-3   This is the phase of the spiritual path where we become aware of our purpose and that we have a particular way or gift that gets developed and unfolds over time. We are spiritually navigating the ocean of life.

HT-4   We discover that there is a way for our soul, unconditional love, and the seeing of beauty to move where it knows that nothing is going to get in the way. Detours are part of the path.

HT-5   We move with conviction toward our interior heart. That includes all the distance that we have already traveled as our empathy and compassion mature. We keep going further inside.

HT-6   We examine all that we have gathered in life and notice that everything was a necessity in life. The tapestry of life includes all of the threads woven together.

HT-7   We can activate the spirit, the Holy Spirit. This is done by opening its door, and through the process of emptying we become empty of unnecessary thoughts, emotions, and concepts.

HT-8   We enter the residence of the sacred by understanding that everything in my life had a purpose for me to grow. I do not have to come back and do it again.

HT-9   I savor what it means to have life and breath. I experience the essence of life and accept life's conditions so that I don't have to do this over again. There is just one breath at a time, and my blueprint becomes smaller without clinging. It's enough to be in presence.

Luo-connecting channel: The luo-connecting channel separates from the Heart 5 point in the wrist, where it connects to the small intestine meridian. It goes back to the heart and up through the root of the tongue (laryngeal artery) to the eye. This channel allows stress and trauma to dissipate out of the body as a mist exiting the skin and forming part of the cloud of Zone B surrounding the body. When trauma cannot dissipate, it is stored in the blood and capillaries. BCVT seeks to re-ignite the instinct for self-healing in the blood and capillaries for dissipation to occur naturally.

Divergent channel: The divergent channel separates from the heart primary channel in the axilla and goes back to the heart. It then goes up along the throat to the face and connects with the small intestine channel at the inner canthus of the eye. This channel deals with latent disorders in the heart and cardiovascular system. Once again, the purpose of BCVT at this level is to re-ignite the client's instinct for self-healing. Cardiometabolic disorders incubate for many years and will need time to heal with the inclusion of lifestyle changes.

Sinew channel: The sinew channel starts at the radial aspect of the little finger and "binds" at the pisiform bone and medial aspect of the elbow. It enters the axilla, where it intersects with the lung sinew channel. At the center of the trunk, it goes down through the diaphragm and terminates at the umbilicus. This channel deals with the myofascial system, especially problems in the upper extremities. This includes side effects from surgeries performed in those areas, especially mastectomies.

As you can see, the eyes are important in three of these channels. In the middle of the brain in the third ventricle is a channel branching from the central channel of the subtle body. Its single root divides into two, which open within the eyes. The doors of this channel in the eyes are the doorways through which the visions of the sacred (the Breath of Life) come from in their connection with the heart inside the heart. From the third ventricle cavity of this channel, the five rainbow lights shine brightly when we visualize them in the heart and in the cosmos.

The Breath of Life wisdom that lives in the heart inside the heart arises as three types of dynamic visions. These visions consist of specific colors, qualities of brightness, shimmering and radiating, and finally beams or rays of light. This threefold dynamism also arises as ways to see the five primary colors wherever we look in nature and all sounds in the environment projected from within the sanctuary of the heart as if the heartbeat itself is the dynamo powering all this beauty. In this way, our eyes allow us to see the Breath of Life and the myriad ways it appears, and inwardly we can sense our heartbeat as the felt power of the universe. We are luminous beings.

The heart channels also connect to the abdomen, especially the small intestine, where blood is built, and the umbilicus, where ancestral fire comes in. Finally, the heart channels connect to the lungs and the great Sea of Chi from our breathing. We will explore all four channels in the three protocols of this chapter, which are devoted to igniting the spiritual heart.

The palpation is based on the three springs discussed earlier in this book with a different orientation. The first is contact with the torsional movement of the vascular tree. The second is synchronizing with the core of stillness in the blood that extends to the horizon. Third are the capillary beds in the skin wherever our hands are located. Our hands are immersed in the blood vascular system at all times. In addition, with each hand position the cycle of attunement shifts slightly. The practitioner lengthens their heart meridian as a way of activating their own heart meridian and lengthens their descending and abdominal aorta. This is done by placing attention on both little fingers once the hands are in place and gently extending the heart meridian as if lengthening the ulnar, brachial, and axillary arteries. Once this horizontal dimension is activated then the vertical dimension of lengthening through the descending and abdominal aorta is sensed. The practitioner is now centered in their blood vascular system and its potential for igniting the spiritual heart.

Acupuncture Points

The protocols in this chapter make use of certain acupuncture points in relation to their proximity to the arteries. These include points associated with the Triple Warmer, or San Janjiao. San Janjiao is responsible for making blood for the heart to distribute, among its other important functions. Stomach points are directly associated with San Janjiao, as the stomach proper is divided into an upper warmer, a middle warmer, and a lower warmer. Small intestine points are also critical because the heart meridian is paired with the small intestine meridian, and one of its functions is building blood. Some European practitioners hold that all cancers are rooted in disorders of the small intestine.

ELEMENTAL CONNECTIONS

Grounding in the five elements, whether of the Indo-Tibetan tradition (space, wind, fire, water, and earth) or the Sino-Tibetan tradition (water, fire, earth, metal, and wood), is an essential preparation. The meridians are directly associated with the Sino-Tibetan elements. The heart is described as having two types of fire. One is spiritual, which manifests as light in the primary channel of the nine acupuncture points. The other is ordinary in the sense of the function of the pericardium to dissipate heat from the core of the body out to the surface of the skin and into Zone B. In essence we are playing with fire and visualizing light, the birthplace of compassion. A biodynamic practitioner is grounded in their respective meanings of burning away impediments and visualizing the home of divinity in the heart. The heart is the path of spiritual realization in all traditions. At the same time, we must have a felt sense of the other elements for igniting the spiritual heart inside the heart.

The wind element in the Indo-Tibetan tradition is directly associated with the movement of all things big and small and is Primary Respiration (PR). There is ordinary sensation and there is subtle extra-ordinary sensation, such as visionary experiences, colors, sound, and a wide variety of non-frightful experience based on the perception of PR. Fear is simply the threshold to such experience and must be respected, as it may need time to transmute.

Embodiment of all five elements is important to maintain balance of the body with the cosmos. For this reason, chapter 27 and 28, which explore the Indo-Tibetan fulcrums of the fire, water, and earth elements, are a prerequisite for exploring the heart at this level.

VISUALIZATION PRACTICE

All visualization practices taught in the previous chapters are equally relevant here. The capacity to sense the spiral of Primary Respiration (PR) coming from its divine wisdom source in the heart as a torsioning radiance moving through the pericardium meridian and exiting Pericardium 8 in the palm of the hand is also an essential part of the practice (see "Heart in Hands," page 450). As the blood spirals, all related vascular structures torsion just as the vascular tree did in the embryo and continues now. And the spiral is reciprocal, as PR spirals back through Pericardium 8 to the heart in an endless cycle of spiritual maturation.

სთ

Inner Spiral Meditation: Synchronizing the Three Dantians

The three dantians manage the flow of potency from the five elements in both systems of elements. This potency is called chi, and there are different kinds of chi from the ancestral chi in the lower dantian, the Great Sea of chi around the heart and spiritual chi (Shen in Taoism) inside the heart (middle dantian) to the heavenly chi in the upper dantian in and around the third ventricle of the brain. This meditation seeks to balance these differentiated potencies, centralizing them in the heart where spirit lives.

1. Attend to your breathing. Notice your inhalation moving down into your lower abdomen. Sense how the transversus abdominus muscle expands during inhalation and recedes during exhalation. Imagine a horizontal line starting at the acupuncture point Du 4 on the second lumbar vertebra and extending anteriorly to a point between the umbilicus and pubic bone. At the middle of that line is the precise location to place the inhalation breath. That point is the lower dantian, the source of the original or source chi. All of creation starts here. Visualize it as a pearl shining as brightly as the moon. The pearl can be any size, from that of a poppyseed to that of the universe. This practice is also called placing your

mind in the Hara. Maintain this breathing regularly in both life and biodynamic practice. The pearl may take on other colors like gold, red, or white.

2. Sense your heartbeat without taking a pulse. It is more readily sensed during an exhalation. While maintaining an upright posture in alignment with the midline or central channel that connects all three dantians, allow the front of your body, especially the central tendon of the diaphragm, to relax into gravity during exhalation. Gravity connects us to the earth element in which the heartbeat can be felt as the front of the body softens. Sensing the heartbeat automatically generates empathy and compassion without the need for elaborate mantras or compassion practices. The heartbeat is the middle dantian. The heart generates heat simply from its constant motion and is infused with spiritual chi from the area of the myocardium adjacent to the dorsal pericardium, the back of the heart at the level of the fifth thoracic vertebra. Thus, the spiritual chi flows throughout the vascular system, reaching every cell in the body. Spiritual chi is incorporated and also enhanced by the heart-to-heart practice with PR. In this way, PR transmutes into spiritual potency.

3. Now imagine the pearl is moving in a clockwise and counterclockwise direction around the inside diameter of the rib cage, pleura, and pericardium at the horizontal level of the midsternum. When the heart contracts, it creates a counterclockwise torsion. This is systole. When the heart relaxes, its muscle fiber moves in a clockwise direction. This is diastole. Allow the pearl to move in both these directions in the tempo of PR. Allow the imagined motion to become real with micromovement of the rib cage. Let this micromovement of counterclockwise-clockwise motion translate into the shoulders and then down the arms and finally into the hands and fingers.

4. The upper dantian is the third ventricle of the brain. This is an important practice used in the protocols below as a way of self-igniting the Breath of Life radiating from the heart and reflected by the third ventricle of the brain out the eyes. Close your eyes and then gently roll up toward the middle of the forehead. This places a gentle stimulus through the optic chiasm into the third ventricle and notice a brief light appearing. Then relax your eyes, keeping them closed. Once your attention is centered on the location of the third ventricle, imagine that the third ventricle is a large bubble of water in the middle of your brain that is full of multicolored lights and potency—an energetic rainbow. Imagine that your eyes are actually located in the third ventricle as a single eye and that you can see the inside of your body and the outside of the client's body, specifically Zone B. Zone B is filled with evaporated biological water that is moving and shape-shifting like a cloud, filled with infrared heat and electricity that is self-generated by the nature of water itself.

5. From the third ventricle, look with this "third eye" and visualize one or more of the five colors of the rainbow manifesting in both your Zone B and especially the client's Zone B. The clear-light pearlescent luminosity of the original chi radiates from the lower dantian and gradually from all the marrow throughout the skeletal system of the body. The marrow starts as an obsidian black color of the void, representing the end of the previous universe, and through the power of the present moment of pearlescent source chi radiating from the lower dantian, it mixes with the spiritual chi from the middle dantian at the level of the capillaries, meridians, and channels. This transforms the marrow as an extension of the lower dantian.

As this clear-light pearlescent luminosity radiates through the skin, it appears as a spectrum of the five colors of the rainbow, all together or individually. Each of the colors represents an aspect of profound wisdom. Nowness (green), openness (white), lightheartedness (blue), impartialness (yellow), and clearness (red). These wisdoms self-arise independently as a function of meditating on the five colors. They are innate, waiting to be activated by loving behavior.

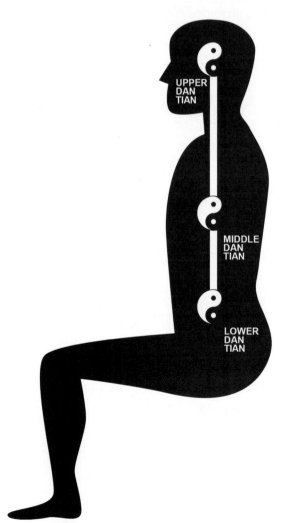

UPPER
DAN
TIAN

MIDDLE
DAN
TIAN

LOWER
DAN
TIAN

Fig. 31.1. The three dantians

The middle dantian allows us to feel this luminosity as a perfect love emotionally. The upper dantian allows us to see this luminosity in ourselves and others directly with our eyes as they are connected to the heart. At the same time we maintain an alignment with the universe by way of connection out through the top of the head via Du 20 to the center of the universe, which the Taoists considered to be the North star in the constellation of the Big Dipper. Internally lengthening the descending and abdominal aorta accomplishes this connection.

6. Now, imagine that your eyes disappear and there is only the bright light of the Breath of Life radiating from your heart to your third ventricle directly in back of your eyes. Now expand your imagination to see this pearlescent brightness in all the dantians. Feel into your vascular tree and allow the cranium, trunk, abdomen, and pelvis to synchronize with this unified torsion under the direction of PR.

Eye Pillow

As much as possible in the following protocols, the client when supine should have their eyes covered with an eye pillow. Periodically check in with your client to determine their comfort level with the eye pillow. As noted, three of the four channels of the heart meridian run to the eyes. Using an eye pillow facilitates the capacity of the client to see the sacred images associated with the Breath of Life and synchronize with the practitioner's visualization practice. It is not a problem if the client does not wish to have an eye pillow, especially on a first session. The offer can be made with each session. The best reason I give to my clients about using the pillow is that it relieves eye strain from too much screen time and enhances the relaxation of the nervous system.

Note: The following three protocols for spiritual heart ignition are intended to be spread out over at least three sessions with a client. They are not designed to be done all in one session with a client.

୧୦

Spiritual Heart Ignition I

I. Pietà Meridian Alignment

This advanced attunement sequence integrates torsioning in order to sense the blood being moved and carrying the virtue and wisdom of PR.

1. Practice a cycle of attunement with the heart-cosmos meditation (page 433).
2. The client is supine and has an eye pillow resting on their eyes if it is comfortable for them. Ask the client to adjust the pillow for their comfort, and offer a Kleenex to be placed under the pillow against the eyes. Begin with the pietà, with your left hand under the right scapula, where points 9 through 15 of the small intestine meridian are located (see fig. 31.2). With your right hand, make contact palm-to-palm with the client's right hand (see fig. 31.3), aligning the Pericardium 8 and Heart 8 points in your palms (see fig. 31.4). Lengthen your heart meridian. Place a little pressure in the backs of the hands into the table. Imagine holding all the blood capillaries in the skin. Sense their torsional movement.

In the cycle of attunement, outwardly a heart-to-heart connection is established with PR. Inwardly, PR moves the blood as the force of Shen, the heavenly spirit residing in the heart as an invisible potential. Shen is a Taoist concept, but it can take any form, such as Jesus or Buddha. The blood is built in the stomach and small intestine. When we fail to ingest real food or to fast for spiritual clarity, our body builds inferior blood. This is because all spiritual virtues associated with Shen are delivered to every cell in the body via the blood.

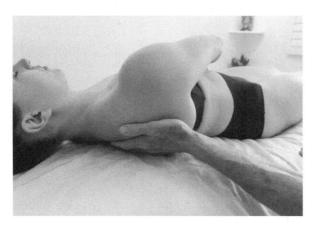

Fig. 31.2. Pietà with focus on scapula

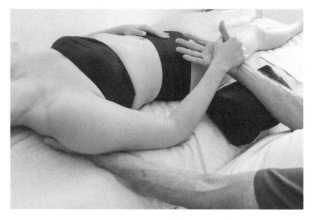

Fig. 31.3. Palm to palm

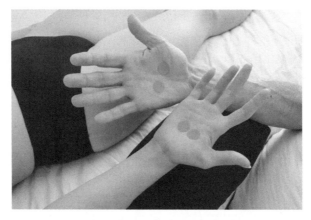

Fig. 31.4. Heart 8 and Pericardium 8

↢ 2. Vascular Tree: Ulnar and Carotid Arteries ↣

1. Approach the vascular tree from the same side as above. Sense its torsional movement with PR. Figure 31.5 shows the location of the heart meridian points 1, 2, 3, 4, 7, and 9 (from the axilla to the little finger). Make contact with the ulnar artery between Heart 5 and 6 (see fig. 31.6). This is where the heart meridian joins the small intestine meridian. With the thumb of your other hand, contact the carotid sinus on the posterior sternocleidomastoid muscle (SCM). This is where you'll also find three acupuncture points lined up horizontally; from posterior to anterior, they are Small Intestine 16, Large Intestine 18, and Stomach 9 (see fig. 31.7).

2. Visualize the vascular tree as a shimmering electric diamond-blue light throughout the meridian and filling the heart where it came from. Which parts of the tree are bright with the Breath of Life?

3. Repeat on the client's other side if necessary.

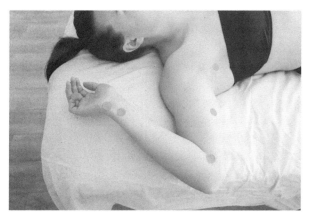

Fig. 31.5. Heart points 1, 2, 3, 4, 7, and 9

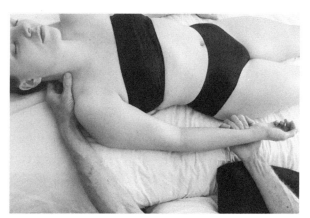

Fig. 31.6. Ulnar and carotid arteries

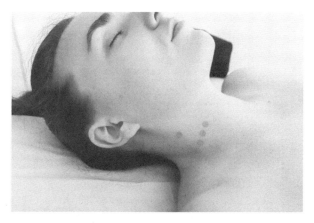

Fig. 31.7. Small Intestine 16, Large Intestine 18, Stomach 9,
San Janjiao 16 (top point)

⚜ 3. Umbilicus and Respiratory Diaphragm ⚜

Approaching the client from the side, place one hand under the diaphragm at the level of T12 and L1. Use your other hand to span the costal arch, with the palm down and Pericardium 8 over the umbilicus (see fig. 31.8). Listen to the rise and fall of the client's breath. Listen to its dimensions from anterior to posterior and lateral to medial. Lengthen your heart meridian.

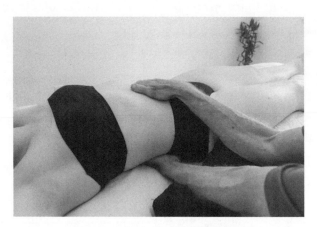

Fig. 31.8. Diaphragm and umbilicus

⚜ 4. Umbilical Zodiac ⚜

1. Standing or sitting by the side of the client, use your thumbs and the pads of your index and middle fingers to palpate the stomach meridian bilaterally on a plane several centimeters above and below the umbilicus. Set the points of contact on the stomach meridian points 21, 23, 25, and 28, which are arranged vertically and horizontally approximately on the bilateral border of the rectus abdominus muscle. Imagine a box with the umbilicus in the center; these points are in the four corners of the box (see figs. 31.9–10).

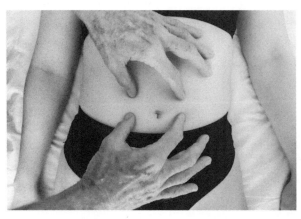

Fig. 31.9. Umbilical zodiac 1

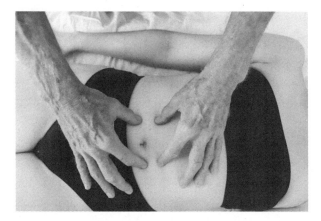

Fig. 31.10. Umbilical zodiac 2

2. Observe the rise and fall of the client's breathing. Does the breath invite closer contact, or is it asking you to move to other points on the box? Play with palpating several millimeters closer to the umbilicus or away from the umbilicus on a diagonal.

3. Then explore the vertical placement of your fingers, moving the points of contact up and down the meridian in several different locations. Pause with each placement.

4. There is a sweet spot unique to each client where both hands synchronize with the client's breath and a heart-to-heart connection with the radiance of the Breath of Life coming from your heart. You may notice it as a torsion motion in the tempo of PR through Pericardium 8 in the palms of the hands. At this sweet spot, place one finger, whether the thumb or the tip of the index finger, gently into the client's umbilicus. Resynchronize with the breath and the Breath of Life. If there is harmony in this position, the unique zodiac arrangement of the client's natal astrology chart as it manifests in this moment is accessed. As PR moves torsionally through the umbilicus, wait for a color to manifest by rolling your eyes up to the middle of your forehead and relaxing them to see the Breath of Life in your third ventricle and heart. Gradually different colors will be seen and can be imagined to fill your body or the client's body.

   Traditional Chinese medicine considers this abdominal region to be a microcosmic reflection of the center of the universe. Thus, the vision is that the microcosmic (metabolic) universe in the body is a mirror of the external universe. The umbilicus is the fulcrum where the cosmos enters the embryo.

5. Place the tip of your index or middle finger in the umbilicus. Place your other hand in contact with the coccyx (see fig. 31.11). Place a gentle drag on the

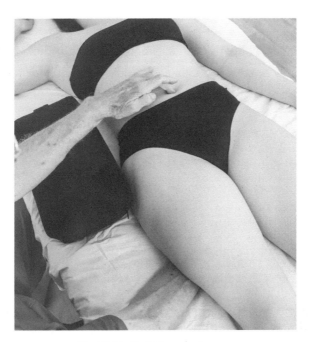

Fig. 31.11. Umbilicus and coccyx

umbilicus toward the heart and then inferiorly away from the heart. Maintain that gentle tension while allowing the client's breath to rise and fall. Now imagine a colored light radiating from the client's lower dantian in the abdomen, filling the client's trunk and upper extremities like a mist spreading upward. Wait for PR to reverse direction and the radiant mist to exit the client's skin, filling zone B. It is like the Trevi Fountain in Rome. Start by visualizing that mist as yellow, white, or crystal clear.

Wait until the trunk, upper extremities, abdomen, and now the whole body to fill with PR and a color radiating from the heart of the client to the center of the universe. Wait for natural dissipation into a stillpoint.

∻ 5. Lung and Scapula ∾

1. Sit at the head of the table and practice a cranial cycle of attunement, as described on page 320, allowing your nervous system to move out of your body backward with PR. Then drop into the Breath of Life in your heart. How bright is it? What color is it now?

2. Make bilateral contact with the client's lung meridian points 1 and 2 (see fig. 31.12). Allow the axillary artery or internal thoracic artery coming from the subclavian artery to touch your fingers.

3. Gently place both hands palm up under the client's scapula (see fig. 31.13). The small intestine has numerous points here, like a constellation of stars in the heavens. Imagine you are holding the universe, and with your eyes gaze above the plane of the horizon into a void stillness at the center of the universe. Make sure you are not breathing onto the face of the client. Lengthen your heart meridian.

4. As your hands are leaving the scapula, allow the client's shoulders to lift slightly toward the ears. This opens the axilla and helps drain the lymph.

5. Ipsilaterally, gently hook your index and middle fingers under the pectoralis major and minor muscles to feel the axillary artery. Check to see if the shoulder can

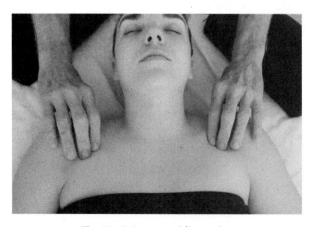

Fig. 31.12. Lung meridian points

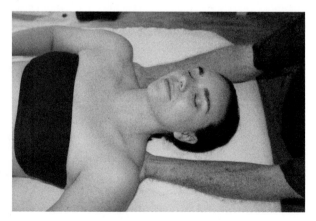

Fig. 31.13. Bilateral scapula

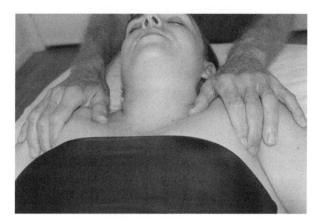

Fig. 31.14. Bilateral axillary artery and Heart 1

be lifted toward the ears by asking the client to shrug their shoulders. Then find the other artery with your other hand in the opposite axilla (see fig. 31.14). This is the general area of Heart 1. From this position, you must determine which side you will continue with. This can be a reflection of the strength of the pulse or an impulse you receive from PR or the client's heart meridian.

∿ 6. Heart Channel ∿

1. Now that you have chosen one side to work with, shift your position to that side of the client. Have the client extend their arm to give access to the axilla. Take a few moments to explore the continuity of the axillary and brachial arteries in the septum of the neurovascular bundle of the humerus. This is a gentle exploration in the system for the location of the artery and the pulse.

2. When you sense the axillary artery in the deep axilla between the latissimus dorsi and pectoralis major (Heart 1), place a single finger from your other hand in the umbilicus to sense the abdominal aorta (see fig. 31.15). Now close your eyes and ignite the Breath of Life by rolling your eyes up to the middle of your forehead.

3. Shift the hand in contact with the umbilicus to Heart 1. Shift your other hand to

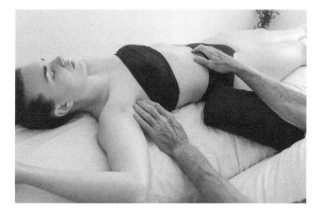

Fig. 31.15. Heart 1 and umbilicus

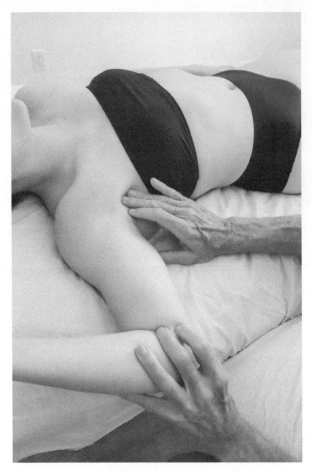

Fig. 31.16. Heart 1 and 3

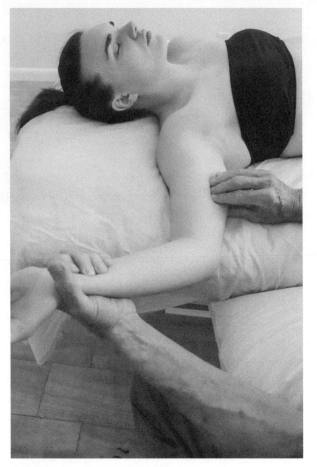

Fig. 31.17. Heart 2 and 4

the elbow and the brachial artery at the level of Heart 3 (see fig. 31.16). Close your eyes and see the client's heart meridian as a tube of electric blue light.

4. Shift the hand at Heart 1 to the mid-humerus in the neurovascular bundle to sense the humoral artery at the level of Heart 2. Shift your other hand to contact the ulnar artery slightly above the crease of the wrist at the level of Heart 4, called Spirit Path (see fig. 31.17). Close your eyes and see the client's heart meridian as a tube of electric blue light.

Consider moving to the other arm at any time during this practice. Your hands may be invited to do so. Similar to fulcrum of the twelve major joints in the water-earth element protocol in chapter 28, in which each side of the body is alternately contacted as if tracing the outline of a constellation in the universe, the heart meridian, too, may need to be contacted on opposite sides of the body in turn. This is rarely a uniform ipsilateral process, however; it needs to be creative for the heavenly home of spirit to enlarge in the heart. In this way the self-development and maturation of the client might move in an optimal direction for the time of life that the client is in in that very moment.

Alternatively, you may receive a signal while contacting the heart meridian to go no further or to finish and leave the contact without going to the other side at all. We are dealing with a double cycle that includes optimizing the void space in the heart where spirit resides while also improving the quality and flow of the blood from the viscera, which is directed by the spirit in the heart in order for the virtues of the spirit to radiate throughout the vascular tree and beyond. This is the territory of becoming a sage or having direct experience of the sacred at will. This is the journey expressed by the heart meridian and its relationships described herein. One entrance to this potency biodynamically is to close one's eyes and ignite the Breath of Life. Radiate the client with the Breath of Life and PR.

⌁ 7. Coccyx and Diaphragm ⌁

Finish this protocol at the coccyx and diaphragm and then the feet as described throughout the preceding chapters. By now, the practitioner can choose their own way of contacting these areas based on the options given in previous chapters.

∞

Spiritual Heart Ignition 2

⌁ 1. Lung Ignition ⌁

The client is supine. Contact the subclavian artery as detailed on page 340. The heart meridian moves through the lungs and the great sea of chi to gather power for radiating virtue throughout the body and the universe. Attune to the client's breathing. Ignite the Breath of Life, center yourself in your vascular tree. Allow the breath to become more full and easy.

⌁ 2. Axillary Artery and Heart Channel Visualization ⌁

1. Gently reach into the client's axilla with the intention to pull the shoulders a centimeter or two up toward the ears, one side at a time (see fig. 31.14, page 509). This opens the lymphatic ducts. Which shoulder moves more easily?
2. With the tips of your fingers in the axilla, palpate for the axillary artery and the sweet spot of Heart 1.
3. Visualize the arteries of the heart meridian as an electric blue diamond light. Wait for the light of the Breath of Life to flow in the meridian and its veins bilaterally.

⌁ 3. Left Ventricle for Broken Heart ⌁

Here we explore the takotsubo pietà. *Takotsubo* is the Japanese word for octopus trap and used as a metaphor for broken heart syndrome. The trap is shaped similar to the left ventricle of the heart that expands during the grieving process. The octopus trap expands when an octopus enters it, just like the human heart expands when filled with grief, which then ferments with the preexisting sorrow to generate great love. This ignites and supports the preexisting love that the spirit radiates from the heart inside the heart.

1. Approach the client from their left side, holding your hands together, palm up, with the edges of the little fingers touching. Place your hands under the spleen. Visualize yourself holding the fulcrum of the left ventricle of the heart between the Heart 8 and Pericardium 8 points on your palms, on the heart's midline alignment from the spleen to the right shoulder (see figs. 31.18–19). Lengthen your heart meridian starting at your little fingers gently pressing down into the table and then lifting your descending and abdominal aorta as if lengthening a midline out the top of the head. Sense the counterclockwise motion of the heart ejecting blood from the left ventricle and the clockwise motion of the ventricle relaxing. Adjust your hands as necessary to be clear about the midline of the left ventricle through the aorta to the right shoulder. Listen to the movement of the client's breathing, respiratory diaphragm, and rib movement. Gently synchronize your breathing with the client's breathing briefly. Wait for the client's heart to show itself to your hands and mind.

2. Now ignite the Breath of Life in yourself. Bring the light to your heart. Offer the Breath of Life to the client's heart by imagining their heart the color white for purification. With every contraction of the left ventricle, the blood moves counterclockwise. Now drop into your heartbeat. With every relaxation of the left ventricle, the blood returns in a clockwise motion.

3. Allow the left ventricle to settle and relax into the palms of your hands. Stay in contact with your own heartbeat, and then synchronize with deep level of PR, the Breath of Life as the motivational force that moves the blood. At the

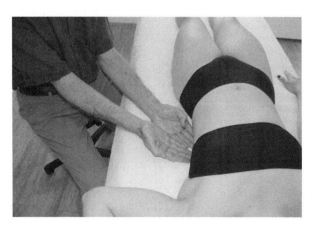

Fig. 31.18. Left ventricle 1

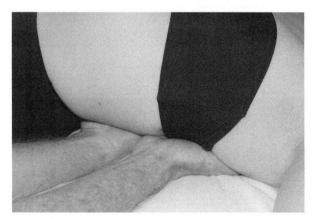

Fig. 31.19. Left ventricle 2

same time, the blood contains the virtuous essence of the spirit residing in the left ventricle and its environment. There is a fulcrum at the center of the heart, which is the location of the atrioventricular (AV) node. It is a space of dynamic stillness. From this fulcrum, the left ventricle is ignited, and the power of the heartbeat generates an enormous amount of heat.

Grief cools the heart so we can expand and relax and fill with love. While we are grieving, the heart must work harder to make sure the blood exits the left ventricle into the aorta. The left ventricle, with its expanding, dilating, and ballooning, is crucial for broken heart syndrome to be metabolized. Grief is a part of the spiritual journey described in the primary heart channel meridian. We are supporting the spiritual journey of our clients with these protocols.

ᔊ 4. Heart Channel ᔊ

1. Make contact with the ulnar and brachial arteries (see fig. 31.20). Sense how the vascular tree as a whole makes a torsional movement in the tempo of PR. Then, tune in to the vascular tree and visualize the tree in one of the five rainbow colors or repeat the image of the electric blue diamond light from above.

2. Using the pads of your index finger and thumb, like plucking a tissue from a Kleenex box, make contact medial to the pisiform bone on the undersurface (Heart 7) and the distal end of the ulnar bone on the top surface (Small Intestine 5; see figs. 31.21–22). Use the pads of the index finger and thumb on your other hand to similarly pluck at the base (lunula) of the client's fingernail of the little finger. The medial edge of the fingernail is Heart 9 (in the cuticle) and the lateral border of the fingernail is Small Intestine 1 (also in the cuticle).

   It does not matter whether the client's hand is palm up or down; it is up to the practitioner to determine the easiest contact with the client.

3. Make a heart-cosmos connection by radiating the Breath of Life from your heart. If the mind is active, turn your thoughts into a prayer. Expand the light of your heart to fill the universe.

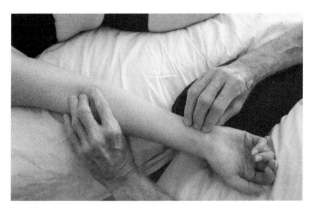

Fig. 31.20. Ulnar and brachial arteries

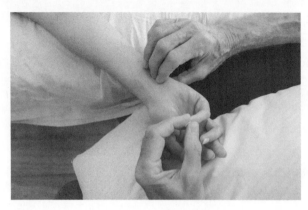

Fig. 31.21. Heart 7 and 9

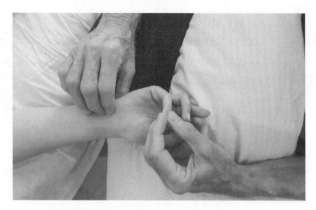

Fig. 31.22. Heart 7 and 9

⌇ 5. Liver Meridian in the Feet ⌇

1. Finish with bilateral contact at Liver 2, which is where the dorsalis pedis artery becomes the arteries arcuate, metatarsals dorsalis, and digitales dorsalis (see figs. 31.23–24). See plate 34 in the color insert for an excellent map of these arteries (note that the names of the arteries in plates 26–35 are in Latin).

2. Then shift to Liver 3, slightly above and still on the dorsalis pedis artery (see fig. 31.25). The liver houses the blood at night and always needs support.

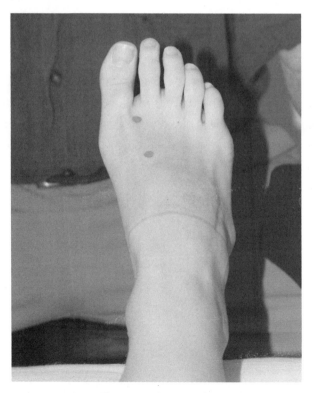

Fig. 31.23. Liver 2 and 3

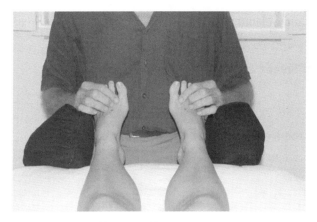

Fig. 31.24. Liver 2 contact

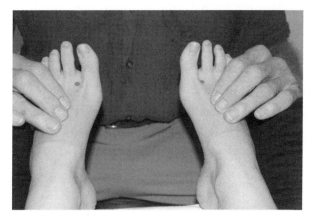

Fig. 31.25. Liver 3 contact

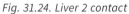

Spiritual Heart Ignition 3

~: 1. Lower Dantian Spiral :~

1. The client is supine. Place the tip of your middle finger into the client's umbilicus. Place your other hand under the low back of the client, contacting the second lumbar vertebra (see fig. 31.26). This contact is for the lower dantian of the client.

2. It is important to sense the spiral torsioning of the blood in the intestines and mesentery. The felt sense of this is a torsion throughout the whole vascular tree. This integrates the ancestral chi, which is spiritual chi.

3. Practice a cycle of attunement with the heart-cosmos meditation (page 433).

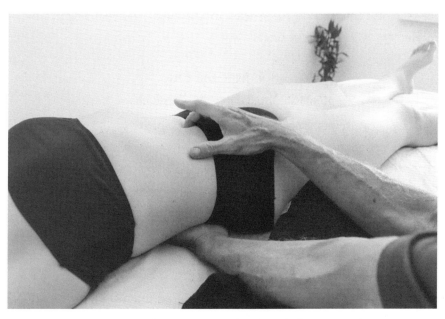

Fig. 31.26. Lower dantian spiral

❧ 2. Celiac Trunk: Hepatic and Splenic Arteries ❧

1. Review the sequence beginning on page 450 in chapter 28, The Third Water-Earth Fulcrums Protocol – The Stomach-Spleen Fulcrum. This is for building the blood.

2. The splenic artery feeds the stomach. The stomach has all three burners for manufacturing and distributing blood to the liver, spleen, and heart. Now visualize colored mists coming from this area, including the liver, filling the heart and vascular tree and then out of the body.

❧ 3. Superior Mesenteric and Renal Arteries ❧

This is a deeper repetition of the "Metabolic Fire" skill found in chapter 27 (page 428). The intention is to make sure the ancestral fire can connect through the right kidney to the heavenly fire of the heart.

1. Line up your index and middle fingers as if they were resting on a piano (see fig. 27.33, page 429). The tips of your index finger should be in contact with the tips of your middle fingers, which are aligned with the renal arteries.

2. Tune in to the client's breathing. Upon exhalation, wait for your fingers to be invited toward the space between the kidneys to sense the superior mesenteric and renal arteries. Remember that the left kidney is more superior than the right, and both kidneys are on the psoas muscle, which may invite your fingers to be on a slight diagonal line.

3. Tune in to PR. Rest in the warmth and heat of your own body and notice temperature variations in yourself. Wait for the client to breathe into your fingertips, or direct them to do so, at least three times. The repelling potency of the fire element will push your fingers out.

❧ 4. Neck and Face:
Stomach–Small Intestine Meridian ❧

With this palpation, remember that the embryonic heart grows against the face of the embryo. This sequence engages the stomach meridian, where the blood begins to be constructed from the food and beverages we consume. It is the work of the three burners of the San Janjiao meridian in the stomach that distributes the raw materials of the blood to the small intestine, liver, spleen, and heart.

1. Sit at the head of the table and practice a cranial cycle of attunement, as described on page 320.

2. Make contact bilaterally at the level of the mid-SCM. Here three acupuncture points are aligned horizontally; from posterior to anterior they are Small

Intestine 16, Large Intestine 18, and Stomach 9 (see fig. 31.7, page 505). These points coincide with the posterior-anterior septum and belly of the mid-SCM for sensing the carotid artery, jugular vein, and vagus nerve. These structures are all located in the carotid sheath under the SCM.

3. Bring your finger pads superiorly halfway to the styloid process while remaining on the posterior septum of the SCM. This is Heaven's Gate, San Janjiao 16 (see figs. 31.7 and 31.27).

4. Make bilateral contact with the facial artery at the level of Small Intestine 18 in the nasal labial fold directly under the lateral corner of the eye (see figs. 31.28–29). The small intestine and San Janjiao (Triple Warmer) meet here.

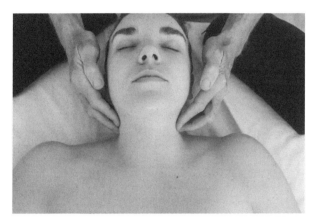
Fig. 31.27. Heaven's Gate

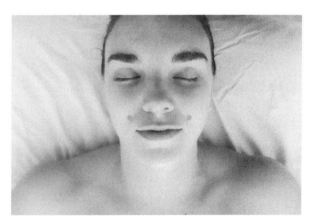
Fig. 31.28. Small Intestine 18

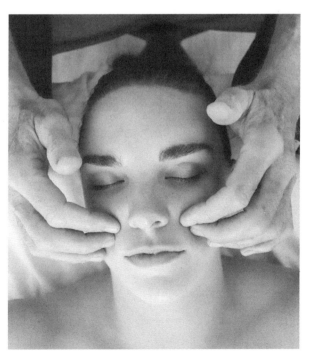
Fig. 31.29. Small Intestine 18

ᴖ 5. The Eyes ᴖ

1. Negotiate permission to contact the corner of the client's eye. Then shift one hand at a time toward the eyes. Let your finger pads make contact with the frontal bone as a way of preparing the client for closer contact with the inner canthus. Then make bilateral contact with the inner canthus of the eyes, using the pad of your index fingers with great gentleness (see figs. 31.30–31). Begin with contact on one eye, wait a few moments and observe how the client responds, such as blinking the eye, and then place the other finger pad on the other inner canthus. It is enough to have the edge of the finger, a millimeter of surface area, touching the inner canthus. The eyes are where the heart's primary and divergent channels meet and end in the face.

2. If the client is comfortable with it, place an eye pillow over their eyes. Make gentle bilateral contact with the center of the eye pillow directly over their eyes (see fig. 31.32). Begin with just several grams of pressure; ask the client if they feel the pressure and if it is comfortable. Ask the client to roll their eyes up to the middle of their forehead for several seconds and then relax. See if your

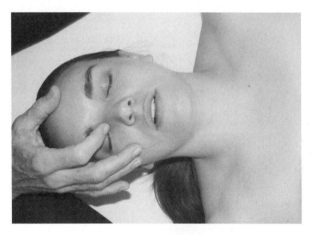

Fig. 31.30. Inner canthus of the eye 1

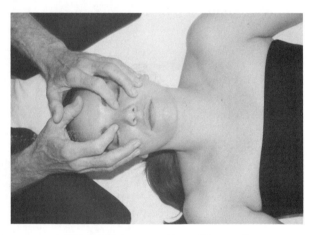

Fig. 31.31. Inner canthus of the eye 2

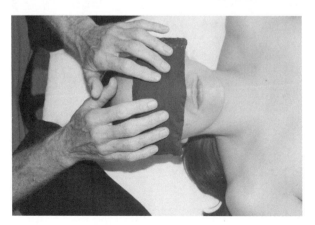

Fig. 31.32. Contact over the eye pillow

fingers can sense the movement of the client's eyes. Repeat several times until you can feel the movement of the client's eyes. Let the client know to relax their eyes.

3. Now bring your attention to your own eyes. Gently roll your eyes up to the middle of your forehead and visualize the Breath of Life as a bright clear light radiating from the heart up the central channel and out your eyes. Relax your eyes periodically and then roll them back up to the middle of your forehead. This is a short three-minute practice.

4. Notice if you feel any activity in the client's eyes, and then repeat the visualization of the Breath of Life. Notice if you can see the light from the client's eyes. Allow your whole hand to sense the potency radiating from the client's third ventricle. At some point this potency will lift your hands off of the client.

   This practice wakes up the branches of the central channel that bifurcate in the third ventricle and come out the eyes. The intention is to recognize the Breath of Life in its deepest wisdom aspect that lives in the heart inside the heart. This potency is strong.

5. Now visualize first your own heart and then the third ventricle of your brain as bright clear light. Then visualize your own eyes as orbs of bright clear light, devoid of any form. While your eyes are closed, bring a gentle attention to your hands and the client's eyes. Notice if the client's eyes appear as a particular color. If so, notice if this color expands to the client's third ventricle, heart and body. This takes only several minutes. The potency will guide your hands.

⁓ 6. The Ears ⁓

Still sitting at the head of the table, make bilateral contact with the maxillary artery several millimeters anterior to the midpoint of the tragus of the ear at Small Intestine 19. Three points are arranged vertically here; from bottom to top they are Gallbladder 2, Stomach 19, and San Janjiao 21 (see figs. 31.33–34). All three points

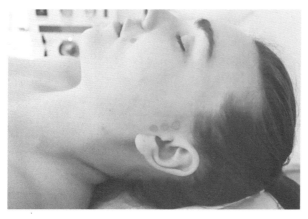

Fig. 31.33. Ear points 1

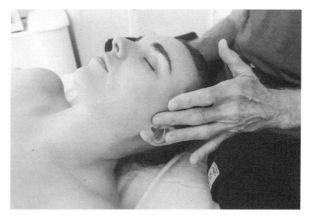

Fig. 31.34. Ear points 2

are being stimulated from the contact and biodynamic perceptual process. The temporomandibular joint here is a gate that allows food and other substances to enter the body. Thus, it is a critical gate for the health of the body and the manufacturing of blood in the stomach, spleen, and small intestine. Try visualizing the client's brain is white as the color of purification.

Practitioner Tip

Small Intestine 19 can be more clearly identified by asking the client to open their mouth slightly, which causes the condyle of the mandible to slide forward; the point is in the depression left when the condyle is forward. Once you have located the point, have the client close their mouth.

∴ 7. Coccyx and Diaphragm ∾

Make contact with the coccyx with one hand, and use the pads of the middle and/ or index fingers of your other hand to contact the respiratory diaphragm posteriorly. This brings the client back to earth and integrates their physiology. Visualize a tube of blue light in front of the spine; it extends out the top of the head and also bifurcates in the third ventricle, exiting through both eyes.

Seated Heart Breathing

At the end of a session, when the client sits up on the edge of the table or has moved to sit in a chair, make sure that their knees are below the plane of their hips and that their feet are on the ground. Stand by the client on their right side. Place your left hand on the back of their ribs, on the left side of their body, approximating the position of the left ventricle of their heart. Then place the palm of your right hand over the coracoid process of the scapula. Just tune in to the client's breathing and imagine holding their entire heart as it fills both of your hands. Synchronize with PR.

I am now finished with the exposition of the biodynamic ministry of laying on of hands, the essence of biodynamic cardiovascular therapy. Whichever protocols you choose to work with, please remember to synchronize with the three spiritual aptitudes of slowness, stillness, and luminosity. Allow your hands to be guided by these three aspects of the sacred. This leads to the wisdom of clarity, openness, and lightheartedness. Allow your mind to become the mind of the heart that lives in sorrow and joy, gratitude and forgiveness, acceptance and resilience. Develop your gift through contemplative skills that are reliable. We all have inglorious moments that pass and do not stay. To know this deeply in our body and mind and heart is great compassion for self and all others.

Postscript

On the title page in the first edition of Osteopathy in the Cranial Field compiled by The Osteopathic Cranial Association, edited by Harold I. Magoun, D.O. as approved by William Garner Sutherland, D.O. (1951), there is a short quote from Alexander Pope's Essay on Criticism written in 1711. It says: "A little learning is a dangerous thing; Drink deep or taste not the Pierian spring." The Pierian spring was a sacred fountain in Greek mythology said to be the source of profound inspiration and supreme knowledge. The spring was created by Pegasus, the winged horse when his hoof hit the ground. The spring was named after the Pierides, the daughters of King Pierus. He challenged the Muses, the goddesses of Song and Art, to a singing contest with his daughters. When the daughters lost the contest, they were turned into magpies. Let us not be turned into magpies by not being reverent and respectful of the sacred that comes from our heart and through our hands blessing the client. We must drink deep from the spring of humility and uncover the gift that the Muses, the Taras, the angelic beings, all divine goddesses and Holy ones have gifted us with through their residence in our human heart. We must drink deep from their fountain of love and compassion and allow it to transform ourselves and for its luminosity to radiate divine essence to all around us. The divine feminine gave me a deep drink of her potency and playfulness appearing in this book and throughout my life as demonstrated herein. I honor the gift of the feminine beyond binary polarization, her magnificence in nourishing me and all others with every breath we collectively take. And above all, the guidance from a living Bodhisattva, His Holiness the Dalai Lama. This is your book too. Thank you all!

Bibliography

Abram, David. 2010. *Becoming Animal: An Earthly Cosmology.* New York: Pantheon Books.

Achard, J.-L. 2017. *The Six Lamps: Secret Dzogchen Instructions of the Bön Tradition.* Boston: Wisdom Publications.

Agrawal, R., E. Noble, L. Vergnes, Z. Ying, K. Reue, and F. Gomez-Pinilla. 2016. "Dietary Fructose Aggravates the Pathobiology of Traumatic Brain Injury by Influencing Energy Homeostasis and Plasticity." *Journal of Cerebral Blood Flow & Metabolism* 36 (5): 941–53.

Aird, William C. 2007. "Phenotypic Heterogeneity of the Endothelium: I. Structure, Function, and Mechanisms." *Circulation Research* 100 (2): 158–73.

Akomolafe, B. 2017. *These Wilds Beyond Our Fences, Letters To My Daughter On Humanity's Search For Home.* New York: Penguin Random House.

Aldridge, D. 1996. "Notes on the Phenomenon of 'Becoming Healthy:' Body, Identity and Lifestyle." *Advances* 12 (1): 51–58.

Allione, T. 2008. *Feeding Your Demons, Ancient Wisdom for Resolving Inner Conflict.* New York: Little, Brown Spark.

Anderson, James G., and Kathleen Abrahamson. 2017. "Your Health Care May Kill You: Medical Errors." Studies in Health Technology and Informatics 234: 13–17.

Andersson, Ola, Barbro Lindquist, Magnus Lindgren, Karin Stjernqvist, Magnus Domellöf, and Lena Hellström-Westas. 2015. "Effect of Delayed Cord Clamping on Neurodevelopment at 4 Years of Age: A Randomized Clinical Trial." *JAMA Pediatrics* 169 (7): 631–38.

Andraweera, Prabha H., and Zohra S. Lassi. 2019. "Cardiovascular Risk Factors in Offspring of Preeclamptic Pregnancies—Systematic Review and Meta-Analysis." *Journal of Pediatrics* 208 (May): 104–113.

Araújo, J., J. Cai, and J. Stevens. 2019. "Prevalence of Optimal Metabolic Health in American Adults: National Health and Nutrition Examination Survey 2009–2016." *Metabolic Syndrome and Related Disorders* 17 (1): 46–52.

Archer, Edward, and Samantha McDonald. 2017. "The Maternal Resources Hypothesis and Childhood Obesity." In *Fetal and Early Postnatal Programming and Its Influence on Adult Health,* by M. S. Patel and J. H. Nielsen, 17–32. CRC Press.

Bansal, V., T. Costantini, L. Kroll, C. Peterson, W. Loomis, B. Eliceiri, A. Baird, P. Wolf, and R. Coimbra. 2009. "Traumatic Brain Injury and Intestinal Dysfunction: Uncovering the Neuro-Enteric Axis." *Journal of Neurotrauma* 26 (8): 1353–59.

Bardacke, N. 2012. *Mindful Birthing: Training the Mind, Body, and Heart for Childbirth and Beyond.* New York: HarperOne.

Batchelor, Stephen. 2000. *Verses from the Center.* New York: Riverhead Books.

Bechera, A., and N. Naqvi. 2004. "Listening to Your Heart; Interoceptive Awareness as a Gateway to Feeling." *Nature Neuroscience* 7 (2): 102–3.

Becker, Rollin E. 2000. *The Stillness of Life: The Osteopathic Philosophy of Rollin E. Becker, D.O.* Edited by Rachel E. Brooks. Portland, Ore: Stillness Press, LLC.

Beebe, B., S. Knoblauch, J. Rustin, and D. Sorter. 2005. *Forms of Intersubjectivity in Infant Research and Adult Treatment.* New York: Other Press.

Bergman, N. 2013. "Breastfeeding and Perinatal Neuroscience." In *Supporting Sucking Skills in Breastfeeding Infants,* 2nd ed., edited by C. Watson Genna, 43–57. Burlington, Mass.: Jones and Bartlett Learning.

Bernstein, J. 2006. *Living in the Borderland: The Evolution of Consciousness and the Challenge of Healing Trauma.* London: Routledge.

Blechschmidt, E. 2012a. *The Beginnings of Human Life.* New York: Springer Science and Business Media.

Blechschmidt, E. 2012b. *The Ontogenetic Basis of Human Anatomy: Biodynamic Approach to Development from Birth to Conception.* Translated by Brian Freeman. Berkeley, CA: North Atlantic Books.

Blechschmidt, E., and R. Gasser. 2012. *Biokinetics and Biodynamics of Human Differentiation: Principles and Applications.* Rev. ed. Berkeley, Calif.: North Atlantic Books.

Blitz, Matthew J., Rachel P. Gerber, Moti Gulersen, Weiwei Shan, Andrew C. Rausch, Lakha Prasannan, Natalie Meirowitz, and Burton Rochelson. 2021. "Preterm Birth among Women with and without Severe Acute Respiratory Syndrome Coronavirus 2 Infection." *Acta Obstetricia et Gynecologica Scandinavica* 100 (12): 2253–59.

Bloom, S. 2013. *Creating Sanctuary: Toward the Evolution of Sane Societies.* New York: Routledge.

Boddy, A. M., A. Fortunato, M. W. Sayres, and A. Aktipis. 2015. "Fetal Microchimerism and Maternal Health: A Review and Evolutionary Analysis of Cooperation and Conflict beyond the Womb." *Bioessays* 37: 1106–37.

Boeldt, D. S., and I. M. Bird. 2017. "Vascular Adaptation in Pregnancy and Endothelial Dysfunction in Preeclampsia." *Journal of Endocrinology* 232 (1): R27.

Bonaz, B., R. D. Lane, M. L. Oshinsky, P. J. Kenny, R. Sinha, E. A. Mayer, and H. D. Critchley. 2021. "Diseases, Disorders, and Comorbidities of Interoception." *Trends in Neuroscience* 44 (1): 39–51.

Bortoft, H. 1996. *The Wholeness of Nature: Goethe's Way toward a Science of Conscious Participation in Nature.* New York: Adonis Press.

Boyd, Andrew. 2002. *Daily Afflictions: The Agony of Being Connected to Everything in the Universe.* New York: W. W. Norton & Company, Inc.

Bryant, Allison S., Ayaba Worjoloh, Aaron B. Caughey, and A. Eugene Washington. 2010. "Racial/Ethnic Disparities in Obstetric Outcomes and Care: Prevalence and Determinants." *American Journal of Obstetrics and Gynecology.* 202 (4): 335–43.

Brennan, Lesley J., Jude S. Morton, and Sandra T. Davidge. 2014. "Vascular Dysfunction in Preeclampsia." *Microcirculation* 21 (1): 4–14.

Brew, Nadine, David Walker, and Flora Y. Wong. 2014. "Cerebral Vascular Regulation and Brain Injury in Preterm Infants." *American Journal of Physiology: Regulatory Integrative and Comparative Physiology* 306 (11).

Brooks, Megan. 2022. "'Lucid Dying': EEG Backs Near-Death Experience during CPR." Medscape (online), November 7, 2022.

Brown, R. P., and P. L. Gerbarg. 2012. *The Healing Power of the Breath.* Boston: Shambhala Press.

Burton, Graham J., and Eric Jauniaux. 2018. "Development of the Human Placenta and Fetal Heart: Synergic or Independent?" *Frontiers in Physiology* 9 (APR): 346187.

Calais-Germain, B. 2006. *Anatomy of Breathing.* Seattle: Eastland Press.

Capobianco, Antony. 2011. "Perinatal Cranial Trauma: Osteopathic Cases and Consideration." *The Cranial Letter* 64 (4): 13–19.

Carneiro, É. M., L. P. Barbosa, J. M. Marson, J. A. Terra Jr., C. J. Martins, D. Modesto, L. A. Resende, and M. F. Borges. 2017. "Effectiveness of Spiritist 'Passe' (Spiritual Healing) for Anxiety Levels, Depression, Pain, Muscle Tension, Well-Being, and Physiological Parameters in Cardiovascular Inpatients: A Randomized Controlled Trial." *Complementary Therapies in Medicine* 30: 73–78.

Carneiro, É. M., G. V. Moraes, and G. A. Terra. 2016. "Effectiveness of Spiritist Passe (Spiritual Healing) on the Psychophysiological Parameters in Hospitalized Patients." Advances in Mind-Body Medicine 30 (3): 4–10.

Carreiro, Jane. 2003. *An Osteopathic Approach to Children.* Churchill Livingstone.

Castanys-Muñoz, Esther, Maria J. Martin, and Enrique Vazquez. 2016. "Building a Beneficial Microbiome from Birth." *Advances in Nutrition* 7 (2): 323–30.

Chang, Fumin, Sheila Flavahan, and Nicholas A. Flavahan. 2016. "Immature Endothelial Cells Initiate Endothelin-Mediated Constriction of Newborn Arteries." *Journal of Physiology* 594 (17): 4933–44.

Channing, A., K. Rosenberg, C. Monk, C. Kleinman, J. Glickstein, S. Levasseur, L. Simson, and I. Williams. 2012. "Maternal Anxiety Associated with Echocardiography." *Open Journal of Pediatrics* 2: 143–49.

Chen, W. G., D. Schloesser, A. M. Arensdorf, J. M. Simmons, C. Cui, R. Valentino, J. W. Gnadt, et al. 2021. "The Emerging Science of Interoception: Sensing, Integrating, Interpreting, and Regulating Signals within the Self." *Trends in Neuroscience* 44 (1): 3–16.

Chodron, P. 1998. "Everybody Loves Something." *Shambhala Sun* (March 1998): 11–12.

Chodron, P. 2011. "Stay with Your Broken Heart." *Tricycle: The Buddhist Review* (Spring 2011): 16.

Chu, Derrick M., Kathleen M. Antony, Jun Ma, Amanda L. Prince, Lori Showalter, Michelle Moller, and Kjersti M. Aagaard. 2016. "The Early Infant Gut Microbiome Varies in Association with a Maternal High-Fat Diet." *Genome Medicine* 8 (1): 1–12.

Combs, H. L., D. T. Berry, T. Pape, J. Babcock-Parziale, B. Smith, R. Schleenbaker, A. Shandera-Ochsner, J. P. Harp, and W. M. High Jr. 2015. "The Effects of Mild Traumatic Brain Injury, Post-Traumatic Stress Disorder, and Combined Mild Traumatic Brain Injury/ Post-Traumatic Stress Disorder on Returning Veterans." *Journal of Neurotrauma* 32 (13): 956–66.

Comeaux, Z. 2002. *Robert Fulford, D.O. and the Philosopher Physician.* Seattle: Eastland Press.

Cosley, B., S. McCoy, L. Saslow, and E. Epel. 2010. "Is Compassion for Others Stress Buffering? Consequences of Compassion and Social Support for Physiological Reactivity to Stress." *Journal of Experimental Social Psychology* 46: 816–32.

Couto, B., A. Salles, L. Sedeño, M. Peradejordi, P. Barttfeld, A. Canales-Johnson, and A. Ibanez. 2014. "The Man Who Feels Two Hearts: The Different Pathways of Interoception." *Social Cognitive Affective Neuroscience* 9 (9): 1253–60.

Cowan, Thomas. 2016. *Human Heart, Cosmic Heart*. White River Junction, Vt.: Chelsea Green Publishing.

Craig, A. 2004. "Human Feelings: Why Are Some More Aware than Others?" *TRENDS in Cognitive Sciences* 8 (6): 239–41.

Craig, A. D. 2009. "How Do You Feel—Now? The Anterior Insula and Human Awareness." *Nature Reviews: Neuroscience* 10 (1): 59–70.

Craig, A. D. 2011. "Significance of the Insula for the Evolution of Human Awareness of Feelings from the Body." *Annals of the New York Academy of Sciences* 1225: 72–82.

Critchley, H., S. Wiens, P. Rotshstein, A. Ohman, and R. Dolan. 2004. "Neural Systems Supporting Interoceptive Awareness." *Nature Neuroscience* 7 (2): 189–95.

Crivellato, Enrico, B. Nico, and D. Ribatti. 2007. "Contribution of Endothelial Cells to Organogenesis: A Modern Reappraisal of an Old Aristotelian Concept." *Journal of Anatomy* 211 (4): 415–27.

Dalai Lama (Tenzin Gyatso). 1994. *A Flash of Lightning in the Dark of the Night: A Guide to the Bodhisattva's Way of Life*. Based on the *Bodhicharyavatara,* an eighth-century treatise by Buddhist philosopher Shantideva. Boston: Shambhala.

Damasio, A. R. 1999. *Feeling of What Happens: Body and Emotion in the Making of Consciousness*. Dallas: Harvest Books.

D'Andrea Meira, I., T. T. Romão, H. J. Pires do Prado, L. T. Krüger, M. Pires, and P. O. da Conceição. 2019. "Ketogenic Diet and Epilepsy: What We Know So Far." *Frontiers in Neuroscience* 13: 5.

Da Silva, Shana Ginar, Mariângela Freitas Da Silveira, Andréa Dâmaso Bertoldi, Marlos Rodrigues Domingues, and Iná Da Silva Dos Santos. 2020. "Maternal and Child-Health Outcomes in Pregnancies Following Assisted Reproductive Technology (ART): A Prospective Cohort Study." *BMC Pregnancy and Childbirth* 20 (1): 1–8.

Dawe, Gavin S., Xiao Wei Tan, and Zhi Cheng Xiao. 2007. "Cell Migration from Baby to Mother." *Cell Adhesion & Migration* 1 (1): 19.

Deadman, P., and M. Al-Khafaji. 2016. *A Manual of Acupuncture*. East Sussex, England: Journal of Chinese Medicine Publications.

de Mause, L. 1996. "Restaging Fetal Traumas in War and Social Violence." *Prenatal and Perinatal Psychology and Health Journal* 10 (4): 229–61.

Desmond, T. 2017. *The Self-Compassion Skills Workbook*. New York: W. W. Norton & Company.

Desoye, Gernot, and Sylvie Hauguel-De Mouzon. 2007. "The Human Placenta in Gestational Diabetes Mellitus: The Insulin and Cytokine Network." *Diabetes Care* 30 (suppl. 2): S120–26.

Doctor, R. M., and F. N. Shiromoto. 2009. "Traumatic Brain Injury (TBI)." Entry in *The Encyclopedia of Trauma and Traumatic Stress Disorders*. New York: Facts On File.

Drews, U. 1995. *Color Atlas of Embryology*. New York: Theime.

Dunham-Snary, Kimberly J., Zhigang G. Hong, Ping Y. Xiong, Joseph C. Del Paggio, Julia E. Herr, Amer M. Johri, and Stephen L. Archer. 2016. "A Mitochondrial Redox Oxygen Sensor in the Pulmonary Vasculature and Ductus Arteriosus." *Pflügers Archiv: European Journal of Physiology* 468 (1): 43–58.

Eliade, M. 1958. *Rites and Symbols of Initiation: The Mysteries of Birth and Rebirth*. New York: Harper and Row.

Eliade, M. 1959. *The Sacred and the Profane: The Nature of Religion.* New York: Harcourt, Brace & World.

Eliade, M. 1960. *Myths, Dreams and Mysteries.* London: Harvill Press.

Eliade, M. 1963. *Myth and Reality.* New York: Harper and Row.

Entringer, Sonja, Karin de Punder, Claudia Buss, and Pathik D. Wadhwa. 2018. "The Fetal Programming of Telomere Biology Hypothesis: An Update." *Philosophical Transactions of the Royal Society B: Biological Sciences* 373 (1741).

Epstein, Franklin H., John R. Vane, Erik E. Änggård, and Regina M. Botting. 1990. "Regulatory Functions of the Vascular Endothelium." *New England Journal of Medicine* 323 (1): 27–36.

Feuda, R., M. Dohrmann, W. Pett, H. Philippe, O. Rota-Stabelli, N. Lartillot, G. Wörheide, and D. Pisani. 2017. "Improved Modeling of Compositional Heterogeneity Supports Sponges as Sister to All Other Animals." *Current Biology* 27 (24): 3864–70.

Fjeldstad, Heidi E.S., Guro M. Johnsen, and Anne Cathrine Staff. 2020. "Fetal Microchimerism and Implications for Maternal Health." *Obstetric Medicine* 13 (3): 112.

Friedman, M. 2022. *Where Spirit Touches Matter: A Journey toward Wholeness.* Durham, N.C., Light Messages Torchflame Books.

Frymann, Viola. 1998. "The Trauma of Birth." In *The Collected Papers of Viola M. Frymann, DO*, edited by Hollis Heaton King, 193–99. Indianapolis: American Academy of Osteopathy.

Fukushima, H., Y. Terasawa, and S. Umeda. 2011. "Association between Interoception and Empathy: Evidence from Heartbeat-Evoked Brain Potential." *International Journal of Psychophysiology* 79 (2): 259–65.

Furst, B. 2020. *The Heart and Circulation: An Integrative Model.* 2nd ed. New York: Springer.

Garfield, James, trans. and comm. 1995. *The Fundamental Wisdom of The Middle Way: Nāgārjuna's Mūlamadhyamakakārikā.* Oxford and New York: Oxford University Press.

Genna, Catherine Watson, and Sharon A. Vallone. 2016. "Hands in Support of Breastfeeding: Manual Therapy." In *Supporting Sucking Skills in Breastfeeding Infants*, 3rd ed., 444. New York: Jones & Bartlett.

Gepshtein, S., A. S. Pawar, S. Kwon, S. Savel'ev, and T. D. Albright. 2022. "Spatially Distributed Computation in Cortical Circuits." *Science Advances* 8 (16).

Gershon, Michael D., M.D. 1998. *The Second Brain: A Groundbreaking New Understanding of the Nervous Disorders of the Stomach and Intestine.* New York: HarperCollins.

Ginsberg, Yuval, Nizar Khatib, Zeev Weiner, and Ron Beloosesky. 2017. "Maternal Inflammation, Fetal Brain Implications and Suggested Neuroprotection: A Summary of 10 Years of Research in Animal Models." *Rambam Maimonides Medical Journal* 8 (2): e0028.

Giordano, K. R., L. M. Rojas-Valencia, V. Bhargava, and J. Lifshitz. 2020. "Beyond Binary: Influence of Sex and Gender on Outcome after Traumatic Brain Injury." *Journal of Neurotrauma* 37 (23): 2454–59.

Gitto, Eloisa, Salvatore Pellegrino, Placido Gitto, Ignazio Barberi, and Russel J. Reiter. 2009. "Oxidative Stress of the Newborn in the Pre- and Postnatal Period and the Clinical Utility of Melatonin." *Journal of Pineal Research* 46 (2): 128–39.

Giussani, Dino A. 2016. "The Fetal Brain Sparing Response to Hypoxia: Physiological Mechanisms." *Journal of Physiology* 594 (5): 1215–30.

Golightly, E., H. N. Jabbour, and J. E. Norman. 2011. "Endocrine Immune Interactions in Human Parturition." *Molecular and Cellular Endocrinology* 335 (1).

Gonzalez, Fernando F., and Donna M. Ferriero. 2009. "Neuroprotection in the Newborn Infant." *Clinics in Perinatology* 36 (4): 859–80.

Gross, E. C., R. J. Klement, J. Schoenen, D. P. D'Agostino, and D. Fischer. 2019. "Potential Protective Mechanisms of Ketone Bodies in Migraine Prevention." *Nutrients* 11 (4): 811.

Grossman, D. 2009. *On Killing: The Psychological Cost of Learning to Kill in War and Society.* New York: Back Bay Books.

Halifax, J. 2005. *Being Met by the Reality Called Mu.* Upaya Institute Chaplain Program handout. Sante Fe: Upaya Institute.

Halifax, J. 2011. "The Precious Necessity of Compassion." *Journal of Symptom and Pain Management* 41 (1): 146–53.

Hanh, Thich Nhat. 2018. "Memories from the Root Temple: Tangerines in Heaven." Post, Plum Village website, November 8, 2018.

Haraway, D. J. 2004. *Crystals, Fabrics and Fields: Metaphors That Shape Embryos.* Berkeley, Calif.: North Atlantic Books.

Hardy, A. C. 1979. *The Spiritual Nature of Man: A Study of Contemporary Religious Experience.* Oxford: Oxford University Press.

Haworth, Sheila G. 2006. "Pulmonary Endothelium in the Perinatal Period." *Pharmacological Reports* 58 (suppl.): 153–64.

Hernandez-Andrade, E., T. Jansson, G. Lingman, K. Liuba, D. Ley, and K. Maršál. 2014. "Blood-Flow Streams in the Fetal Inferior Vena Cava: Experimental Animal Study Using Ultrasound Contrast Agent." *Ultrasound in Obstetrics & Gynecology* 43 (3): 353–54.

Heydrich, L., F. Walker, L. Blättler, B. Herbelin, O. Blanke, and J. E. Aspell. 2021. "Interoception and Empathy Impact Perspective Taking." *Frontiers in Psychology* 11: 599429.

Hill, Lee, Ruchika Sharma, Lara Hart, Jelena Popov, Michal Moshkovich, and Nikhil Pai. 2021. "The Neonatal Microbiome in Utero and beyond: Perinatal Influences and Long-Term Impacts." *Journal of Laboratory Medicine* 45 (6): 275–91.

Hillman, J. 1993. *We've Had a Hundred Years of Psychotherapy, and the World's Getting Worse.* Rev. ed. New York: HarperOne.

Hillman, Noah H., Suhas G. Kallapur, and Alan H. Jobe. 2012. "Physiology of Transition from Intrauterine to Extrauterine Life." *Clinics in Perinatology* 39 (4): 769–83.

Ho, D. H., and W. W. Burggren. 2010. "Epigenetics and Transgenerational Transfer: A Physiological Perspective." *Journal of Experimental Biology* 213 (1): 3–16.

Hofmann, S., P. Grossman, and D. Hinton. 2011. "Loving-Kindness and Compassion Meditation: Potential for Psychological Interventions." *Clinical Psychology Review* 31: 1126–32.

Hooper, Stuart Brian, Graeme Roger Polglase, and Charles Christoph Roehr. 2015. "Cardiopulmonary Changes with Aeration of the Newborn Lung." *Paediatric Respiratory Reviews* 16 (3): 147–50.

Ikkyu. 2000. *Crow with No Mouth: Ikkyu 15th Century Zen Master.* Versions by Stephen Berg. Copper Canyon Press.

Illich, I. 1976. *Medical Nemesis: The Expropriation of Health.* New York: Pantheon Books.

Ives, Christopher W., Rachel Sinkey, Indranee Rajapreyar, Alan T.N. Tita, and Suzanne Oparil. 2020. "Preeclampsia—Pathophysiology and Clinical Presentations: JACC State-of-the-Art Review." *Journal of the American College of Cardiology* 76 (14): 1690–702.

Jealous, J. 1996. *Around the Edges*. Tide *(An Osteopathic Newsletter)*. Spring 1996.

Jealous, J. S. 2001. "Biodynamics of Osteopathy: Phase IV." (Course Materials: Emergence of Originality). Direction of Ease, LLC.

Jenkinson, Stephen. 2015. *Die Wise: A Manifesto for Sanity and Soul*. Berkeley, Calif.: North Atlantic Books.

Jinpa, T. 2015. *A Fearless Heart: How the Courage to Be Compassionate Can Transform Our Lives*. New York: Hudson Street Press.

Kaczynski, Andrew T., Jan M. Eberth, Ellen W. Stowe, Marilyn E. Wende, Angela D. Liese, Alexander C. McLain, Charity B. Breneman, and Michele J. Josey. 2020. "Development of a National Childhood Obesogenic Environment Index in the United States: Differences by Region and Rurality." *International Journal of Behavioral Nutrition and Physical Activity* 17 (1): 1–11.

Kallenbach, L. R., K. L. Johnson, and D. W. Bianchi. 2011. "Fetal Cell Microchimerism and Cancer: A Nexus of Reproduction, Immunology, and Tumor Biology." *Cancer Research* 71 (1): 8–13.

Kalsched, D. 1996. *The Inner World of Trauma: Archetypal Defenses of the Personal Spirit*. New York: Routledge.

Khong, T. Yee, Janine H. C. Tee, and Andrew J. Kelly. 1997. "Absence of Innervation of the Uteroplacental Arteries in Normal and Abnormal Human Pregnancies." *Gynecologic and Obstetric Investigation* 43 (2): 89–93.

Kirby, Margaret Loewy. 2007. *Cardiac Development*. New York: Oxford University Press.

Kiserud, Torvid. 2005. "Physiology of the Fetal Circulation." *Seminars in Fetal and Neonatal Medicine* 10 (6): 493–503.

Kok, B., and B. Fredrickson. 2010. "Upward Spirals of the Heart: Autonomic Flexibility, as Indexed by Vagal Tone, Reciprocally and Respectively Predicts Positive Emotions and Social Connectedness." *Biological Psychology* 85 (3): 432–36.

Kolacz, J. and S. W. Porges. 2018. "Chronic Diffuse Pain and Functional Gastrointestinal Disorders after Traumatic Stress: Pathophysiology through a Polyvagal Perspective." *Frontiers in Medicine* 5 (145).

Kroener, Lindsay, Erica T. Wang, and Margareta D. Pisarska. 2016. "Predisposing Factors to Abnormal First Trimester Placentation and the Impact on Fetal Outcomes." *Seminars in Reproductive Medicine* 34 (1): 27–35.

Kuban, Karl C. K., T. Michael O'Shea, Elizabeth N. Allred, Nigel Paneth, Deborah Hirtz, Raina N. Fichorova, and Alan Leviton. 2014. "Systemic Inflammation and Cerebral Palsy Risk in Extremely Preterm Infants." *Journal of Child Neurology* 29 (12): 1692.

Lakshminrusimha, Satyan, and Martin Keszler. 2015. "Persistent Pulmonary Hypertension of the Newborn." *NeoReviews* 16 (12): e680–94.

Lamott, Anne. 2017. "12 Truths I Learned from Life and Writing." TED Talk, Vancouver, BC.

Larre, C., and E. R. de la Vallée. 2012. *The Heart: In Ling Shu Chapter 8*. N.p.: Monkey Press.

Leddy, Meaghan A, Michael L Power, and Jay Schulkin. 2008. "The Impact of Maternal Obesity on Maternal and Fetal Health." *Reviews in Obstetrics and Gynecology* 1 (4): 170.

Ledoux, A. A., R. J. Webster, A. E. Clarke, D. B. Fell, B. D. Knight, W. Gardner, P. Cloutier, C. Gray, M. Tuna, and R. Zemek. 2022. "Risk of Mental Health Problems in Children and Youths following Concussion." *JAMA Network Open* 5 (3): e221235.

Le Huërou-Luron, Isabelle, Sophie Blat, and Gaëlle Boudry. 2010. "Breast- v. Formula-Feeding: Impacts on the Digestive Tract and Immediate and Long-Term Health Effects." *Nutrition Research Reviews* 23 (1): 23–36.

Lewis, John. 2012. *A. T. Still: From the Dry Bone to the Living Man.* Blaenau Ffestiniog, Wales: Dry Bone Press.

Lindsay, Karen L., Claudia Buss, Pathik D. Wadhwa, and Sonja Entringer. 2019. "The Interplay between Nutrition and Stress in Pregnancy: Implications for Fetal Programming of Brain Development." *Biological Psychiatry* 85 (2): 135.

Loori, J. D. 1996. *The Stillpoint: A Beginner's Guide to Zen Meditation.* Mt. Tremper, N.Y.: Dharma Communications.

Lustig, Robert H. 2022. *Metabolical: The Lure and the Lies of Processed Food, Nutrition, and Modern Medicine.* New York: HarperCollins.

Mahmood, U., and K. O'Donoghue. 2014. "Microchimeric Fetal Cells Play a Role in Maternal Wound Healing after Pregnancy." *Chimerism* 5 (2): 40–52.

Markin, R. D., and S. Zilcha-Mano. 2018. "Cultural Processes in Psychotherapy for Perinatal Loss: Breaking the Cultural Taboo against Perinatal Grief." *Psychotherapy* 55 (1): 20–26.

Marshall, Nicole E., Barbara Abrams, Linda A. Barbour, Patrick Catalano, Parul Christian, Jacob E. Friedman, William W. Hay, et al. 2022. "The Importance of Nutrition in Pregnancy and Lactation: Lifelong Consequences." *American Journal of Obstetrics and Gynecology* 226 (5): 607–32.

Martin, A. K., A. J. Petersen, H. W. Sesma, M. B. Koolmo, K. M. Ingram, K. B. Slifko, V. N. Nguyen, R. C. Doss, and A. M. Linabery. 2020. "Concussion Symptomology and Recovery in Children and Adolescents with Pre-existing Anxiety." *Journal of Neurology, Neurosurgery and Psychiatry* 91 (10): 1060–66.

McCraty, R., and F. Shaffer. 2015. "Heart Rate Variability: New Perspectives on Physiological Mechanisms, Assessment of Self-Regulatory Capacity, and Health Risk." *Global Advances in Health and Medicine* 4 (1): 46–61.

Meier, T. B., P. S. Bellgowan, R. Singh, R. Kuplicki, D. W. Polanski, and A. R. Mayer. 2015. "Recovery of Cerebral Blood Flow following Sports-Related Concussion." *JAMA Neurology* 72(5): 530–38.

Mez, J., D. H. Daneshvar, P. T. Kiernan, et al. 2017. "Clinicopathological Evaluation of Chronic Traumatic Encephalopathy in Players of American Football." *JAMA* 318 (4): 360–70.

Moeckel, Eva, and Noori Mitha. 2008. "Birth and Treating the Baby." In *Textbook of Pediatric Osteopathy*, 43–78. Churchill Livingstone.

Mollayeva, T., S. Mollayeva, and A. Colantonio. 2018. Traumatic Brain Injury: Sex, Gender and Intersecting Vulnerabilities." *Nature Reviews Neurology* 14 (12): 711–22.

Mollayeva, T., V. Amodio, S. Mollayeva, A. D'Souza, H. Colquhoun, E. Quilico, H. L. Haag, and A. Colantonio. 2019. "A Gender-Transformative Approach to Improve Outcomes and Equity among Persons with Traumatic Brain Injury." *BMJ Open* 9 (5): e024674.

Morris, D. 1998. "Illness and Health in the Post Modern Age." *Advances* 14 (4): 237–64.

Mulkey, Sarah B., and Adre dú Plessis. 2018. "The Critical Role of the Central Autonomic Nervous System in Fetal-Neonatal Transition." *Seminars in Pediatric Neurology* 28 (December): 29–37.

Murphy, Peter J. 2005. "The Fetal Circulation." *Continuing Education in Anaesthesia Critical Care & Pain* 5 (4): 107–12.

Murphy, Vanessa E., Roger Smith, Warwick B. Giles, and Vicki L. Clifton. 2006. "Endocrine Regulation of Human Fetal Growth: The Role of the Mother, Placenta, and Fetus." *Endocrine Reviews* 27 (2): 141–69.

Nair, Jayasree, Sylvia F. Gugino, Lori C. Nielsen, Michael G. Caty, and Satyan Lakshminrusimha. 2016. "Fetal and Postnatal Ovine Mesenteric Vascular Reactivity." *Pediatric Research* 79 (4): 575–82.

Newburg, David S., and W. Allan Walker. 2007. "Protection of the Neonate by the Innate Immune System of Developing Gut and of Human Milk." *Pediatric Research* 61 (1): 2–8.

Nobrega Cruz, Nayara Azinheira, Danielle Stoll, Dulce Elena Casarini, and Mariane Bertagnolli. 2021. "Role of ACE2 in Pregnancy and Potential Implications for COVID-19 Susceptibility." *Clinical Science* 135 (15): 1805–24.

Norbu, Thinley. 1999. *Magic Dance: The Display of the Self-Nature of the Five Wisdom Dakinis.* Boulder: Shambhala.

Nyima, C., and D. R. Schlim. 2015. *Medicine and Compassion: A Tibetan Lama and an American Doctor on How to Provide Care with Compassion and Wisdom.* Boston: WisdomNPublications.

O'Donohue, J. 1997. *Anam Cara: Spiritual Wisdom from the Celtic World.* New York: Bantam.

O'Donohue, John. 2008. *To Bless the Space between Us: A Book of Blessings.* New York: Doubleday.

O'Hearn Meghan, Brianna N. Lauren, John B. Wong, David D. Kim, and Dariush Mozaffarian. 2022. "Trends and Disparities in Cardiometabolic Health Among U.S. Adults, 1999–2018." *Journal of the American College of Cardiology* 80 (2): 138–151.

O'Rahilly, R., and F. Muller. 2001. *Human Embryology and Teratology.* 3rd ed. New York: Wiley-Liss.

Panksepp, J., and L. Biven. 2012. *The Archaeology of Mind: Neuroevolutionary Origins of Human Emotions.* New York: W.W. Norton & Company.

Papaiconomou, C., R. Bozanovic-Sosic, A. Zakharov, and M. Johnston. 2002. "Does Neonatal Cerebrospinal Fluid Absorption Occur via Arachnoid Projections or Extracranial Lymphatics?" *American Journal of Physiology: Regulatory Integrative and Comparative Physiology* 283 (4): 52–54.

Patterson, Z. R., and M. R. Holahan. 2012. "Understanding the Neuroinflammatory Response following Concussion to Develop Treatment Strategies." *Frontiers in Cellular Neuroscience* 6: 58.

Paul, A. M. 2011. *Origins: How the Nine Months before Birth Shape the Rest of Our Lives.* New York: Freepress.

Paulus, S. 1999. "The Breath of Life: The Fundamental Principle of Osteopathy." *Inter Linea Journal of Osteopathic Philosophy* 1 (1): 6–8.

Pavlov, V. A., and K. J. Tracey. 2012. "The Vagus Nerve and the Inflammatory Reflex: Linking Immunity and Metabolism." *Nature Reviews Endocrinology* 8 (12): 743–54.

Pert, C. 1997. *Molecules of Emotion.* New York: Random House.

Peterson, C., and M. Seligman. 2004. *Character Strengths and Virtues: A Handbook of Classifications.* New York: Oxford University Press.

Phoswa, Wendy N., and Olive P. Khaliq. 2021. "The Role of Oxidative Stress in Hypertensive Disorders of Pregnancy (Preeclampsia, Gestational Hypertension) and Metabolic Disorder of Pregnancy (Gestational Diabetes Mellitus)." *Oxidative Medicine and Cellular Longevity* 2021.

Pichler, Gerhard, Georg M. Schmölzer, and Berndt Urlesberger. 2017. "Cerebral Tissue Oxygenation during Immediate Neonatal Transition and Resuscitation." *Frontiers in Pediatrics* 5 (February): 29.

Piver, S. 2012. *The Mindful Way through Pregnancy.* Boston: Shambhala.

Podvoll, E. M. 1983. "The History of Sanity in Contemplative Psychotherapy." *Naropa Institute Journal of Psychology* 2: 11–32.

Poeppelman, Rachel Stork, and Joseph D. Tobias. 2018. "Patent Ductus Venosus and Congenital Heart Disease: A Case Report and Review." *Cardiology Research* 9 (5): 330.

Polglase, Graeme R., Suzanne L. Miller, Samantha K. Barton, Martin Kluckow, Andrew W. Gill, Stuart B. Hooper, and Mary Tolcos. 2014. "Respiratory Support for Premature Neonates in the Delivery Room: Effects on Cardiovascular Function and the Development of Brain Injury." *Pediatric Research* 75 (6): 682–88.

Popkin, B. M., S. Du, W. D. Green, M. A. Beck, T. Algaith, C. H. Herbst, R. F. Alsukait, M. Alluhidan, N. Alazemi, and M. Shekar. 2020. "Individuals with Obesity and COVID-19: A Global Perspective on the Epidemiology and Biological Relationships." *Obesity Reviews* 21 (11): e13128.

Porges, S. W. 1998. "Love: An Emergent Property of the Mammalian Autonomic Nervous System." *Psychoneuroendocrinology* 23 (8): 837–61.

Porges, S. W. 2001. "The Polyvagal Theory: Phylogenetic Substrates of a Social Nervous System." *International Journal of Psychophysiology* 42 (2): 123–46.

Porges, S. W. 2004. "Neuroception: A Subconscious System for Detecting Threats and Safety." *Zero to Three* 24 (5): 19–24.

Porges, S. W. 2007. "The Polyvagal Perspective." *Biological Psychology* 74 (2): 116–43.

Porges, S. W. 2009. "The Polyvagal Theory: New Insights into Adaptive Reactions of the Autonomic Nervous System." *Cleveland Clinic Journal of Medicine* 76 (suppl. 2): S86.

Porges, S. W. 2011. *The Polyvagal Theory: Neurophysiological Foundations of Emotions, Attachment, Communication, and Self-Regulation.* New York: W. W. Norton.

Porges, S. W. 2017. "Vagal Pathways: Portals to Compassion." In *The Oxford Handbook of Compassion Science,* by E. M. Seppälä, E. Simon-Thomas, S. L. Brown, M. C. Worline, C. D. Cameron, and J. R. Doty. New York: Oxford University Press.

Porges, S. W. 2023. "The Vagal Paradox: A Polyvagal Solution." *Comprehensive Psychoneuroendocrinology* 16: 100200.

Porges, S. W. 2024a. "Disorders of Gut-Brain Interaction (DGBI) through the Lens of Polyvagal Theory." *Neurogastroenterology and Motility.*

Porges, S. W. 2024b. *Polyvagal Perspectives, Interventions, and Strategies.* New York: Norton.

Purser, R. E. 2019. *McMindfulness: How Mindfulness Became the New Capitalist Spirituality.* New York: Repeater.

Quigley, K. S., S. Kanoski, W. M. Grill, L. F. Barrett, and M. Tsakiris. 2021. "Functions of Interoception: From Energy Regulation to Experience of the Self." *Trends in Neuroscience* 44 (1): 29–38.

Rabe, Heike, Judith Mercer, and Debra Erickson-Owens. 2022. "What Does the Evidence Tell Us? Revisiting Optimal Cord Management at the Time of Birth." *European Journal of Pediatrics* 181 (5): 1797–807.

Radoš, Milan, Matea Živko, Ante Periša, Darko Orešković, and Marijan Klarica. 2021. "No Arachnoid Granulations—No Problems: Number, Size, and Distribution of Arachnoid

Granulations from Birth to 80 Years of Age." *Frontiers in Aging Neuroscience* 13: 698865.

Rajan, Radhika Ravi. 2013. "Our Navel: The Root of Our Consciousness." *Speaking Tree* blog, November 13, 2013.

Ramcharan, Khedar S., Gregory Y. H. Lip, Paul S. Stonelake, and Andrew D. Blann. 2011. "The Endotheliome: A New Concept in Vascular Biology." *Thrombosis Research* 128 (1): 1–7.

Reich, W. 1945. *Character Analysis*. New York: Touchstone Book.

Reich, W. 1980. *The Mass Psychology of Fascism*. 3rd ed. New York: Farrar, Straus and Giroux.

Reynolds, D. K. 1982. *The Quiet Therapies: Japanese Pathways to Personal Growth*. Honolulu: University of Hawaii Press.

Ribatti, Domenico, Roberto Tamma, and Tiziana Annese. 2021. "The Role of Vascular Niche and Endothelial Cells in Organogenesis and Regeneration." *Experimental Cell Research* 398 (1): 112398.

Ricard, Matthieu. 2004. "Working with Desire: Three Approaches from Tibetan Buddhism." *Tricycle: The Buddhist Review* (Summer 2004).

Rijnink, E. C., M. E. Penning, R. Wolterbeek, S. Wilhelmus, M. Zandbergen, S. G. van Duinen, J. Schutte, J. A. Bruijn, and I. M. Bajema. 2015. "Tissue Microchimerism Is Increased during Pregnancy: A Human Autopsy Study." *Molecular Human Reproduction* 21 (11): 857–64.

Rogers, Lynette K., and Markus Velten. 2011. "Maternal Inflammation, Growth Retardation, and Preterm Birth: Insights into Adult Cardiovascular Disease." *Life Sciences* 89 (13–14): 417–21.

Romeu-Mejia, R., C. C. Giza, and J. T. Goldman. 2019. "Concussion Pathophysiology and Injury Biomechanics." *Current Reviews in Musculoskeletal Medicine* 12 (2): 105–16.

Rosenberg, L. 1998. "The Art of Doing Nothing." *Tricycle: The Buddhist Review* 7 (3): 40-47.

Roshi, S. 2011. *Zen Mind, Beginner's Mind, Informal Talks on Zen Meditation and Practice*. Boulder: Shambhala.

Roth, G. 1992. *When Food Is Love: Exploring the Relationship between Eating and Intimacy*. New York: Plume.

Roth, G. 2011. *Women, Food and God: An Unexpected Path to Almost Everything*. New York: Scribner.

Rushton, C. H. 2018. *Moral Resilience: Transforming Moral Suffering in Healthcare*. New York: Oxford University Press.

Sakka, L., G. Coll, and J. Chazal. 2011. "Anatomy and Physiology of Cerebrospinal Fluid." *European Annals of Otorhinolaryngology, Head and Neck Diseases* 128 (6): 309–16.

Salk Institute. 2022. "An Ocean in Your Brain: Interacting Brain Waves Key to How We Process Information." Salk Institute news release (online), April 22, 2022.

Schleip, R. 2014. "Interoception Some Suggestions for Manual and Movement Therapies." *Terra Rosa* 15 (Dec. 4, 2014).

Schlitz, M., E. Taylor, and N. Lewis. 1998. "Toward a Noetic Model of Medicine." *Ions: Noetic Sciences Review* 47: 44–63.

Scott, Jim, trans. 1997. "Eight Cases of Basic Goodness Not to Be Shunned." Originally composed by Gyalwa Gotsangpa (thirteenth century CE). Translation and arrangement by Jim Scott, under the guidance of Khenpo Tsultrim Gyamtso Rinpoche, Karme Choling, Barnet, Vermont, August 1997.

Selhub, Eva M., and Alan C. Logan. 2012. *Your Brain on Nature: The Science of Nature's Influence on Your Health, Happiness, and Vitality.* Mississauga, Ontario: John Wiley & Sons.

Seppälä, E. M., E. Simon-Thomas, S. L. Brown, M. C. Worline, C. D. Cameron, and J. R. Doty. 2017. *The Oxford Handbook of Compassion Science.* New York: Oxford University Press.

Sergueef, Nicette. 2007. *Cranial Osteopathy for Infants, Children and Adolescents: A Practical Handbook.* Churchill Livingstone.

Siegel, D. J. 1999. *The Developing Mind: How Relationships and the Brain Interact to Shape Who We Are.* New York: Guilford Press.

Siegel, D. J. 2012a. *The Developing Mind: How Relationships and the Brain Interact to Shape Who We Are.* 2nd ed. New York: Guilford Press.

Siegel, D. J. 2012b. *Pocket Guide to Interpersonal Neurobiology.* New York: W.W. Norton.

Signoretti, S., G. Lazzarino, B. Tavazzi, and R. Vagnozzi. 2011, "The Pathophysiology of Concussion." *PM & R: The Journal of Injury, Function, and Rehabilitation* 3 (10; suppl. 2): S359–68.

Simionescu, M., and F. Antohe. 2006. "Functional Ultrastructure of the Vascular Endothelium: Changes in Various Pathologies." *Handbook of Experimental Pharmacology* 176 (part 1): 41–69.

Smith, Caitlin J., and Kelli K. Ryckman. 2015. "Epigenetic and Developmental Influences on the Risk of Obesity, Diabetes, and Metabolic Syndrome." *Diabetes, Metabolic Syndrome and Obesity: Targets and Therapy* 8 (June): 295.

Sobrevia, Luis, Rocío Salsoso, Bárbara Fuenzalida, Eric Barros, Lilian Toledo, Luis Silva, Carolina Pizarro, et al. 2016. "Insulin Is a Key Modulator of Fetoplacental Endothelium Metabolic Disturbances in Gestational Diabetes Mellitus." *Frontiers in Physiology* 7: 119.

Stern, D. 2004. *The Present Moment in Psychotherapy and Everyday Life.* New York: W. W. Norton & Company.

Still, Andrew T. 2015. *Philosophy of Osteopathy.* Createspace Indepenent Publishing Platform.

Stock, Sarah J., Jade Carruthers, Clara Calvert, Cheryl Denny, Jack Donaghy, Anna Goulding, Lisa E. M. Hopcroft, et al. 2022. "SARS-CoV-2 Infection and COVID-19 Vaccination Rates in Pregnant Women in Scotland." *Nature Medicine* 28 (3): 504–12.

Sulemanji, Mustafa, and Khashayar Vakili. 2013. "Neonatal Renal Physiology." *Seminars in Pediatric Surgery* 22 (4): 195–98.

Sutherland, W. G. 1967. "Untitled Talk in 1944 at Des Moines Still College of Osteopathy." In *Contributions of Thought,* 101–15. Fort Worth, Tex.: Sutherland Cranial Teaching Foundation.

Sutherland, W. G. 1993. *Teachings in the Science of Osteopathy.* Fort Worth, Tex: Rudra Press.

Sütterlin, S., S. M. Schulz, T. Stumpf, P. Pauli, and C. Vögele. 2013. "Enhanced Cardiac Perception Is Associated with Increased Susceptibility to Framing Effects." *Cognitive Science* 37 (5): 922–35.

Sweet, David G., Virgilio Carnielli, Gorm Greisen, Mikko Hallman, Eren Ozek, Arjan Te Pas, Richard Plavka, et al. 2019. "European Consensus Guidelines on the Management of Respiratory Distress Syndrome—2019 Update." *Neonatology* 115 (4): 432.

Swinburn, Boyd A., Gary Sacks, Kevin D. Hall, Klim McPherson, Diane T. Finegood, Marjory L. Moodie, and Steven L. Gortmaker. 2011. "The Global Obesity Pandemic: Shaped by Global Drivers and Local Environments." *Lancet* 378 (9793): 804–14.

Szejer, M. 2005. *Talking to Babies: Healing with Words on a Maternity Ward.* Boston: Beacon Press.

Tarrant, J. 1999. *The Light inside the Dark: Zen, Soul, and the Spiritual Life.* New York: Perennial.

Tata, Mathew, Christiana Ruhrberg, and Alessandro Fantin. 2015. "Vascularisation of the Central Nervous System." *Mechanisms of Development* 138 (November): 26.

Thaler, Israel, Dorit Manor, Joseph Itskovitz, Shraga Rottem, Nathan Levit, Ilan Timor-Tritsch, and Joseph M. Brandes. 1990. "Changes in Uterine Blood Flow during Human Pregnancy." *American Journal of Obstetrics and Gynecology* 162 (1): 121–25.

Tóth-Heyn, Péter, Alfred Drukker, and Jean Pierre Guignard. 2000. "The Stressed Neonatal Kidney: From Pathophysiology to Clinical Management of Neonatal Vasomotor Nephropathy." *Pediatric Nephrology* (Berlin, Germany) 14 (3): 227–39.

Thurman, Robert, and Nida Chenagtsang. 2022. "Wisdom is Bliss." Lecture given in Los Angeles.

Vadakke-Madathil, Sangeetha, and Hina W. Chaudhry. 2021. "Chimerism as the Basis for Organ Repair." *Annals of the New York Academy of Sciences* 1487 (1): 12–20.

Valdesolo, P., and D. DeSteno. 2011. "Synchrony and the Social Tuning of Compassion." *Emotion* 11 (2): 262–66.

Valera, E. M., A. C. Joseph, K. Snedaker, M. J. Breiding, C. L. Robertson, A. Colantonio, H. Levin, et al. 2021. "Understanding Traumatic Brain Injury in Females: A State-of-the-Art Summary and Future Directions." *Journal of Head Trauma Rehabilitation* 36 (1): E1–E17.

van der Bie, G. 2001. *Embryology: Early Development from a Phenomenological Point of View.* Nijmegen, Netherlands: Louis Bolk Institute.

van der Burg, Jelske W., Sarbattama Sen, Virginia R. Chomitz, Jaap C. Seidell, Alan Leviton, and Olaf Dammann. 2016. "The Role of Systemic Inflammation Linking Maternal BMI to Neurodevelopment in Children." *Pediatric Research* 79 (1–1): 3–12.

Vanderploeg, R. D., H. G. Belanger, and G. Curtiss. 2009. "Mild Traumatic Brain Injury and Posttraumatic Stress Disorder and Their Associations with Health Symptoms." *Archives of Physical Medicine and Rehabilitation* 90 (7): 1084–93. Erratum in *Archives of Physical Medicine and Rehabilitation* 91 (6; 2010): 967–69.

van der Post, L. 1980. *The Heart of the Hunter: Customs and Myths of the African Bushman.* New York: Harcourt Brace Jovanovich.

Verny, Thomas, M.D., and John Kelly. 1981. *The Secret Life of the Unborn Child.* New York: Dell Publishing.

Vieten, C. 2009. *Mindful Motherhood: Practical Tools for Staying Sane during Pregnancy and Your Child's First Year.* Oakland, Calif.: New Harbinger Publications, Inc.

Vrachnis, Nikolaos, Fotodotis M. Malamas, Stavros Sifakis, Panayiotis Tsikouras, and Zoe Iliodromiti. 2012. "Immune Aspects and Myometrial Actions of Progesterone and CRH in Labor." *Clinical & Developmental Immunology* 2012.

Wales, A. 1953. The Management, Reactions and Systemic Effects of Fluctuations of Cerebrospinal Fluid. *Journal of the Osteopathic Cranial Association*, 35–47.

Wang, Y., L. D. Nelson, A. A. LaRoche, A. Y. Pfaller, A. S. Nencka, K. M. Koch, and M. A. McCrea. 2016. "Cerebral Blood Flow Alterations in Acute Sport-Related Concussion." *Journal of Neurotrauma* 33 (13): 1227–36.

Wang, Y., and S. Zhao. 2010. *Vascular Biology of the Placenta*. San Rafael, Calif.: Morgan & Claypool Life Sciences.

Watanabe, Atsuyuki, Jun Yasuhara, Masao Iwagami, Yoshihisa Miyamoto, Yuji Yamada, Yukio Suzuki, Hisato Takagi, and Toshiki Kuno. 2022. "Peripartum Outcomes Associated with COVID-19 Vaccination During Pregnancy: A Systematic Review and Meta-Analysis." *JAMA Pediatrics* 176 (11): 1098–106.

Wegela, K. K. 1988. "'Touch & Go' in Clinical Practice: Some Implications of the View of Intrinsic Health for Psychotherapy." *Journal of Contemplative Psychotherapy* 5: 3–24.

Wegela, K. K. 1997. *How to Be a Help Instead of a Nuisance*. Boston: Shambhala.

Weihong, Yuan, Jed A. Diekfuss, Kim D. Barber Foss, Jonathan A. Dudley, James L. Leach, Megan E. Narad, Christopher A. DiCesare, et al. 2021. "High School Sports-Related Concussion and the Effect of a Jugular Vein Compression Collar: A Prospective Longitudinal Investigation of Neuroimaging and Neurofunctional Outcomes." *Journal of Neurotrauma* 38 (20): 2811–21.

Weinstein, A. W. 2016. *Prenatal Development and Parents' Lived Experiences: How Early Events Shape Our Psychophysiology and Relationships*. New York: Norton.

Wells, Jana, Arun Swaminathan, Jenna Paseka, and Corrine Hanson. 2020. "Efficacy and Safety of a Ketogenic Diet in Children and Adolescents with Refractory Epilepsy-A Review." *Nutrients* 12 (6): 1809.

Weng, H. Y., J. L. Feldman, L. Leggio, V. Napadow, J. Park, and C. J. Price. 2021. "Interventions and Manipulations of Interoception." *Trends in Neuroscience* 44 (1): 52–62.

Wilber, K. 1997. "An Integral Theory of Consciousness." *Journal of Consciousness Studies* 4 (1): 71–92.

Wilson, W. S., trans. 2015. *The Pocket Samurai*. Boulder: Shambhala.

World Health Organization (WHO), UNICEF, UNFPA, World Bank Group, and the United Nations Population Division. 2015. *Trends in Maternal Mortality: 1990 to 2015*. Geneva: World Health Organization.

World Obesity Federation. n.d. "Data Tables: Prevalence of Adult Overweight & Obesity." World Obesity Federation Global Obesity Observatory (online). Accessed June 25, 2023.

Wu, Tai Wei, Timur Azhibekov, and Istvan Seri. 2016. "Transitional Hemodyamics in Preterm Neonates: Clinical Relevance. *Pediatrics and Neonatology* 57 (1): 7–18.

Yamasaki, Z. A. 2024. *Trauma-Informed Yoga Flip Chart: A Tool for Teaching Professionals*. New York: Norton.

Yeganeh Kazemi, Nazanin, Bohdana Fedyshyn, Shari Sutor, Yaroslav Fedyshyn, Svetomir Markovic, and Elizabeth Ann L. Enninga. 2021. "Maternal Monocytes Respond to Cell-Free Fetal DNA and Initiate Key Processes of Human Parturition." *Journal of Immunology* 207 (10): 2433–44.

Zhang, A. L., D. C. Sing, C. M. Rugg, B. T. Feeley, and C. Senter. 2016. "The Rise of Concussions in the Adolescent Population." *Orthopaedic Journal of Sports Medicine* 4 (8).

Zhou, Y., A. Kierans, D. Kenul, Y. Ge, J. Rath, J. Reaume, R. I. Grossman, and Y. W. Lui. 2013. "Mild Traumatic Brain Injury: Longitudinal Regional Brain Volume Changes." *Radiology* 267 (3): 880–90.

Resources

HOW TO REACH THE SHEAS

You may reach Michael Shea, Ph.D., online at **SheaHeart.com**.

You may reach out to Cathy Shea for guidance and coaching through her website, **www.cathysheaschool.com.** She offers National Board Certification for professionals wanting to practice the SheaWay Colon Hydrotherapy, including the gentle SloFill Method.

ORGANIZATIONS

Biodynamic Craniosacral Therapy Association of North America (BCTA/NA): a nonprofit professional organization supporting students, practitioners, and teachers of the biodynamic model of craniosacral therapy

Center for Compassion and Altruistic Research and Education (CCARE) at Stanford University: excellent contemplative research

Center for Healthy Minds at the University of Wisconsin: excellent research on contemplative neuroscience

Greater Good Science Center and the University of California, Berkeley: excellent contemplative research

Turtle Back Craniosacral Education in Chatham, New York: Michael Shea taught the biodynamic cardiovascular therapy model with Turtle Back for many years.

PRACTITIONERS

Dale G. Alexander, Ph.D. MA, BSEd, LMT, is the author of *The Inside-Out Paradigm*. He brings more than forty-five years of clinical experience in resolving chronic somatic difficulties to his teaching, writing, and daily work with clients. He practices out of Lake Worth Beach and Key West, Florida.

Almut Althaus is a healing practitioner offering shiatsu and biodynamic craniosacral therapy. She has practiced since 1990 in Kassel, Germany, where she lives with her family. She is Michael Shea's European course manager.

Zach Bush, M.D., is an international authority on the microbiome as it relates to health, disease, and food systems. He can be reached via his personal website.

K. Michelle Doyle, MSN, BCST, CNM, NYS LM, FACNM, was called to midwifery as a small child and has worked in women's health for decades. In Los Angeles, she was a midwife assistant, childbirth educator, labor and delivery nurse, and perinatal bereavement counselor. She became a certified nurse midwife (CNM) and a licensed midwife (LM) in New York in 1999. Since then, she has worked with multitudes of women and caught well over 1,400 babies. After ten years of being employed by medical practices and attending births in Rensselaer County hospitals, Michelle started her own midwifery practice. Established in 2009, Local Care Midwifery (LCM) was the first Capital District practice to offer planned home birth services with a licensed midwife. The beginning of LCM also marked the birth of Michelle's craniosacral career. Training with Margery Chessare and Michael Shea, Michelle incorporates both BCST and BCVT into her daily life and work. Michelle continues to answer her call to midwifery by providing high-quality, loving, and attentive health care to women, birthing families, babies, and more.

Bill Harvey is a Rolfing, biodynamic craniosacral therapy, and biodynamic cardiovascular therapy practitioner. His interest lies in combining these three approaches as well as visceral manipulation. He is the author of *Breathing, Mudras and Meridians* (2021), for which Michael Shea wrote the foreword. This book provides a basic training on how to become aware of our physiological functioning and its interplay with our feelings.

Andraly Horn, farmer, LMT, BCST, practices in Rhode Island and is one of the finest biodynamic practitioners and teachers in North America. Website: search for Open Farms Retreat online.

Joachim Lichtenberg, based in Germany, offers advanced craniosacral courses for the viscera, the cardiovascular system, the cranial nerves, the brain, and for working with children and their families.

Robert Lustig, M.D., is a pediatric neuroendocrinologist and an international authority on the danger of sugar in the diet. He also started the Real Food movement to improve the health of school lunch programs. He can be reached via his personal website.

Todd McLaughlin is a master Ashtanga Yoga Instructor and owns the Native Yoga Studio along with his wife Tamara in Juno Beach, Florida. His podcast called Toddcast is a gem of yogic information.

Mary Monro is an osteopath based in Edinburgh, Scotland. She has twenty-five years of experience and particularly enjoys working with the health issues of pregnancy, birth, and infancy. She can be reached via her personal website.

Elizabeth Newman is a certified Instructor from the BCTA-NA and a long time assistant and co-teacher with Michael Shea. She lives and practices in Los Angeles, California. She runs health care missions on the Hopi Indian reservation and other Native American groups. She is an expert in Trauma Informed Care.

Holly Pinto is the director of the Pinto-Shea Cranial Institute located in The Body Therapy Center and School of Massage in Swansea, Illinois. She is the principal instructor and co-teacher with Michael Shea. She is a certified Instructor with the BCTA-NA. Thomas Rau, M.D., is a practitioner of biological medicine at the BioMed Center Sonnenberg in Switzerland. Michael and Cathy Shea teach his model in their clinic and course offerings.

Carlos Rodeiro Barreiro teaches biodynamic cardiovascular therapy all over Europe. He is a brilliant teacher. Together with Mar Ximenis, he developed the BioStillness International School, which is now a referent in the teaching of the cranial field.

Jörg Schürpf is an excellent instructor of biodynamic manual therapy and Chi Nei Tsang. He practices in Switzerland and can be contacted via his personal website.

Ann Diamond Weinstein, Ph.D., is a preconception, prenatal, and early parenting specialist who offers consultation and education to individuals and professionals on trauma-sensitive approaches to preconception, pregnancy, birth, perinatal loss, and early parenting. She is the author of *Prenatal Development and Parents' Lived Experiences: How Early Events Shape Our Psychophysiology and Relationships* and the blog *From the Beginning: Prenatal Origins of the Parent-Child Relationship*.

Many other practitioners were named in the acknowledgment section at the beginning of this book. They are all excellent and of course there are many I have not named or remembered at this point in time while finishing this book. I apologize to all those I neglected to mention because the number of special people who have supported me on my journey is vast. I love all of you and could not be here and now with this book without you.

Index

Page numbers in *italics* refer to illustrations.

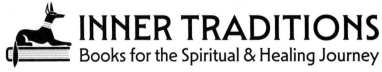